Bibliography for Training in Child and Adolescent Mental Health

For Training in Child Psychiatry, Child Psychology, Social Work, and Child and Adolescent Psychiatric Nursing

Editor
Irving N. Berlin, M.D.

Associate Editor
Bennett L. Leventhal, M.D.

With Sections on Films, Videotapes, and Books to Help Children, Adolescents, and Parents

UNIVERSITY OF NEW MEXICO PRESS: ALBUQUERQUE

Library of Congress Cataloging-in-Publication Data

Bibliography for training in child and adolescent mental health: for training in child psychiatry, child psychology, social work, and child and adolescent psychiatric nursing / editor, Irving N. Berlin; associate editor, Bennett L. Leventhal.—3rd ed.

p. cm.

Rev. ed. of: Bibliography of child psychiatry and child mental health with a selected list of films / edited by Irving N. Berlin. [2nd ed.]. c1976.

Previous ed. cataloged under: Berlin, Irving N., 1917–

Includes indexes.

Supported by grant no. 1TO1MH17682-02 from the National Institute of Mental Health, Psychiatry Training Branch.

ISBN 0–8263–1275–6 (CL)

1. Child psychiatry—Bibliography. 2. Child mental health—Bibliography. 3. Adolescent psychiatry—Bibliography. 4. Teenagers—Mental health—Bibliography. I. Berlin, Irving N., 1917– . II. Leventhal, Bennett. III. National Institute of Mental Health (U.S.) Psychiatry Training Branch. IV. Bibliography of child psychiatry and child mental health with a selected list of films.

[DNLM: 1. Adolescent Psychiatry—bibliography. 2. Adolescent Psychology—bibliography. 3. Child Psychiatry—bibliography. 4. Child Psychology—bibliography. 5. Mental Disorders—in adolescence. 6. Mental Disorders—in infancy & childhood. ZWS 350
B5814]
Z6671.52.P78B53 1991
[RJ449]
016.61892'89—dc20
DNLM/DLC
for Library of Congress

91–11973
CIP

Funding for the preparation of the Bibliography was provided by a Grant from the National Institute of Mental Health, Psychiatry Training Branch #1TO1MH17682-02

Third edition

Contents

Part II: Development 52

Part III: Psychopathology: Disease and Disorder (continued)

Part III: Psychopathology: Disease and Disorder (continued)

Part III: Psychopathology: Disease and Disorder (continued)

Part III: Psychopathology: Disease and Disorder (continued)

Part III: Psychopathology: Disease and Disorder (continued)

Part IV Therapeutics (continued)

Part IV Therapeutics (continued)

Part IV Therapeutics (continued)

Part XI Films and Videos with Commentary (continued)

Part XII Suggested Reading for Children, Adolescents, and Parents (continued)

Contributors

Professional position and affiliation are listed in each section.

Paul Adams, M.D.
Marc Amaya, M.D.
Thomas Anders, M.D.
George Anderson, Ph.D.
Richard Angell, M.D.
E. J. Anthony, M.D.
Eugene L. Arnold, M.D.
William Arroyo, M.D.
George Awad, M.D.
Lawrence Bender, M.D.
Elissa P. Benedek, M.D.
Irving N. Berlin, M.D.
Sidney Berman, M.D.
Efrain Bleiberg, M.D.
Eli M. Bower, Ph.D.
Joel Bregman, M.D.
Christine Broden, M.D.
Patrick Butterfield, M.D.
Justin Call, M.D.
Magda Campbell, M.D.
Ian Canino, M.D.
Dennis Cantwell, M.D.
Donald J. Carek, M.D.
Charles D. Casat, M.D.
Donald J. Cohen, M.D.
Deane L. Critchley, Ph.D., R.N.
Robert Emde, M.D.
Norbert Enzer, M.D.
Spencer Eth, M.D.
Ken Farley, M.D.
Carl Feinstein, M.D.
Jo Ann B. Fineman, M.D.
Charles Fischer, M.D.
Joseph Fischoff, M.D.
Lois T. Flaherty, M.D.
Steven Forness, Ed.D.
Fred Frankel, Ph.D.
Gregory Fritz, M.D.
Eleanor Galenson, M.D.
I. Lee Gislason, M.D.
Paul N. Graffagnino, M.D.
Arthur Green, M.D.
Stanley Greenspan, M.D.
Robert Harmon, M.D.
William Harris, M.D.
Saul I. Harrison, M.D.
Thomas Haslip, M.D.
Christoph M. Heinicke, Ph.D.
Lionel Hersov, M.D.
David Inwood, M.D.
Linda H. Jackson, M.D.
Wendell E. Jeffrey, Ph.D.
Michael G. Kalogerakis, M.D.
Connie Kasasi
Charles Keith, M.D.
Paulina K. Kernberg, M.D.
S. Peter Kim, M.D.
William Klykylo, M.D.
Annaliese F. Korner, Ph.D.
Irvin A. Kraft, M.D.
Paul Laybourne, M.D.
James F. Leckman, M.D.
Nadine Levinson, D.D.S.
Michael Lewis, Ph.D.
Lewis Lipsitt, Ph.D.
John Looney, M.D.
Alexander P. Lucas, M.D.
Henry C. Maier, Ph.D.
Richard C. Marohn, M.D.
Edward A. Mason, M.D.
David Scott May, M.D.
Brian McConville, M.D.
Elizabeth McCullough, M.D.
John J. McDermott, Jr., M.D.
John Meeks, M.D.
Eric K. Milliner, M.D.
Carlos Mocedo, M.D.
Spyros J. Monopolis, M.D.
Joseph D. Noshpitz, M.D.
S. Wendell Obetz, M.D.
Joy Osofsky, Ph.D.
Arthur H. Parmelee, M.D.
David Pauls, Ph.D.
Richard Perry, M.D.
Theodore Petti, M.D.
Cynthia Pfeffer, M.D.
Carl M. Pfeifer, M.D.
David B. Pruitt
Andres Pumariega, M.D.
Mark Riddle, M.D.
Graham Rogeness, M.D.
Andrew Russell, M.D.
S. Mark Sacher, D.O.
Richard M. Sarles, M.D.
Lewis Saunder, M.D.
Diane Schetky, M.D.
John Schowalter, M.D.
David Shaffer, M.D.
Pirooz Sholevar, M.D.
Marian Sigman, Ph.D.
Larry Silver, M.D.
Arthur M. Small, M.D.
Albert Solnit, M.D.
John Stevenson, M.D.
Peter E. Tanguay, M.D.
Jay Tarnow, M.D.
Peter Toscano, M.D.
Kenneth Towbin, M.D.
Alexander Tymchuck, Ph.D.
Phyllis Tyson, Ph.D.
Robert Tyson, M.D.
Mario Valente, M.D.
Larry Vitulano, Ph.D.
Fred Volkmar, M.D.
Hulse Wagner, M.D.
Lloyd A. Wells, Ph.D., M.D.
Henry Work, M.D.
Harry H. Wright, M.D., M.B.A.
Alayne Yates, M.D.
Gwen Zahnes, Ph.D.
Kenneth J. Zucker, Ph.D.

Dedication

To Reginald S. Lourie, M.D.--We are grieved at his death and are determined to make his commitment to Prevention real. Reg Lourie has been a particular friend and mentor and, with his quiet example of effectiveness, has provided me and many others with a model of a colleague, leader, and researcher. His early work in infancy and early childhood was especially inspiring. He has influenced many individuals by his patience and inspiration as a teacher and by his gentle but firm supervision. As a psychoanalyst, he was never doctrinaire, but always at the forefront of using careful observation to delineate the etiology, the developmental impact of any psychopathology, or the effect of psychosocial stressors on children, adolescents, and families. He recognized early that treatment had to include not only the affected patient, but also parents and significant others in the environment. He also recognized, taught, and wrote that treatment was provided by a variety of people in contact with a family if their purpose was to help with the integration and improvement of family function. Thus, welfare workers, teachers, and public health nurses, as well as child mental health specialists, were all involved in helping the child and family to more functional behavior and improved mental health.

I had my most intensive experience with Reg Lourie during the Congressional Commission on Child Mental Health. As president of the Commission, he helped set its direction and emphasis on fact-finding and on trying to discover how prevention could be utilized to reduce psychopathology and make later treatment or rehabilitation less necessary. As a member of the Board of Directors of the Commission, I worked closely with Reg, helping to edit certain sections of the report.

As President of the Academy of Child Psychiatry, Reg provided a benevolent leadership in times of stress, which helped us think more fully about the necessary changes in our organization.

When Reg Lourie retired as Professor and Director of Psychiatry at Children's Hospital in Washington, D.C., he immediately became involved with the National Institute of Mental Health's Intramural Program on prevention and early interventions in disturbances of infancy and early childhood.

Reg will be sorely missed by all of us who looked to his work as a model of devotion to scientific inquiry that contributed to reducing the mental health problems of infancy and childhood. His modest self-references as the recipient, two year ago, of the first Academy of Child and Adolescent Psychiatry's Simon-Weil Award for contributions to liaison child psychiatry and his encyclopedic knowledge of the history of pediatric-child psychiatry relations were typical of Reg and endearing to all.

Reg was at once a beloved and inspirational colleague and teacher and an example of a productive researcher and user of research in treatment and early interventions and especially in nationwide prevention programs.

Acknowledgements

We are all indebted to Carol Miller, M.A., R.N., and Robert Hines, M.D., formerly of the Children's Ward of the McAuley Neuropsychiatric Institute of Saint Mary's Hospital in San Francisco, for allowing us to use their list of therapeutic fairy tales.

I am especially grateful and indebted to my lovely and meticulous wife, Deane L. Critchley, without whom this bibliography would not have been completed. She spent many hours making sure that the format was consistent and that each section and subsection editor was credited and placed correctly. Her help in checking the completeness of all the sections and subsections, as well as ensuring the accuracy of the table of contents and proofing this enormous bibliography, permitted its final completion. I cannot thank her sufficiently.

We appreciate the support and encouragement provided by the Society of Professors of Child and Adolescent Psychiatry. Many of the section and subsection editors are members of the society.

A. History of Child Mental Health: Concerns and Activities

Section Editor:

Joseph D. Noshpitz, M.D.
Clinical Professor of Child Psychiatry
Children's Hospital
and
George Washington University School of Medicine
Washington, D.C.

Associate Editors:

Irving N. Berlin, M.D.
Professor of Psychiatry and Pediatrics
University of New Mexico School of Medicine
Albuquerque, New Mexico

Larry Silver, M.D.
Clinical Professor of Psychiatry
Georgetown University
Washington, D.C.
and
Director of Training
The Division of Child and Adolescent Psychiatry
Georgetown University
Washington, D.C.

Hulse Wagner, M.D.
Wichita Falls, Texas

Henry Work, M.D.
Clinical Professor of Psychiatry
Georgetown University School of Medicine
Washington, D.C.

1. History of Concern with Children and Psychotherapies Used with Children

Anthony, E. J. (1986). A brief history of child psychoanalysis. Introduction. Journal of the American Academy of Child Psychiatry 25, 8-11.

Aries, P. (1962). Centuries of childhood: A social history of family life. New York: Knopf.

Blanton, R. L. (1975). Historical perspectives on classification of mental retardation. In N. Hobbs (Ed.), Issues in the classification of children. San Francisco: Jossey-Bass.

Blumin, S. M. (1975). Rip Van Winkle's grandchildren: Family and household in the Hudson Valley, 1800-1869. Journal of Urban History 1, 293-315.

Bremner, R. (1970-1971). Children and youth in America. Cambridge: Harvard University Press.

Brody, S. (1974). Contributions to child analysis. In R. S. Eissler, et al. (Eds.), Psychoanalytic study of the child (Vol. 29, pp 13-20). New York: International Universities Press.

Burke, N. H. M., & Miller, E. (1929). Child mental hygiene-- its history, methods, and problems. British Journal of Medical Psychology 9,218-242.

Calhoun, A. C. (1960). A social history of the American family. Volume 1: Colonial period. New York: Barnes and Noble.

Campbell, C. M. (1917). A survey of the school population in the Locust Point district of Baltimore. Mental Hygiene 1, 96-147.

Dreyer, B. A. (1976). Adolf Meyer and mental hygiene: An ideal for public health. American Journal of Public Health 66, 998-1003.

Eisenberg, L. (1977). Child psychiatry perspectives: The cultivation of children. Journal of the American Academy of Child Psychiatry 16, 529-539.

Faust, F. L., & Brantingham, P. J. (1974). The era of the 'socialized' juvenile court--1899-1967. In F. L. Faust (Ed.), Juvenile justice philosophy: Readings, cases and comments. St. Paul, Minn.: West Pub.

Flicker, B. D. (1977). The historical development of the juvenile justice system. In B. D. Iheker (Ed.), Standards for juvenile justice: A summary and analysis (pp. 27-51). Cambridge, Mass.: Ballinger.

Gordon, M. (1973). The American family in social-historical perspective. New York: St. Martin's Press.

Greven, P. J. (1973). Family structure in seventeenth century Andover, Massachusetts. In S. N. Green (Ed.), The American family in social-historical perspective. New York: St. Martin's Press.

Grotberg, E. H. (1967). Two hundred years of children. Washington, D.C.: U.S. Department of Health, Education, and Welfare.

Haareven, T. K. (1975). Family time and industrial time: Family and work in a planned corporation town, 1900-1924. Journal of Urban History 1(3), 365-389.

Hardy, S. C., & Allen, V. R. (1975). The influence of Robert Burton and Clifford Whittingham Beers on the development of psychiatry. Journal - Oklahoma State Medical Association 68, 185-188.

Kahn, J. (1978). Tribute to Emanuel Miller. Journal of Child Psychology and Psychiatry and Allied Disciplines 19, 305-308.

Kern, S. (1973). Freud and the birth of child psychiatry. Journal of the History of the Behavioral Science 9, 360-368.

Lambert, J. P. (1977). William S. Langford, M.D. 1906-1976. Journal of the American Academy of Child Psychiatry 16: 347.

Lipman-Blumen, J. (1975). A crisis framework applied to macrosociological family changes: Marriage, divorce, and occupational trends associated with World War II. Journal of Marriage and the Family 37(4), 889-894.

Lowery, L. G., & Sloan, V. (1948). Orthopsychiatry, 1923-1948: Retrospect and prospect. Menasha, Wis.: Banta.

Lowery, L. G., & Smith, G. (1933). The institute for child guidance. New York: The Commonwealth Fund.

McPeak, W. R. (1975). Family interactions as etiological factors in mental disorders: An analysis of The American Journal of Insanity, 1844-1848. American Journal of Psychiatry 132, 1327-1329.

Mora, G., & Brand, J. L. (1970). Psychiatry and its history: Methodological problems in research. Springfield, Ill.: Charles C. Thomas.

Rachman, A. W., & Raubolt, R. R. (1984). The pioneers of adolescent group psychotherapy. International Journal of Group Psychotherapy 34, 387-413.

Rosenthal, D. (1974). Introduction to Manfred Bleuler's "The offspring of schizophrenics." Schizophrenia Bulletin 6, 91-93.

Schlossman, S. L. (1977). Love the American delinquent: The theory and practice of "progressive juvenile justice," 1825-1920 (pp. 303-341). Chicago: University of Chicago Press.

Scull, A. T. (1975). Cyclical trends in psychiatric practice: The case of Bettelheim and Tuke. Social Science and Medicine 9, 633-640.

Sears, R. R. (1975). Your ancients revisited: A history of child development. Chicago: University of Chicago Press.

Slaff, B. (1981). The history of adolescent psychiatry. In S. C. Feinstein, et al. (Eds.), Adolescent psychiatry: Developmental and clinical studies (Vol. 9, pp. 7-21). Chicago: University of Chicago Press.

Solnit, A. J. (1975). Presentation of the C. Anderson Aldrich Award to Anna Freud. Pediatrics 56, 330-331.

Steinhauer, P. D. (1982). The Canadian Academy of Child Psychiatry. The development of child psychiatry in Canada. Journal of the American Academy of Child Psychiatry 21, 217-218.

Stevenson, G. S., & Smith, G. (1934). The child guidance clinic--a quarter century of development. New York: The Commonwealth Fund.

Trainor, D. (1979). Bowlby reviews 30 years of child development study. Journal of Asthma Research 16, 45-49.

Truitt, R. P., Lowery, L. G., Hoffman, C. W., Connor, W. L., Taylor, E., & Kendel, F. R. (1928). The child guidance clinic in the community. New York: The Commonwealth Fund.

Wiener, J. M., & Jaffe, S. (1977). History of drug therapy in childhood and adolescent psychiatric disorders. In J. M. Wiener (Ed.), Psychopharmacology in childhood and adolescence (pp. 9-40). New York: Basic Books.

Wilkerson, A. E. (1973). The rights of children. Philadelphia: Temple University Press.

2. History of Legal, Governmental, and Social Concerns with Children

Abbott, G. (1938). The child and the state. Chicago: University of Chicago Press.

Barger, A., Lundberg, E., & Emmo, O. (1927). Handbook for the use of boards of directors, superintendents, and staffs of institutions for dependent children. Washington, D.C.: Children's Bureau.

Beck, R. (1973). White House conference on children: An historical perspective. Harvard Educational Review 43, 653-668.

Bernard, J. (1957). Social problems at midcentury. New York: Rinehart and Winston, Inc.

Billingsley, A., & Giovanni, J. M. (1972). Children of the storm: Black children and American children welfare. New York: Harcourt, Brace, Jovanovich, Inc.

Brace, C. L. (1892). The dangerous classes of New York and twenty years' work among them. New York: Wynkoop and Hallenbeck.

Bradbury, D. E. (1962). Five decades of action for children: A history of the children's bureau. Washington, D.C.: Department of Health, Education, and Welfare.

Bremner, R. (1970-1971). Children and youth in America. Cambridge: Harvard University Press.

Brown, J. (1960). Child welfare classics. Social Service Review 34, 195-202.

Caulfield, E. (1931). The infant welfare movement of the eighteenth century. New York: Paul Hocker.

Chambers, C. A. (1963). Seedtime of reform: American social service and social action, 1918-1933. Minneapolis: University of Minnesota Press.

Deutsch, A. (1950). Our rejected children. Boston: Little, Brown.

Fleming, V. (1976). America's children, 1976: A bicentennial assessment. Washington, D.C.: National Council of Organization for Children and You.

Folks, H. (1902). The care of destitute, neglected, and dependent children. New York: Macmillan.

Fox, S. J. (1970). Juvenile justice reform: An historical perspective. Stanford Law Review 22, 1187-1239.

Hart, H. (1910). Preventive treatment of neglected children. New York: Charities Publication Committee.

Hunter, R. (1965). The child. In (Ed.), Poverty: Social conscience in the progressive era. New York: Harper and Row.

Infausto, F. (1969). Perspectives on adoption. Annals of the American Academy of Political and Social Sciences 383, 1-12.

Jernegan, M. W. (1931). Laboring and dependent classes in colonial America: 1607-1783. Chicago: University of Chicago Press.

Kraus, H. D. (1971). Illegitimacy: Law and social policy. Indianapolis: Bobbs-Merrill.

Levenson, I. (1975). Poverty and public policy. New York: Hudson Institute.

Levine, M., & Levine, A. (1970). A social history of helping services. New York: Appleton-Century-Crofts.

Light, R. J. (1973). Abused and neglected children in America: A study of alternative policies. Harvard Educational Review 43, 556-598.

Lundberg, E. (1947). Unto the least of these: Social services for children. New York: Appleton-Century-Crofts.

Mencher, S. (1967). Poor law to poverty program. Pittsburgh: University of Pittsburgh Press.

Payne, G. H. (1916). The child in human progress. New York: G. Putnam's Sons.

Pickett, R. S. (1969). House of refuge: Origins of juvenile reform in New York State, 1815-1857. Syracuse: Syracuse University Press.

Rodham, H. (1973). Children under the law. Harvard Education Review 43, 487-514.

Rothman, D. J. (1971). The discovery of the asylum: Social order and disorder in the New Republic. Boston: Little, Brown.

Sirault, G. (1963). The needs of children: A survey of the needs of children in developing countries. New York: Free Press of Glencoe.

Snapper, K. J. (1975). The status of children 1975. Washington: George Washington University.

Spargo, J. (1906). The bitter cry of the children. New York: Macmillan.

Thurston, H. W. (1930). The dependent child. New York: Columbia University Press.

Trattner, W. I. (1970). Crusade for the children: A history of the national child labor committee and child labor reform in America. Chicago: Quadrangle Books, Inc.

Trattner, W. I. (1974). From poor to welfare state: A history of social welfare in America. New York: The Free Press.

Whittaker, J. K. (1951). Colonial child care institutions: Our heritage of care. Child Welfare 50, 396-400.

3. History of Development of Various Clinical Specialties in the Treatment of Children

Adamson, W. C. (1968). History of child psychiatry. I: Frederick H. Allen, M.D., child psychiatrist. Transactions and Studies of the College of Physicians of Philadelphia 36, 96-103.

Allen, F. H. (1955). Symposium, 1955: Progress in orthopsychiatry. Psychiatry. American Journal of Orthopsychiatry 25, 479-491.

Allen, F. H. (1963). From the founders of child psychiatry: Child psychiatry comes of age. Journal of the American Academy of Child Psychiatry 2, 187-198.

Anthony, E. J. (1970). The emergence of child psychiatry as an academic discipline. Child Psychiatry and Human Development 1, 4-15.

Axelrod, S. (1955). Symposium, 1955: Progress in orthopsychiatry. Allied disciplines. American Journal of Orthopsychiatry 25, 524-538.

Barhash, A. Z., et al. (1951). Appraising the contribution of the mental hygiene clinic to its community. 3. Discussion. American Journal of Orthopsychiatry 21, 94-104.

Beck, S. J. (1959). Clinical psychology: A discipline--quantitative and humanist. In S. J. Beck & H. B. Molish (Eds.), Reflexes to intelligences (pp. 482-495). Glencoe, Ill.: Free Press.

Berkman, T. D. (1955). Symposium, 1955: Progress in orthopsychiatry. Psychiatric social work. American Journal of Orthopsychiatry 25, 511-524.

Cameron, K. (1956). Past and present trends in child psychiatry. Journal of Mental Science 102, 599-603.

Coleman, J. V. (1951). Appraising the contribution of the mental hygiene clinic to its community. 2. In the promotion of mental health. American Journal of Orthopsychiatry 21, 83-93.

Crutcher, R. (1943). Child psychiatry: A history of its development. Psychiatry 6, 191-201.

Eisenberg, L. (1969). Child psychiatry: The past quarter century. American Journal of Orthopsychiatry 39, 389-401.

French, L. A. M. (1940). Psychiatric social work. New York: The Commonwealth Fund.

Freud, A. (1966). A short history of child analysis. In R. S. Eissler, et al. (Eds.), Psychoanalytic study of the child (Vol. 21, pp. 7-14). New York: International Universities Press.

Freud, S. (1955). Analysis of a phobia in a five-year-old boy (1909). In E. Jones (Ed.), The standard edition of the complete works of Sigmund Freud (pp. 5-149). New York and London: Hogarth Press.

Gardner, G. E. (1951). Appraising the contribution of the mental hygiene clinic to its community. 1. In psychiatric treatment, training, and research. American Journal of Orthopsychiatry 21, 74-82.

Gardner, G. E. (1972). William Healy (1869-1963). Journal of the American Academy of Child Psychiatry 11, 1-29.

Ginsburg, E. L. (1948). Psychiatric social work. In L. G. Lowrey (Ed.), Orthopsychiatry 1923-1948: Retrospect and prospect (pp. 471-483). New York: American Orthopsychiatric Association.

Healy, W., & Bronner, A. F. (1948). The child guidance clinic: Birth and growth of an idea. In L. G. Lowrey (Ed.), Orthopsychiatry 1923-1948: Retrospect and prospect (pp. 14-49). New York: American Orthopsychiatric Association.

Hunt, D. (1970). Parents and children in history. New York: Basic Books.

Kanner, L. (1960a). Arnold Gesell's place in the history of developmental psychology and psychiatry. In E. Shagass & B. Pasamanick (Eds.), Child development and child psychiatry (pp. 1-9). Washington, D.C.: American Psychiatric Association.

Kanner, L. (1960b). Child psychiatry. Retrospect and prospect. American Journal of Psychiatry 117, 15-22.

Kanner, L. (1973a). The birth of early infantile autism. Journal of Autism and Childhood Schizophrenia 3, 93-95.

Kanner, L. (1973b). Historical perspective on developmental deviations. Journal of Autism and Childhood Schizophrenia 3, 187-198.

Levine, M., & Levine A. (1970). A social history of helping services: Clinic, court, school and community. New York: Appleton-Century-Crofts.

Levy, D. M. (1968). Beginnings of the child guidance movement. American Journal of Orthopsychiatry 38, 799-804.

Liss, E. (1964). From the founders of child psychiatry: The vicissitudes of a hybrid. Journal of the American Academy of Child Psychiatry 3, 762-768.

Lowrey, L. G. (1944). Psychiatry for children. A brief history of developments. American Journal of Psychiatry 101, 375-388.

Lowrey, L. G. (1948). The birth of orthopsychiatry. In L. G. Lowrey (Ed.), Orthopsychiatry 1923-1948: Retrospect and prospect (pp. 190-208). New York: American Orthopsychiatry Association.

Lowrey, L. G. (1955). The contribution of orthopsychiatry to psychiatry: Brief historical note. American Journal of Orthopsychiatry 25, 475-478.

Lurie, H. L. (1957). The development of social welfare programs in the United States. Social Work Year Book (Vol. 13, pp. 19-44). Silver Springs, Md.: National Association of Social Work Publication Department.

MacMillan, M. B. (1960). Extra-scientific influences in the history of childhood psychopathology. American Journal of Psychiatry 116, 1091-1096.

Marx, O. M. (1970). What is the history of psychiatry? American Journal of Orthopsychiatry 40, 593-605.

Moore, M. U. (1948). Contributions of orthopsychiatry to family casework. In L. G. Lowrey (Ed.), Orthopsychiatry 1923-1948: Retrospect and prospect (pp. 310-322). New York: American Orthopsychiatry Association.

Murphy, G. (1930). An historical introduction to modern psychology (rev. ed.). New York: Harcourt, Brace.

Rae-Grant, Q. A. F. (1970). Symposium: Child psychiatry. Adult and child psychiatry--one or two nations? Canadian Psychiatric Association Journal 15, 247-251.

Rexford, E. N. (1962). Child psychiatry and child analysis in the United State today. Journal of the American Academy of Child Psychiatry 1, 365-384.

Rexford, E. N. (1969). Children, child psychiatry, and our brave new world. Archives of General Psychiatry 20, 25-37.

Richmond, J. B. (1968). Future projection of orthopsychiatry. American Journal of Orthopsychiatry 38, 809-813.

Selesnick, S. T. (1967). Historical perspectives in the development of child psychiatry. International Journal of Psychiatry 3, 368-382.

Senn, M. J. E. (1971). The bequest of Frederick H. Allen to child psychiatry. Journal of the American Academy of Child Psychiatry 10, 589-602.

Shakow, D. (1948). Clinical psychology: An evaluation. In L. G. Lowrey (Ed.), Orthopsychiatry 1923-1948: Retrospect and prospect (pp. 231-247). New York: American Orthopsychiatry Association.

Shakow, D. (1968). The contributions of Levy, Menninger, and Stevenson. American Journal of Orthopsychiatry 38, 804-809.

Solnit, A. J. (1966). Who deserves child psychiatry? A study in priorities. Journal of the American Academy of Child Psychiatry 5, 1-16.

Watson, R. I. (1953). A brief history of clinical psychology. Psychological Bulletin 50, 321-346.

Watson, R. I. (1955). Symposium, 1955: Progress in orthopsychiatry. Psychology. American Journal of Orthopsychiatry 25, 491-510.

Watson, R. I. (1959). History of the study of the child. In R. I. Watson (Ed.), Psychology of the child (pp. 3-37). New York: Wiley.

Witmer, H. L. (1940). Psychiatric clinics for children. New York: The Commonwealth Fund.

4. History of Concerns with Child Development

Ball, R. S. (1977). The Gesell developmental schedules: Arnold Gesell (1880-1961). Journal of Abnormal Child Psychology 5, 233-239.

Cooper, M. G. (1977). Observational studies of children from diary to ethnogram. A century of progress. Child: Care, Health and Development 3, 283-292.

Drell, M. J. (1982). Hermine Hug-Hellmuth, a pioneer in child analysis. Bulletin of the Menninger Clinic 46, 139-150.

Elkind, D. (1981). Jean Piaget (1896-1980). American Psychologist 36, 911-913.

Esman, A. H. (1982). The study of lives: Discussion of Tashjian and Shaw. In S. C. Feinstein, et al. (Eds.), Adolescent psychiatry: Developmental and clinical studies (Vol. 10, pp. 99-105). Chicago: University of Chicago Press.

Friedman, R. M. (1975). The child psychology of Maurice Merleau-Ponty. Psychoanalytic Review 62, 469-480.

Jackson, D. J. (1984). Contributions to the history of psychology: XXXV. Dorothy Burlingham. Psychological Reports 54, 855-863.

Jackson, D. J. (1986). Contributions to the history of psychology: XL. The Hampstead wartime nurseries. Psychological Reports 58, 127-130.

Lomax, E. (1977). The Laura Spelman Rockefeller Memorial: Some of its contributions to early research in child development. Journal of the History of the Behavioral Sciences 13, 283-293.

Lystad, M. (1984). The world according to Dr. Seuss. Children Today 13, 19-22.

Matthews, R. M. (1980). Permissiveness and Dr. Blatz: Where did society's ideas on child-raising go wrong? Canadian Medical Association Journal 122, 99-101.

Palermo, D. S. (1982). The history of the Boyd R. McCandless young scientist awards: The first recipients. Advances in Child Development and Behavior 16, 1-6.

Pinkham, J. R. (1982). The dentist and child-patient encounter: An Adlerian analysis. ASDC Journal of Dentistry for Children 49, 266-272.

Rachman, A. W., & Raubolt, R. R. (1984). The pioneers of adolescent group psychotherapy. International Journal of Group Psychotherapy 34, 387-413.

Senn, M. J. (1975). Insights on the child development movement in the United States. Monographs of the Society for Research in Child Development (Vol. 40, pp. 1-107). Chicago: University of Chicago Press.

Siegel, A. W., & White, S. H. (1982). The child study movement: Early growth and development of the symbolized child. Advances in Child Development and Behavior 17, 233-285.

Sigman, M., & Parmelee, A. H. (1977). Child psychology, 1877. American Journal of Diseases of Children 131, 908.

Sprung, H., & Sprung, L. (1984). [William Thierry Preyer (1841-1897) as methodologist and methodic]. Zeitschrift fur Psychologie mit Zeitschrift fur Angewandte Psychologie 192, 170-181.

B. Cultural Aspects of Child Mental Health

Section Coeditors:

Irving N. Berlin, M.D.
Professor of Psychiatry and Pediatrics
University of New Mexico School of Medicine
Albuquerque, New Mexico

S. Peter Kim, M.D.
Professor of Psychiatry and Pediatrics
Director, Child, Adolescent and Family Psychiatry
University of Georgia School of Medicine
Augusta, Georgia

Harry H. Wright, M.D., M.B.A.*
Associate Professor
University of South Carolina School of Medicine
Columbia, South Carolina

Subsection Editor:

Ian Canino, M.D.
Clinical Associate Professor
Department of Psychiatry
Columbia University College of Physicians and Surgeons
New York, New York

Associate Editors:

William Arroyo, M.D.
Assistant Professor
University of Southern California School
of Medicine
Los Angeles, California

Patrick Butterfield, M.D.
Professor
University of South Carolina School of Medicine
Columbia, South Carolina

***I want to acknowledge Dr. Harry H. Wright's major contributions to many of the subsections of this section.**

--Irving N. Berlin

Linda H. Jackson, M.D.
Highland Hospital
Ashville, North Carolina

Elizabeth McCullough, M.D.
Assistant Professor
University of South Carolina School of Medicine
Columbia, South Carolina

Alayne Yates, M.D.
Professor of Psychiatry and Pediatrics
University of Arizona School of Medicine
Tucson, Arizona

1. Historical References

Brody, S. (1956). Maternal behavior: The literature. In S. Brody, Patterns of mothering (pp. 28-72). New York: International Universities Press.

Erikson, E. H. (1945). Childhood and tradition in two American Indian tribes. In R. S. Eissler, et al. (Eds.), Psychoanalytic study of the child (Vol 1, pp. 319-350). New York: International Universities Press.

Kaffman, M. (1961). Evaluation of emotional disturbance in 403 Israeli kibbutz children. American Journal of Psychiatry 117, 732-738.

Kaffman, M. (1972). Toilet-training by multiple caretakers: Enuresis among kibbutz children. Israel Annals of Psychiatry and Related Disciplines 10, 341-365.

Kiev, A. (1964). Magic, faith, and healing: Studies in primitive psychiatry today. New York: The Free Press.

Kline, C. L., & Lee, N. (1974). A transcultural study of dyslexia: Analysis of language disabilities in 277 Chinese children simultaneously learning to read and write in English and in Chinese. In S. Chess & A. Thomas (Eds.), (1973). Annual progress in child psychiatry and child development (pp. 297-320). New York: Brunner/Mazel.

Leighton, A. H. (1965). Cultural change and psychiatric disorder. In A. V. S. DeReuck & R. Porter (Eds.), Transcultural psychiatry (pp. 216-228). London: Churchill.

Mead, M. (1956). The implications of culture change for personality development. In D. G. Haring (Ed.), Personal character and cultural milieu (3rd ed., pp. 623-636). Syracuse: Syracuse University Press.

Mead, M. (1957). Changing patterns of parent-child relations in an urban culture. International Journal of Psycho-Analysis 38, 369-378.

Murphy, J. M., & Leighton, A. H. (Eds.). (1965). Approaches to cross-cultural psychiatry. Ithaca: Cornell University Press.

Rollins, N. (1972). Child psychiatry in the Soviet Union: preliminary observations. Cambridge: Harvard University Press.

Rubel, A. J. (1960). Concepts of disease in Mexican-American culture. American Anthropologist 62, 795-814.

Spiro, M. E. (1965). Religious systems as culturally constituted defense mechanisms. In M. E. Spiro (Ed.), Context and meaning in cultural anthropology (pp. 100-113). New York: The Free Press.

Valentine, C. A. (1963). Men of anger and men of shame: Lakalai ethnopsychology and its implications for sociopsychological theory. Ethnology 2, 441-447.

Weinstein, E. A. (1962). Cultural aspects of delusion: A psychiatric study of the Virgin Islands. New York: Free Press of Glencoe.

2. Self-Concept, Social Identity, and Culture

Abu-Saad, H. (1984). Cultural group indicators of pain in children. Maternal-Child Nursing Journal 13, 187-196.

August, G. J., & Felker, D. W. (1977). Role of affective meaningfulness and self-concept in the verbal learning styles of white and black children. Journal of Educational Psychology 69, 253-260.

Barclay, A., Yater, A., & Lamp, R. (1982). Heterogeneity of intellectual performance by disadvantaged children within a metropolitan area. Perceptual and Motor Skills 55, 781-782.

Beratis, S., Kolb, R., Sperling, E., & Stein, R. E. (1981). Development of a child with long-lasting deprivation of oral feeding. Journal of the American Academy of Child Psychiatry 20, 53-64.

Bird, H. R. (1982). The cultural dichotomy of colonial people. Journal of the American Academy of Psychoanalysis 10, 195-209.

Boat, B. W., Campbell, F. A., & Ramey, C. T. (1986). Preventive education and birth order as co-determinants of IQ in disadvantaged 5-year-olds. Child: Care, Health and Development 12, 25-36.

Bolling, J. L. (1974). The changing self-concept of black children. The black identity test. Journal of the National Medical Association 66, 28-31, 34.

Brown, N. W. (1977). Personality characteristics of black adolescents. Adolescence 12, 81-87.

Bruneau, O. J. (1984). Comparison of behavioral characteristics and self-concepts of American Indian and Caucasian preschoolers. Psychological Reports 54, 571-574.

Calhoun, G., Sheldon, S. R., Serrano, R., & Cooke, D. (1978). An ethnic comparison of self-esteem in Portuguese-, Mexican-, and Anglo-American pupils. Psychology 98, 11-14.

Carrier, J. M. (1985). Mexican male bisexuality. Journal of Homosexuality 11, 78-85.

Davey, A. G. (1977). Racial awareness and social identity in young children. Mental Health and Society 4, 255-262.

Davids, A. (1973). Self-concept and mother-concept in black and white preschool children. Child Psychiatry and Human Development 4, 30-43.

deVries, M. W., & Sameroff, A. J. (1984). Culture and temperament: Influences on infant temperament in three East African societies. American Journal of Orthopsychiatry 54, 83-96.

Di Angi, P. (1976). Erikson's theory of personality development as applied to the black child. Perspectives in Psychiatric Care 14, 184-185.

Dinges, N. G., & Hollenbeck, A. R. (1978). The effect of instructional set on the self-esteem of Navajo children. Journal of Social Psychology 104, 9-13.

EchoHawk, M., & Parsons, O. R. (1977). Leadership vs. behavioral problems and belief in personal control among American Indian youth. Journal of Social Psychology 102, 47-54.

Gadpaille, W. J. (1978). Psychosexual developmental tasks imposed by pathologically delayed childhood: A cultural dilemma. In S. C. Feinstein, et al. (Eds.), Adolescent psychiatry: Developmental and clinical studies (Vol. 6, pp. 136-155). Chicago: University of Chicago Press.

Goldmeier, H. (1982). Children of the gilded ghetto in revolt: The early years, 1967-1974. Adolescence 17, 881-894.

Goldwert, M. (1985). Mexican machismo: The flight from femininity. Psychoanalytic Review 72, 161-169.

Grossman, B., Wirt, R., & Davids, A. (1985). Self-esteem, ethnic identity, and behavioral adjustments among Anglo and Chicano adolescents in West Texas. Journal of Adolescence 8, 57-68.

Henggeler, S. W., & Tavormina, J. B. (1978). The children of Mexican-American migrant workers: A population at risk? Journal of Abnormal Child Psychology 6, 97-106.

Hurley, O. L., Hirshoren, A., Kavale, K., & Hunt, J. T. (1978). Intercorrelations among tests of general mental ability and achievement for black and white deaf children. Perceptual and Motor Skills 46, 1107-1113.

Kaltsounis, B., & Higdon, G. (1977). Black teachers' perceptions of the ideal pupil. Perceptual and Motor Skills 45, 1071-1075.

Katz, I., Cole, O. J., & Baron, R. M. (1976). Self-evaluation, social reinforcement, and academic achievement of black and white schoolchildren. Child Development 47, 368-374.

Korn, S. J., & Gannon, S. (1983). Temperament, cultural variation and behavior disorder in preschool children. Child Psychiatry and Human Development 13, 203-212.

Kuo, H. K., & Marsella, A. J. (1977). The meaning and measurement of Machiavellianism in Chinese and American college students. Journal of Social Psychology 101, 165-173.

Lyles, M. R., Yancey, A., Grace, C., & Carter, J. H. (1985). Racial identity and self-esteem: Problems peculiar to biracial children. Journal of the American Academy of Child Psychiatry 24, 150-153.

Milgram, R. M., & Feingold, S. (1977). Concrete and verbal reinforcement in creative thinking of disadvantaged children. Perceptual and Motor Skills 45, 675-678.

Miyake, K., Chen, S. J., & Campos, J. J. (1985). Infant temperament, mother's mode of interaction, and attachment in Japan: An interim report. Monographs of the Society for Research in Child Development (Vol. 50, pp. 276-297). Chicago: University of Chicago Press.

Moore, T. L., & Baltes, P. B. (1975). Training of white adolescents to accurately simulate black adolescent personality. Adolescence 10, 231-239.

Olowu, A. A. (1983). A cross-cultural study of adolescent self-concept. Journal of Adolescence 6, 263-274.

Parish, T. S., Fleetwood, R. S., & Lentz, K. J. (1975). Effect of neutral conditioning on racial attitudes of children. Perceptual and Motor Skills 40, 695-701.

Powell, G. J. (1985). Self-concepts among Afro-American students in racially isolated minority schools: Some regional differences. Journal of the American Academy of Child Psychiatry 24, 142-149.

Roberts, A., Mosley, K. Y., & Chamberlain, M. W. (1975). Age differences in racial self-identity of young black girls. Psychological Reports 37, 1263-1266.

Ross, M. W. (1983). Femininity, masculinity, and sexual orientation: Some cross-cultural comparisons. Journal of Homosexuality 9, 27-36.

Sheikh, A. A., & Twerski, M. (1974). Future-time perspective in Negro and White adolescents. Perceptual and Motor Skills 39, 308.

Spencer, M. B. (1984). Black children's race awareness, racial attitudes and self-concept: A reinterpretation. Journal of Child Psychology and Psychiatry and Allied Disciplines 25, 433-441.

Tyler, J. D., & Holsinger, D. N. (1975). Locus of control differences between rural American Indian and white children. Journal of Social Psychology 95, 149-155.

Verkuyten, M. (1986). The impact of ethnic and sex differences on happiness among adolescents in the Netherlands. Journal of Social Psychology 126, 259-260.

Weissbluth, M. (1982). Chinese-American infant temperament and sleep duration: An ethnic comparison. Journal of Developmental and Behavioral Pediatrics 3, 99-102.

3. Cultural Differences in Development and Mental Disorders

Alzate, H. (1982). Effect of formal sex education on the sexual knowledge and attitudes of Colombian medical students. Archives of Sexual Behavior 11, 201-214.

Anderson, J., & Chung, J. (1982). Culture and illness: Parents' perceptions of their child's long term illness. Nursing Papers 14, 40-52.

Armiger, B. (1971). Critique of "Developing a psychometric instrument for the use of children's drawings in cross-cultural research: Problems, procedures, and potentials." Communicating Nursing Research 4, 151-158.

Bryant, C. A. (1982). The impact of kin, friend and neighbor networks on infant feeding practices. Cuban, Puerto Rican and Anglo families in Florida. Social Science and Medicine 16, 1757-1765.

Burke, A. W. (1980). A cross cultural study of delinquency among West Indian boys. International Journal of Social Psychiatry 26, 81-87.

Choi, E. S., & Hamilton, R. K. (1986). The effects of culture on mother-infant interaction. Journal of Obstetric, Gynecologic, and Neonatal Nursing 15, 256-261.

Coll, C. G., Spekoski, C., & Lester, B. M. (1981). Cultural and biomedical correlates of neonatal behavior. Developmental Psychobiology 14, 147-154.

Copeland, D. R., Silberberg, Y., & Pfefferbaum, B. (1983). Attitudes and practices of families of children in treatment for cancer. A cross-cultural study. American Journal of Pediatric Hematology/Oncology 5, 65-71.

Danna, J. J. (1980). Migration and mental illness: What role do traditional childhood socialization practices play? Culture, Medicine and Psychiatry 4, 25-42.

deVries, M. W., & Sameroff, A. J. (1984). Culture and temperament: Influences on infant temperament in three East African societies. American Journal of Orthopsychiatry 54, 83-96.

Dinges, N. G., & Hollenbeck, A. R. (1978). The effect of instructional set on the self-esteem of Navajo children. Journal of Social Psychology 104, 9-13.

Ekblad, S. (1984). Children's thoughts and attitudes in China and Sweden: Impacts of a restrictive versus a permissive environment. Acta Psychiatrica Scandinavica 70, 578-590.

Field, T., & Pawlby, S. (1980). Early face-to-face interactions of British and American working- and middle-class mother-infant dyads. Child Development 51, 250-253.

Furnham, A., & Kirris, R. (1983). Self-image disparity, ethnic identity and sex-role stereotypes in British and Cypriot adolescents. Journal of Adolescence 6, 275-292.

Gonzales-Tamayo, E. (1974). Dogmatism, self-acceptance, and acceptance of others among Spanish and American students. Journal of Social Psychology 94, 15-25.

Heckel, R. V., & Rajagopal, J. (1975). Future time perspective in Indian and American college students. Journal of Social Psychology 95, 131-132.

Holborow, P., & Berry, P. (1986). A multinational, cross-cultural perspective on hyperactivity. American Journal of Orthopsychiatry 56, 320-322.

Hollos, M. (1975). Logical operations and role-taking abilities in two cultures: Norway and Hungary. Child Development 46, 638-649.

Hong, K. M., & Townes, B. D. (1976). Infants' attachment to inanimate objects. A cross-cultural study. Journal of the American Academy of Child Psychiatry 15, 49-61.

Jahoda, G. (1981). Sex differences in retention of verbal and spatial characteristics of stimuli: A cross-cultural replication. Journal of Experimental Child Psychology 31, 424-429.

Kagan, J., Klein, R. E., Finley, G. E., Rogoff, B., & Nolan E. (1979). A cross-cultural study of cognitive development. Monographs of the Society for Research in Child Development (Vol. 44, pp. 1-77). Chicago: University of Chicago Press.

Kagan, S., & Zahn, G. L. (1975). Field dependence and the school achievement gap between Anglo-American and Mexican-American children. Journal of Educational Psychology 67, 643-650.

Kempe, C. H. (1982). Cross-cultural perspectives in child abuse. Pediatrics 69, 497-498.

Kilpatrick, W. (1974). Identity, youth and the dissolution of culture. Adolescence 9, 407-412.

Kitamura, A. (1983-1985). Suicide and attempted suicide among children and adolescents. A transcultural study. Pediatrician 12, 73-79.

Korbin, J. E., & Johnston, M. (1982). Steps toward resolving cultural conflict in a pediatric hospital. Clinical Pediatrics 21, 259-263.

Krener, P. G., & Sabin, C. (1985). Indochinese immigrant children: Problems in psychiatric diagnosis. Journal of the American Academy of Child Psychiatry 24, 453-458.

Magen, Z. (1983). Re-forming the boundaries: A trans-cultural comparison of positive experiences among adolescent males and females. Adolescence 18, 851-858.

Margalit, M. (1981). Cultural differences in the hyperactive syndrome rated in the Conners abbreviated scale. Journal of Learning Disabilities 14, 330-331.

McClain, E. W. (1975). An Eriksonian cross-cultural study of adolescent development. Adolescence 10, 527-541.

Minde, K. K., & Cohen, N. J. (1978). Hyperactive children in Canada and Uganda. Journal of the American Academy of Child Psychiatry 17, 476-487.

Olowu, A. A. (1983). A cross-cultural study of adolescent self-concept. Journal of Adolescence 6, 263-274.

Perlman, D., Josephson, W., Tai Hwang, W., Begum, H., & Thomas, T. L. (1978). Cross-cultural analysis of students' sexual standards. Archives of Sexual Behavior 7, 545-548.

Powell, G. J., & Gaines, R. (1982). An in-progress research report of perceptual-cognitive development of young black children in three cultures. Journal of the National Medical Association 74, 115-123.

Richmond, B. O., Sukemune, S., Ohnoto, M., Kawamoto, H., & Zamazaki, T. (1984). Anxiety among Canadian, Japanese, and American children. Journal of Psychology 116, 3-5.

Riesman, P. (1983). On the irrelevance of child rearing practices for the formation of personality. An analysis of childhood, personality, and values in two African communities. Culture, Medicine and Psychiatry 7, 103-129.

Seefeldt, C. (1984). Children's attitudes toward the elderly: A cross-cultural comparison. International Journal of Aging and Human Development 19, 319-328.

Snarey, J. R. (1985). Cross-cultural universality of social-moral development: A critical review of Kohlbergian research. Psychological Bulletin 97, 202-232.

Solheim, J. S. (1982). A cross-cultural examination of use of corporal punishment on children: A focus on Sweden and the United States. Child Abuse and Neglect 6, 147-154.

Solomons, H. C. (1982). Standardization of the Denver developmental screening test on infants from Yucatan, Mexico. International Journal of Rehabilitation Research 5, 179-189.

Stevenson, H. W., Parker, T., Wilkinson, A., Bonnevaux, B., & Gonzales, M. (1978). Schooling, environment, and cognitive development: A cross-cultural study. Monographs of the Society for Research in Child Development (Vol. 43, pp. 1-92). Chicago: University of Chicago Press.

Stevenson, H. W., Stigler, J. W., Lee, S. Y., Lucker, G. W., Kitamura, S., & Hsu, C. C. (1985). Cognitive performance and academic achievement of Japanese, Chinese, and American children. Child Development 56, 718-734.

Stevenson, H. W., Stigler, J. W., Lucker, G. W., Lee, S., Hsu, C., & Kitamura, S. (1982). Reading disabilities: The case of Chinese, Japanese, and English children. Child Development 53, 1164-1181.

Stoker, D. H. (1974). Cultural differences in child guidance clinic patients. International Journal of Social Psychiatry 20, 186-202.

Stone, E. J., & Crouch, A. (1979). Children's perceptions of vulnerability to health problems from a cross-cultural perspective. Journal of School Health 49, 347-350.

Strong, P. M., & Davis, A. G. (1977). Roles, role formats and medical encounters: A cross-cultural analysis of staff-client relationships in children's clinics. Sociological Review 25, 775-800.

Takahashi, T. (1980). Adolescent symbiotic psychopathology. A cultural comparison of American and Japanese patterns and resolutions. Bulletin of the Menninger Clinic 44, 272-288.

van der Ploeg, H. M., & Hulshof, R. E. (1984). Cross-cultural study of the relationship among academic performance, test anxiety, intelligence, and sex. Psychological Reports 55, 343-346.

Vaughn, G. M., & Cattell, R. B. (1976). Personality differences between young New Zealanders and Americans. Journal of Social Psychology 99, 3-12.

Whitam, F. L. (1980). The prehomosexual male child in three societies: The United States, Guatemala, Brazil. Archives of Sexual Behavior 9, 87-99.

Wiig, E. H., Becker-Redding, U., & Semel, E. M. (1983). A cross-cultural, cross-linguistic comparison of language abilities of 7- to 8- and 12- to 13-year-old children with learning disabilities. Journal of Learning Disabilities 16, 576-585.

Wilks, J., Callan, V. J., & Forsyth, S. J. (1985). Cross-cultural perspectives on teenage attitudes to alcohol. International Journal of the Addictions 20, 547-561.

4. Cultural Aspects of Mental Health and Illness

Berlin, I. N. (1984). Suicide among American Indian adolescents. Linkages for Indian child welfare programs (pp. 1-8). Washington, D. C.: National American Indian Court Judges Association.

Berlin, I. N. (1985). Prevention of adolescent suicide among some Native American tribes. In S. C. Feinstein, J. G. Looney, A. Z. Schwartzberg, & A. D. Sorosky (Eds.), Adolescent psychiatry: Developmental and clinical studies (pp. 77-93). Chicago: University of Chicago Press.

Bourne, P. G. (1975). The Chinese student-acculturation and mental illness. Psychiatry 38(3), 269-277.

Canino, I., Gould, M., Prupis, S., & Schaffer, D. (1986). Hispanic vs. black children in an outpatient mental health clinic. Journal of the American Academy of Child Psychiatry 25, 254-259.

Cochrane, R. (1979). Psychological and behavioral disturbances in West Indians, Indians and Pakistanis in Britain: A comparison of rates among child and adults. British Journal of Psychiatry 34, 201-210.

Comer, J. (1985). Black children and child psychiatry. American Journal of Child Psychiatry 24(2), 129-133.

Kim, S. P. (1980). Behavioral symptoms in three transracially adopted Asian Children: Diagnosis dilemma. Child Welfare 59(4), 213-224.

Kim, S. P., Hong, S., & Kim, B. S. (1979). Adoption of Korean children by New York area couples: A preliminary study. Child Welfare 58(7), 419-427.

Knight, G. P. (1978). Acculturation of second and third generation Mexican American children. Journal of Cross-Cultural Psychology 9(1), 87-97.

Powell, J. (1983). Coping with adversity: The psychosocial development of Afro-American children. In J. Powell (Ed.), The psychosocial development of minority group children (pp. 49-76). New York: Brunner/Mazel.

Quinton, D. (1980). Cultural and community influences. In M. Rutter (Ed.), Scientific foundations of developmental psychiatry (pp. 77-91). London: William Heinemann Med. Bks.

Sauna, V. D. (1981). Familial and sociocultural antecedents in psychopathology. In H. Triandis & J. Draguns (Eds.), Handbook of cross-cultural psychology-pathology (pp. 175-236). Boston: Allyn & Bacon.

Singer, K., Ney, P. G., & Lieh-Mak, F. (1978). A cultural perspective on child psychiatric disorders. Comprehensive Psychiatry 19(6), 533-540.

Sue, S., Wagner, N., Ja, D., Margullis, C., & Lew, L. (1976). Conceptions of mental illness among Asian- and Caucasian-American students. Psychological Reports 38, 703-708.

Weisner, T. (1981). Cities, stress, and children: A review of some cross-cultural questions. In R. Munroe, R. Munroe, & B. Whiting (Eds.), Handbook of cross-cultural human development (pp. 783-808). New York: Garland STPM Press.

Werner, E. E., & Smith, R. S. (1982). Vulnerable but invincible: A study of resilient children. New York: McGraw-Hill.

5. Cross-Cultural Attitudes toward Mental Illness and Therapy

Barbarian, O. A. (1984). Racial themes in psychotherapy with blacks: Effects of training on the attitudes of black and white psychiatrists. American Journal of Social Psychiatry 4, 13-20.

Bourne, P. G. (1975). The Chinese student--acculturation and mental illness. Psychiatry 38(3), 269-277.

Greenblatt, M., & Norman, M. (1982). Hispanic mental health and use of mental health services: A critical review of the literature. American Journal of Social Psychiatry 2(3), 25-31.

Jackson, J. F. (1986). Characteristics of black infant attachment behaviors. American Journal of Social Psychiatry 4(1), 32-35.
Kim, S. P. (1980). Behavioral symptoms in three transracially adopted Asian children: Diagnosis dilemma. Child Welfare 59(4), 213-224.
Kim, S. P., Hong, S., & Kim, B. S. (1979). Adoption of Korean children by New York area couples: A preliminary study. Child Welfare 58(7), 419-427.
Ratnavale, D. N. (1983). The mental health needs of refugees and other victims of disaster. American Journal of Social Psychiatry 3(3), 39-46.
Sue, S., Wagner, N., Ja, D., Margullis, C., & Lew, L. (1976). Conceptions of mental illness among Asian- and Caucasian-American students. Psychological Reports 38, 703-708.
Yamamoto, J., Koretsune, S., & Reece, S. (1982). The applicability of the psychiatric status schedule to the Japanese and Japanese-American psychiatric patients in Los Angeles. American Journal of Social Psychiatry 2(2), 24-27.

6. Cross-Cultural Use of Mental Health Services

Barbarian, O. A. (1984). Racial themes in psychotherapy with blacks: Effects of training on the attitudes of black and white psychiatrists. American Journal of Social Psychiatry 4, 13-20.
Greenblatt, M., & Norman, M. (1982). Hispanic mental health and use of mental health services: A critical review of the literature. American Journal of Social Psychiatry 2(3), 25-31.
Jackson, J. F. (1986). Characteristics of black infant attachment behaviors. American Journal of Social Psychiatry 4(1), 32-35.
Ratnavale, D. N. (1983). The mental health needs of refugees and other victims of disaster. American Journal of Social Psychiatry 3(3), 39-46.
Yamamoto, J., Koretsune, S., & Reece, S. (1982). The applicability of the psychiatric status schedule to the Japanese and Japanese-American psychiatric patients in Los Angeles. American Journal of Social Psychiatry 2(2), 24-27.

7. Cultural Aspects of Divorce and Custody and Single Parent Families

Adams, P. L., & Horovitz, J. H. (1980). Psychopathology and fatherlessness in poor boys. Child Psychiatry and Human Development 10, 135-143.
Adams, W. J. (1985). The missing triad: The case of two-child families. Family Process 24, 409-413.
Ahrons, C. R., & Arnn, S. (1981). When children from divorced families are hospitalized: Issues for staff. Health and Social Work 6, 21-28.
Atwell, A. E., Moore, U. S., & Nowell, C. S. (1982). The role of stepparents in child custody disputes. Bulletin of the American Academy of Psychiatry and the Law 10, 211-217.
Benedek, E. P., & Schetky, D. H. (1985). Custody and visitation. Problems and perspectives. Psychiatric Clinics of North America 8, 857-873.

Bergmann, M. V. (1985). The effect of role reversal on delayed marriage and maternity. In A. Solnit, et al. (Eds.), Psychoanalytic study of the child (Vol. 40, pp. 197-219). New Haven: Yale University Press.

Braxton, E. T. (1976). Structuring the black family for survival and growth. Perspectives in Psychiatric Care 14, 165-173.

Browning, D. H., & Boatman, B. (1977). Incest: Children at risk. American Journal of Psychiatry 134, 69-72.

Buxton, M. (1976). Applying the guidelines of beyond the best interest of the child. Child Psychiatry and Human Development 7, 94-102.

Chabassol, D. J. (1978). Fear of success in high school girls as related to family composition. Psychological Reports 42, 889-90.

Chavis, W. M., & Lyles, G. J. (1975). Divorce among educated black women. Journal of the National Medical Association 67, 128-134.

Chess, S., Thomas, A., Korn, S., Mittelman, M., & Cohen, J. (1983). Early parental attitudes, divorce and separation, and young adult outcome: Findings of a longitudinal study. Journal of the American Academy of Child Psychiatry 22, 47-51.

Chethik, M., & Kalther, N. (1980). Developmental arrest following divorce: The role of therapist as a developmental facilitator. Journal of the American Academy of Child Psychiatry 19, 281-288.

Coles, R. (1977). Privileged American children. Pediatrics 60, 381-382.

Coombs, L. C., & Freedman, R. (1979). Some roots of preference: Roles, activities and familial values. Demography 16, 359-376.

Critchley, D. L. (1981). The child as patient: Assessing the effects of family stress and disruption on the mental health of the child. Perspectives in Psychiatric Care 19, 144-155.

Derdeyn, A. P. (1975). Child custody consultation. American Journal of Orthopsychiatry 45, 791-801.

Derdeyn, A. P. (1983). The family in divorce: Issues of parental anger. Journal of the American Academy of Child Psychiatry 22, 385-391.

Earls, F. (1981). Parenting in urban America. Journal of the National Medical Association 73, 99-100.

Emery, R. E., & O'Leary, K. D. (1982). Children's perceptions of marital discord and behavior problems of boys and girls. Journal of Abnormal Child Psychology 10, 11-24.

Escalona, S. K. (1975). Children in a warring world. American Journal of Orthopsychiatry 45, 765-772.

Escalona, S. K. (1982). Babies at double hazard: Early development of infants at biologic and social risk. Pediatrics 70, 670-676.

Farran, D. C., & Ramey, C. T. (1980). Early face-to-face interactions of British and American working- and middle-class mother-infant dyads. Child Development 51, 250-253.

Field, T. M., Widmayer, S.M., Stringer, S., & Ignatoff, E. (1980). Teenage, lower-class, black mothers and their preterm infants: An intervention and developmental follow-up. Child Development 51, 426-436.

Fischer, D. G. (1984). Family size and delinquency. Perceptual and Motor Skills 58, 527-534.

Fosarelli, P. D. (1984). Latchkey children. Journal of Developmental and Behavioral Pediatrics 5, 173-177.

Futterman, E. H. (1980). Child psychiatry perspectives. After the "civilized" divorce. Journal of the American Academy of Child Psychiatry 19, 525-530.

Gardner, R. A. (1978). Social, legal and therapeutic changes that should lessen the traumatic effects of divorce on children. Journal of the American Academy of Psychoanalysis 6, 231-247.

Garman, A. R., Chinn, S., & Rona, R. J. (1982). Comparative growth of primary school children from one and two parent families. Archives of Disease in Childhood 57, 453-458.

Goldzband, M. G. (1983). Current trends affecting family law and child custody. A psychiatrist's perspective. Psychiatric Clinics of North America 6, 683-694.

Golombok, S., Spencer, A., & Rutter, M. (1983). Children in lesbian and single-parent households: Psychosexual and psychiatric appraisal. Journal of Child Psychology and Psychiatry and Allied Disciplines 24, 551-572.

Grotevant, H. D. (1979). Environmental influences on vocational interest development in adolescents from adoptive and biological families. Child Development 50, 854-860.

Hanson, S. (1981). Single custodial fathers and the parent-child relationship. Nursing Research 30, 202-204.

Hardy-Brown, K., Plomin, R., Greenhalgh, J., & Jax, K. (1980). Selective placement of adopted children: Prevalence and effects. Journal of Child Psychology and Psychiatry and Allied Disciplines 21, 143-152.

Hendricks, L. E., & Montgomery, T. (1983). A limited population of unmarried adolescent fathers: A preliminary report of their views on fatherhood and the relationship with the mothers of their children. Adolescence 18, 201-210.

Hershorn, M., & Rosenbaum, A. (1985). Children of marital violence: A closer look at the unintended victims. American Journal of Orthopsychiatry 55, 260-266.

Kalter, N., & Plunkett, J. W. (1984). Children's perceptions of the causes and consequences of divorce. Journal of the American Academy of Child Psychiatry 23, 326-334.

Kalter, N., & Rember, J. (1981). The significance of a child's age at the time of parental divorce. American Journal of Orthopsychiatry 51, 85-100.

Kellam, S. G., Ensminger, M. E., & Turner, R. J. (1977). Family structure and the mental health of children. Concurrent and longitudinal community-wide studies. Archives of General Psychiatry 34, 1012-1022.

Lindblad-Goldberg, M., & Dukes, J. L. (1985). Social support in black, low-income, single-parent families: Normative and dysfunctional patterns. American Journal of Orthopsychiatry 55, 42-58.

Martin, H. P., Burgess, D., & Crnic, L. S. (1984). Mothers who work outside of the home and their children: A survey of health professionals' attitudes. Journal of the American Academy of Child Psychiatry 23, 472-478.

Offord, D. R., Allen, N., & Abrams, N. (1978). Parental psychiatric illness, broken homes, and delinquency. Journal of the American Academy of Child Psychiatry 17, 224-238.

Peters, L. C., & Esses, L. M. (1985). Family environment as perceived by children with a chronically ill parent. Journal of Chronic Diseases 38, 301-308.

Plionis, E. M. (1977). Family functioning and childhood accident occurrence. American Journal of Orthopsychiatry 47, 250-263.

Porter, B., & O'Leary, K. D. (1980). Marital discord and childhood behavior problems. Journal of Abnormal Child Psychology 8, 287-295.

Prinz, R. J., Myers, D. R., Holden, E. W., Tarnowski, K. J., & Roberts, W. A. (1983). Marital disturbance and child problems: A cautionary note regarding hyperactive children. Journal of Abnormal Child Psychology 11, 393-399.

Rickel, A. U., & Langner, T. S. (1985). Short- and long-term effects of marital disruption on children. American Journal of Community Psychology 13, 599-611.

Rivara, F. P., Sweeney, P. J., & Henderson, B.F. (1985). A study of low socioeconomic status, black teenage fathers and their nonfather peers. Pediatrics 75, 648-656.

Rutter, M. (1978). Family, area and school influences in the genesis of conduct disorders. Journal of Child Psychology and Psychiatry and Allied Disciplines 19, 95-113.

Seegmiller, B. R. (1980). Sex-role differentiation in preschoolers: Effects of maternal employment. Journal of Psychology 104, 185-189.

Siegel, A. E. (1984). Working mothers and their children. Journal of the American Academy of Child Psychiatry 23, 486-488.

Small, G. W., & Nicholi, A. M. (1982). Mass hysteria among schoolchildren. Early loss as a predisposing factor. Archives of General Psychiatry 39, 721-724.

Wallerstein, J. S. (1985). Children of divorce: Preliminary report of a ten-year follow-up of older children and adolescents. Journal of the American Academy of Child Psychiatry 24, 545-553.

Young, J. L., & Griffith, E. E. (1985). Psychiatric consultation in Catholic annulment proceedings. Hospital and Community Psychiatry 36, 346-347.

8. Effects of War and Catastrophe on Children of Different Cultures

Arroyo, W., & Eth, S. (1985). Children traumatized by Central American warfare. In S. Eth & R. S. Pynoos (Eds.), Post-traumatic stress disorder. Washington D.C.: American Psychiatric Press.

Ayalon, O. (1980). Coping with terrorism. In S. Breznitz (Ed.), Stress in Israel. New York: Van Nostrand Reinhold.

Ayalon, O. (1982). Children as hostages. The Practitioner 226, 1773-1781.

Burlingham, D., & Freud, A. (1942). Young children in wartime. London: Allen & Unwin.

Cairns, E., Hunter, D., & Herring, L. (1980). Young children's awareness of violence in Northern Ireland: The influence of Northern Irish television in Scotland and Northern Ireland. British Journal of Social Psychology 19, 3-6.

Carlin, J. E. (1979). The catastrophically uprooted child: Southeast Asian refugee children. In J. Noshpitz (Ed.), Basic handbook of child psychiatry. New York: Basic Books.

Carlin, J. E., & Sokoloff, B. Z. (1985). Mental health treatment issues for Southeast Asian refugee children. In T. C. Owan (Ed.), Southeast Asian mental health: Treatment, prevention, services, training, and research. Washington, D.C.: Department of Health and Human Services.

Chen, M., et al. (1982). Volunteering behavior and its correlates in adolescent males during the Yom Kippur War. In C. D. Spielberger, I. G. Sarason, & N. A. Milgram (Eds.), Stress and anxiety. Washington, D.C.: Hemisphere.

Cohen, R. E. (1985). Coping and adaptation: Adolescent refugee camps. In J. Szapocnik, R. Cohen, & R. Hernandez (Eds.), Coping with adolescent refugees--the Mariel boatlift. New York: Praeger.

Coromina, J. (1943). Repercussions of the war on children as observed during the Spanish Civil War. The Nervous Child 2, 324-337.

Dahl, B. B., McCubbin, H. I., and Ross, K. L. (1977). Second generational effects of war-induced separations: Comparing the adjustment of children in reunited and non-reunited families. Military Medicine 142, 146-147, 150-151.

Day, R. C., & Sadek, S. N. (1982). The effect of Benson's relaxation response on the anxiety levels of Lebanese children under stress. Journal of Experimental Child Psychology 34, 350-356.

Freud, A., & Burlingham, D. (1943). War and children. New York: Medical War Books.

Geleerd, E. R. (1942). Psychiatric care of children in wartime. American Journal of Orthopsychiatry 12, 587-593.

Hefez, A. (1985). The role of the press and the medical community in the epidemic of "mysterious gas poisoning" in the Jordan West Bank. American Journal of Psychiatry 142, 833-837.

Hellman, I. (1983). Work in the Hampstead war nurseries. International Journal of Psycho-Analysis 64, 435-439.

Jackson, D. J. (1986). Contributions to the history of psychology: XL. The Hampstead wartime nurseries. Psychological Reports 58, 127-130.

Jackson, H. C. (1982). Moral nihilism: Developmental arrest as a sequel to combat stress. In S. C. Feinstein, J. G. Looney, A. Z. Schwartzberg, & A. D. Sorosky (Eds.), Adolescent psychiatry: Developmental and clinical studies. Chicago: University of Chicago Press.

Lin, K. M., Tazuma, L., & Masuda, M. (1979). Adaptational problems of Vietnamese refugees. I. Health and mental health status. Archives of General Psychiatry 36, 955-961.

Looney, J., et al. (1979). Consulting to children in crisis. Child Psychiatry and Human Development 10, 5-14.

Lyons, H. A. (1971). Psychiatric sequelae of the Belfast riots. British Journal of Psychiatry 118, 265-273.

McHan, E. J. (1985). Imitation of aggression by Lebanese children. Journal of Social Psychology 125, 613-617.

Mercier, M. D., & Despert, J. L. (1942). Psychological effects of the war on French children. Psychosomatic Medicine 5, 266-272.

Milgram, N. A. (1982). War related stress in Israeli children and youth. In L. Goldberger & S. Breznitz (Eds.), Handbook of stress. New York: The Free Press.

Milgram, R. M., & Milgram, N. A. (1976). The effect of the Yom Kippur War on anxiety level in Israeli children. Journal of Psychology 94, 107-113.

Newcombe, N., & Lerner, J. C. (1982). Britain between the wars: The historical context of Bowlby's theory of attachment. Psychiatry 45, 1-12.

Perez, M. M. (1984). Exile--the Chilean experience. International Journal of Social Work 30, 157-161.

Rambaut, R. D., & Rambaut, B. G. (1976). The family in exile: Cuban expatriates in the United States. American Journal of Psychiatry 133, 395-399.

Raviv, A., & Klingman, A. (1980). Children under stress. In S. Breznitz (Ed.), Stress in Israel (pp. 138-180). New York: Van Nostrand Reinhold.

Solantaus, T., Rimpela, M., & Taipale, V. (1984). The threat of war in the minds of 12-18-year-olds in Finland. Lancet 1, 784-785.

Solnit, A. J., & Newman, L. M. (1984). Anna Freud: The child expert. Psychoanalytical Study of the Child 39, 45-63.

Terr, L. C. (1984). Children at acute risk: Psychic trauma. In L. Grinspoon (Ed.), Psychiatry update (pp. 104-120). Washington, D.C.: American Psychiatric Press.

Tobin, J. J., & Friedman, J. (1984). Intercultural and developmental stresses confronting Southeast Asian refugee adolescents. Journal of Operational Psychiatry 15, 39-45.

Williams, C. L., & Westermeyer, J. (1983). Psychiatric problems among adolescent Southeast Asian refugees: A descriptive study. Journal of Nervous and Mental Disease 171, 79-85.

Ziv, A., & Israeli, R. (1973). Effects of bombardment on the manifest anxiety level of children living in kibbutzim. Journal of Consulting and Clinical Psychology 40, 287-291.

Ziv, A., Kruglanski, A. W., & Shulman, S. (1974). Children's psychological reactions to wartime stress. Journal of Personality and Social Psychology 30, 24-30.

9. Poverty as a Cultural Variable

Allen, W. (1978). Black family research in the United States, review, assessment, extension. Journal of Comparative Family Studies 9, 167-190.

Alvarez, G. (1982). The neurology of poverty. Social Science and Medicine 16, 945-950.

Brown, S. V. (1982). Early childbearing and poverty: Implications for social services. Adolescence 17, 397-408.

Crisp, A. D. (1980). Making substance abuse prevention relevant to low-income black neighborhoods. Journal of Psychedelic Drugs 12, 13-19.

Ferry, P. C. (1981). On giving new neurones: Are early intervention programs effective? Pediatrics 67, 38-41.

Fischman, S. H., & Palley, H. A. (1978). Adolescent unwed motherhood: Implications for a national family policy. Health and Social Work 3, 30-46.

Furnham, A. (1982). The perception of poverty among adolescents. Journal of Adolescence 5, 135-147.

Gispert, M., Brinich, P., Wheeler, K., & Frieger, L. (1984). Predictors of repeat pregnancies among low-income adolescents. Hospital and Community Psychiatry 35, 719-723.

Goldensohn, S. S. (1981). Psychotherapy for the economically disadvantaged: Contributions from the social sciences. Journal of the American Academy of Psychoanalysis 9, 291-302.

Guerin, L. S. (1977). Hospitalization as a positive experience for poverty children: Observations on children from low-income multi-problem families. Clinical Pediatrics 16, 509-513.

Heacock, D. R. (1976). The black slum child and the problem of aggression. American Journal of Psychoanalysis 36, 219-226.

Johnson, C. L. (1974). Adolescent pregnancy: Intervention into the poverty cycle. Adolescence 9, 391-406.

Lawrence, M. M. (1982). Psychoanalytic psychotherapy among poverty populations and the therapist's use of the self. Journal of the American Academy of Psychoanalysis 10, 241-255.

Lee, J. A. (1980). The helping professional's use of language in describing the poor. American Journal of Orthopsychiatry 50, 580-584.

Lindblad-Goldberg, M., & Dukes, J. L. (1985). Social support in black, low-income, single-parent families: Normative and dysfunctional patterns. American Journal of Orthopsychiatry 55, 42-58.

Piuck, C. L. (1975). Child-rearing patterns of poverty. American Journal of Psychotherapy 29, 485-502.

Rockwell, R. C., & Elder, G. H. (1982). Economic deprivation and problem behavior: Childhood and adolescence in the great depression. Human Development 25, 57-64.

Ross, G. S. (1984). Home intervention for premature infants of low-income families. American Journal of Orthopsychiatry 54, 263-270.

Rutter, M. (1980). Long term effects of early experience. Medical Child Neurology 22, 800.

Sandler, I. N. (1980). Social support resources, stress, and maladjustment of poor children. American Journal of Community Psychology 8, 41-52.

Stacey, B. G., & Singer, M. S. (1985). The perception of poverty and wealth among teenagers. Journal of Adolescence 8, 231-241.

Williams, K. R. (1984). Economic sources of homicide: Reestimating the effects of poverty and inequality. American Sociological Review 49, 283-289.

Zigler, E., Abelson, W. D., Trickett, P. K., & Seitz, V. (1982). Is an intervention program necessary in order to improve economically disadvantaged children's IQ scores? Child Development 53, 340-348.

10. Effects of Immigration on Mental Health

Bradley, S., & Sloman, L. (1975). Elective mutism in immigrant families. Journal of the American Academy of Child Psychiatry 14, 510-514.

Earls, F. (1982). Cultural and national differences in the epidemiology of behavior problems of preschool children. Culture, Medicine and Psychiatry 6, 45-56.

Earls, F., & Richman, N. (1980). The prevalence of behavior problems in three year old children of West Indian born parents. Journal of Child Psychology and Psychiatry and Allied Disciplines 20, 99-107.

Earls, F., & Richman, N. (1980). Behavior problems in pre-school children of West Indian born parents: A reexamination of family and social factors. Journal of Child Psychology and Psychiatry and Allied Disciplines 21, 107-117.

Marcos, L. R. (1982). Adults' recollection of their language deprivation as immigrant children. American Journal of Psychiatry 139, 607-610.

Minde, K., & Minde, R. (1976). Children of immigrants. The adjustment of Ugandan Asian primary-school children in Canada. Canadian Psychiatric Association Journal 21, 371-381.

Nicol, A. R. (1971). Psychiatric disorder in the children of Caribbean immigrants. Journal of Child Psychology and Psychiatry and Allied Disciplines 12, 271-287.

Queralt, M. (1984). Understanding Cuban immigrants: A cultural perspective. Social Work 29, 115-120.

Rutter, M., Yule, B., Morton, J., & Bagley, C. (1975). Children of West Indian immigrants. III. Home circumstances and family patterns. Journal of Child Psychology and Psychiatry and Allied Disciplines 16, 105-123.

Rutter, M., Yule, W., Berger, M., Yule, B., Morton, J., & Bagley, C. (1974). Children of West Indian immigrants. I. Rates of behavioural deviance and of psychiatric disorder. Journal of Child Psychology and Psychiatry and Allied Disciplines 15, 241-262.

Steinhausen, H. C. (1985). Psychiatric disorders in children and family dysfunction. A study of migrant workers' families. Social Psychiatry 20, 11-16.

Szapocznik, J., et al. (1978). Theory and practice in matching treatment to the special characteristics and problems of Cuban immigrants. Journal of Community Psychology 6, 112-122.

Wintrob, R. M. (1973). The influence of others: Witchcraft and rootwork and explanations of behavior disturbances. Journal of Nervous and Mental Disease 156, 318-326.

11. Asian Children, Adolescents, and Families: Mental Health Issues

Abbott, K. A., & Abbott, E. L. (1968). Juvenile delinquency in San Francisco's Chinese-American community. 1961-1966. Journal of Sociology 4, 45-56.

Arkoff, A., & Weaver, H. (1966). Body image and body dissatisfaction in Japanese-Americans. Journal of Social Psychology 68(2), 323-330.

Aybe, H. I. (1971). Deference and ethnic differences in voice levels. Journal of Social Psychology 85, 181-185.

Bourne, P. G. (1973). Suicide among Chinese in San Francisco. American Journal of Public Health 63(8), 744-750.

Bourne, P. G. (1975). The Chinese student--acculturation and mental illness. Psychiatry 38(3), 269-277.

Chang, T. S. (1975). The self-concept of children in ethnic groups: Black-American and Korean-American. Elementary School Journal 76, 52-58.

Egawa, J., & Tashima, N. (1981). Alternative service delivery models in Pacific/Asian American communities (p. 59). San Francisco: Pacific Asian Mental Health Research Project.

Egawa, J., & Tashima, N. (1982). Indigenous healers in Southeast Asian refugee communities (p. 50). San Francisco: Pacific Asian Mental Health Research Project.

Ewing, J. A., Rouse, B. A., & Pellizzari, E. D. (1974). Alcohol sensitivity and ethnic background. American Journal of Psychiatry 131(2), 206-210.

Hanna, J. M. (1978). Metabolic responses of Chinese, Japanese and Europeans to alcohol. Alcoholism: Clinical and Experimental Research 2(2), 89-92.

Hurh, W. M. (1980). Towards a Korean-American ethnicity: Some theoretical models. Ethnic and Racial Studies 3(2), 444-464.

Hurh, W. M., & Kim, K. C. (1981). Methodological problems in cross-cultural research: A Korean immigrant study. California Sociologist 4, 17-32.

Hurh, W. M., & Kim, K. C. (1982). Race relations paradigm and Korean American research. In E. Y. Yu, E. H. Phillips, & E. S. Yang (Eds.), Korean in Los Angeles (pp. 219-245). Los Angeles: Center for Korean-American and Korean Studies, California State University.

Hurh, W. M., & Kim, K. C. (1983). Korean immigrants in America: Ethnic confinement & adhesive adaptation. Madison, N.J.: Fairleigh Dickinson University Press.

Ito, K. L., & So, A. Y. (1982). Asian-American field survey: Re-analysis of health data. Health Care Alternatives of Asian American Women Research Project.

Kih, S. D., Sakauy, K., Koh, T. H., & Murata, A. (1983). A reflection on the study of Asian American elderly by Asian American researchers. Journal of Asian American Psychological Association 8, 22-33.

Kim, S. P. (1983). Self-concept, English language acquisition, and school adaptation in recently immigrated Asian children. Journal of Children in Contemporary Society 15(3), 71-79.

Kim, S. P., Siomopoulos, G., & Cohen, R. J. (1977). Verbal abstraction and culture: An exploratory study with proverbs. Psychological Reports 41, 967-972.

Kitano, H. H. L. (1961). Differential childrearing attitudes between first and second generation Japanese in the US. Journal of Social Psychology 53, 13-19.

Kitano, H. H. L. (1964). Intra- and intergenerational differences in maternal attitudes toward child rearing. Journal of Social Psychology 63(2), 215-220.

Kitano, H. H. L. (1967). Japanese-American crime delinquency. Journal of Psychology 66(2), 253-263.

Kuo, E. C. (1974). The family bilingual socialization: A sociolinguistic study of a sample of Chinese children in the US. Journal of Social Psychology 92, 181-191.

Levine, G. N., & Montero, D. M. (1973). Socioeconomic mobility among three generations of Japanese Americans. Journal of Social Issues 20(2), 33-48.

Levine, G. N., & Rhodes, R. C. (1981). The Japanese-American community: A three-generation study. New York: Praeger.

Lewis, H. P., & Lewis, E. R. (1965). Written language performance of sixth-grade children of low socio-economic status from bilingual and monolingual backgrounds. Journal of Experimental Education 33(3), 237-242.

Lott, J. T. (1976). Migration of mentality: The Philipino community. Social Casework 57(3), 165-172.

Marsella, A. J., Kinzie, D., & Gordon, P. (1973). Ethnic variations in the expression of depression. Journal of Cross-Cultural Psychology 4(4), 435-458.

Marsella, A. J., Sanborn, K. O., Kameoka, V., Shizuru, L., & Brennan, J. (1975). Cross-validation of self-report measures of depression among normal populations of Japanese, Chinese and Caucasian ancestry. Journal of Clinical Psychology 31(2), 281-287.

Marsella, A. J., Walker, E., & Johnson, F. (1973). Personality correlates of depressive disorders in female college students of different ethnic groups. International Journal of Social Psychiatry 19, 77-81.

Nishio, K. (1982). Characteristics of cultural therapeutic issues of Japanese clients in Japanese-American clients in the US (p. 31). San Francisco: Pacific Asian Mental Health Research Project.

Schwitters, S. Y., Johnson, R. C., McClearn, G. E., & Wilson, J. R. (1982). Alcohol use and the flushing response in different racial/ethnic groups. Journal of Studies on Alcohol 43, 1259-1262.

Sue, S., & Morishima, J. K. (1982). The mental health of Asian Americans. San Francisco: Jossey-Bass.

Sue, S., Wagner, N., Ja, D., Margullis, C., & Lew, L. (1976). Conceptions of mental illness among Asian- and Caucasian-American students. Psychological Reports 38, 703-708.

Sue, S., Zane, N., & Ito, J. (1979). Alcohol drinking patterns among Asian and Caucasian Americans. Journal of Cross-Cultural Psychology 10, 41-56.

Tanka-Matsumi, J., & Marsella, A. (1976). Cross-cultural variations in the phenomenal experience of depression: Word association studies. Journal of Cross-Cultural Psychology 7, 379-396.

Tashima, E., & Ito, K. (1982). Asian American self-concept: Preliminary thoughts on illness expression and the role of women. Health Care Alternatives of Asian American Women Research Project.

Wilson, R. A., & Hosokawa, B. (1980). East to America: A history of the Japanese in the US. New York: William A. Morrow.

Yee, L. Y., & LaFiorge, R. (1974). Relationship between mental abilities, social class, and exposure to English in Chinese fourth graders. Journal of Educational Psychology 66, 826-834.

12. Hispanic Children, Adolescents, and Families: Mental Health Issues

Acosta, F. X. (1979). Barriers between mental health services and Mexican Americans: An examination of a paradox. American Journal of Community Psychology 7, 503-520.

Alvellar, J., & Kagan, S. (1976). Development of competitive behaviors in Anglo-American and Mexican-American children. Psychological Reports 39, 191-198.

Anchor, K. N., & Anchor, F. N. (1974). School failure and parental school involvement in an ethnically mixed school. Journal of Comparative Psychology 2, 265-267.

Anderson, J. G., & Evans, F. B. (1976). Family socialization and educational achievement in two cultures: Mexican-American and Anglo-American. Sociometry 39, 209-222.

Arce, A. A. (1982). Psychiatric training issues: The Puerto Rican perspective. American Journal of Psychiatry 139, 461-465.

Badaines, J. (1976). Identification, imitation and sex role preference in father-present and father-absent black and Chicano boys. Journal of Psychology 92, 15-24.

Bird, H. R., et al. (1982). The Puerto Rican family: Cultural factors and family intervention strategies. Journal of the American Academy of Psychoanalysis 10, 257-268.

Bloom, D., & Padilla, A. M. (1979). A peer-interviewer model in conducting surveys among Mexican-American youth. Journal of Comparative Psychology 7, 129-136.

Brosnan, F. L. (1983). Overrepresentation of low socioeconomic minority students in special education programs in California. Learning Disabilities Quarterly 6, 517-525.

Bryant, B., & Meadow, A. (1976). School-related problems of Mexican-American adolescents. Journal of School Psychology 14, 139-150.

Buriel, R., Loya, P., Gonda, T., & Klessen, K. (1979). Child abuse and neglect referral patterns of Anglo and Mexican-Americans. Hispanic Journal of Behavioral Science 1, 215-227.

Canino, G., & Canino, I. A. (1982). Culturally syntonic family therapy for migrant Puerto Ricans. Hospital and Community Psychiatry 33, 299-303.

Canino, I. A., et al. (1986). A comparison of symptoms and diagnoses in Hispanic and black children in an outpatient mental health clinic. Journal of the American Academy of Child and Adolescent Psychiatry 25, 254-259.

Cauce, A. M., et al. (1980). Implicit and incorrect assumptions concerning the assessment of the Latino in the United States. American Journal of Community Psychology 9, 571-586.

Chesney, A. P., et al. (1980). Mexican-American folk medicine: Implications for the family physician. Journal of Family Practice 11, 567-574.

Cohen, R. E., & Fernandez, C. L. (1974). Ethnic identity and psychocultural adaptation of Spanish-speaking families. Child Welfare 53, 413-521.

Comas-Diaz, L. (1981). Puerto Rican espiritismo and psychotherapy. American Journal of Orthopsychiatry 51, 636-645.

Concha, P., Garcia, L., & Perez, A. (1975). Cooperation versus competition: Comparison of Anglo-American and Cuban-American youngsters in Miami. Journal of Social Psychology 95, 273-274.

Constantino, G., Malgady, R. G., & Rogler, L. H. (1984). Cuentos folkloricos as a therapeutic modality with Puerto Rican children. Hispanic Journal of Behavioral Science 6, 169-178.

Dembo, R., Schmeidler, J., & Burgos, W. (1979). Factors in the drug involvement of inner city junior high school youths: A discriminant analysis. International Journal of Social Psychiatry 25, 92-103.

Diaz-Guerrero, R. (1977). A Mexican psychology. American Psychologist 32, 934-944.

Fernandez-Pol, B. (1980). Culture and psychopathology: A study of Puerto Ricans. American Journal of Psychiatry 137, 724-726.

Ford, J. G., & Graves, J. R. (1977). Differences between Mexican-American and white children in interpersonal distance and social touching. Perceptual and Motor Skills 45, 779-785.

Gaviria, M., & Wintrob, R. M. (1976). Supernatural influence in psychopathology--Puerto Rican folk beliefs about mental illness. Canadian Psychiatric Association Journal 21, 361-369.

Gibson, G. (1978). An approach to identification and prevention for developmental difficulties among Mexican-American children. American Journal of Orthopsychiatry 48, 96-113.

Gilman, R. A. (1975). A selective annotated bibliography of bibliographies and other sources of information and resources potentially useful in Mexican-American bilingual-bicultural education. San Francisco: Mexican Language Association Forum on Bilingual Bibliographies and Information.

Gray, E., & Cosgrove, J. (1985). Ethnocentric perception of childrearing practices in protective services. Child Abuse and Neglect 9, 389-396.

Green, J. M., Trankina, F. J., & Chavez, N. (1976). Therapeutic intervention with Mexican-American children. Psychiatric Annals 6, 60-75.

Guinn, B. (1985). Emotions and obesity among Mexican-American children. Journal of School Health 55, 113-115.

Guinn, R. (1975). Characteristics of drug use among Mexican-American students. Journal of Drug Education 5, 235-241.

Guinn, R. (1978). Alcohol use among Mexican-American youth. Journal of School Health 48, 90-91.

Hardy-Fanta, C. & Montana, P. (1982). The Hispanic female adolescent: A group therapy model. International Journal of Group Psychotherapy 32, 351-366.

Jacobson, C. K. (1977). Separatism, integrationism, and avoidance among black, white, and Latin adolescents. Social Forces 55, 1011-1127.

Kagan, S., & Carlson, H. (1975). Development of adaptive assertiveness in Mexican and United States children. Developmental Psychology 11, 71-78.

Kagan, S., & Ender, P. B. (1975). Maternal response to success and failure of Anglo-American, Mexican-American, and Mexican children. Child Development 46, 452-458.

Keefe, S., Padilla, A., & Carlos, M. (1979). The Mexican-American extended family as an emotional support system. Human Organization 38, 144-152.

Knight, G. P., Kagan, S., Nelson, W., & Gumbiner, J. (1978). Acculturation of second- and third-generation Mexican-American children: Field independence, locus of control, self-esteem, and school achievement. Journal of Cross-Cultural Psychology 9, 87-97.

Korn, S. J., & Gannon, S. (1985). Temperament, cultural variation, and behavior disorder in preschool children. In S. Chess & A. Thomas (Eds.), Annual progress in child psychiatry and child development (pp. 401-410). New York: Brunner/Mazel.

Langgulung, H., & Torrance, R. P. (1972). The development of causal thinking of children in Mexico and the United States. Journal of Cross-Cultural Psychology 3, 315-320.

Laosa, L. M. (1975). Bilingualism in three United States Hispanic groups: contextual use of language by children and adults in their families. Journal of Educational Psychology 67, 617-627.

Laosa, L. M., Swartz, J. D., & Diaz-Guerrero, R. (1974). Perceptual-cognitive and personality development of Mexican and Anglo-American children as measured by human figure drawing. Developmental Psychology 10, 131-139.

Lasky, R. E., Klein, R. E., Yarbrough, C., & Kallio, K. D. (1981). The predictive validity of infant assessments in rural Guatemala. Child Development 52, 847-856.

Lecorgne, L. L., & Laosa, L. M. (1976). Father absence in low-income Mexican-American families: Children's social adjustment and conceptual differentiation of sex-role attributes. Developmental Psychology 12, 470-471.

Levine, E. S., & Bartz, K. W. (1979). Comparative child-rearing attitudes among Chicano, Anglo and black parents. Hispanic Journal of Behavioral Science 1, 165-178.

Littlefield, R. P. (1974). Self-disclosure among some Negro, white and Mexican-American adolescents. Journal of Counseling Psychology 21, 133-136.

Martinez, R., & Norman, R. D. (1984). Effects of acculturation on field independence among Chicano children. Hispanic Journal of Behavioral Science 6, 113-126.

Martinez, R., Norman, R. D., & Delaney, H. D. (1984). A children's Hispanic background scale. Hispanic Journal of Behavioral Science 6, 103-112.

Mendelberg, H. E. (1986). Identity conflict in Mexican-American adolescents. Adolescence 21, 215-224.

Moore, D. S., & Erickson, P. I. (1985). Age, gender and ethnic differences in sexual and contraceptive knowledge, attitudes, and behaviors. Family and Community Health 8, 38-51.

Morales, A., Ferguson, Y., & Munford, P. R. (1983). The juvenile justice system and minorities. In G. J. Powell (Ed.), The psychosocial development of minority group children. New York: Brunner/Mazel.

Mull, J. D., & Mull, D. S. (1981). Residents' awareness of folk medicine beliefs of their Mexican patients. Journal of Medical Education 56, 520-522.

Newton, F. C. R., Olmedo, E. L., & Padilla, A. M. (1982). Hispanic mental health research--a reference guide. Berkeley: University of California Press.

Padilla, E. R., Padilla, A. M., Morales, A., Olmedo, E. L., & Ramirez, R. (1979). Inhalant, marijuana, and alcohol abuse among barrio children and adolescents. International Journal of the Addictions 14, 945-964.

Pumariega, A. J. (1986). Acculturation and eating attitudes in adolescent girls: A comparative and correlational study. Journal of the American Academy of Child and Adolescent Psychiatry 2, 276-279.

Ramirez, M., & Price-Williams, D (1974). Cognitive styles of children of three ethnic groups in the United States. Journal of Cross-Cultural Psychology 5, 212-219.

Raymond, J. S., et al. (1980). The relative impact of family and social involvement on Chicano mental health. American Journal of Community Psychology 8, 557-569.

Rice, A. S., Ruiz, R. A., & Padilla, A. M. (1974). Person perception, self-identity, and ethnic group preference in Anglo, black, and Chicano preschool and third-grade children. Journal of Cross-Cultural Psychology 5, 100-108.

Rueda, R., & Smith, D. C. (1983). Interpersonal tactics and communicative strategies of Anglo-American and Mexican-American mildly mentally retarded and nonretarded students. Applied Research in Mental Retardation 4, 153-161.

Ruiz, P. (1976). Folk healers as associate therapists. Current Psychiatric Therapies 16, 269-275.

Schneer, H. I., Perlstein, A., & Brosovsky, M. (1975). Hospitalized suicidal adolescents: Two generations. Journal of the American Academy of Child and Adolescent Psychiatry 14, 268-280.

Stybel, L. J. (1977). Psychotherapeutic options in the treatment of child and adolescent hydrocarbon inhalers. American Journal of Psychotherapy 31, 525-532.

Szapocznik, J., Scopetta, M. A., & King, O. E. (1978). Theory and practice in matching treatment to the special characteristics and problems of Cuban immigrants. Journal of Community Psychology 6, 112-122.

Tans, E. J. (1983). Cuban unaccompanied minors program: The Wisconsin experience. Child Welfare 62, 269-279.

Trankina, F. J. (1983). Clinical issues and techniques in working with Hispanic children and their families. In G. J. Powell (Ed.), The psychosocial development of minority group children. New York: Brunner/Mazel.

Vigil, D. (1979). Adaptation strategies and cultural life styles of Mexican-American adolescents. Hispanic Journal of Behavioral Science 1, 375-392.

Wright, P., & Santa Cruz, R. (1983). Ethnic composition of special education programs in California. Learning Disabilities Quarterly 6, 387-394.

Zimmering, P., Toolan, J., Safrin, R., & Wortis, S. B. (1951). Heroin addiction in adolescent boys. Journal of Nervous and Mental Disease 11, 19-34.

13. American Indian and Native Alaskan: Mental Health Issues

Aase, J. M. (1981). The fetal alcohol syndrome in American Indians: A high risk group. Neurobehavioral Toxicology and Teratology 3, 153-156.

Ablon, J., Metcalf, A., & Miller, D. (1967). An overview of mental health problems of Indian children. Report to the joint commission on the mental health of children. New York: Harper and Row.

Attneave, C. L. (1979). The American Indian child. In J. B. Noshpitz (Ed.), Basic handbook of child psychiatry (Vol. 1, pp. 239-248). New York: Basic Books.

Beauvais, F., & LaBoueff, S. (1985). Drug and alcohol abuse intervention in American Indian communities. International Journal of the Addictions 20, 139-171.

Beiser, M., & Attneave, C. L. (1982). Mental disorders among Native American children: Rates and risk periods for entering treatment. American Journal of Psychiatry 139, 193-198.

Berlin, I. N. (1978). Anglo adoption of Native Americans: Repercussions in adolescence. Journal of the American Academy of Child Psychiatry 17(2), 387-388.

Berlin, I. N. (1983). Prevention of emotional problems among Native American children: Overview of developmental Issues. In S. Chess & A. Thomas (Eds.), Annual progress in child psychiatry and child development. New York: Brunner/Mazel.

Berlin, I. N. (1984). Suicide among American Indian adolescents. In N. Gale (Ed.), Linkages for Indian welfare programs. Washington, D. C.: National American Indian Court Judges Association. pp. 1-8.

Berlin, I. N. (1986). Psychopathology and its antecedent among American Indian adolescents. In B. B. Lahey (Ed.), Advances in clinical child psychology (pp. 125-152). New York: Plenum Press.

Berry, J. W. (1979). Acculturation as varieties of adaption. In A. M. Padilla (Ed.), Acculturation: Theory, models and some new findings. Boulder, Colo.: Westview Press.

Broudy, D. W. & May, P. A. (1983). Demographic and epidemiologic transition among the Navajo Indians. Social Biology 30, 1-16.

Brunneau, O. J. (1984). Comparison of behavioral characteristics and self-concepts of American Indian and Caucasian preschoolers. Psychological Reports 54, 571-574.

Byler, W. (1977). The destruction of American Indian families. In S. Unger (Ed.), The destruction of the American Indian family (pp. 34-61). New York: Association on American Indian Affairs.

Cockerham, W. C. (1975). Drinking attitudes and practices among Wind River Reservation youth. Quarterly Journal of Studies on Alcohol 36, 321-326.

Cockerham, W. C. (1976). Patterns of alcohol and multiple drug use among white and American Indian adolescents. International Journal of the Addictions 11, 209-220.

Deloria, V. (1979). Speaking of Indians. Vermillion, S. Dak.: The Dakota Press.

Department of Health and Human Services (1981). Report of the Third National Indian Child Conference: The Indian family--foundations for future. Albuquerque: Indian Health Service, Office of Mental Health Programs.

Dinges, N., Trimble, J. E., & Hollenbeck, A. R. (1979). American Indian adolescent socialization: A review of the literature. Journal of Adolescence 2, 259-296.

Dinges, N., Yazzie, M., & Tollefson, G. D. (1974). Developmental intervention for Navajo family mental health. Personnel and Guidance Journal 52, 390-395.

Dizmang, L. H., Watson, J., May, P. A., & Bopp, J. (1974). Adolescent suicide at an Indian reservation. American Journal of Orthopsychiatry 44(1), 43-49.

EchoHawk, M., & Parsons, O. R. (1977). Leadership vs. behavioral problems and belief in personal control among American Indian youth. Journal of Social Psychology 102, 47-54.

Goldstein, G. S. (1974). The model dormitory. Psychiatric Annals 4, 85-92.

Green, B. E., Sack, W. H., & Pambrun, A. (1981). A review of child psychiatric epidemiology with special reference to American Indian and Alaska native children. White Cloud Journal 2(2), 23-36.

Green, H. J. (1983). Risks and attitudes associated with extra-cultural placement of American Indian children: A critical review. Journal of American Academy of Child Psychiatry 22, 63-67.

Hammerschlag, C., Alderfer, C. P., & Berg, D. (1973). Indian education: A human systems analysis. American Journal of Psychology 130, 1098-1102.

Holmgren, C., Fitzgerald, B. J., & Carman, R. S. (1983). Alienation and alcohol use by American Indian and Caucasian high school students. Journal of Social Psychology 120, 139-140.

Johnson, D. L., & Johnson, C. A. (1965). Totally discouraged: A depressive syndrome of the Dakota Sioux. Transcultural Research 1, 141-143.

Jones, K. L., Smith, D. W., Ulleland, C. M., & Streissguth, A. P. (1973). Pattern of malformation in offspring of chronic alcoholic mothers. Lancet 1, 1267-1271.

Kaufman, A. (1973). Gasoline sniffing among children in a pueblo Indian village. Pediatrics 51, 1060-1064.

Kleinfeld, J. (1982). Getting it together at adolescence: Case studies of positive socializing environments for Eskimo youth. In S. M. Manson (Ed.), New directions in prevention among American Indian and Alaska native communities (pp. 341-367). Portland: Oregon Health Sciences University.

Kleinfeld, J., & Bloom, J. (1977). Boarding schools: Effects on the mental health of Eskimo adolescents. American Journal of Psychology 134(4), 441-447.

Krause, R. F., & Buffler, P. A. (1979). Sociocultural stress and the American native in Alaska: An analysis of changing patterns of psychiatric illness and alcohol abuse among the Alaska natives. Culture, Medicine and Psychiatry 3, 11-151.

Krush, T. P., & Bjork, J. (1965). Mental health factors in an Indian boarding school. Mental Hygiene 49, 94-103.

Krush, T. P., Bjork, J., Sindell, P. S., & Nelle, J. (1966). Some thoughts on the formation of personality disorder: Study of the Indian boarding population. American Journal of Psychology 122, 868-876.

Leighton, A. (1971). Cosmos and the Gallup city dump. In B. H. Kaplan (Ed.), Psychiatric disorder and the urban environment. New York: Behavioral Publications.

May, P. A. (1982). Substance abuse and American Indians: Prevalence and susceptibility. International Journal of the Addictions 17, 1185-1209.

May, P. A., & Dizmang, L. H. (1974). Suicide in the American Indian. Psychiatric Annals 4, 22-27.

May, P. A., Hymbaugh, K. J., Aase, J. M., & Samet, J. M., (1979). Epidemiology of fetal alcohol syndrome among American Indians of the Southwest. Social Biology 30, 374-387.

McIntosh, J. L. (1983-1984). Suicide among Native Americans: Further tribal data considerations. Omega 14, 215-229.

Medicine, G. (1981). Native American resistance to integration: Contemporary confrontations and religious revitalization. Plains Anthropologist 94, 277-286.

Mesteth, L. (1968). Gas and glue sniffing among the school age population. Pine Ridge Research Bulletin 4, 36-40.

Mindell, C., & Gurwitt, A. (1977). The placement of American Indian children: The need for change. In S. Unger (Ed.), The destruction of the American Indian family. New York: Association on American Indian Affairs.

Mindell, C., & Maynard, E. (1967). Ambivalence towards education among Indian high school students. Pine Ridge Research Bulletin 1, 26-31.

Nelson, I. (1977). Alcoholism in Zuni, New Mexico. Preventive Medicine 6, 152-166.

Oetting, E. R., & Dinges, N. (1982). Evaluation of the Toyei model dormitory project. Final report to the Office of Mental Health Programs, Indian Health Service. Washington, D.C.: Indian Health Service.

Peters, R. (1981). Suicidal behavior among Native Americans: An annotated bibliography. White Cloud Journal 2(3), 9-20.

Red Horse, Y. (1982). A cultural network model: Perspectives for adolescent services and paraprofessional training. In S. M. Manson (Ed.), New directions in prevention among American Indians and Alaska native communities (pp. 173-188). Portland: Oregon Health Sciences University.

Saslow, H. L., & Harrover, M. J. (1968). Research on psychological adjustment of Indian youth. American Journal of Psychiatry 125, 224-231.

Schottstaedt, M. F., & Bjork, J. (1977). Inhalant abuse in an Indian boarding school. American Journal of Psychology 134, 1290-1293.

Shore, J. H. (1975). American Indian suicide--fact and fantasy. Psychiatry 38, 86-91.

Shore, J. H., Bopp, J. F., Waller, T. R., & Dawes, J. W. (1972). Suicide prevention center on an Indian reservation. American Journal of Psychology 128(9), 76-81.

Shore, J. H., Kinzie, J. D., Pattison, E. M., & Hampson, J. (1973). Psychiatric epidemiology of and Indian village. Psychiatry 36, 70-81.

Shore, J. H., & Manson, S. M. (1981). Cross-cultural studies of depression among American Indians and Alaska natives. White Cloud Journal 2(2), 5-12.

Shure, M., Spivack, G., & Jaeger, M. (1971). Problem-solving thinking and adjustment among disadvantaged preschool children. Child Development 42, 1791-1803.

Stratton, R., Zeiner, A., & Paredes, A. (1978). Tribal affiliations and prevalence of alcohol problems. Journal of Studies on Alcohol 39, 1166-1177.

Streissguth, A. P. (1977). Maternal drinking and the outcome of pregnancy: Implications for child mental health. American Journal of Othopsychiatry 47, 422-431.

Topper, M. D. (1974). Drinking patterns, culture change, sociability, and Navajo adolescents. Addictive Disease: An International Journal 1, 97-116.

Townsley, H. C., & Goldstein, G. S. (1977). One view of the etiology of depression in the American Indian. Public Health Reports 92(5), 458-461.

Van Winkle, N. W., & May, P. A. (1986). Native American suicide in New Mexico 1967-1979--a comparative study. Human Organization 45(4), 296-309.

Ward, J. A. (1984). Preventive implications of a native Indian mental health focus on suicide and violent death. Journal of Preventive Psychiatry 2, 371-386.

Westermeyer, J. (1977). Cross-racial foster home placement among Native American psychiatric patients. Journal of the National Medical Association 69, 231-236.

Westermeyer, J., Walker, D., & Benton, E. (1981). A review of some methods for investigating substance abuse epidemiology among American Indians and Alaska natives. White Cloud Journal 2(2), 13-21.

Westermeyer, J., & Neider, J. (1985). Cultural affiliation among American Indian alcoholics: Correlations and change over a ten-year period. Journal of Operational Psychiatry 16, 17-23.

14. Black Children, Adolescents, and Families: Mental Health Issues

Barbarin, O. A. (1984). Racial themes in psychotherapy with blacks: Effects of training on the attitudes of black and white psychiatrists. American Journal of Social Psychiatry 4, 13-20.

Beiser, M., & Attneave, C. L. (1982). Mental disorders among Native American children: Rates and risk periods for entering treatment. American Journal of Psychiatry 139, 193-198.

Berlin, I. N. (1983). Prevention of emotional problems among Native-American children: Overview of developmental issues. In S. Chess & A. Thomas (Eds.), Annual progress in child psychiatry and child development. New York: Brunner/Mazel.

Bernard, V. W. (1953). Psychoanalysis and members of minority groups. Journal of the American Psychoanalytic Association 1, 256-269.

Bernard, V. W. (1972). Interracial practice in the midst of change. American Journal of Psychiatry 128, 96-97.

Berry, J. W. (1979). Acculturation as varieties of adaption. In A. M. Padilla (Ed.), Acculturation: Theory, models and some new findings. Boulder, Colo.: Westview Press.

Billingsley, A. (1968). Black families in white America. Englewood Cliffs, N.J.: Prentice-Hall.

Brunneau, O. J. (1984). Comparison of behavioral characteristics and self-concepts of American Indian and Caucasian preschoolers. Psychological Reports 54, 571-574.

Calneck, M. (1970). Racial factors in the countertransference: The black therapist and the black client. American Journal of Orthopsychiatry 40, 39-46.

Carter, J. H. (1979). Frequent mistakes made with black patients in psychotherapy. Journal of the National Medical Association 71, 1007-1009.

Carter, H. J., & Haizlip, T. M. (1972). Race and its relevance to transference. American Journal of Orthopsychiatry 42, 865-871.

Green, H. J. (1983). Risks and attitudes associated with extra-cultural placement of American Indian children: A critical review. Journal of the American Academy of Child Psychiatry 22, 63-67.

Hill, R. B. (1971). The strengths of black families. New York: Emerson Hall.

Holmgren, C., Fitzgerald, B. J., & Carman, R. S. (1983). Alienation and alcohol use by American Indian and Caucasian high school students. Journal of Social Psychology 120, 139-140.

Kellam, S. G., Ensminger, M. E., & Turner, R. J. (1977). Family structure and the mental health of children. Archives of General Psychiatry 4, 1012-1022.

Kendrick, E. A., McMillan, M. F., & Pinderhughes, C. A. (1983). A racial minority: Black Americans and mental health care. American Journal of Social Psychiatry 3, 11-18.

LaVietes, R. L. (1974). Crisis intervention for ghetto children: Contraindications and alternative considerations. American Journal of Orthopsychiatry 6, 57-61.

May, P. A., & Dizmang, L. H. (1974). Suicide in the American Indian. Psychiatric Annals 4, 22-27.

McAdoo, H. (1981). The black family. Beverly Hills: Sage.

McIntosh, J. L. (1983-1984). Suicide among Native Americans: Further tribal data and considerations. Omega 14, 215-229.

Meers, D. R. (1973). Psychoanalytic research and intellectual functioning of ghetto-reared black children. Psychoanalytical Study of the Child 28, 395-417.

Richmond, B. O., Sukemune, S., Ohmoto, M., Kawamoto, H., & Hamazaki, T. (1984). Anxiety among Canadian, Japanese, and American children. Journal of Psychology 116, 3-6.

Saslow, H. L., & Harrover, M. J. (1968). Research on psychosocial adjustment of Indian youth. American Journal of Psychiatry 125, 224-231.

Shervington, W. (1986). The black family: Clinical overview. American Journal of Social Psychiatry 6, 6-10.

Spurlock, J. (1985). Assessment and therapeutic intervention of black children. Journal of the American Academy of Child Psychiatry 24, 168-174.

Spurlock, J. (1986). Development of self-concept in Afro-American children. Hospital and Community Psychiatry 37, 67-70.

Stack, C. B. (1974). All our kin. New York: Harper and Row.

Taylor, R. L. (1976). Psychosocial development among black children and youth: A reexamination. American Journal of Orthopsychiatry 46, 4-19.

Thomas, A., & Chess, S. (1984). Genesis and evolution of behavioral disorder from infancy to early adult life. American Journal of Psychiatry 141, 1-9.
Thomas, A., & Sillen, S. (1972). Racism and psychiatry. New York: Brunner/Mazel.
Varghese, F. (1983). The racially different psychiatrist--implications for psychotherapy. Australian and New Zealand Journal of Psychiatry 17, 329-333.
Wallace, H. M. (1972). The health of American Indian children. Health Services 87, 867-876.
Werner, E. E., & Smith, R. S. (1979). An epidemiologic perspective on some antecedents and consequences of childhood mental health problems and learning disabilities. Journal of the American Academy of Child Psychiatry 18, 292-306.
Westermeyer, J. (1977). Cross-racial foster home placement among Native American psychiatric patients. Journal of the National Medical Association 69, 231-236.
Westermeyer, J., & Neider, J. (1985). Cultural affiliation among American Indian alcoholics: Correlations and change over a ten-year period. Journal of Operational Psychiatry 16, 17-23.
Wilking, V. (1982). The protean shape and form of the black family. Psychiatric Annals 12, 855-861.

15. Culture and the Development of Psychometric Instruments

Adler, I., & Kandel, D. B. (1981). Cross-cultural perspectives on developmental stages in adolescent drug use. Journal of Studies on Alcohol 42, 701-715.
Alzate, H. (1982). Effect of formal sex education on the sexual knowledge and attitudes of Colombian medical students. Archives of Sexual Behavior 11, 201-214.
Anderson, J., & Chung, J. (1982). Culture and illness: Parents' perceptions of their child's long term illness. Nursing Papers 14, 40-52.
Armiger, B. (1971). Critique of "Developing a psychometric instrument for the use of children's drawings in cross-cultural research: problems, procedures, and potentials." Communicating Nursing Research 4, 151-158.
Becker, T. (1976). Self and social responsibility: A comparative view of American and Israeli youth. American Journal of Psychoanalysis 36, 155-162.
Bekenan, P., Sapp, G. L., & Noisuwane, T. (1975). The utility of verbal models in changing self-esteem of institutionalized Thai and American adolescents. Journal of Social Psychology 96, 155-161.
Bowd, A. D. (1975). Note on conservation differences for Indian and white children. Perceptual and Motor Skills 41, 361-362.

16. Cultural Aspects of Psychopathology and Treatment

Acosta, F. X., Yamamoto, J., Evans, L. A., & Skilbeck, W. M. (1983). Preparing low-income Hispanic, black, and white patients for psychotherapy: Evaluation of a new orientation program. Journal of Clinical Psychology 39, 872-877.
Adler, I., & Kandel, D. B. (1981). Cross-cultural perspectives on developmental stages in adolescent drug use. Journal of Studies on Alcohol 42, 701-715.

Akinsola, H. A., & Fryers, T. (1986). A comparison of patterns of disability in severely mentally handicapped children of different ethnic origins Psychological Medicine 16, 127-133.

Aloia, G. F., Maxwell, J. A., & Aloia, S. D. (1981). Influence of a child's race and the EMR label on initial impressions of regular-classroom teachers. American Journal of Mental Deficiency 85, 619-623.

Beiser, M., & Attneave, C. L. (1982). Mental disorders among Native American children: Rates and risk periods for entering treatment. American Journal of Psychiatry 139, 193-198.

Bird, H. R., & Canino, I. (1981). The sociopsychiatry of espiritismo: Findings of a study of psychiatric populations of Puerto Rican and other Hispanic children. Journal of the American Academy of Child Psychiatry 20, 725-740.

Bourne, P. G. (1975). The Chinese student--acculturation and mental illness. Psychiatry 38, 269-277.

Cockerham, W. (1976). Drug use among white and American Indian high school youth. International Journal of the Addictions 11, 209-220.

Cockerham, W. C. (1977). Patterns of alcohol and multiple drug use among rural white and American Indian adolescents. International Journal of the Addictions 12, 271-285.

Davids, L. (1982). Ethnic identity, religiosity, and youthful deviance: The Toronto Computer Dating Project--1979. Adolescence 17, 673-684.

De Figueiredo, J. M. (1980). Some methodological remarks on transcultural interviewing on psychopathology. International Journal of Social Psychiatry 26, 280-292.

Fernandez-Pol, B., Bluestone, H., Morales, G., & Mizruchi, M. (1985). Cultural influences and alcoholism: A study of Puerto Ricans. Alcoholism 9, 443-446.

Giovacchini, P. L. (1980). Sociocultural factors, life- style, and adolescent psychopathology. In S. C. Feinstein, et al. (Eds.), Adolescent psychiatry: Developmental and clinical studies (Vol. 8, pp. 65-78). Chicago: University of Chicago Press.

Glass, J. (1983). Cultural factors complicating diagnosis and treatment of an African college student. Hospital and Community Psychiatry 34, 550-552.

Hahn, R. A. (1985). Culture-bound syndromes unbound. Social Science and Medicine 21, 165-171.

Hall, L. E., & Tucker, C. M. (1985). Relationships between ethnicity, conceptions of mental illness, and attitudes associated with seeking psychological help. Psychological Reports 57, 907-916.

Harding, R. K., & Looney, J. G. (1977). Problems of Southeast Asian children in a refugee camp. American Journal of Psychiatry 134, 407-411.

Lawson, W. B. (1986). Chronic mental illness and the black family. American Journal of Social Psychiatry 4(1), 57-61.

Maddahian, E., Newcomb, M. D., & Bentler, P. M. (1985). Single and multiple patterns of adolescent substance use: Longitudinal comparisons of four ethnic groups. Journal of Drug Education 15, 311-326.

Margalit, M. (1979). Ethnic differences in expressions of shame feeling by mothers of severely handicapped children. International Journal of Social Psychiatry 25, 79-81.

Meile, R. L., & Whitt, H. P. (1981). Cultural consensus and definition of mental illness. Social Science and Medicine [A] 15, 231-242.

Parra, F., & So, A. Y. (1983). The changing perceptions of mental illness in a Mexican-American community. International Journal of Social Psychiatry 29, 95-100.

Reynolds, C. R., & Paget, K. D. (1981). Factor analysis of the revised Children's Manifest Anxiety Scale for blacks, whites, males, and females with a national normative sample. Journal of Consulting and Clinical Psychology 49, 352-359.

Rodriguez-Andrew, S. (1985). Inhalant abuse: An emerging problem among Mexican-American adolescents. Children Today 14, 23-25.

Sanua, V. D. (1983). Infantile autism and childhood schizophrenia: Review of the issues from the sociocultural point of view. Social Science and Medicine 17, 1633-1651.

Schneider, B. A., Schneider, E. L., Hardesty, A. S., & Burdock, E. I. (1978). Interrelations of psychiatric diagnosis, psychological profile and ethnic background. Psychological Reports 43, 55-61.

Singer, K., Ney, P. G., & Lieh-Mak, F. (1978). A cultural perspective on child psychiatric disorders. Comprehensive Psychiatry 19, 533-540.

Whorton, J. E., & Wilson, R. M. (1983). Comparison of discrepancies in reading by black and white educable mentally retarded students. Psychological Reports 52, 488-490.

Williams, C. L., & Westermeyer, J. (1983). Psychiatric problems among adolescent Southeast Asian refugees. A descriptive study. Journal of Nervous and Mental Disease 171, 79-85.

Winfree, L. T., & Griffiths, C. T. (1983). Youth at risk: Marijuana use among Native American and Caucasian youths. International Journal of the Addictions 18, 53-70.

17. Treatment of Children, Adolescents, and Families from Various Cultures

Acosta, F. X., Yamamoto, J., Evans, L. A., & Skilbeck, W. M. (1983). Preparing low-income Hispanic, black, and white patients for psychotherapy: Evaluation of a new orientation program. Journal of Clinical Psychology 39, 872-877.

Arce, A. A., & Torres-Matrullo, C. (1982). Application of cognitive behavioral techniques in the treatment of Hispanic patients. Psychiatric Quarterly 54, 230-236.

Bernal y del Rio, V. (1982). Peculiarities of psychoanalytic treatment in a bicultural bilingual situation. Journal of the American Academy of Psychoanalysis 10, 173-193.

Bird, H. R., & Canino, G. (1982). The Puerto Rican family: Cultural factors and family intervention strategies. Journal of the American Academy of Psychoanalysis 10, 257-268.

Bluestone, H., & Vela, R. M. (1982). Transcultural aspects in the psychotherapy of the Puerto Rican poor in New York City. Journal of the American Academy of Psychoanalysis 10, 269-283.

Bradshaw, W. H. (1978). Training psychiatrists for working with blacks in basic residency programs. American Journal of Psychiatry 135, 1520-1524.

Canino, G., & Canino, I. A. (1982). Culturally syntonic family therapy for migrant Puerto Ricans. Hospital and Community Psychiatry 33, 299-303.

Chen, C. C. (1984). Group therapy with Chinese school children. International Journal of Group Psychotherapy 34, 485-501.

Chwast, J. (1977). Psychotherapy of disadvantaged acting-out adolescents. American Journal of Psychotherapy 31, 216-226.

Cole, J., & Pilisuk, M. (1976). Differences in the provision of mental health services by race. American Journal of Orthopsychiatry 46, 510-525.

Danieli, Y. (1981). The Group Project for holocaust survivors and their children. Children Today 10, 11, 33.

Dansky, J. L. (1980). Cognitive consequences of sociodramatic play and exploration training for economically disadvantaged preschoolers. Journal of Child Psychology and Psychiatry and Allied Disciplines 21, 47-58.

Fogelman, E., & Savran, B. (1979). Therapeutic groups for children of holocaust survivors. International Journal of Group Psychotherapy 29, 211-235.

Golden, K. M. (1982). Voodoo in the hospital: A diagnostic and treatment dilemma. American Journal of Social Psychiatry 2(3), 39-42.

Hardy-Fanta, C., & Montana, P. (1982). The Hispanic female adolescent: A group therapy model. International Journal of Group Psychotherapy 32, 351-366.

Jackson, A. M., Farley, G. K., Zimet, S. G., & Waterman, J. M. (1978). Race and sex as variables for children involved in treatment. Psychological Reports 43, 883-886.

Jason, L. A., Gesten, E., & Yock, T. (1976). Relational and behavioral interventions with economically disadvantaged toddlers. American Journal of Orthopsychiatry 46, 270-278.

Katz, P. (1981). Psychotherapy with native adolescents. Canadian Journal of Psychiatry 26, 455-459.

Knudson, K. H., & Kagan, S. (1977). Visual perspective role-taking and field-independence among Anglo-American and Mexican-American children of two ages. Journal of Genetic Psychology 131, 243-253.

LaVietes, R. L. (1974). Crisis intervention for ghetto children: Contraindications and alternative considerations. American Journal of Orthopsychiatry 44, 720-727.

McDermott, J. G., Char, W. F., Robillard, A. B., Hsu, J., Tseng, W. S., & Ashton, G. C. (1983). Cultural variations in family attitudes and their implications for therapy. Journal of the American Academy of Child and Adolescent Psychiatry 22, 454-458.

Munoz, J. A. (1986). Countertransference and its implementation in the treatment of a Hispanic adolescent boy. Psychiatry 49, 160-179.

Perkowski, S. (1974). Some observations concerning black children living in a residential care agency. International Journal of Social Psychiatry 20, 89-93.

Pinderhughes, E. B. (1984). Teaching empathy: Ethnicity, race and power at the cross-cultural treatment interface. American Journal of Social Psychiatry 4(1), 5-12.

Ruiz, P. (1976). Folk healers as associate therapists. Current Psychiatric Therapies 16, 269-275.

Schaefer, C., & Brown, S. (1976). Investigating ethnic prejudice among boys in residential treatment. Journal of Social Psychology 100, 317-318.

Spurlock, J. (1985). Assessment and therapeutic intervention of black children. Journal of the American Academy of Child and Adolescent Psychiatry 24, 168-174.

Vander Kolk, C. J. (1978). Physiological reactions of black, Puerto Rican, and white students in suggested ethnic encounter. Journal of Social Psychology 104, 107-114.

Yamamoto, J., & Acosta, F. X. (1982). Treatment of Asian Americans and Hispanic Americans: Similarities and differences. Journal of the American Academy of Psychoanalysis 10, 585-607.

18. Cross-Cultural Research

Bryant, C. A. (1982). The impact of kin, friend and neighbor networks on infant feeding practices. Cuban, Puerto Rican and Anglo families in Florida. Social Science and Medicine 16, 1757-1765.

Burke, A. W. (1980). A cross cultural study of delinquency among West Indian boys. International Journal of Social Psychiatry 26, 81-87.

Choi, E. S., & Hamilton, R. K. (1986). The effects of culture on mother-infant interaction. Journal of Obstetric, Gynecologic, and Neonatal Nursing 15, 256-261.

Coll, C. G., Spekoski, C., & Lester, B. M. (1981). Cultural and biomedical correlates of neonatal behavior. Developmental Psychobiology 14, 147-154.

Copeland, D. R., Silberberg, Y., & Pfefferbaum, B. (1983). Attitudes and practices of families of children in treatment for cancer. A cross-cultural study. American Journal of Pediatric Hematology/Oncology 5, 65-71.

Danna, J. J. (1980). Migration and mental illness: What role do traditional childhood socialization practices play? Culture, Medicine and Psychiatry 4, 25-42.

deVries, M. W., & Sameroff, A. J. (1984). Culture and temperament: Influences on infant temperament in three East African societies. American Journal of Orthopsychiatry 54, 83-96.

Dinges, N. G., & Hollenbeck, A. R. (1978). The effect of instructional set on the self-esteem of Navajo children. Journal of Social Psychology 104, 9-13.

Ekblad, S. (1984). Children's thoughts and attitudes in China and Sweden: Impacts of a restrictive versus a permissive environment. Acta Psychiatrica Scandinavica 70, 578-590.

Field, T., & Pawlby, S. (1980). Early face-to-face interactions of British and American working- and middle-class mother-infant dyads. Child Development 51, 250-253.

Furnham, A., & Kirris, R. (1983). Self-image disparity, ethnic identity and sex-role stereotypes in British and Cypriot adolescents. Journal of Adolescence 6, 275-292.

Gonzales-Tamayo, E. (1974). Dogmatism, self-acceptance, and acceptance of others among Spanish and American students. Journal of Social Psychology 94, 15-25.

Heckel, R. V., & Rajagopal, J. (1975). Future time perspective in Indian and American college students. Journal of Social Psychology 95, 131-132.

Holborow, P., & Berry, P. (1986). A multinational, cross-cultural perspective on hyperactivity. American Journal of Orthopsychiatry 56, 320-322.

Hollos, M. (1975). Logical operations and role-taking abilities in two cultures: Norway and Hungary. Child Development 46, 638-649.

Hong, K. M., & Townes, B. D. (1976). Infants' attachment to inanimate objects. A cross-cultural study. Journal of the American Academy of Child and Adolescent Psychiatry 15, 49-61.

Jahoda, G. (1981). Sex differences in retention of verbal and spatial characteristics of stimuli: A cross-cultural replication. Journal of Experimental Child Psychology 31, 424-429.

Kagan, J., Klein, R. E., Finley, G. E., Rogoff, B., & Nolan, E. (1979). A cross-cultural study of cognitive development. Monographs of the Society for Research in Child Development (Vol. 44, pp. 1-77). Chicago: University of Chicago Press.

Kagan, S., & Zahn, G. L. (1975). Field dependence and the school achievement gap between Anglo-American and Mexican-American children. Journal of Educational Psychology 67, 643-650.

Kempe, C. H. (1982). Cross-cultural perspectives in child abuse. Pediatrics 69, 497-498.

Kilpatrick, W. (1974). Identity, youth and the dissolution of culture. Adolescence 9, 407-412.

Kitamura, A. (1983-1985). Suicide and attempted suicide among children and adolescents. A transcultural study. Pediatrician 12, 73-79.

Korbin, J. E., & Johnston, M. (1982). Steps toward resolving cultural conflict in a pediatric hospital. Clinical Pediatrics 21, 259-263.

Krener, P. G., & Sabin, C. (1985). Indochinese immigrant children: Problems in psychiatric diagnosis. Journal of the American Academy of Child and Adolescent Psychiatry 24, 453-458.

Magen, Z. (1983). Re-forming the boundaries: A trans-cultural comparison of positive experiences among adolescent males and females. Adolescence 18, 851-858.

Margalit, M. (1981). Cultural differences in the hyperactive syndrome rated in the Conners abbreviated scale. Journal of Learning Disabilities 14, 330-331.

McClain, E. W. (1975). An Eriksonian cross-cultural study of adolescent development. Adolescence 10, 527-541.

Minde, K. K., & Cohen, N. J. (1978). Hyperactive children in Canada and Uganda. Journal of the American Academy of Child Psychiatry 17, 476-487.

Olowu, A. A. (1983). A cross-cultural study of adolescent self-concept. Journal of Adolescence 6, 263-274.

Perlman, D., Josephson, W., Tai Hwang, W., Begum, H., & Thomas, T. L. (1978). Cross-cultural analysis of students' sexual standards. Archives of Sexual Behavior 7, 545-548.

Powell, G. J., & Gaines, R. (1982). An in-progress research report of perceptual-cognitive development of young black children in three cultures. Journal of the National Medical Association 74, 115-123.

Richmond, B. O., Sukemune, S., Ohnoto, M., Kawamoto, H., & Hamazaki, T. (1984). Anxiety among Canadian, Japanese, and American children. Journal of Psychology 116, 3-6.

Riesman, P. (1983). On the irrelevance of child rearing practices for the formation of personality. An analysis of childhood, personality, and values in two African communities. Culture, Medicine and Psychiatry 7, 103-129.

Seefeldt, C. (1984). Children's attitudes toward the elderly: A cross-cultural comparison. International Journal of Aging and Human Development 19, 319-328.

Snarey, J. R. (1985). Cross-cultural universality of social-moral development: A critical review of Kohlbergian research. Psychological Bulletin 97, 202-232.

Solheim, J. S. (1982). A cross-cultural examination of use of corporal punishment on children: A focus on Sweden and the United States. Child Abuse and Neglect 6, 147-154.

Solomons, H. C. (1982). Standardization of the Denver Developmental Screening Test on infants from Yucatan, Mexico. International Journal of Rehabilitation Research 5, 179-189.

Stevenson, H. W., Parker, T., Wilkinson, A., Bonnevaux, B., & Gonzales, M. (1978). Schooling, environment, and cognitive development: A cross-cultural study. Monographs of the Society for Research in Child Development (Vol. 43, pp. 1-92). Chicago: University of Chicago Press.

Stevenson, H. W., Stigler, J. W., Lee, S. Y., Lucker, G. W., Kitamura, S., & Hsu, C. C. (1985). Cognitive performance and academic achievement of Japanese, Chinese, and American children. Child Development 56, 718-734.

Stevenson, H. W., Stigler, J. W., Lucker, G. W., Lee, S., Hsu, C., & Kitamura, S. (1982). Reading disabilities: The case of Chinese, Japanese, and English. Child Development 53, 1164-1181.

Stoker, D. H. (1984). Cultural differences in child guidance clinic patients. International Journal of Social Psychiatry 20, 186-202.

Stone, E. J., & Crouch, A. (1979). Children's perceptions of vulnerability to health problems from a cross-cultural perspective. Journal of School Health 49, 347-350.

Strong, P. M., & Davis, A. G. (1977). Roles, role formats and medical encounters: A cross-cultural analysis of staff-client relationships in children's clinics. Sociological Review 25, 775-800.

Takahashi, T. (1980). Adolescent symbiotic psychopathology. A cultural comparison of American and Japanese patterns and resolutions. Bulletin of the Menninger Clinic 44, 272-288.

van der Ploeg, H. M., & Hulshof, R. E. (1984). Cross-cultural study of the relationship among academic performance, test anxiety, intelligence, and sex. Psychological Reports 55, 343-346.

Vaughn, G. M., & Cattell, R. B. (1976). Personality differences between young New Zealanders and Americans. Journal of Social Psychology 99, 3-12.

Whitam, F. L. (1980). The prehomosexual male child in three societies: The United States, Guatemala, Brazil. Archives of Sexual Behavior 9, 87-99.

Wiig, E. H., Becker-Redding, U., & Semel, E. M. (1983). A cross-cultural, cross-linguistic comparison of language abilities of 7- to 8- to 12- to 13-year-old children with learning disabilities. Journal of Learning Disabilities 16, 576-585.

Wilks, J., Callan, V. J., & Forsyth, S. J. (1985). Cross-cultural perspectives on teenage attitudes to alcohol. International Journal of the Addictions 20, 547-561.

19. Training in Multicultural Mental Health

Barbarin, O. A. (1984). Racial themes in psychotherapy with blacks: Effects of training on the attitudes of black and white psychiatrists. American Journal of Social Psychiatry 4, 13-20.

Beiser, M., & Attneave, C. L. (1982). Mental disorders among Native American children: Rates and risk periods for entering treatment. American Journal of Psychiatry 139, 193-198.

Berlin, I. N. (1983). Prevention of emotional problems among Native-American children: Overview of developmental issues. In S. Chess & A. Thomas (Eds.), Annual progress in child psychiatry and child development. New York: Brunner/Mazel.

Bernard, V. W. (1972). Interracial practice in the midst of change. American Journal of Psychiatry 128, 96-97.

Bourne, P. G. (1975). The Chinese student--acculturation and mental illness. Psychiatry 38, 269-277.

Brunneau, O. J. (1984). Comparison of behavioral characteristics and self-concepts of American Indian and Caucasian preschoolers. Psychological Reports 54, 571-574.

Calneck, M. (1970). Racial factors in the countertransference: the black therapist and the black client. American Journal of Orthopsychiatry 40, 39-46.

Carter, J. H. (1979). Frequent mistakes made with black patients in psychotherapy. Journal of the National Medical Association 71, 1007-1009.

Carter, J. H., & Haizlip, T. M. (1972). Race and its relevance to transference. American Journal of Orthopsychiatry 42, 865-871.

Cockerham, W. (1976). Drug use among white and American Indian high school youth. International Journal of the Addictions 11, 209-220.

Cockerham, W. C. (1977). Patterns of alcohol and multiple drug use among rural white and American Indian adolescents. International Journal of the Addictions 12, 271-285.

Davids, L. (1982). Ethnic identity, religiosity, and youthful deviance: The Toronto Computer Dating Project--1979. Adolescence 17, 673-684.

De Figueiredo, J. M. (1980). Some methodological remarks on transcultural interviewing on psychopathology. International Journal of Social Psychiatry 26, 280-292.

Fernandez-Pol, B., Bluestone, H., Morales, G., & Mizruchi, M. (1985). Cultural influences and alcoholism: A study of Puerto Ricans. Alcoholism 9, 443-446.

Green, H. J. (1983). Risks and attitudes associated with extra-cultural placement of American Indian children: A critical review. Journal of the American Academy of Child and Adolescent Psychiatry 22, 63-67.

Hill, R. B. (1971). The strengths of black families. New York: Emerson Hall.

Holmgren, C., Fitzgerald, B. J., & Carman, R. S. (1983). Alienation and alcohol use by American Indian and Caucasian high school students. Journal of Social Psychology 120, 139-140.

Kellam, S. G., Ensminger, M. E., & Turner, R. J. (1977). Family structure and the mental health of children. Archives of General Psychiatry 4, 1012-1022.

Kendrick, E. A., McMillan, M. F., & Pinderhughes, C. A. (1983). A racial minority: Black Americans and mental health care. American Journal of Social Psychiatry 3, 11-18.

Lawson, W. B. (1986). Chronic mental illness and the black family. American Journal of Social Psychiatry 4(1), 57-61.

Maddahian, E., Newcomb, M. D., & Bentler, P. M. (1985). Single and multiple patterns of adolescent substance use: Longitudinal comparisons of four ethnic groups. Journal of Drug Education 15, 311-326.

Margalit, M. (1979). Ethnic differences in expressions of shame feeling by mothers of severely handicapped children. International Journal of Social Psychiatry 25, 79-81.

Meile, R. L., & Whitt, H. P. (1981). Cultural consensus and definition of mental illness. Social Science and Medicine [A] 15, 231-242.

Padilla, E. R., Padilla, A. M., Morales, A., Olmedo, E. L., & Ramirez, R. (1979). Inhalant, marijuana, and alcohol abuse among barrio children and adolescents. International Journal of the Addictions 14, 945-964.

Parra, F., & So, A. Y. (1983). The changing perceptions of mental illness in a Mexican-American community. International Journal of Social Psychiatry 29, 95-100.

Powell, G. J. (Ed.). (1983). The psychosocial development of minority group children. New York: Brunner/Mazel.

Reynolds, C. R., & Paget, K. D. (1981). Factor analysis of the revised Children's Manifest Anxiety Scale for blacks, whites, males, and females with a national normative sample. Journal of Consulting and Clinical Psychology 49, 352-359.

Rodriguez-Andrew, S. (1985). Inhalant abuse: An emerging problem among Mexican-American adolescents. Children Today 14, 23-25.

Sanua, V. D. (1983). Infantile autism and childhood schizophrenia: Review of the issues from the sociocultural point of view. Social Science and Medicine 17, 1633-1651.

Schneider, B. A., Schneider, E. L., Hardesty, A. S., & Burdock, E. I. (1978). Interrelations of psychiatric diagnosis, psychological profile and ethnic background. Psychological Reports 43, 55-61.

Schottstaedt, M. D., & Bjork, J. W. (1977). Inhalant abuse in an Indian borading School. American Journal of Psychiatry 134, 1290-1293.

Singer, K., Ney, P. G., & Lieh-Mak, F. (1978). A cultural perspective on child psychiatric disorders. Comprehensive Psychiatry 19, 533-540.

Whorton, J. E., & Wilson, R. M. (1983). Comparison of discrepancies in reading by black and white educable mentally retarded students. Psychological Reports 52, 488-490.

Williams, C. L., & Westermeyer, J. (1983). Psychiatric problems among adolescent Southeast Asian refugees. A descriptive study. Journal of Nervous and Mental Disease 171, 79-85.

Winfree, L. T., & Griffiths, C. T. (1983). Youth at risk: Marijuana use among Native American and Caucasian youths. International Journal of the Addictions 18, 53-70.

20. Miscellaneous References

Acosta, F. X., Yamamoto, J., Evans, L. A., & Skilbeck, W. M. (1983). Preparing low-income Hispanic, black, and white patients for psychotherapy: Evaluation of a new orientation program. Journal of Clinical Psychology 39, 872-877.

Allen, W. (1978). Black family research in the United States, review, assessment, extension. Journal of Comparative Family Studies 9, 167-190.

Alvarez, G. (1982). The neurology of poverty. Social Science and Medicine 16, 945-950.

Anchor, K. N., & Anchor, F. N. (1974). School failure and parental school involvement in an ethnically mixed school. Journal of Community Psychology 2, 265-267.

Anderson, J. G., & Evans, F. B. (1976). Family socialization and educational achievement in two cultures: Mexican-American and Anglo-American. Sociometry 39, 209-222.

Arce, A. A. (1982). Psychiatric training issues: The Puerto Rican perspective. American Journal of Psychiatry 139, 461-465.

Arce, A. A., & Torres-Matrullo, C. (1982). Application of cognitive behavioral techniques in the treatment of Hispanic patients. Psychiatric Quarterly 54, 230-236.

Badaines, J. (1976). Identification, imitation and sex role preference in father-present and father-absent black and Chicano boys. Journal of Psychology 92, 15-24.

Benjamin, G. A., Kalin, M. W., & Sales, B. D. (1984). Developmental differences in infants and policy on undocumented Mexican-American parents. Hispanic Journal of Behavioral Science 6, 103-112.

Bernal, G. (1982). Cuban families. In M. McGoldrick, J. K. Pearce, & J. Giordano (Eds.), Ethnicity and family therapy. New York: Guilford Press.

Bloom, J., Mendelsohn, B., & Richards, W. (1976). Experiences and statements of Alaskan native high school students. Journal of Clinical Psychology 32, 362-366.

Bolling, J. L. (1974). The changing self-concept of black children. The black identity test. Journal of the National Medical Association 66, 28-31, 34.

Brown, N. W. (1977). Personality characteristics of black adolescents. Adolescence 12, 81-87.

Brown, S. V. (1982). Early childbearing and poverty: Implications for social services. Adolescence 17, 397-408.

Carrier, J. M. (1985). Mexican male bisexuality. Journal of Homosexuality 11, 75-85.

Cochrane, R. (1979). Psychological and behavioral disturbances in West Indians, Indians and Pakistanis in Britain: A comparison of rates among child and adults. British Journal of Psychiatry 34, 201-210.

Comer, J. (1985). Black children and child psychiatry. American Journal of Child Psychiatry 24(2), 129-133.

Crisp, A. D. (1980). Making substance abuse prevention relevant to low-income black neighborhoods. Journal of Psychedelic Drugs 12, 13-19.

Fischman, S. H., & Palley, H. A. (1978). Adolescent unwed motherhood: Implications for a national family policy. Health and Social Work 3, 30-46.

Furnham, A. (1982). The perception of poverty among adolescents. Journal of Adolescence 5, 135-147.

Gispert, M., Brinich, P., Wheeler, K., & Krieger, L. (1984). Predictors of repeat pregnancies among low-income adolescents. Hospital and Community Psychiatry 35, 719-723.

Glover, J. A. (1976a). Comparative levels of creative ability among elementary school children. Journal of Genetic Psychology 129, 131-135.

Glover, J. A. (1976b). Comparative levels of creative ability in black and white college students. Journal of Genetic Psychology 128, 95-99.

Goldensohn, S. S. (1981). Psychotherapy for the economically disadvantaged: Contributions from the social sciences. Journal of the American Academy of Psychoanalysis 9, 291-302.

Goldmeier, H. (1982). Children of the gilded ghetto in revolt: The early years, 1967-1974. Adolescence 17, 881-894.

Goldwert, M. (1985). Mexican machismo: The flight from femininity. Psychoanalytic Review 72, 161-169.

Guerin, L. S. (1977). Hospitalization as a positive experience for poverty children: Observations on children from low-income multi-problem families. Clinical Pediatrics 16, 509-513.

Hardy-Fanta, C., & Montana, P. (1982). The Hispanic female adolescent: A group therapy model. International Journal of Group Psychotherapy 32, 351-366.

Heacock, D. R. (1976). The black slum child and the problem of aggression. American Journal of Psychoanalysis 36, 219-226.

Healy, G. W., & DeBlassie, R. R. (1974). A comparison of Negro, Anglo, and Spanish-American adolescents' self-concepts. Adolescence 9, 15-24.

Johnson, C. L. (1974). Adolescent pregnancy: Intervention into the poverty cycle. Adolescence 9, 391-406.

Jrsella, A. J. (1977). The meaning and measurement of Machiavellianism in Chinese and American College students. Social Psychology 101, 165-173.

Knight, G. P. (1978). Acculturation of second and third generation Mexican American children. Journal of Cross-Cultural Psychology 9(1), 87-97.

Lawrence, M. M. (1982). Psychoanalytic psychotherapy among poverty populations and the therapist's use of the self. Journal of the American Academy of Psychoanalysis 10, 241-255.

Lee, J. A. (1980). The helping professional's use of language in describing the poor. American Journal of Orthopsychiatry 50, 580-584.

Lindblad-Goldberg, M., & Dukes, J. L. (1985). Social support in black, low-income, single-parent families: Normative and dysfunctional patterns. American Journal of Orthopsychiatry 55, 42-58.

Powell, J. (1983). Coping with adversity: The psychosocial development of Afro-American children. In J. Powell (Ed.), The psychosocial development of minority group children. New York: Brunner/Mazel.

Quinton, D. (1980). Cultural and community influences. In M. Rutter (Ed.), Scientific foundations of developmental psychiatry. London: William Heinemann Med. Bks.

Sauna, V. D. (1981). Familial and sociocultural antecedents in psychopathology. In H. Triandis & J. Draguns (Eds.), Handbook of cross-cultural psychology-pathology. Boston: Allyn & Bacon.

Schofield, J. W. (1978). An exploratory study of the draw-a-person as a measure of racial identity. Perceptual and Motor Skills 46, 311-321.

Sheldon, S. R., Serrano, R., & Joke, D. (1978). An ethnic comparison of self-esteem in Portuguese-, Mexican-, and American pupils. Psychology 98, 11-14.

Singer, K., Ney, P. G., & Lieh-Mak, F. (1978). A cultural perspective on child psychiatric disorders. Comprehensive Psychiatry 19(6), 533-540.

Spencer, M. B. (1984). Black children's race awareness, racial attitudes and self-concept: A reinterpretation. Journal of Child Psychology and Psychiatry and Allied Disciplines 25, 433-441.

Spurlock, J. (1986). Development of self-concept in Afro-American children. Hospital and Community Psychiatry 37, 67-70.

Taylor, R. L. (1976). Psychosocial development among black children and youth: A reexamination. American Journal of Orthopsychiatry 46, 4-19.

Taylor, R. L. (1976). Erikson's theory of personality development as applied to the child. Journal of Perspectives in Psychiatric Care 14, 184-185.

Weisner, T. (1981). Cities, stress, and children: A review of some cross-cultural questions. In R. Munroe, R. Munroe, & B. Whiting (Eds.), Handbook of cross-cultural human development. New York: Garland STPM Press.

Werner, E. E., & Smith, R. S. (1982). Vulnerable but invincible: A study of resilient children. New York: McGraw-Hill.

PART II

DEVELOPMENT

A. Infant and Neonatal Development

Section Editor:

Justin Call, M.D.
Professor of Psychiatry and Pediatrics
Director, Division of Child and Adolescent Psychiatry
University of California School of Medicine
Irvine, California

Subsection Editors:

Paul Adams, M.D.
Professor of Psychiatry
University of Texas School of Medicine
Galveston, Texas

Stanley Greenspan, M.D.
Chief, Mental Health Study Center
Director, Clinical Infant Development Programs
National Institute of Mental Health
Rockville, Maryland

Adolescent Development:

Brian McConville, M.D.
Associate Professor of Psychiatry
University of Cincinnati School of Medicine
Cincinnati, Ohio

Associate Editors:

Christine Broden, M.D.
Assistant Clinical Professor of Psychiatry
University of California School of Medicine
Irvine, California

Dennis Cantwell, M.D.
Professor of Psychiatry
Director, Division of Child and Adolescent Psychiatry
University of California School of Medicine
Los Angeles, California

Robert Emde, M.D.
Professor of Psychiatry
University of Colorado School of Medicine
Denver, Colorado

Jo Ann B. Fineman, M.D.
Clinical Professor of Psychiatry
University of Arizona
School of Medicine
Tucson, Arizona

Eleanor Galenson, M.D.
Clinical Professor of Psychiatry
Mt. Sinai School of Medicine
New York, New York

I. Lee Gislason, M.D.
Associate Adjunct Professor of Psychiatry
University of California School of Medicine
Irvine, California

Robert Harmon, M.D.
Professor of Psychiatry
Director, Division of Child and Adolescent Psychiatry
University of Colorado School of Medicine
Denver, Colorado

Christoph M. Heinicke, Ph.D.
Clinical Professor of Psychiatry
University of California School of Medicine
Los Angeles, California

Wendell E. Jeffrey, Ph.D.
Department of Psychiatry
University of California School of Medicine
Los Angeles, California

Anneliese F. Korner, Ph.D.
Professor of Psychiatry
Stanford University School of Medicine
Palo Alto, California

Development

Nadine Levinson, D.D.S.
Assistant Clinical Professor of Psychiatry
University of California School of Medicine
Irvine, California

Michael Lewis, Ph.D.
Institute for Research in Human Development
Education Testing Service
Princeton, New Jersey

Lewis Lipsitt, Ph.D.
Professor and Director, Child Study Center
Brown University
Providence, Rhode Island

Joseph D. Noshpitz, M.D.
Professor of Child Psychiatry
George Washington University School of Medicine
Washington, D.C.

Joy Osofsky, Ph.D.
Professor of Psychiatry and Pediatrics
Louisiana State University School of Medicine
New Orleans, Louisiana

Arthur H. Parmelee, M.D.
Professor of Pediatrics
University of California School of Medicine
Los Angeles, California

Lewis Saunder, M.D.
Professor of Psychiatry
University of Colorado School of Medicine
Denver, Colorado

Albert Solnit, M.D.
Professor of Psychiatry and Pediatrics
Yale Child Study Center
Yale University School of Medicine
New Haven, Connecticut

Phyllis Tyson, Ph.D.
Clinical Instructor of Psychiatry
University of California School of Medicine
San Diego, California

Robert Tyson, M.D.
Clinical Professor of Psychiatry
University of California School of Medicine
Irvine, California

Fellows in Child Psychiatry:

Lawrence Bender, M.D.
University of California School of Medicine
Irvine, California

S. Mark Sacher, D.O.
University of California School of Medicine
Irvine, California

1. History of Infant Development

Ainsworth, M., Andry, R. G., Harlow, R. G., Lebovici, S., Mead, M., Prugh, D., & Wootton, B. (1962). Deprivation of maternal care: A reassessment of its effects. Monograph 14. Geneva: World Health Organization.

Ainsworth, M., Bell, S. M., & Stayton, D. (1974). Infant-mother attachment and social development: Socialization as a product of reciprocal responsiveness to signals. In M. Richards (Ed.), The integration of the child into a social world. Cambridge: Cambridge University Press.

Ainsworth, M., Blehar, M., Waters, E., & Wall, S. (1978). Patterns of attachment. Hillsdale, N.J.: Erlbaum.

Ainsworth, M., & Wittig, B. (1969). Attachment and exploratory behavior of one year olds in a strange situation. In B. M. Foss (Ed.), Determinants of infant behavior (Vol. 4). New York: Wiley.

Alpert, A. (1959). Reversibility of pathological fixations associated with maternal depression in infancy. In R. S. Eissler, et al. (Eds.), Psychoanalytic study of the child (Vol. 14, pp. 169-185). New York: International Universities Press.

Als, H., Tronick, E., & Brazelton, T. B. (1980). The achievement of affective reciprocity and the beginnings of the development of autonomy: The study of a blind infant. Journal of the American Academy of Child Psychiatry 19, 22-40.

Als, H., Tronick, E., Lester, B., & Brazelton, T. B. (1979). The Brazelton neonatal behaviroal assessment scale (BNBAS). In J. Osofsky (Ed.), Handbook of infant development. New York: Wiley.

Barrera, M., & Maurer, D. (1981). The perception of facial expressions by the three month old. Child Development 52, 203-206.

Bayley, N. (1969). Bayley scales of infant development. New York: The Psychological Corporation.

Bayley, N., & Schaefer, E. S. (1964). Correlation of maternal and child behaviors with the development of mental abilities: Data from the Berkeley growth study. Chicago: Child Development Publications.

Development

Bell, S. M. (1970). The development of the concept of the object as related in infant-mother attachment. Child Development 41, 291-311.

Benjamin, J. (1961). Some developmental observations relating to the theory of anxiety. Journal of the American Psychoanalytic Association 9, 652-668.

Bergman, P., & Escalona, S. K. (1949). Unusual sensitivities in very young children. In R. S. Eissler, et al. (Eds.), Psychoanalytic study of the child (Vol. 31, pp. 333-352). New York: International Universities Press.

Bowlby, J. (1969). Attachment and loss. Vol. 1: Attachment. New York: Basic Books.

Brazelton, T. B. (1962a). Crying in infancy. Pediatrics 29, 588-597.

Brazelton, T. B. (1962b). Observations of the neonate. Journal of the Academy of Child Psychiatry 1, 38.

Brazelton, T. B. (1973). Neonatal assessment scale. London and Philadelphia: Spastics International Medical Publishers.

Brazelton, T. B. (1980). Neonatal assessment. In S. Greenspan & G. Pollock (Eds.), The course of life. Vol. 1. Infancy and early childhood (DHHS Publication No. ADM 80-999). Washington, D.C.: Government Printing Office.

Brazelton, T. B. (1983). Precursors for the development of emotions in early infancy. In R. Plutchik & H. Kellerman (Eds.), Emotions in early development. Vol. 2: The emotions. New York: Academic Press.

Brazelton, T. B., Scholl, M. L., & Robey, J. S. (1966). Visual responses in the new born. Pediatrics 37, 284-290.

Brazelton, T. B., Young, G. G., & Bullowa, M. (1982). Inception and resolution of early developmental pathology: A case history. Journal of the Academy of Child Psychiatry 10, 124.

Brody, S. (1956). Patterns of mothering. New York: International Press.

Brody, S., & Axelrod, S. (1966). Anxiety, socialization and ego formation in infancy. International Journal of Psycho-Analysis 47, 218-229.

Brody, S., & Axelrod, S. (1970). Anxiety and ego formation in infancy. New York: International Universities Press.

Bronson, G. W., & Pankey, W. (1977). On the distinction between fear and wariness. Child Development 48, 1167-1183.

Brown, A., Matheny, A., & Wilson, R. (1973). Baldwin's kindness concept measure as related to children's cognition and temperament: A twin study. Child Development 44, 193-195.

Buckley, P. (1989). Fifty years after Freud: Dora, the Rat Man, and the Wolf-Man. American Journal of Psychiatry 146 (11), 1394-1403.

Burlingham, D. (1961). Some notes on the development of the blind. In R. S. Eissler, et al. (Eds.), Psychoanalytic study of the child (Vol. 16, pp 121-145). New York: International Universities Press.

Burns, P., Sander, L., Stechler, G., & Julia, H. (1972). Distress in feeding, short-term effects of caretaker environment on the first 10 days. Journal of the American Academy of Child Psychiatry 11, 427-439.

Call, J. (1964). Newborn approach behavior and early ego development. International Journal of Psycho-Analysis 45, 286-294.

Caplan, G., Mason, E. A., & Kaplan, D. M. (1965). Four studies of crisis in parents of prematures. Community Mental Health Journal 1, 149-161.

Caplan, H., Bibace, R., & Rabinovitch, M. S. (1963). Paranatal stress, cognitive organization and ego function: A controlled follow-up study of children born prematurely. Journal of the American Academy of Child Psychiatry 2, 434-450.

Carmichael, L. (1970). The onset and early development of behavior. In L. Carmichael (Ed.), Manual of child psychology (3rd ed.) (pp. 447-563). New York: Wiley.

Chess, S. (1973). Temperament in the normal infant. In S. G. Sapir & A. C. Nitzburg (Eds.), Children with learning problems: Readings in a developmental-interaction approach (pp. 291-307). New York: Brunner/Mazel.

Cohen, D. J., Allen, M. G., Pollin, W., Inoff, G., Werner, M., & Dibble, E. (1972). Personality development in twins: Competence in the newborn and preschool periods. Journal of the American Academy of Child Psychiatry 11, 625-644.

Condon, W. S., & Sander, L. W. (1974). Neonate movement is synchronized with adult speech: Interactional participation and language acquisition. Science 183, 99-101.

Connolly, K. (1974). Learning and the concept of critical periods in infancy. In S. Chess & A. Thomas (Eds.), Annual progress in child psychiatry and child development: 1973 (pp. 115-127). New York: Brunner/Mazel.

Dudek, S. (1972). Longitudinal study of Piaget's developmental stages and the concept of regression, II. Journal of Personality Assessment 36, 468-478.

Dudek, S., & Dyer, S. (1972). A longitudinal study of Piaget's developmental stages and the concept of regression. Journal of Personality Assessment 36, 1025-1034.

Eisenberg, R. (1969). Auditory behavior in the human neonate: Functional properties of sound and their ontogenic implications. International Audiology 8, 34.

Elmer, E., & Gregg, G. (1967). Developmental characteristics of abused children. Pediatrics 40, 596-602.

Emde, R., Gaensbauser, T., & Harmon, R. (1976). Emotional expression in infancy: A biobehavioral study. Psychological Issues, Monograph 37 (Vol. 10). New York: International Universities Press.

Engel, G., Reichsman, F., & Monica, F. K. (1979). A 25 year longitudinal study of the consequence of trauma in infancy, reported by Milton Vederman. Journal of the American Psychoanalytic Association 27, 127-144.

Erikson, E. H. (1937). Configuration in play--clinical notes. Psychoanalytic Quarterly 6, 139-214.

Erikson, E. H. (1950). Childhood and society. New York: Norton.

Erikson, E. H. (1970). The theory of infantile sexuality. In E. H. Erikson (Ed.), Childhood and society (rev. ed., pp. 48-108). New York: Norton.

Erikson, E. H. (1980). Elements of a psychoanalytic theory of psychosocial development in infancy and early childhood. In S. Greenspan & G. Pollock (Eds.), The course of life, Vol. 1. Infancy and early childhood (DHHS Publication No. ADM 80-999). Washington, D.C.: Government Printing Office.

Escalona, S. K. (1968). The roots of individuality: Normal patterns of development in infancy. Chicago: Aldine.

Evans, J. (1961). Rocking at night. Journal of Child Psychology and Psychiatry and Allied Disciplines 2, 71-85.

Fish, B. (1963). The maturation of arousal and attention in the first months of life. Journal of the American Academy of Child Psychiatry 2, 253-270.

Fraiberg, S. (1959). The magic years: Understanding and handling the problems of early childhood. New York: Scribner's.

Fraiberg, S. (1974a). Blind infants and their mothers. An examination of the sign system. In M. Lewis & L. Rosenblum (Eds.), The effect of the infant on its caregiver. New York: Wiley.

Fraiberg, S. (1974b). The clinical dimension of baby games. Journal of the American Academy of Child Psychiatry 13, 202-220.

Fraiberg, S. H., & Freedman, D. A. (1964). Studies in ego development of the congenitally blind child. In R. S. Eissler, et al. (Eds.), Psychoanalytic study of the child (Vol. 19, pp. 113-169). New York: International Universities Press.

Freedman, D. A., Fox-Kolendal, B. J., Margileth, D. A., & Miller, D. H. (1969). The development of the use of sound as a guide to affective and cognitive behavior: A two phase process. Child Development 40, 1099-1105.

Freud, A. (1965). Normality and pathology in childhood. The writings of Anna Freud (Vol. 6). New York: International Universities Press.

Freud, A., & Burlingham, D. (1973). Infants without families. Reports on the Hampstead nurseries, 1939-1945. In A. Freud, The collected writings of Anna Freud (Vol. 3). New York: International Universities Press.

Fries, M. E. (1946). The child's ego development and the training of adults in his environment. In R. S. Eissler, et al. (Eds.), Psychoanalytic study of the child (Vol. 2, pp. 85-112). New York: International Universities Press.

Fries, M. E., & Woolf, P. J. (1953). Some hypotheses on the role of congenital activity type in personality development. In R. S. Eissler, et al. (Eds.), Psychoanalytic study of the child (Vol. 8, pp. 48-632). New York: International Universities Press.

Gaensbauer, T., & Emde, R. N. (1973). Wakefulness and feeding in human newborns. Archives of General Psychiatry 28, 894-987.

Gaensbauer, T., & Sands, S. (1979). Distorted affective communication in abused/neglected infants and their potential impact on caretakers. Journal of the American Academy of Child Psychiatry 18, 236-250.

Garmezy, N. (1974). The study of competence in children at risk for severe psychopathology. In E. J. Anthony & C. Koupernik (Eds.), The child in his family: Children at psychiatric risk (Vol. 3). New York: Wiley.

Geschwind, N. (1970). The organization of language and the brain. Science 170, 940-952.

Gesell, A. L., & Amatruda, C. (1945). The embryology of behavior: The beginnings of the human mind. New York: Harper.

Gewirtz, J. L. (1969). Levels of conceptual analysis in environment-infant interaction research. Merrill-Palmer Quarterly 15, 9.

Greenacre, P. C (1960). Considerations regarding the parent-infant relationship. International Journal of Psycho-Analysis 1, 571-584.

Greenspan, S. I. (1979). Intelligence and adaptation: An integration of psychoanalytic and Piagetian developmental psychology. Psychological Issues, Monographs 47-48. New York: International Universities Press.

Greenspan, S. I., & Pollock, G. H. (Eds.) (1980). The course of life: Psychoanalytic contributions toward understanding personality development, Vol. 1, Infancy and early childhood (DHHS Publication No. ADM 80-999). Washington, D.C.: Government Printing Office.

Harlow, H. F. (1958). The nature of love. American Psychologist 13, 673-685.

Hartmann, H., Kris, E., & Loewenstein, R. M. (1946). Comments on the formation of psychic structure. In R. S. Eissler, et al. (Eds.), Psychoanalytic study of the child (Vol. 2, pp. 11-38). New York: International Universities Press.

Hoffer, W. (1949). Mouth, hand, and ego integration. In R. S. Eissler, et al. (Eds.), Psychoanalytic study of the child (Vols. 3/4, pp. 49-56). New York: International Universities Press.

Hollos, M., & Cowan, P. (1973). Social isolation and cognitive development: Logical operations and role-taking abilities in three Norwegian social settings. Child Development 44, 630-641.

Hunt, J. M. (1941). Infants in an orphanage. Journal of Abnormal and Social Psychology 36, 338.

Illingworth, R. S., & Lister, J. (1964). The critical or sensitive period, with special reference to certain feeding problems in infants and children. Journal of Pediatrics 65, 839-848.

Inhelder, B., & Piaget, J. (1958). The growth of logical thinking from childhood to adolescence. New York: Basic Books.

Josselyn, I. M. (1962). Concepts related to child Development: 1. The oral stage. Journal of the American Academy of Child Psychiatry 1, 209-224.

Kanner, L. (1949). Autistic disturbance of affective contact. The Nervous Child 2, 217-250.

Kaplan, D. M., & Mason, E. A. (1960). Maternal reactions to premature birth viewed as an acute emotional disorder. American Journal of Orthopsychiatry 30, 539-547.

Katan, A. (1972). The infant's first reaction to strangers: Distress or anxiety? International Journal of Psycho-Analysis 53, 501-503.

Kennell, J. H., & Bergen, M. E. (1966). Early childhood separation. Pediatrics 37, 291-298.

Klaus, M. H., Jerauld, R., Kreger, N. C., McAlpine, W., Steffa, M., & Kennell, J. H. (1972). Maternal attachment, importance of the first postpartum days. New England Journal of Medicine 286, 460-463.

Korner, A. (1964). Some hypotheses regarding the significance of individual differences at birth for later development. In R. S. Eissler, et al. (Eds.), Psychoanalytic study of the child (Vol. 19, pp. 58-72). New York: International Universities Press.

Development

Korner, A., & Thoman, E. (1970). Visual alertness in neonates as evoked by maternal care. Journal of Experimental Child Psychology 10, 67.

Lewis, M., & Rosenblum, L. A. (1974). The effect of the infant on its caregiver. New York: Wiley.

Lipsitt, L. (1966). Learning processes of newborns. Merrill-Palmer Quarterly 12, 45.

Lipton, E. L., Steinsschneider, A., & Richmond, J. D. (1960). Autonomic function in the neonate. Psychosomatic Medicine 22, 57-65.

Lourie, R. S. (1971). The first three years of life: An overview of a new frontier of psychiatry. American Journal of Psychiatry 127, 1457-1463.

Lowrey, L. G. (1940). Personality distortion and early institutional Care. American Journal of Orthopsychiatry 10, 546.

Mahler, M. S. (1958). On two crucial phases of integration of the sense of identity: Separation-individuation and bisexual identity. Abstract in panel on problems of identity. 1957, rep. D. L. R. Rubintine. Journal of the American Psychoanalytic Association 6, 131-142.

Mahler, M. S. (1965). On the significance of the normal separation-individuation phase. In M. Schur (Ed.), Drive, affects, behavior (Vol. 2, pp. 161-169). New York: International Universities Press.

Mahler, M. S. (1972). Rapprochement subphase of the separation-individuation process. Psychoanalytic Quarterly 41, 487-506.

Mahler, M., Pine, F., & Bergman, P. (1975). The psychological birth of the infant: Symbiosis and individuation. New York: Basic Books.

Matas, L., Arend, R., & Sroufe, L. A. (1978). Continuity of adaptation in the second year: The relationship between quality of attachment and later competent functioning. Child Development 489, 547-556.

McCall, R. B. (1972). Smiling and vocalization in infants as indices of perceptual-cognitive processes. Merrill-Palmer Quarterly 18, 341-347.

McCall, R. B., Hogarty, P. S., & Hurlburt, N. (1974). Transitions in infant sensorimotor development and the prediction of childhood IQ. In S. Chess & A. Thomas (Eds.), Annual progress in child psychiatry and child development: 1973 (pp. 50-83). New York: Brunner/Mazel.

Meadow, K. (1975). The development of deaf children. In E. M. Heterington (Ed.), Review of child deveopment research (Vol. 5). Chicago: University of Chicago Press.

Meltzoff, A., & Moore, K. (1977). Imitation of facial and manual gestures by human neonates. Science 198, 75-78.

Muir, D., & Field, J. (1979). Newborn infants orient to sound. Child Development 50, 431-436.

Murphy, L. B., & Moriarty, A. E. (1976). Vulnerability, coping and growth. New Haven: Yale University Press.

Osofsky, J., & Danziger, B. (1974). Relationships between neonatal characteristics and mother infant interaction. Developmental Psychology 16, 124.

Paine, R. S. (1965). The contribution of developmental neurology to child psychiatry. Journal of the American Academy of Child Psychiatry 4, 353-386.

Parmelee, A. H., Wenner, W. H., & Schulz, H. R. (1964). Infant sleep patterns: From birth to 16 weeks of age. Journal of Pediatrics 65, 576-582.

Pasamanick, B., & Knobloch, H. (1956). Pregnancy experience and the development of behavior disorder in children. American Journal of Psychiatry 112(8), 613-618.

Piaget, J. (1952). The origins of intelligence in children. New York: Norton.

Piaget, J. (1954). The construction of reality in the child. New York: Basic Books.

Piaget, J. (1962a). Play, dreams and imitation in children. New York: Norton.

Piaget, J. (1962b). The stages in the intellectual development of the child. In S. Harrison & J. McDermott (Eds.), Childhood psychopathology. New York: International Universities Press.

Piaget, J. (1981). Intelligence and affectivity: Their relationship during child development [1954]. Palo Alto: Annual Reviews.

Piaget, J., & Inhelder, B. (1969). The psychology of the child. New York: Basic Books.

Provence, S., & Lipton, R. C. (1962). Infants in institutions. New York: International Universities Press.

Richmond, J. B., & Caldwell, B. M. (1963). Child-rearing practices and their consequences. In A. J. Solnit & S. A. Provence (Eds.), Modern perspectives in child development. (pp. 627-654). New York: International Universities Press.

Ritvo, S., McCollum, A. T., Omwake, E., Provence, S. A., & Solnit, A. J. (1963). Some relations of constitution, environment and personality as observed in a longitudinal study of child development. In A. Solnit & S. A. Provence S. (Eds.), Modern perspectives in child development. New York: International Universities Press.

Ritvo, S., & Solnit, A. J. (1958). Influence of early mother child interaction on identification processes. Discussion by R. Loewenstein, J. Arlow, and R. Knight. In R. S. Eissler, et al. (Eds.), Psychoanalytic study of the child (Vol. 13, pp. 64-91). New York: International Universities Press.

Robson, K. (1967). The role of eye-to-eye contact in maternal-infant attachment. Journal of Child Psychology and Psychiatry and Allied Disciplines 8, 13-25.

Rodman, F. R. (Ed.). (1987). The spontaneous gesture: Selected letters of D. W. Winnicott. Cambridge and London: Harvard University Press.

Rubin, K. (1973). Egocentrism in childhood: A unitary construct? Child Development 44, 102-110.

Rutter, M., Korn, S., & Birch, H. G. (1963). Genetic and environmental factors in the development of "primary reaction patterns." British Journal of Social and Clinical Psychology 2, 161-173.

Sander, L. (1962). Issues in early mother child interaction. Journal of the American Academy of Child Psychiatry 1, 141.

Sander, L. (1975). Infant and caretaking environment. In E. J. Anthony (Ed.), Explorations in child psychiatry (pp. 129-166). New York: Plenum Press.

Sander, L. (1976). Primary prevention and some aspects of temporal organization in early infant caretaker interaction. In E. Rexford, L. Sander, & T. Shapiro (Eds.),

Infant psychiatry: A new syntheses (pp. 187-204). New Haven: Yale University Press.

Sander, L., Julia, H., Stechler, G., & Burns, P. (1972). Continuous 24 hour interactional monitoring in infants reared in two caretaking environments. Psychosomatic Medicine 34, 20-282.

Sandler, J., & Rosenblatt, B. (1962). The concept of the representational world. In R. S. Eissler, et al. (Eds.), Psychoanalytic study of the child (Vol. 1, pp. 128-145). New York: International Universities Press.

Scarr, S., & Salapatek, P. (1970). Patterns of fear development during infancy. Merrill-Palmer Quarterly 16, 53-90.

Schlesinger, H., & Meadow, J. (1972). Sound and sign: childhood deafness and mental health. Berkeley: University of California Press.

Silberstein, R. M., Blackman, S., & Mandell, W. (1966). Auto-erotic head banging: A reflection on the opportunism of infants. Journal of the American Academy of Child Psychiatry 5, 235-242.

Sommerfeld, D. P. (1989). The origins of mother blaming: Historical perspectives on childhood and motherhood. Infant Mental Health Journal 10(1), 14-24.

Spitz, R. (1946). Anaclitic depression. In R. S. Eissler, et al. (Eds.), Psychoanalytic study of the child (Vol. 11, pp. 313-342). New York: International Universities Press.

Spitz, R. A. (1946). Hospitalism: An inquiry into the genesis of psychiatric conditions in early childhood. In R. S. Eissler, et al. (Eds.), Psychoanalytic study of the child (Vol. 12, pp. 53-74). New York: International Universities Press.

Spitz, R. A. (1959). A genetic field theory of ego formation. New York: International Universities Press.

Spitz, R. A. (1965). The first year of life. New York: International Universities Press.

Spitz, R., & Wolf, M. (1946). The smiling response. Genetic Psychology Monographs 34, 57-125.

Spock, B. (1963). The striving for autonomy and regressive object relationship. In R. S. Eissler, et al. (Eds.), Psychoanalytic study of the child (Vol. 18, pp. 340-343). New York: International Universities Press.

Spock, B. (1965). Innate inhibition of aggressiveness in infancy. In R. S. Eissler, et al. (Eds.), Psychoanalytic study of the child (Vol. 20, pp. 340-343). New York: International Universities Press.

Sroufe, L., Waters, E., & Matas, L. (1977). Attachment as an organizational construct. Child Development 48, 1184.

Sroufe, L., & Wunsch, J. (1977). The development of laughter in the first year of life. Child Development 43, 1326-1344.

Sroufe, L. A. (1979). The coherence of individual development: Early care, attachment, and subsequent developmental issues. American Psychologist 34, 834-841.

Stechler, G., & Latz, E. (1966). Some observations on attention and arousal in the human infant. Journal of the Academy of Child Psychiatry 5, 517.

Stern, D. (1971). A micro-analysis of mother-infant interactions: Behavior regulating social contact between a mother and her 3 1/2 month old twins. Journal of the American Academy of Child Psychiatry 10, 501-517.

Stern, D. (1974). The goal and structure of mother-infant play. Journal of the American Academy of Child Psychiatry 13, 402-421.

Stevenson, O. (1954). The first treasured possession: A study of the part played by specially loved objects and toys in the lives of certain children. In R. S. Eissler, et al. (Eds.), Psychoanalytic study of the child (Vol. 9, pp. 199-217). New York: International Universities Press.

Thomas, A., & Chess, S. (1977). Temperament and development. New York: Brunner/Mazel.

Thomas, A., Chess, S., & Birch, H. (1968). Temperament and behavior disorders in children. New York: New York University Press.

Traisman, A. S., & Traisman, H. S. (1958). Thumb- and finger-sucking: A study of 2,650 infants and children. Journal of Pediatrics 53, 566-572.

Tronick, E., Als, H., Adamson, L., Wise, S., & Brazelton, T. B. (1978). The infant's response to entrapment between contradictory messages in face-to-face interaction. Journal of the American Academy of Child Psychiatry 17, 1-13.

Vygotsky, L. (1962). Thought and language. Boston: MIT Press.

Waddington, C. H. (1966). Principles of development and differentiation. New York: Macmillan.

Werner, E. E., Bierman, J. M., French, F. E. (1971). The children of Kauai. Honolulu: University of Hawaii Press.

White, R. W. (1960). Competence and the psychosexual stages of development. Nebraska Symposium on Motivation 8, 97-141.

Winick, M. (1973). Effects of prenatal nutrition upon pregnancy risk. Clinical Obstetrics and Gynecology 16, 1.

Winnicott, D. W. (1953). Transitional objects and transitional phenomena: A study of the first not-me possession. International Journal of Psycho-Analysis 34, 89-97.

Winnicott, D. W. (1958). Collected works, through pediatrics to psychoanalysis. New York: Basic Books.

Winnicott, D. W. (1960). Transitional objects and transitional phenomena. International Journal of Psycho-Analysis. 1953. Reprinted in Collected papers: Through pediatrics to psychoanalysis (pp. 229-242). New York: Basic Books.

Winnicott, D. W. (1962). The maturational processes and the facilitating environment. New York: International Universities Press.

Wolf, K. M. (1952). Observations of individual tendencies in the first year of life. In M. Senn (Ed.), Problems of infancy and childhood. New York: Josiah Macy Foundation.

Wolff, P. H. (1966). The causes, controls, and organizations of behavior in the neonate. Psychological Issues, Monograph #17. New York: International Universities Press.

Wolff, P. H., & Feinbloom, R. L. (1969). Critical periods and cognitive development. Pediatrics 44, 999.

Wolff, P. H., & White, B. L. (1965). Visual pursuit and attention in young infants. Journal of the American Academy of Child Psychiatry 4, 473-484.
Yarrow, L. J. (1964). Separation from parents during early childhood. In M. Hoffman & L. Hoffman (Eds.), Review of child development research (Vol. 1). New York: Russell Sage Foundation.
Yarrow, L. J., Rubenstein, J. L., Pedersen, F. A., & Jankowski, J. J. (1974). Dimensions of early stimulation and their differential effects on infant development. In S. Chess & A. Thomas (Eds.), Annual progress in child psychiatry and child development: 1973 (pp. 3-17). New York: Brunner/Mazel.
Yorke, C., Kennedy, H., & Wiseberg, S. (1980). Some clinical and theoretical aspect of two development lines. In S. Greenspan & G. Pollock (Eds.), The course of life. Vol. 1. Infancy and early childhood (DHHS Publication No. ADM 80-999). Washington, D.C.: Government Printing Office.
Zahn-Waxler, C., Radke-Yarrow, M., & King, R. A. (1979). Childrearing and children's prosocial initiations towards victims of distress. Child Development 50, 319-330.

2. Factors Influencing Early Development

Abe, K., Oda, N., & Amatomi, M. (1984). Natural history and predictive significance of head-banging, head-rolling and breath-holding spells. Developmental Medicine and Child Neurology 26, 644-648.
Allen, D. V., & Robinson, D. O. (1984). Middle ear status and language development in preschool children. ASHA 26, 33-37.
Andrews, S. R., Blumenthal, J. B., Johnson, D. L., Kahn, A. J., Ferguson, C. J., Lasater, T. M., Malone, P. E. & Wallace, D. B. (1982). The skills of mothering: A study of parent child development center. Monographs of the Society for Research in Child Development (Vol. 47, pp. 1-83). Chicago: University of Chicago Press.
Arend, R., Gove, F. L., & Sroufe, L. A. (1979). Continuity of individual adaptation from infancy to kindergarten: A predictive study of ego-resiliency and curiosity in preschoolers. Child Development 50, 950-959.
Ayres, A. J., & Mailloux, Z. (1981). Influence of sensory integration procedures on language development. American Journal of Occupational Therapy 35, 383-390.
Baker, L., & Cantwell, D. P. (1982). Developmental, social and behavioral characteristics of speech and language disordered children. Child Psychiatry and Human Development 12, 195-206.
Bee, H. L., Barnard, K. E., Eyres, S. J., Gray, C. A., Hammond, M. A., Spietz, A. L., Snyder, C., & Clark, B. (1982). Prediction of IQ and language skill from perinatal status, child performance, family characteristics, and mother-infant interaction. Child Development 53, 1134-1136.
Beiser, H. R. (1984). President's plenary address. On curiosity: A developmental approach. Journal of the American Academy of Child Psychiatry 23, 517-526.
Birtchnell, J. (1980). Women whose mothers died in childhood: An outcome study. Psychological Medicine 10, 699-713.

Bornstein, M. H. (1985). How infant and mother jointly contribute to developing cognitive competence in the child. Proceedings of the National Academy of Sciences of the United States of America 82, 7470-7473.

Bornstein, M. H., & Sigman, M. D. (1986). Continuity in mental development from infancy. Child Development 57, 251-274.

Bradley, R. H., & Caldwell, B. M. (1984). The relation of infants' home environments to achievement test performance in first grade: A follow-up study. Child Development 55, 803-809.

Brodzinsky, D. M., Singer, L. M., & Braff, A. M. (1984). Children's understanding of adoption. Child Development 55, 869-878.

Capute, A. J., Shapiro, B. K., Palmer, F. B., Ross, A. & Wachtel, R. C. (1985). Cognitive-motor interactions. The relationship of infant gross motor attainment to IQ at 3 years. Clinical Pediatrics 24, 671-675.

Carey, W. B. (1985). Clinical use of temperament data in pediatrics. Journal of Developmental and Behavioral Pediatrics 6, 137-142.

Chess, S., Thomas, A., Korn, S., Mittelman, M., & Cohen, J. (1983). Early parental attitudes, divorce and separation, and young adult outcome: Findings of a longitudinal study. Journal of the American Academy of Child Psychiatry 22, 47-51.

Clarke, A. D., & Clarke, A. M. (1984). constancy and Change in the growth of human characteristics. Journal of Child Psychology and Psychiatry and Allied Disciplines 25, 191-210.

Coffey, B., Shader, R. I., & Greenblatt, D. J. (1983). Pharmacokinetics of benzodiazepines and psychostimulants in children. Journal of Clinical Psychopharmacology 3, 217-225.

Colombo, J. (1982). The critical period concept: Research, methodology, and theoretical issues. Psychological Bulletin 91, 260-275.

Cotton, N. S. (1984). Childhood play as an analog to adult capacity to work. Child Psychiatry and Human Development 14, 135-144.

Davis, J. M., Elfenbein, J., Schum, R., & Bentler, R. A. (1986). Effects of mild and moderate hearing impairments on language, educational, and psychosocial behavior of children. Journal of Speech and Hearing Disorders 51, 53-62.

Deinard, A. S., List, A., Lindgren, B., Hunt, J.V., & Chang, P. N. (1986). Cognitive deficits in iron-deficient and non iron-deficient anemic children. Journal of Pediatrics 108, 681-689.

Dowling, S. (1980). Going forth to meet the environment: A developmental study of seven infants with esophageal atresia. Psychosomatic Medicine 42, 153-161.

Drucker, J., & Shapiro, C. B. (1979). First scribbles: The emergence of an ego function. Journal of the American Academy of Child Psychiatry 18, 628-646.

Eisenberg, L. (1981). Social context of child development. Pediatrics 68, 705-712.

Escalona, S. K. (1982). Babies at double hazard. Early development of infants at biologic social risk. Pediatrics 70, 670-676.

Fergusson, D. M., Beautrais, A. L., & Silva, P. A. (1982). Breast-feeding and cognitive development in the first seven years of life. Social Science and Medicine 16, 1705-1708.

Ferry, P. C. (1981). On growing new neurons: Are early intervention programs effective. Pediatrics 67, 38-41.

Field, T., Gewirtz, J. L., Cohen, D., Garcia, R., Greenberg, R., & Collins, K. (1984). Leave-taking and reunions of infants, toddlers, preschoolers, and their parents. Child Development 55, 628-635.

Frankenburg, W. K., & Coons, C. E. (1986). Home screening questionnaire: Its validity in assessing home environment. Journal of Pediatrics 108, 624-626.

Frankenburg, W. K., Fandal, A. W., Sciarillo, W., & Burgess, D. (1981). The newly abbreviated and revised Denver developmental screening test. Journal of Pediatrics 99, 995-999.

Freedman, D. A. (1981). The effects of sensory and other deficits in children on their experience of people. Journal of the American Psychoanalytic Association 29, 831-867.

Frodi, A. M., & Lamb, M. E. (1980). Child abusers' responses to infant smiles and cries. Child Development 51, 238-241.

Furrow, D., & Nelson, K. (1984). Environmental correlates of individual differences in language acquisition. Journal of Child Language 11, 523-534.

Gaines, R., & Powell, G. J. (1981). Children's color perception in relation to habitat and skin color. Child Development 52, 914-920.

Garmezy, N., Masten, A. S., & Tellegen, A. (1984). The study of stress and competence in children: A building block for developmental psychopathology. Child Development 55, 97-111.

Goldin-Meadow, S., & Mylander, C. (1983). Gestural communication in deaf children: Noneffect of parental input on language development. Science 221, 372-374.

Goldin-Meadow, S., & Mylander, C. (1984). Gestural communication in deaf children: The effects and noneffects of parental input on early language development. Monographs of the Society for Research in Child Development (Vol. 49, pp. 1-151). Chicago: University of Chicago Press.

Granrud, C. E. (1986). Binocular vision and spatial perception in 4- and 5-month-old infants. Journal of Experimental Psychology: Human Perception and Performance 12, 36-49.

Greenspan, S, I., & Porges, S. W. (1984). Psychopathology in infancy and early childhood: Clinical perspectives on the organization of sensory and affective-thematic experience. Child Development 55, 49-70.

Gullo, D. F., Bersani, C., & Conlin, S. (1983). Changes in peer interaction during the first three years of life. Psychological Reports 52, 708.

Gunnar, M. R., Senior, K., & Hartup, W. W. (1984). Peer presence and the exploratory behavior of eighteen- and thirty-month-old children. Child Development 55, 1103-1109.

Heinicke, C. M. (1984). The role of pre-birth parent characteristics in early family development. Child Abuse and Neglect 8, 169-181.

Hunt, J., & Rudden, M. (1986). Gender differences in the psychology of parenting: Psychoanalytic and feminist perspectives. Journal of the American Academy of Psychoanalysis 14, 213-226.

Hunziker, U. A., & Barr, R. G. (1986). Increased carrying reduces infant crying: A randomized controlled trial. Pediatrics 77, 641-648.

Jenkins, S., Owen, C., Bax, M., & Hart, H. (1984). Continuities of common behaviour problems in preschool children. Journal of Child Psychology and Psychiatry and Allied Disciplines 25, 75-89.

Kagan, J. (1979). The form of early development. Continuity and discontinuity in emergent competences. Archives of Genetic Psychiatry 36, 1047-1054.

Kagan, J. (1982). Canalization of early psychological development. Pediatrics 70, 474-783.

Kagan, J., Lapidus, D. R., & Moore, M. (1978). Infant antecedents of cognitive functioning: A longitudinal study. Child Development 49, 1005-1023.

Kaiser, M. K., & Proffitt, D. R. (1984). The development of sensitivity to causally relevant dynamic information. Child Development 55, 1614-1624.

Kamhi, A. G. (1982). The effect of self-initiated and other-initiated actions on linguistic performance. Journal of Speech and Hearing Research 25, 177-183.

Kennedy, H., Moran, G., Wiseberg, S., & Yorke, C. (1985). Both sides of the barrier. Some reflections on childhood fantasy. In A. Solnit, et al. (Eds.), Psychoanalytic study of the child (Vol. 40, pp. 275-283). New Haven: Yale University Press.

Klein, R. P., & Durfee, J. T. (1979). Prediction of preschool social behavior from social-emotional development at one year. Child Psychiatry and Human Development 9, 145-151.

Krueger, D. W. (1983). Childhood parent loss: Developmental impact and adult psychopathology. American Journal of Psychotherapy 37, 582-592.

Kurtines, W., & Greif, E. B. (1974). The development of moral thought: Review and evaluation of Kohlberg's approach. Psychological Bulletin 81, 453-470.

Largo, R. H., & Howard, J. A. (1979). Developmental progression in play behavior of children between nine and thirty months: II: Spontaneous play and language development. Developmental Medicine and Child Neurology 21, 492-503.

Largo, R. H., & Stutzle, W. (1977a). Longitudinal study of bowel and bladder control by day and at night in the first six years of life. I: Epidemiology and interrelations between bowel and bladder control. Developmental Medicine and Child Neurology 19, 598-606.

Largo, R. H., & Stutzle, W. (1977b). Longitudinal study of bowel and bladder control by day and at night in the first six year of life. II: The role of potty training and the child's initiative. Developmental Medicine and Child Neurology 19, 607-613.

Lepper, M. R., Ross, L., & Lau, R. R. (1986). Persistence of inaccurate beliefs about the self: Perseverance effects in the classroom. Journal of Personality and Social Pychology 50, 482-491.

Lien, N. M., Meyer, K. K., & Winick, M. (1977). Early malnutrition and "late" adoption: A study of their effects on the development of Korean orphans adopted into American families. American Journal of Clinical Nutrition 30, 1734-1739.

Development

Lowe, M. (1975). Trends in the development of representational play in infants from one to three years--an observational study. Journal of Child Psychology and Psychiatry and Allied Disciplines 16, 33-47.

Lynch, A., Mychalkiw, W., & Hutt, S. J. (1978). Prenatal progesterone. I. Its effect on development and on intellectual and academic achievement. Early Human Development 2, 305-322.

Mahalski, P. A., Silva, P. A., & Spears, G. F. (1985). Children's attachment to soft objects at bedtime, child rearing, and child development. Journal of the American Academy of Child Psychiatry 24, 442-446.

Marcus, D. E., & Overton, W. F. (1978). The development of cognitive gender constancy and sex role preferences. Child Development 49, 434-444.

Marschark, M., & Nall, L. (1985). Metaphoric competence in cognitive and language development. Advances in Child Development and Behavior 19, 49-81.

McGee, R., Silva, P. A., & Williams, S. (1984). Perinatal, neurological, environmental and developmental characteristics of seven-year-olds children with stable behaviour problems. Journal of Child Psychology and Psychiatry and Allied Disciplines 25, 573-586.

Miller, P. H. (1985). Children's reasoning about the causes of human behavior. Journal of Experimental Child Psychology 39, 343-362.

Modarressi, T., & Kenny, T. (1977). Children's response to their true and distorted mirror images. Child Psychiatry and Human Development 8, 94-101.

Newson, J., Newson, E., & Mahalski, P. A. (1982). Persistent infant comfort habits and their sequelae at 11 and 16 years. Journal of Child Psychology and Psychiatry and Allied Disciplines 23, 421-436.

Offer, D., & Sabshin, M. (Eds.). (1984). Normality and the life cycle. New York: Basic Books.

Parmelee, A. H. (1986). Children's illnesses: Their beneficial effects on behavioral development. Child Development 57, 1-10.

Petersen, G. A., & Sherrod, K. B. (1982). Relationship of maternal language to language development and language delay of children. American Journal of Mental Deficiency 86, 391-398.

Provence, S., & Solnit, A. J. (1983). Development-promoting aspects of the sibling experience. Vicarious mastery. In A. Solnit, et al. (Eds.), Psychoanalytic study of the child (Vol. 38, pp. 337-351). New Haven: Yale University Press.

Ramey, C. T., Yeates, K. O., & Short, E. J. (1984). The plasticity of intellectual development: Insights from preventive intervention. Child Development 55, 1913-1925.

Ratner, H. H. (1984). Memory demands and the development of young children's memory. Child Development 55, 2173-2191.

Rees, K. (1978). The child's understanding of his past: Cognitive factors in reconstruction with children. In A. Solnit, et al. (Eds.), Psychoanalytic study of the child (Vol. 33, pp. 237-259). New Haven: Yale University Press.

Roth, F. P. (1984). Accelerating language learning in young children. Journal of Child Language 11, 89-107.

Rutter, M. (1979). Maternal deprivation, 1972-1978: New findings, new concepts, new approaches. Child Development 50, 283-305.

Rutter, M. (1980). The long-term effects of early experience. Developmental Medicine and Child Neurology 22, 800-815.

Rutter, M. (1981). Social-emotional consequences of day care for preschool children. American Journal of Orthopsychiatry 51, 4-28.

Sherman, M., & Hertzig, M. E. (1983). Treasured object use--a cognitive and developmental marker. Journal of the American Academy of Child Psychiatry 22, 541-544.

Silva, P. A., McGee, R., & Williams, S. (1982). The predictive significance of slow walking and slow talking: a report form the Dunedin Multidisciplinary Child Development Study. British Journal of Disorders of Communication 127, 133-139.

Simonds, J. F., & Parraga, H. (1982). Prevalence of sleep disorders and sleep behaviors in children and adolescents. Journal of the American Academy of Child Psychiatry 21, 383-388.

Spohr, H. L., & Steinhausen, H. C. (1984). Clinical, psychopathological and developmental aspects in children with the fetal alcohol syndrome: A four-year follow-up study. Ciba Foundation Symposium 105, 197-217.

St. James-Roberts, I. (1979). Neurological plasticity, recovery from brain insult, and child development. Advances in Child Development and Behavior 14, 253-319.

Staley, A. A., & O'Donnell, J. P. (1984). A developmental analysis of mothers' reports of normal children's fears. Journal of Genetic Psychology 144, 165-178.

Stoller, R. J. (1978). Boyhood gender aberrations: Treatment issues. Journal of the American Psychoanalytic Association 26, 541-558.

Streissguth, A. P., Clarren, S. K., & Jones, K. L. (1985). Natural history of the fetal alcohol syndrome: A 10-year-follow-up of eleven patients. Lancet 2, 85-91.

Taylor, M., & Flavell, J. H. (1984). Seeing and believing: Children's understanding of the distinction between appearance and reality. Child Development 55, 1710-1720.

Teele, D. W., Klein, J. O., & Rosner, B. A. (1984). Otitis media with effusion during the first three years of life and development of speech and language. Pediatrics 74, 282-287.

Terr, L. C. (1987). Childhood trauma and the creative product: A look at the early lives and later works of Poe, Wharton, Magritte, Hitchcock and Berman. In A. Solnit, et al. (Eds.), Psychoanalytic study of the child (Vol. 42, pp. 545-572). New Haven: Yale University Press.

Tyson, R. L. (1986). The roots and psychopathology and our theories of development. Journal of the American Academy of Child Psychiatry 25, 12-22.

Ullman, D. G., & Kausch, D. F. (1979). Early identification of developmental strengths and weaknesses in preschool children. Exceptional Children 46, 8-13.

Vaughn, B. E., Kopp, C. B., & Krakow, J. B. (1984). The emergence and consolidation of self-control from eighteen to thirty months of age: Normative trends and individual differences. Child Development 55, 990-1004.

3. Factors Related to Adaptation in Various Periods of Development

Amsterdam, B. (1972). Mirror self-image reactions before age two. Developmental Psychobiology 5, 297-305.

Amsterdam, B., & Greenberg, L. M. (1977). Self-conscious behavior of infants: A videotape study. Developmental Psychobiology 10, 1-6.

Amsterdam, B. K., & Levitt, M. (1980). Consciousness of self and painful self-consciousness. In A. Solnit, et al. (Eds.), Psychoanalytic study of the child (Vol. 35, pp. 67-83). New Haven: Yale University Press.

Anderson, J. R. (1984). The development of self-recognition: A review. Development Psychobiology 17, 35-49.

Arend, R., Gove, F. L., & Sroufe, L. A. (1979). Continuity of individual adaptation from infancy to kindergarten: A predictive study of ego-resiliency and curiosity in preschoolers. Child Development 50, 950-959.

Bauman, S. (1981). Physical aspects of the self. A review of some aspects of boy image development in childhood. Psychiatric Clinics of North America 4, 455-470.

Berman, P. W., Smith, V. L., & Goodman, V. (1983). Development of sex differences in response to an infant and to the caretaker role. Journal of Genetic Psychology 143, 283-284.

Birtchnell, J. (1974). The effect of early parent loss upon the direction and degree of sexual identity. British Journal of Medical Psychology 47, 129-137.

Blos, P. (1985). Intergenerational separation-individuation. Treating the mother-infant pair. In A. Solnit, et al. (Eds.), Psychoanalytic study of the child (Vol. 40, pp. 41-56). New Haven: Yale University Press.

Busch-Rossnagel, N. A., & Peters, D. L. (1980). Parental development in first-time mothers of handicapped, at-risk and normal children. International Journal of Rehabilitation Research 3, 229-231.

Calderone, M. S. (1985). Adolescent sexuality: Elements and genesis. Pediatrics 76, 699-703.

Campbell, S. B. (1979). Mother-infant interaction as a function of maternal ratings of temperament. Child Psychiatry and Human Development 10, 67-76.

Carey, W. B., & McDevitt, S. C. (1978). Stability and change in individual temperament diagnoses from infancy to early childhood. Journal of the American Academy of Child Psychiatry 17, 331-337.

Clarke, A. D., & Clarke, A. M. (1984). Constancy and change in the growth of human characteristics. Journal of Child Psychology and Psychiatry and Allied Disciplines 25, 191-210.

Cohen, D. J., Caparulo, B. K., & Wetstone, H. (1981). The emergence of meanings and intentions. Mothers' dialogue with normal and language-impaired children. Psychiatric Clinics of North America 4, 489-508.

Dare, C., & Holder, A. (1981). Developmental aspects of the interaction between narcissism, self-esteem and object relations. International Journal of Psycho-Analysis 62, 323-337.

deVries, M. W., & Sameroff, A. J. (1984). Culture and temperament: Influences on infant temperament in three East African societies. American Journal of Orthopsychiatry 54, 83-96.

Dewald, P. A., & Kramer, S. (1976). Dialogue on the role of family life in child development. International Journal of Psycho-Analysis 57, 403-409.

Di Angi, P. (1976). Erikson's theory of personality development as applied to the black child. Perspectives in Psychiatric Care 14, 184-185.

Dibble, E. D., & Cohen, D. J. (1981). Personality development in identical twins. The first decade of life. In A. Solnit, et al. (Eds.), Psychoanalytic study of the child (Vol. 36, pp. 45-70). New Haven: Yale University Press.

Emde, R. N. (1983). The prerepresentational self and its affective core. In A. Solnit, et al. (Eds.), Psychoanalytic study of the child (Vol. 38, pp. 165-192). New Haven: Yale University Press.

Fagot, B. I., & Leinbach, M. D. (1985). Gender identity: Some thoughts on an old concept. Journal of the American Academy of Child Psychiatry 24, 684-688.

Feder, L. (1980). Preconceptive ambivalence and external reality. International Journal of Psycho-Analysis 61, 161-178.

Feiring, C. (1984). Behavioral styles in infancy and adulthood: The work of Karen Horney and attachment theorists collaterally considered. American Journal of Psychoanalysis 44, 197-208.

Frankel, S., & Sherick, I. (1977). Observations on the development of normal envy. In A. Solnit, et al. (Eds.), Psychoanalytic study of the child (Vol. 32, pp. 257-281). New Haven: Yale University Press.

Freud, A. (1981). Insight. Its presence and absence as a factor in normal development. In A. Solnit, et al. (Eds.), Psychoanalytic study of the child (Vol. 36, pp. 241-249). New Haven: Yale University Press.

Fries, M. E., Nelson, M. C., & Woolf, P. J. (1980). Developmental and etiological factors in the treatment of character disorders with archaic ego function. Psychoanalytic Review 67, 337-352.

Fullard, W., McDevitt, S. C., & Carey, W. B. (1984). Assessing temperament in one- to three-year-old children. Journal of Pediatric Psychology 9, 205-217.

Furman, E. (1985). On fusion, integration, and feeling good. In A. Solnit, et al. (Eds.), Psychoanalytic study of the child (Vol. 40, pp. 81-110). New Haven: Yale University Press.

Gaddini, R. (1977). The pathology of the self as a basis of psychosomatic disorders. Psychotherapy and Psychosomatics 32, 16-26.

Gaddini, R. (1984). On the origins of the battered child syndrome: Abuse as acting out of preverbal events. Child Abuse and Neglect 8, 41-45.

Gislason, I. L., & Call, J. D. (1982). Dog bite in infancy: Trauma and personality development. Journal of the American Academy of Child Psychiatry 21, 203-207.

Goethals, G. W. (1976). The evolution of sexual and genital intimacy: A comparison of the views of Erik H. Erikson and Harry Stack Sullivan. Journal of the American Academy of Psychoanalysis 4, 529-544.

Goldman, R., & Goldman, J. (1983). Children's perceptions of sex differences in babies and adolescents: A cross-national study. Archives of Sexual Behavior 12, 277-294.

Greenspan, S., & Lourie, R. S. (1981). Developmental structuralist approach to the classification of adaptive and pathologic personality organizations: Infancy and early childhood. American Journal of Psychiatry 138, 725-735.

Grotstein, J. S. (1982-1983). The significance of Kleinian contributions to psychoanalysis. III. The Kleinian theory of ego psychology and object relations. International Journal of Psychoanalytic Psychotherapy 9, 487-510.

Harkness, S., & Super, C. M. (1985). The cultural context of gender segregation in children's peer groups. Child Development 56, 219-224.

Haugh, S. S., Hoffman, C. D., & Cowan, G. (1980). The eye of the very young beholder: Sex typing of infants by young children. Child Development 51, 598-600.

Henderson, J. (1982). The role of the father in separation-individuation. Bulletin of the Menninger Clinic 46, 231-254.

Himmelfarb, S., Hock, E., and Wenar, C. (1985). Infant temperament and non compliant behavior at four years: A longitudinal study. Genetic Society of General Psychology Monograph 111, 7-21.

Jacobson, J. G. (1983). The structural theory and the representational world: Developmental and biological considerations. Psychoanalytic Quarterly 52, 543-563.

Kaplan, L. J. (1974). The concept of the family romance. Psychoanalytic Review 61, 169-202.

Kennedy, J. H., & Bakeman, R. (1984). The early mother-infant relationship and social competence with peers and adults at three years. Journal of Psychology 116, 23-34.

Kestenberg, J. S. (1980). The three faces of femininity. Psychoanalytic Review 67, 313-335.

Lamb, M. E. (1977). A re-examination of the infant social world. Human Development 20, 65-85.

Lamb, M. E. (1982). Paternal influences on early socio-emotional development. Journal of Child Psychology and Psychiatry and Allied Disciplines 23, 185-190.

Lehrer, S. (1984). Modern correlates of Freudian psychology. Infant sexuality and the unconscious. American Journal of Medicine 77, 977-980.

Leichtman, M. (1985). The influence of an older sibling on the separation-individuation process. In A. Solnit, et al. (Eds.), Psychoanalytic study of the child (Vol. 40, pp. 111-161). New Haven: Yale University Press.

Lester, E. P. (1976). On the psychosexual development of the female child. Journal of the American Academy of Psychoanalysis 4, 515-527.

Lester, E. P. (1983). Separation-individuation and cognition. Journal of the American Psychoanalytic Association 31, 127-156.

Lewis, H. B. (1985). Depression vs. paranoia: Why are there sex differences in mental illness? Journal of Personality 53, 150-178.

Lewis, M. (1975). Early sex differences in the human: Studies of socioemotional development. Archives of Sexual Behavior 4, 329-335.

Lustman, J. (1977). On splitting. In A. Solnit, et al. (Eds.), Psychoanalytic study of the child (Vol. 32, pp. 119-154). New Haven: Yale University Press.

Mahler, M. S. (1981). Aggression in the service of separation-individuation. Case study of a mother-daughter relationship. Psychoanalytic Quarterly 50, 625-638.

Mahler, M.S., & McDevitt, J. B. (1982). Thoughts on the emergence of the sense of self, with particular emphasis on the body self. Journal of the American Psychoanalytic Association 30, 827-848.

Martinson, F. M. (1976). Eroticism in infancy and childhood. Journal of Sexual Research 12, 251-262.

McDevitt, J. B. (1979). The role of internalization in the development of object relations during the separation-individuation phase. Journal of the American Psychoanalytic Association 27, 327-343.

McDonagh, M. J. (1976). Creative process and its relation to sense of self, separateness, and reality. Perspectives in Psychiatric Care 14, 68-74.

McHale, S. M., & Huston, T. L. (1984). Men and women as parents: Sex role orientations, employment, and parental roles with infants. Child Development 55, 1349-1361.

Mordock, J. B. (1979). The separation-individuation process and developmental disabilities. Exceptional Children 46, 176-184.

Plaut, E. A. (1984). Ego instincts. A concept whose time has come. In A. Solnit, et al. (Eds.), Psychoanalytic study of the child (Vol. 39, pp. 235-258). New Haven: Yale University Press.

Pridham, K. F., & Chang, A. S. (1985). Parents' beliefs about themselves as parents of a new infant: Instrument development. Research in Nursing and Health 8, 19-29.

Rinsley, D. B. (1981). Dynamic and developmental issues in borderline and related "spectrum" disorders. Psychiatric Clinics of North America 4, 117-132.

Sadler, L. S., & Catrone, C. (1983). The adolescent parent: A dual developmental crisis. Journal of Adolescent Health Care 4, 100-105.

Shill, M. (1981). TAT measures gender identity (castration anxiety) in father-absent males. Journal of Personality Assessment 45, 136-146.

Shopper, M. (1978). The role of audition in early psychic development, with special reference to the use of the putt-toy in the separation-individuation phase. Journal of the American Psychoanalytic Association 26, 283-310.

Solnit, A. J. (1982). Developmental perspectives on self and object constancy. In A. Solnit, et al. (Eds.), Psychoanalytic study of the child (Vol. 37, pp. 201-218). New Haven: Yale University Press.

Spieler, S. (1984). Preoedipal girls need fathers. Psychoanalytic Review 71, 63-80.

Stoller, R. J., & Herdt, G. H. (1982). The development of masculinity: A cross-cultural contribution. Journal of the American Psychoanalytic Association, 30 29-59.

Sutherland, J. D. (1980). The British object relations theorists: Balint, Winnicott, Fairbairn, Guntrip. Journal of the American Psychoanalytic Association 28, 829-860.

Terhune, C. B. (1979). The role of hearing in early ego organization. In A. Solnit, et al. (Eds.), Psychoanalytic study of the child (Vol. 34, pp. 371-383). New Haven: Yale University Press.

Tolpin, M. (1978). Self-objects and oedipal objects: A Crucial developmental distinction. In A. Solnit, et al. (Eds.), Psychoanalytic study of the child (Vol. 33, pp. 167-184). New Haven: Yale University Press.

Tyson, P. (1982). A developmental line of gender identity, gender role, and choice of love object. Journal of the American Psychoanalytic Association 30, 61-86.

van der Velde, C. D. (1985). Body images of one's self and of others: Developmental and clinical significance. American Journal of Psychiatry 142, 527-537.

Weisz, J. R., & Stipek, D. J. (1982). Competence, contingency, and the development of perceived control. Human Development 25, 250-281.

Werner, E. E. (1986). Resilient offspring of alcoholics: A longitudinal study from birth to age 18. Journal of Studies on Alcohol 47, 34-40.

Wilson, R. S. (1981). Synchronized developmental pathways for infant twins. Progress in Clinical and Biological Research 69(B), 199-209.

Ziegler, R. G., & Musliner, P. J. (1977). Persistent themes: A naturalistic study of personality development in the family. Family Process 16, 293-305.

4. Psychodynamic Aspects of Development

Abelson, A. G. (1979). Development of psychosexual concepts in relation to expressive language performance. Psychiatry 42, 274-279.

Anthony, W. S. (1977). Activity in the learning of Piagetian operational thinking. British Journal of Educational Psychology 47, 18-24.

Arend, R., Gove, F. L., & Sroufe, L. A. (1979). Continuity of individual adaptation from infancy to kindergarten: A predictive study of ego-resiliency and curiosity in preschoolers. Child Development 50, 950-959.

Bauman, S. (1981). Physical aspects of the self. A review of some aspects of body image development in childhood. Psychiatric Clinics of North America 4, 455-470.

Belsky, J., Rovine, M., & Taylor, D. G. (1984). The Pennsylvania infant and family development project, III: The origins of individual differences in infant-mother attachment: Maternal and infant contributions. Child Development 55, 718-728.

Bemporad, J. R. (1980). Review of object relations theory in the light of cognitive development. Journal of the American Academy of Psychoanalysis 8, 57-75.

Bemporad, J. R. (1984). From attachment to affiliation. American Journal of Psychoanalysis 44, 79-97.

Brazelton, T. B., & Als, H. (1979). Four early stages in the development of mother-infant interaction. In A. Solnit, et al. (Eds.), Psychoanalytic study of the child (Vol. 34, pp. 349-369). New Haven: Yale University Press.

Bruner, J. (1984). Interaction, communication, and self. Journal of the American Academy of Child Psychiatry 23, 1-7.

Busch, F., & McKnight, J. (1973). Parental attitudes and the development of the primary transitional object. Child Psychiatry and Human Development 4, 12-20.

Call, J. D. (1980). Some prelinguistic aspects of language development. Journal of the American Psychoanalytic Association 28, 259-289.

Colarusso, C. A. (1979). The development of time sense--from birth to object constancy. International Journal of Psycho-Analysis 60, 243-251.

Drucker, J., & Shapiro, C.B. (1979). First scribbles: the emergence of an ego function. Journal of the American Academy of Child Psychiatry 18, 628-646.

Egeland, B., & Farber, E. A. (1984). Infant-mother attachment: Factors related to its development and changes over time. Child Development 55, 753-771.

Egeland, B., & Sroufe, L. A. (1981). Attachment and early maltreatment. Child Development 52, 44-52.

Erlich, H. S. (1978). Adolescent suicide: Maternal longing and cognitive development. In A. Solnit, et al. (Eds.), Psychoanalytic study of the child (Vol. 33, pp. 261-277). New Haven: Yale University Press.

Freud, A. (1976). Psychopathology seen against the background of normal development. The forty-ninth Maudsley Lecture, delivered before the Royal College of Psychiatrists, 21 November 1975. British Journal of Psychiatry 129, 401-406.

Freud, A. (1981a). The concept of developmental lines. Their diagnostic significance. In A. Solnit, et al. (Eds.), Psychoanalytic study of the child (Vol. 36, pp. 129-136). New Haven: Yale University Press.

Freud, A. (1981b). Insight. Its presence and absence as a factor in normal development. In A. Solnit, et al. (Eds.), Psychoanalytic study of the child (Vol. 36, pp. 241-249). New Haven: Yale University Press.

Gordon, A. H., & Jameson, J. C. (1979). Infant-mother attachment in patients with nonorganic failure to thrive syndrome. Journal of the American Academy of Child Psychiatry 18, 251-259.

Gottschalk, L. A. (1981). Psychoanalytic contributions to the generation of creativity in children. Psychiatry 44, 210-229.

Hong, K. M. (1978). The transitional phenomena: A theoretical integration. In A. Solnit, et al. (Eds.), Psychoanalytic study of the child (Vol. 33, pp. 47-79. New Haven: Yale University Press.

Kramer, J. A., Hill, K. T., & Cohen, L. B. (1975). Infants' development of object permanence: A refined methodology and new evidence of Piaget's hypothesized ordinality. Child Development 46, 149-155.

Lipton, E. L. (1976). Psychoanalytic child development research and the practice of general psychiatry. International Journal of Psycho-Analysis 57, 113-126.

Litt, C. J. (1981). Children's attachment to transitional objects: A study of two pediatric populations. American Journal of Orthopsychiatry 51, 131-139.

Mahalski, P. A., Silva, P. A., & Spears, G. F. (1985). Children's attachment to soft objects at bedtime, child rearing, and child development. Journal of the American Academy of Child Psychiatry 24, 442-446.

McDevitt, J. B. (1979). The role of internalization in the development of object relations during the separation-individuation phase. Journal of the American Psychoanalytic Association 27, 327-343.

Modarressi, T. (1977). The mutative object. A contribution to the theory of object relationships. Journal of the American Academy of Child Psychiatry 16, 208-217.

Neubauer, P. B. (1984). Anna Freud's concept of developmental lines. In A. Solnit, et al. (Eds.), Psychoanalytic study of the child (Vol. 39, pp. 15-27). New Haven: Yale University Press.

Noam, G. G., Hauser, S. T., Santostefano, S., Garrison, W., Jacobson, A. M., Powers, S. I., & Mead, M. (1984). Ego development and psychopathology: A study of hospitalized adolescents. Child Development 55, 184-194.

Ornstein, A. (1981). Self-pathology in childhood: Developmental and clinical considerations. Psychiatric Clinics of North America 4, 435-453.

Pine, F. (1982). The experience of self. Aspects of its formation, expansion, and vulnerability. In A. Solnit, et al. (Eds.), Psychoanalytic study of the child (Vol. 37, pp. 143-167). New Haven: Yale University Press.

Schwartz, P. (1983). Length of day-care attendance and attachment behavior in eighteen-month-old infants. Child Development 54, 1073-1078.

Shane, M., & Shane, E. (1984-1985). Change and integration in psychoanalytic developmental theory. International Journal of Psychoanalytic Psychotherapy 10, 457-471.

Sherman, M., & Hertzig, M. E. (1983). Treasured object use--a cognitive and developmental theory. Journal of the American Adademy of Child Psychiatry 22, 541-544.

Smillie, D. (1982). Rethinking Piaget's theory of infancy. Human Development 25, 282-294.

Stingle, S. F., & Cook, H. (1985). Age and sex differences in the cooperative and noncooperative behavior of pairs of American children. Journal of Psychology 119, 335-345.

Taylor, M., & Flavell, J. H. (1984). Seeing and believing: Children's understanding of the distinction between appearance and reality. Child Development 55, 1710-1720.

Tyson, R. L. (1986). The roots of psychopathology and our theories of development. Journal of the American Academy of Child Psychiatry 25, 12-22.

5. Psychological Aspects of Development

Barton, S. S. (1980). How does the child know? Origins of the symbol in the theories of Piaget and Werner. Journal of the American Academy of Psychoanalysis 8, 77-94.

Bates, E., Bretherton, I., Beeghly-Smith, M., & McNew, S. (1982). Social bases of language development: A reassessment. Advances in Child Development and Behavior 16, 7-75.

Bauman, S. (1981). Physical aspects of the self. A review of some aspects of body image development in childhood. Psychiatric Clinics of North America 4, 455-470.

Blatt, S. J., Brenneis, C.B., & Schimek, J. G. (1976). Normal development and psychopathological impairment of the concept of the object on the Rorschach. Journal of Abnormal Psychology 85, 364-373.

Call, J. D. (1980). Some prelinguistic aspects of language development. Journal of the American Psychoanalytic Association 28, 259-289.

Crockenberg, S. B. (1981). Infant irritability, mother responsiveness, and social support influences on the security of infant-mother attachment. Child Development 52, 857-865.

Dent, K. A. (1982). Two daughters of a deaf mute mother: Implications for ego and cognitive development. Journal of the American Academy of Psychoanalysis 10, 427-441.

Elkind, D. (1982). Piagetian psychology and the practice of child psychiatry. Journal of the American Academy of Child Psychiatry 21, 435-445.

Emde, R. N. (1985). The affective self: Continuities and transformations from infancy. In J. D. Call, E. Galenson, & R. L. Tyson (Eds.), Frontiers of infant psychiatry. New York: Basic Books.

Freud, A. (1981). Insight. Its presence and absence as a factor in normal development. In A. Solnit, et al. (Eds.), Psychoanalytic study of the child (Vol. 36, pp. 137-145). New Haven: Yale University Press.

Gottschalk, L. A. (1981). Psychoanalytic contributions to the generation of creativity in children. Psychiatry 44, 210-229.

Grellert, E. A. (1982). Childhood play behavior of homosexual and heterosexual men. Psychological Reports 51, 606-610.

Grotstein, J. (1980-1981). The significance of Kleinian contributions to psychoanalysis. II. Freudian and Kleinian conceptions of early mental development. International Journal of Psychoanalytic Psychotherapy 8, 393-428.

Herzog, D.B., & Rathbun, J. M. (1982). Childhood depression. Development considerations. American Journal of Diseases of Children 136, 115-120.

Holinger, P. C. (1989). A developmental perspective on psychotherapy and psychoanalysis. American Journal of Psychiatry 146(11), 1404-1412.

Holmes, J. (1982). Obsessional phenomena and the development of imaginative competence. British Journal of Medical Psychology 55, 147-158.

Kagan, J. (1986). Continuity and discontinuity in development. In J. Noshpitz (Ed.), Basic handbook of child psychiatry (Vol. 5, pp. 33-37). New York: Basic Books.

Kashani, J. H., Orvaschel, H., Rosenberg, T. K., & Reid, J. D. (1989). Psychopathology in a community sample of children and adolescents: A developmental perspective. Journal of the American Academy of Child and Adolescent Psychiatry 28(5), 701-706.

Kashani, J. H., Rosenberg, T. K., & Reid, J. D. (1989). Developmental perspectives in child and adolescent depressive symptoms in a community sample. American Journal of Psychiatry 146(7), 871-875.

McDevitt, J. B. (1986). Separation-individuation and the beginning emergence of the sense of self. In J. Noshpitz, (Ed.), Basic handbook of child psychiatry (Vol. 5, pp. 38-80). New York: Basic Books.

Lamb, M. E. (1982). Individual differences in infant sociability: Their origins and implications for cognitive development. Advances in Child Development and Behavior 16, 213-239.

Liben, L. S., & Belknap, B. (1981). Intellectual realism: Implications for investigations of perceptual perspective taking in young children. Child Development 52, 921-924.

Litt, C. J. (1981). Children's attachment to transitional objects. A study of two pediatric populations. American Journal of Orthopsychiatry 51, 131-139.

Mangham, C. A. (1981). Insight. Pleasurable affects associated with insight and their origins in infancy. In A. Solnit, et al. (Eds.), Psychoanalytic study of the child (Vol. 36, pp. 271-277). New Haven: Yale University Press.

Milrod, D. (1982). The wished-for self image. In A. Solnit, et al. (Eds.), Psychoanalytic study of the child (Vol. 37, pp. 95-120). New Haven: Yale University Press.

Nachman, P. A., & Stern, D. N. (1985). Affect retrieval: A form of recall memory in prelinguistic infants. In J. D. Call, E. Galenson, & R. L. Tyson (Eds.), Frontiers of infant psychiatry. New York: Basic Books.

Ornstein, A. (1981). Self-pathology in childhood: Developmental and clinical considerations. Psychiatric Clinics of North America 4, 435-453.

Pine, F. (1982). The experience of self. Aspects of its formation, expansion, and vulnerability. In A. Solnit, et al. (Eds.), Psychoanalytic study of the child (Vol. 37, pp. 143-167). New Haven: Yale University Press.

Rubenstein, J. L., Howes, C., & Boyle, P. (1981). A two-year follow-up of infants in community-based day care. Journal of Child Psychology and Psychiatry and Allied Disciplines 22, 209-218.

Rutter, M. (1981). Social-emotional consequences of day care for preschool children. American Journal of Orthopsychiatry 51, 4-28.

Schwartz, P. (1983). Length of day-care attendance and attachment behavior in eighteen-month-old infants. Child Development 54, 1073-1078.

Segal, H. (1982). Early infantile development as reflected in the psychoanalytical process: Steps in integration. International Journal of Psycho-Analysis 63, 15-22.

Sherman, M., & Hertzig, M. E. (1983). Treasured object use--a cognitive and developmental marker. Journal of the American Academy of Child Psychiatry 22, 541-544.

Solnit, A. J. (1982). Early psychic development as reflected in the psychoanalytic process. International Journal of Psycho-Analysis 63, 23-37.

Stern, D. N., Barnett, R. K., & Spieker, S. (1983). Early transmission of affect: Some research issues. In J. D. Call, E. Galenson, & R. L. Tyson (Eds.), Frontiers of infant psychiatry. New York: Basic Books.

6. Historic References in General Personality Development

Baldwin, A. L. (Ed.). (1966a). Theories of child development. New York: Wiley.

Baldwin, A. L. (1966b). Toward an integrated theory of child development. In A. L. Baldwin (Ed.), Theories of child development (pp. 579-599). New York: Wiley.

Bandura, A., & Walters, R. H. (1963). Social learning and personality development. New York: Holt, Rinehart, and Winston.

Becker, W. C., & Krug, R. S. (1964). A circumplex model for social behavior in children. Child Development 36, 329-365.

Benedek, T. (1970). The family as a psychological field. In E. J. Anthony & T. Benedek (Eds.), Parenthood: Its psychology and psychopathology (pp. 109-136). Boston: Little, Brown.

Birch, H. G. (1974). Malnutrition, learning, and intelligence. In S. Chess & A. Thomas (Eds.), Annual progress in child psychiatry and child development: 1973 (pp. 321-346). New York: Brunner/Mazel.

Bloom, B. S. (1964). Stability and change in human characteristics. New York: Wiley.

Bowlby, J. (1951). Maternal care and mental health. Geneva: World Health Organization.

Bowlby, J. (1958). The nature of the child's tie to his mother. International Journal of Psycho-Analysis 39, 350-373.

Bowlby, J. (1969). Attachment and loss. Vol. 1. Attachment. New York: Basic Books.

Bronson, W. C. (1966a). Central orientations: A study of behavior organization from childhood to adolescence. Child Development 37, 125-155.

Bronson, W. C. (1966b). Early antecedents of emotional expressiveness and reactivity control. Child Development 37, 793-810.

Chomsky, N. (1973). Recent contributions to the theory of innate ideas. In S. G. Sapir & A. C. Nitzburg (Eds.), Children with learning problems: Readings in a developmental-interaction approach (pp. 99-108). New York: Brunner/Mazel.

Clausen, J. A. (1966). Family structure, socialization, and personality. Review of Child Development Research 2, 1-53.

Coles, R. (1967). The meaning of race. In R. Coles (Ed.), Children of crisis: A study of courage and fear (pp. 45-272). Boston: Little, Brown.

Cravioto, J., et al. (1966). Nutrition, growth, and neurointegrative development: An experimental and ecologic study. Evanston, Ill.: American Academy of Pediatrics.

Deutsch, C. P. (1973). Social class and child development. In B. M. Caldwell & H. N. Ricciuti (Eds.), Review of child development research. Vol. 3. Child development and social policy (pp. 233-282). Chicago: University of Chicago Press.

Dubin, R., & Dubin, E. R. (1965). Children's social perceptions: A review of research. Child Development 36, 809-838.

Emmerich, W. (1968). Personality development and concepts of structure. Child Development 39, 671-690.

Development

Erikson, E. H. (Ed.). (1959a). Identity and the life cycle. New York: International Universities Press.

Erikson, E. H. (1959b). Growth and crises of the healthy personality. In E. H. Erikson (Ed.), Identity and the life cycle (pp. 50-100). New York: International Universities Press.

Erikson, E. H. (1963). The theory of infant sexuality. In E. H. Erikson (Ed.), Childhood and society (pp. 48-108). New York: Norton.

Flavell, J. H. (1963). The developmental psychology of Jean Piaget. Princeton, N.J.: Van Nostrand.

Freud, A. (1966). The assessment of normality in childhood. In A. Freud (Ed.), Normality and pathology in childhood (pp. 54-107). London: Hogarth Press.

Freud, S. (1964). The dissection of the psychical personality (1933). In E. Jones (Ed.), Collected papers. Standard edition (pp. 57-80). New York and London: Hogarth Press.

Gillespie, W. H. (1968). The psychoanalytic theory of child development. In E. Miller (Ed.), Foundations of child psychiatry (pp. 51-69). Oxford: Pergamon.

Gilmore, J. B. (1966). The role of anxiety and cognitive factors in children's play behavior. Child Development 37, 397-416.

Harlow, H. F., & Harlow, M. K. (1962). Social deprivation in monkeys. Scientific American 207, 136-146.

Harlow, H. F., Harlow, M. K., & Hansen, E. W. (1963). The maternal affectional system of rhesus monkeys. In H. L. Rheingold (Ed.), Maternal behavior in mammals (pp. 254-281). New York: Wiley.

Hartmann, H. (1958). Ego psychology and the problem of adaptation. New York: International Universities Press.

Hatfield, J. S., Ferguson, L. R., & Alpert, R. (1967). Mother-child interaction and the socialization process. Child Development 38, 365-414.

Herzog, E., & Sudia, C. E. (1973). Children in fatherless families. In B. M. Caldwell & H. N. Rucciuti (Eds.), Review of child development research. Vol. 3. Child Development and social policy (pp. 141-232). Chicago: University of Chicago Press.

Hess, E. H. (1970). Ethology and developmental psychology. In L. Carmichael (Ed.), Manual of child psychology (3rd ed., pp. 1-38). New York: Wiley.

Hess, R. D. (1970). Social class and ethnic infuences upon socialization. In L. Carmichael (Ed.), Manual of child psychology (3rd ed., pp. 457-557). New York: Wiley.

Hoffman, M. L. (1970). Moral development. In L. Carmichael (Ed.), Manual of child psychology (3rd ed.) (pp. 261-359). New York: Wiley.

Huttenlocher, J. (1964). Development of formal reasoning on concept formation problems. Child Development 35, 1233-1242.

Jones, M. C., Bayley, N., et al. (Eds.) (1971). The course of human development; selected papers from the longitudinal studies. Waltham, Mass.: Xerox College Pub.

Josselyn, I. M. (1968). Passivity. Journal of the American Academy of Child Psychiatry 7, 569-588.

Kagan, J. (1973). Impulsive and reflective children: Significance of conceptual tempo. In S. G. Sapir & A. C. Nitzburg (Eds.), Children with learning problems: Readings in a developmental-interaction approach (pp. 308-317). New York: Brunner/Mazel.

Kagan, J. (1987). Continuity and discontinuity in development. [Introduction by J. D. Call.] In J. D. Noshpitz (Ed.), Basic handbook of child psychiatry (Vol. 5, pp. 33-38). New York: Basic Books.

Kagan, J., & Moss, H. A. (1960). The stability of passive and dependent behavior from childhood through adulthood. Child Development 31, 577-591.

Kamii, C. K., & Radin, N. L. (1967). Class differences in the socialization practices of Negro mothers. Journal of Marriage and the Family 29, 302-310.

Khan, M. M. R. (1963). The concept of cumulative trauma. In R. S. Eissler, et al. (Eds.), Psychoanalytic study of the child (Vol. 18, pp. 286-306). New York: International Universities Press.

Klein, M. (1948). The development of a child. In M. Klein (Ed.), Contributions to psychoanalysis: 1921-1945 (pp. 13-67). London: Hogarth Press.

Korner, A. F., & Grobstein, R. (1966). Visual alertness as related to soothing in neonates: Implications for maternal stimulation and early deprivation. Child Development 37, 867-876.

Krech, D., Rosenzweig, M. R., & Bennett, E. L. (1966). Environmental impoverishment, social isolation and changes in brain chemistry and anatomy. Physiology and Behavior 1, 99-104.

Kuhn, D. Z., Madsen, Jr., C. H., & Becker, W. C. (1967). Effects of exposure to an aggressive model and "frustration" on children's aggressive behavior. Child Development 38, 739-745.

Lipsitt, L. P. (1967). Learning in the human infant. In H. W. Stevenson, E. H. Hess, & H. L. Rheingold (Eds.), Early behavior: Comparative and developmental approaches (pp. 225-247). New York: Wiley.

Lytton, H. (1971). Observation studies of parent-child interaction: A methodological review. Child Development 42, 651-684.

Macnamara, J. (1974). Cognitive basis of language learning in infants. In S. Chess & A. Thomas (Eds.), Annual progress in child psychiatry and child development: 1973 (pp. 265-284). New York: Brunner/Mazel.

Maier, H. W. (1969). Three theories of child development: The contributions of Erik H. Erikson, Jean Piaget, and Robert R. Sears, and their applications (rev. ed.). New York: Harper and Row.

Mittler, P. (1969). Genetic aspects of psycholinguistic abilities. Journal of Child Psychology and Psychiatry and Allied Disciplines 10, 165-176.

Nash, J. (1965). The father in contemporary culture and current psychological literature. Child Development 36, 261-297.

Parson, T., & Bales, R. F. (1954). Family socialization and interaction process. Glencoe, Ill.: The Free Press.

Phillips, R. H. (1960). The nature and function of children's formal games. Psychoanalytic Quarterly 29, 200-207.

Piaget, J. (1952). The origins of intelligence in children. New York: International Universities Press.

Piaget, J. (1959). The language and thought of the child (3rd ed.). New York: international Universities Press.

Piaget, J. (1970). Piaget's theory. In L. Carmichael (Ed.), Manual of child psychology (3rd ed.) (pp. 703-732). New York: Wiley.

Piaget, J., & Inhelder, B. (1969). The psychology of the child. New York: Basic Books.

Rexford, E. N. (1963). A developmental concept of the problems of acting out. Journal of the American Academy of Child Psychiatry 2, 6-21.

Rosenblith, J. F. (1966). Prognostic value of neonatal assessment. Child Development 37, 623-631.

Rutter, M. (1971). Normal psychosexual development. Journal of Child Psychology and Psychiatry and Allied Disciplines 11, 259-283.

Scott, J. P. (1962). Critical periods in behavioral development. Science 138, 949-958.

Sears, R. R., Rau, L., & Alpert, R. (1965). Identification and child rearing. Stanford: Stanford University Press.

Simmel, M. L. (1966). Developmental aspects of the body scheme. Child Development 37, 83-95.

Spitz, R. A., Emde, R. N., & Metcalf, D. R. (1970). Further prototypes of ego formation: A working paper from a research project on early development. In R. S. Eissler, et al. (Eds.), Psychoanalytic study of the child (Vol. 25, pp. 417-441). New York: International Universities Press.

Sullivan, H. S. (1953). The interpersonal theory of psychiatry. New York: Norton.

Szurek, S. A. (1969). The child's needs for his emotional health. In J. G. Howells (Ed.), Modern perspectives in international child psychiatry (pp. 157-199). Edinburgh: Oliver and Boyd.

Walters, J., Connor, R., & Zunich, M. (1964). Interaction of mothers and children from lower-class families. Child Development 35, 433-440.

Werner, E. E. (1974). Infants around the world: Cross-cultural studies of psychomotor development from birth to two years. In S. Chess & A. Thomas (Eds.), Annual progress in child psychiatry and child development: 1973 (pp. 84-112). New York: Brunner/Mazel.

Whiteman, P. H., & Kosier, K. P. (1964). Development of children's moralistic judgments: Age, Sex, IQ, and certain personal-experimental variables. Child Development 35, 843-850.

Winnicott, D. W. (1965). Growth and development in immaturity. In D. W. Winnicott (Ed.), The family and individual development (pp. 21-29). London: Tavistock.

7. General Personality Development: Various Theories

Abelin, E. L. (1975). Some further observations and comments on the earliest role of the father. International Journal of Psycho-Analysis 56, 293-302.

Abelson, A. G. (1979). Development of psychosexual concepts in relation to expressive language performance. Psychiatry 42, 274-279.

Aleksandrowicz, M. K., & Aleksandrowicz, D. R. (1975a). The molding of personality: A newborn's innate characteristics in interaction with parents' personalities. Child Psychiatry and Human Development 5, 231-241.

Aleksandrowicz, M. K., & Aleksandrowicz, D. R. (1975b). Precursors of ego in neonates. Factor analysis of Brazelton scale data. Journal of the American Academy of Child Psychiatry 15, 257-268.

Allen, M. G., Greenspan, S. I., & Pollin, W. (1976). The effect of parental perceptions on early development in twins. Psychiatry 39, 65-71.

Amsterdam, B., & Greenberg, L. M. (1977). Self-conscious behavior of infants: A videotape study. Developmental Psychobiology 10, 1-6.

Anderson, J. R. (1984). The development of self-recognition: A review. Developmental Psychobiology 17, 35-49.

Andresen, J. J. (1980). Conflict and the origins of identification. Psychoanalytic Review 67, 25-43.

Anthony, E. J. (1977). Nonverbal and verbal systems of communication. A study in complementarity. In A. Solnit, et al. (Eds.), Psychoanalytic study of the child (Vol. 32, pp. 307-325). New Haven: Yale University Press.

Archer, J. (1984). Gender roles as developmental pathways. British Journal of Social Psychology 23, 245-256.

Arend, R., Gove, F. L., & Sroufe, L. A. (1979). Continuity of individual adaptation from infancy to kindergarten: A predictive study of ego-resiliency and curiosity in preshcoolers. Child Development 50, 950-959.

Baker, S. W. (1980). Psychosexual differentiation in the human. Biology of Reproduction 22, 61-72.

Bauman, S. (1981). Physical aspects of the self. A review of some aspects of body image development in childhood. Psychiatric Clinics of North America 4, 455-470.

Behrends, R. S., & Blatt, S. J. (1985). Internalization and psychological development throughout the life cycle. In A. Solnit, et al. (Eds.), Psychoanalytic study of the child (Vol. 40, pp. 11-39). New Haven: Yale University Press.

Benedek, E. P., Poznanski, E., & Mason, S. (1979). A note on the female adolescent's psychological reactions to breast development. Journal of the American Academy of Child Psychiatry 18, 537-545.

Beratis, S., Kolb, R., Sperling, E., & Stein, R. E. (1981). Development of a child with long-lasting deprivation of oral feeding. Journal of the American Academy of Child Psychiatry 20, 53-64.

Beratis, S., Miller, R., & Galenson, E. (1982-1983). Separation-individuation and transitional objects in a four-year-old psychotic child. International Journal of Psychoanalytic Psychotherapy 9, 561-582.

Berman, P. W., Smith, V. L., & Goodman, V. (1983). Development of sex differences in response to an infant and to the caretaker role. Journal of Genetic Psychology 143, 283-284.

Binnie-Dawson, J. L., & Cheung, Y. M. (1982). The effects of different types of neonatal feminization and environmental stimulation on changes in sex-associated activity/spatial learning skills. Biological Psychology 15, 109-140.

Blasi, A., & Hoeffel, E. C. (1974). Adolescence and formal operations. Human Development 17, 344-363.

Bleiberg, E., Jackson, L., & Ross, J. L. (1986). Gender identity disorder and object loss. Journal of the American Academy of Child Psychiatry 25, 58-67.

Block, J. H. (1983). Differential premises arising from differential socialization of the sexes: Some conjectures. Child Development 54, 1335-1354.

Bloom-Feshbach, S., Bloom-Feshbach, J., & Gaughran, J. (1980). The child's tie to both parents: Separation patterns and nursery school adjustment. American Journal of Orthopsychiatry 50, 505-521.

Blos, P., Jr. (1985). Intergenerational separation-individuation. Treating the mother-infant pair. In A. Solnit, et al. (Eds.), Psychoanalytic study of the child (Vol. 40, pp. 41-56). New Haven: Yale University Press.

Bouras, M., & Raimbault, G. (1977). Personality development in children after renal transplantation. Archives of French Pediatrics 34, 665-670.

Bowker, L. H., & Klein, M. W. (1983). The etiology of female juvenile delinquency and gang membership: A test of psychological and social structural explanations. Adolescence 18, 739-751.

Bowlby, J. (1977). The making and breaking of affectional bonds. I. Aetiology and psychopathology in the light of attachment theory. An expanded version of the Fiftieth Maudsley Lecture, delivered before the Royal College of Psychiatrists, 19 November 1976. British Journal of Psychiatry 130, 201-210.

Brantley, H. T., & Clifford, E. (1979). Cognitive, self-concept, and body image measures of normal, cleft palate, and obese adolescents. Cleft Palate Journal 16, 177-182.

Brickman, A. S. (1983). Pre-oedipal development of the superego. International Journal of Psycho-Analysis 64(1), 83-92.

Brinich, P. M. (1980). Some potential effects of adoption on self and object representations. In A. Solnit, et al. (Eds.), Psychoanalytic study of the child (Vol. 35, pp. 107-133). New Haven: Yale University Press.

Bruneau, O. J. (1984). Comparison of behavioral characteristics and self-concepts of American Indian and Caucasian preschoolers. Psychological Reports 54, 571-574.

Burns, W. J., & Zweig, A. R. (1980). Self-concepts of chronically ill children. Journal of Genetic Psychology 137, 179-190.

Calderone, M. S. (1985). Adolescent sexuality: Elements and genesis. Pediatrics 76, 699-703.

Calef, V., Weinshel, E. M., Renik, O., & Mayer, E. L. (1980). Enureses: A functional equivalent of a fetish. International Journal of Psycho-Analysis 61, 295-305.

Calhoun, G., Jr., Connley, S., & Bolton, J. A. (1984). comparison of delinquents and nondelinquents in ethnicity, ordinal position, and self-perception. Journal of Clinical Psychology 40, 323-328.

Campbell, S. B. (1979). Mother-infant interaction as a function of maternal ratings of temperament. Child Psychiatry and Human Development 10, 67-76.

Carey, W. B., & McDevitt, S. C. (1978). Stability and change in individual temperament diagnoses from infancy to early childhood. Journal of the American Academy of Child Psychiatry 17, 331-337.

Cattell, R. B., Schuerger, J. M., & Klein, T. W. (1982). Heritabilities of ego strength (factor C), super ego strength (factor G), and self-sentiment (factor Q3) by multiple abstract variance analysis. Journal of Clinical Psychology 38, 769-779.

Champion, V. L., Austin, J. K., & Tzeng, O. (1982). Assessment of relationship between self-concept and body image using multivariate techniques. Issues in Mental Health Nursing 4, 299-315.

Clarke, A. D., & Clarke, A. M. (1984). Constancy and change in the growth of human characteristics. Journal of Child Psychology and Psychiatry and Allied Disciplines 25, 191-210.

Clarke, B. A. (1983). Improving adolescent parenting through participant modeling and self-evaluation. Nursing Clinics of North America 18, 303-311.

Cohen, D. J., Dibble, E., & Grawe, J. M. (1977). Parental style. Mothers' and fathers' perceptions of their relations with twin children. Archives of General Psychiatry 34, 445-451.

Cohen, K. N., & Clark, J. A. (1984). Transitional object attachments in early childhood and personality characteristics in later life. Journal of Personality and Social Psychology 46, 106-111.

Coleman, J. M. (1985). Achievement level, social class, and the self-concepts of mildly handicapped children. Journal of Learning Disabilities 18, 26-30.

Colonna, A. B., & Friedmann, M. (1984). Prediction of development. In A. Solnit, et al. (Eds.), Psychoanalytic study of the child (Vol. 39, pp. 509-526). New Haven: Yale University Press.

Connor, J. M., Dann, L N., & Twentyman, C. T. (1982). A self-report measure of assertiveness in young adolescents. Journal of Clinical Psychology 38, 101-106.

Dewald, P. A., & Kramer, S. (1976). Dialogue on "the role of family life in child development." International Journal of Psycho-Analysis 57, 403-409.

Dibble, E. D., & Cohen, D. J. (1981). Personality development in identical twins. The first decade of life. In A. Solnit, et al. (Eds.), Psychoanalytic study of the child (Vol. 36, pp. 45-70). New Haven: Yale University Press.

Dien, D. S. (1983). Big me and little me: A Chinese perspective on self. Psychiatry 46, 281-286.

Donnellan, G. J. (1980). Conceptual models and symbol formation during the latency period. Psychoanalytic Review 67, 291-312.

Dowling, S. (1977). Seven infants with esophageal atresia. A developmental study. In A. Solnit, et al. (Eds.), Psychoanalytic study of the child (Vol. 32, pp. 215-256). New Haven: Yale University Press.

Drotar, D., Owens, R., & Gotthold, J. (1980). Personality adjustment of children and adolescents with hypopituitarism. Child Psychiatry and Human Development 11, 59-66.

Development

Drucker, J., & Shapiro, C. B. (1979). First scribbles: The emergence of an ego function. Journal of the American Academy of Child Psychiatry 18, 628-646.

Dunn, J., & Kendrick, C. (1980). Studying temperament and parent-child interaction: Comparison of interview and direct observation. Developmental Medicine and Child Neurology 22, 484-496.

Egeland, B., Sroufe, L. A., & Erickson, M. (1983). The developmental consequence of different patterns of maltreatment. Child Abuse and Neglect 7, 459-469.

Ehrhardt, A. A., Ince, S, E., & Meyer-Bahlburg, H. F. (1981). Career aspiration and gender role development in young girls. Archives of Sexual Behavior 10, 281-299.

Ehrhardt, A. A., & Meyer-Bahlburg, H. F. (1981). Effects of prenatal sex hormones on gender-related behavior. Science 211, 1312-1318.

Elkind, D. (1976). Cognitive adaptation in latency. The construction of social reality. Canadian Psychiatric Association Journal 21, 186-191.

Emde, R. N. (1983). The prerepresentational self and its affective core. In A. Solnit, et al. (Eds.), Psychoanalytic study of the child (Vol. 38, pp. 165-192). New Haven: Yale University Press.

Emde, R. N., Johnson, W. F., & Easterbrooks, M. A. (1988). The do's and don'ts of early moral development: Psychoanalytic tradition and current research. In J. Kagan & S. Lamb (Eds.), The emergency of morality. Chicago: University of Chicago Press.

Escalona, S. K. (1982). Growing up with the threat of nuclear war: Some indirect effects on personality development. American Journal of Orthopsychiatry 52, 600-607.

Escalona, S. K. (1984). Social and other environmental influences on the cognitive and personality development of low birthweight infants. American Journal of Mental Deficiency 88, 508-512.

Fagot, B. I., & Leinbach, M. D. (1985). Gender identity: Some thoughts on an old concept. Journal of the American Academy of Child Psychiatry 24, 684-688.

Feiring, C. (1984). Behavioral styles in infancy and adulthood: The work of Karen Horney and attachment theorists collaterally considered. American Journal of Psychoanalysis 44, 197-208.

Finegan, J. K., Zucker, K. J., Bradley, S. J., & Doering, R. W. (1982). Patterns of intellectual functioning and spatial ability in boys and gender identity disorder. Canadian Journal of Psychiatry 27, 135-139.

Freud, A. (1981). Insight. Its presence and absence as a factor in normal development. In A. Solnit, et al. (Eds.), Psychoanalytic study of the child (Vol. 36, pp. 241-249). New Haven: Yale University Press.

Fries, M. E. (1977). Longitudinal study: Prenatal period to parenthood. Journal of the American Psychoanalytic Association 25, 115-132.

Fullard, W., McDevitt, S. C., & Carey, W. B. (1984). Assessing temperament in one- to three-year-old children. Journal of Pediatric Psychology 9, 205-217.

Galenson, E., & Roiphe, H. (1980). The preoedipal development of the boy. Journal of the American Psychoanalytic Association 28, 805-826.

Gilberg, A. L. (1978). Adolescence: The interface of neurophysiology and cultural determinants. American Journal of Psychoanalysis 38, 87-90.

Gilligan, C. (1980). The effects of social institutions on the moral development of children and adolescents. Bulletin of the Menninger Clinic 44, 498-523.

Gislason, I. L., & Call, J. D. (1982). Dog bite in infancy: Trauma and personality development. Journal of the American Academy of Child Psychiatry 21, 203-207.

Goldman, R., & Goldman, J. (1983). Children's perceptions of sex differences in babies and adolescents: A cross-national study. Archives of Sexual Behavior 12, 277-294.

Gordon, M., Crouthamel, C., Post, E. M., & Richman, R. A. (1982). Psychosocial aspects of constitutional short stature: Social competence, behavior problems, self-esteem, and family functioning. Journal of Pediatrics 101, 477-480.

Green, R. (1985). Gender identity in childhood and later sexual orientation: Follow-up of 78 males. American Journal of Psychiatry 142, 339-341.

Greenspan, S. I. (1988). The development of the ego: Insights from clinical work with infants and children. Journal of the American Psychoanalytic Association 36 (Supplement), 3-55.

Greenspan, S. I. (1989). Biological and environmental specificity and the psychopathological developmental process: A new hypothesis on the role of early sensory-affective experience in the genesis of thought disorders. Journal of the American Psychoanalytic Association 37, 605-638.

Harvey, D. H., & Greenway, A. P. (1984). The self-concept of physically handicapped children and their non-handicapped siblings: An empirical investigation. Journal of Child Psychology and Psychiatry and Allied Disciplines 25, 273-284.

Henderson, J. (1982). The role of the father in separation-individuation. Bulletin of the Menninger Clinic 46, 231-254.

Himmelfarb, S., Hock, E., & Wenar, C. (1985). Infant temperament and noncompliant behavior at four years: A longitudinal study. Genetic, Social, and General Psychology Monographs 111, 7-21.

The influence of early deficits on later development (1985). Panel report. Journal of the American Psychoanalytic Association 33, 631-644.

Janus, S. S., & Bess, B. E. (1976). Latency: Fact or fiction? American Journal of Psychoanalysis 36, 339-346.

Kay, P. (1980). The imaginary companion: Review of the literature. Maternal-Child Nursing Journal 9, 7-11.

Kestenberg, J. S. (1980). The three faces of femininity. Psychoanalytic Review 67, 313-335.

Khantzian, E. J., & Mack, J. E. (1983). Self-preservation and the care of the self. Ego instincts reconsidered. In A. Solnit, et al. (Eds.), Psychoanalytic study of the child (Vol. 38, pp. 209-232). New Haven: Yale University Press.

Kitahara, M. (1983). Female puberty rites: Reconsideration and speculation. Adolescence 18, 957-964.

Klinger, E., & McNelly, F. W., Jr. (1976). Self starts and performances of preadolescent boys carrying out leadership roles inconsistent with their social status. Child Development 47, 126-137.

Lamb, M. E. (1982). Paternal influences on early socio-emotional development. Journal of Child Psychology and Psychiatry and Allied Disciplines 23, 185-190.

Lazarus, P. J. (1982). Correlation of shyness and self-esteem for elementary school children. Perceptual and Motor Skills 55, 8-10.

Ledingham, J. E., Younger, A., Schwartzman, A., & Bergeron, G. (1982). Agreement among teacher, peer, and self-ratings of children's aggression, withdrawal, and likability. Journal of Abnormal Child Psychology 10, 363-372.

Lee, G. (1982). Relationship of self-concept during late pregnancy to neonatal perception and parenting profile. Journal of Obstetric, Gynecologic, and Neonatal Nursing 11, 186-190.

Lefley, H. P. (1975). Differential self-concept in American Indian children as a function of language and examiner. Journal of Personality and Social Psychology 31, 36-41.

Leichtman, M. (1985). The influence of an older sibling on the separation-individuation precess. In A. Solnit, et al. (Eds.), Psychoanalytic study of the child (Vol. 40, pp. 111-161). New Haven: Yale University Press.

Lester, E. P. (1983). Separation-individuation and cognition. Journal of the American Psychoanalytic Association 31, 127-156.

Lewis, M. (1977). Language, cognitive development, and personality. A synthesis. Journal of the American Academy of Child Psychiatry 16, 646-661.

Lidz, T. (1979). Family studies and changing concepts of personality development. Canadian Journal of Psychiatry 24, 621-632.

Lotterman, A. (1981). Superman as a male latency stage myth. Bulletin of the Menninger Clinic 45, 491-498.

Lyles, M. R., Yancey, A., Grace, C., & Carter, J. H. (1985). Racial identity and self-esteem: Problems peculiar to biracial children Journal of the American Academy of Child Psychiatry 24, 150-153.

Lytton, H., & Watts, D. (1981). The social development of twins in longitudinal perspective: How stable is genetic determination over age 2 to 9? Progress in Clinical and Biological Research 69(B), 255-259.

Mahler, M. S. (1974). Symbiosis and individuation. The psychological birth of the human infant. In R. S. Eissler, et al. (Eds.), Psychoanalytic study of the child (Vol. 29, pp. 89-106). New York: International Universities Press.

Mahler, M. S. (1981). Aggression in the service of separation-individuation. Case study of a mother-daughter relationship Psychoanalytic Quarterly 50, 625-638.

Mahler, M. S., & McDevitt, J. B. (1982). Thoughts on the emergence of the sense of self, with particular emphasis on the body of self. Journal of the American Psychoanalytic Association 30, 827-848.

Manaster, G. J., Saddler, C. D., & Wukasch, L. (1977). The ideal self and cognitive development in adolescence. Adolescence 12, 547-558.

Mangham, C. A. (1981). Insight. Pleasurable affects associated with insight and their origins in infancy. In A. Solnit, et al. (Eds.), Psychoanalytic study of the child (Vol. 36, pp. 271-277). New Haven: Yale University Press.

Massie, H. N., Bronstein, A., Afterman, J., Campbell, B. K. (1988). Inner themes and outer behaviors in early child development. In A. Solnit, et al. (Eds.), Psychoanalytic study of the child (Vol. 43, pp. 213-242). New Haven: Yale University Press.

McHale, S. M., & Huston, T. L. (1984). Men and women as parents: Sex role orientations, employment, and parental roles with infants. Child Development 55, 1349-1361.

Neubauer, P. B., & Flapan, D. (1976). Developmental groupings in latency children. Journal of the American Academy of Child Psychiatry 15, 646-664.

Norbeck, J. S. (1981). Young children's ability to conserve facial identity when facial emotion varies. Nursing Research 30, 329-333.

Oates, R. K. (1984). Personality development after physical abuse. Archives of Disease in Childhood 59, 147-150.

Ornitz, E. M., & Pynoos, R. S. (1989). Startle modulation in children with post-traumatic stress disorder. American Journal of Psychiatry 146(7), 866-870.

Parmelee, A. H. (1986). Children's illnesses: Their beneficial effects on their behavioral development. Child Development 57, 1-10.

Phillips, D. (1984). The illusion of incompetence among academically competent children. Child Development 55, 2000-2016.

Rae-Grant, Q. (1976). New family structures and the latency child. Canadian Psychiatric Association Journal 21, 197-198.

Richardson, S. A., Koller, H., & Katz, M. (1986). Factors leading to differences in the school performance of boys and girls. Journal of Developmental and Behavioral Pediatrics 7, 49-55.

Riesman, P. (1983). On the irrelevance of child rearing practices for the formation of personality. An analysis of childhood, personality, and values in two African communities. Culture, Medicine and Psychiatry 7, 103-129.

Rosenthal, B. G. (1974). Development of self-identification in relation to attitudes towards the self in the Chippewa Indians. Genetic Psychology Monographs 90, 43-141.

Sadler, L. S., & Catrone, C. (1983). The adolescent parent: A dual developmental crisis. Journal of Adolescent Health Care 4, 100-105.

Sandler, J., & Sandler, A. M. (1978). On the development of object relationships and affects. International Journal of Psycho-Analysis 59, 285-296.

Shapiro, T., & Perry, R. (1976). Latency revisited. The age 7 plus or minus 1. In R. S. Eissler, et al. (Eds.), Psychoanalytic study of the child (Vol. 31, pp. 79-105). New York: International Universities Press.

Sherick, I., Greenman, G., & Legg, C. (1976). Some comments on the significance and development of midline behavior during infancy. Child Psychiatry and Human Development 6, 170-183.

Simmons, C. H., & Parsons, R. J. (1983). Developing internality and perceived competence: The empowerment of adolescent girls. Adolescence 18, 917-922.

Solnit, A. J. (1982). Developmental perspectives on self and object constancy. In A. Solnit, et al. (Eds.), Psychoanalytic study of the child (Vol. 37, pp. 201-218). New Haven: Yale University Press.

Spencer, M. B. (1984). Black children's race awareness, racial attitudes and self-concept: A reinterpretation. Journal of Child Psychology and Psychiatry and Allied Disciplines 25, 433-441.

Spurlock, J. (1986). Development of self-concept in Afro-American children. Hospital and Community Psychiarty 37, 66-70.

Standley, K., Soule, A. B., Copans, S. A., & Klein, R. P. (1978). Multidimensional sources of infant temperament. Genetic Psychology Monographs 98, 203-231.

Stoller, R. J., & Herdt, G. H. (1982). The development of masculinity: A cross-cultural contribution. Journal of the American Psychoanalytic Association 30, 29-59.

Suter, B., Seegmiller, B. R., & Dunivant, N. (1980). Effects of age, sex, and income level on sex-role differentiation in preschoolers. Journal of Psychology 104, 217-220.

Sutherland, J. D. (1980). The British object relations theorists: Balint, Winnicott, Fairbairn, Guntrip. Journal of the American Psychoanalytic Association 28, 829-860.

Tashjian, L. D. (1982). Aspects of internalization and individuation: James Joyce's portrait of the artist as a young man. In S. C. Feinstein, et al. (Eds.), Adolescent psychiatry: Developmental and clinical studies (Vol. 10, pp. 75-84). Chicago: University of Chicago Press.

Taylor, M., & Flavell, J. H. (1984). Seeing and believing: Children's understanding of the distinction between appearance and reality. Child Development 55, 1710-1720.

Terhune, C. B. (1979). The role of hearing in early ego organization. In A. Solnit, et al. (Eds.), Psychoanalytic study of the child (Vol. 34, pp. 371-383). New Haven: Yale University Press.

Tishler, C. L., & McKenry, P. C. (1982). Parental negative self and adolescent suicide attempts. Journal of the American Academy of Child Psychiatry 21, 404-408.

Trupin, E. W. (1976). Correlates of ego-level and agency-communion in stage REM dreams of 11-13 year old children. Journal of Child Psychology and Psychiatry and Allied Disciplines 17, 169-180.

Tyson, P. (1978). Transference and developmental issues in the analysis of a prelatency child. In A. Solnit, et al. (Eds.), Psychoanalytic study of the child (Vol. 33, pp. 213-236). New Haven: Yale University Press.

Tyson, P. (1980). The gender of the analyst: In relation to transference and countertransference manifestations in prelatency children. In A. Solnit, et al. (Eds.), Psychoanalytic study of the child (Vol. 35, pp. 321-338). New Haven: Yale University Press.

Tyson, P., & Tyson, R. L. (1984). Narcissism and superego development. Journal of the American Psychoanalytic Association 32, 75-98.

van der Velde, C. D. (1985). Body images of one's self and of others: Developmental and clinical significance. American Journal of Psychiatry 142, 527-537.
Williams, K., Goodman, M., & Green, R. (1985). Parent-child factors in gender role socialization in girls. Journal of the American Academy of Child Psychiatry 24, 720-731.
Zeanah, C. H. (1989). Adaptation following perinatal loss: A critical review. Journal of the American Academy of Child and Adolescent Psychiatry 28, 467-480.
Zeanah, C. H., Anders, T. F., Seifer, R., & Stern, D. N. (1989). Implications of research on infant development for psychodynamic theory and practice. Journal of the American Academy of Child and Adolescent Psychiatry 28(5), 657-668.
Zucker, K. J., Finegan, J. A., Doering, R. W., & Bradley, S. J. (1983). Human figure drawings of gender-problem children: A comparison to sibling, psychiatric, and normal controls. Journal of Abnormal Child Psychology 11, 287-298.
Zuger, B. (1978). Effeminate behavior present in boys from childhood: Ten additional years of follow-up. Comprehensive Psychiatry 19, 363-369.

8. Development of Affect

Barden, R. C., Zelko, F. A., Duncan, S. W., & Masters, J. C. (1980). Children's consensual knowledge about the experiential determinants of emotion. Journal of Personality and Social Psychology 39, 968-976.
Bauer, D. H. (1976). An exploratory study of developmental changes in children's fears. Journal of Child Psychology and Psychiatry and Allied Disciplines 17, 69-74.
Birtchnell, J. (1980). Women whose mothers died in childhood: An outcome study. Psychological Medicine 10, 699-713.
Boesch, E. E. (1984). The development of affective schemata. Human Development 27, 173-183.
Cummings, E. M., Zahn-Waxler, C., & Radke-Yarrow, M. (1984). Developmental changes in children's reactions to anger in the home. Journal of Child Psychology and Psychiatry and Allied Disciplines 25, 63-74.
Emde, R.N., Gaensbauer, T. J., & Harmon, R. J. (1976). Emotional expression in infancy: A biobehavioral study. Psychological Issues 10, 1-200.
Freedman, D. A. (1979). The sensory deprivations. An approach to the study of the emergence of affects and the capacity for object relations. Bulletin of the Menninger Clinic 43, 29-68.
Freedman, D. A., Montgomery, J. R., Wilson, R., Bealmear, P. M., & South, M. A. (1976). Further observations on the effect of reverse isolation from birth on cognitive and affective development. Journal of the American Academy of Child Psychiatry 15, 593-603.
Furman, R. A. (1978). Some developmental aspects of the verbalization of affects. In A. Solnit, et al. (Eds.), Psychoanalytic study of the child (Vol. 33, pp. 187-211). New Haven: Yale University Press.

Development

Harmon, R. J., Morgan, G. A., & Glicken, A. D. (1984). Continuities and discontinuities in affective and cognitive-motivational development. Child Abuse and Neglect 8, 157-167.

Malatesta, C. Z., Grigoryev, P., Lamb, C., Albin, M., & Culver, C. (1986). Emotion socialization and expressive development in preterm and full-term infants. Child Development 57, 316-330.

Mangham, C. A. (1981). Insight. Pleasurable affects associated with insight and their origins in infancy. In A. Solnit, et al. (Eds.), Psychoanalytic study of the child (Vol. 36, pp. 271-277). New Haven: Yale University Press.

Osofsky, J. D., & Eberhart-Wright, A. (1988). Affective exchanges between high risk mothers and infants. International Journal of Psycho-Analysis 69, 221-231.

Pine, F. (1979). On the expansion of the affect array. A developmental description. Bulletin of the Menninger Clinic 43, 79-95.

Porges, S. W. (1989). Vagal tone: A mediator of affect. In J. A. Garber & K. A. Dodge (Eds.), The development of affect regulation and dysregulation. New York: Cambridge University Press.

Prawat, R. S. (1976). Mapping the affective domain in young adolescents. Journal of Educational Psychology 68, 566-572.

Sroufe, L. A., & Waters, E. (1976). The ontogenesis of smiling and laughter: A perspective on the organization of development in infancy. Psychological Review 83, 173-189.

Staley, A. A., & O'Donnell, J. (1984). A developmental analysis of mothers' reports of normal children's fears. Journal of Genetic Psychology 144, 165-178.

Tronick, E. (1989). Emotions and emotional communication in infants. American Psychologist 44, 112-119.

Webb, T. E., & Van Devere, C. A. (1981). Continuities in the structural expression of affectivity: A developmental comparison. Child Psychiatry and Human Development 12, 40-45.

Wilson, B. J., & Cantor, J. (1985). Developmental differences in empathy with a television protagonist's fear. Journal of Experimental Child Psychology 39, 284-299.

9. Psychosocial and Psychophysiological Aspects of Infancy

Galenson, E. (1987). Gender identity. [Introduction by J. D. Call]. In J. D. Noshpitz (Ed.), Basic handbook of child psychiatry (Vol. 5, pp. 61-66). New York: Basic Books.

Hakamada, S., Watanabe, K., Hara, K., & Miyazaki, S. (1980). The evolution of some EEG features in normal and abnormal infants. Brain Development 2, 373-377.

Harding, C. G. (1982). Development of the intention to communicate. Human Development 25, 140-151.

Harmon, R. J., Morgan, G. A., & Glicken, A. D. (1984). Continuities and discontinuities in affective and cognitive-motivational development. Child Abuse and Neglect 8, 157-167.

Harriman, A. E., & Lukosius, P. A. (1982). On why Wayne Dennis found Hope infants retarded in age at onset of walking. Perceptual and Motor Skills 55, 79-86.

Hart, H., Bax, M., & Jenkins, S. (1978). The value of a developmental history. Developmental Medicine and Child Neurology 20, 442-452.

Hartley, X. Y. (1986). A summary of recent research into the development of children with Down's syndrome. Journal of Mental Deficiency Research 30, 1-14.

Hartmann, H. (1981). A review of twins: A study of three pairs of identical twins by Dorothy Burlingham. In A. Solnit, et al. (Eds.), Psychoanalytic study of the child (Vol. 36, pp. 147-150). New Haven: Yale University Press.

Harvey, D., Prince, J., Bunton, J., Parkinson, C., & Campbell, S. (1982). Abilities of children who were small-for-gestational-age babies. Pediatrics 69, 296-300.

Haskins, R. (1985). Public school aggression among children with varying day-care experience. Child Development 56, 689-703.

Hay, D. F., Nash, A., & Pedersen, J. (1981). Responses of six-month-olds to distress of their peers. Child Development 52, 1071-1075.

Heinicke, C. M. (1980). Continuity and discontinuity of task orientation. Journal of the American Academy of Child Psychiatry 19, 637-653.

Henry, G. (1984). Reflections on infant observation and its applications. Journal of Analytic Psychology 29, 155-169.

Herzog, D. B., & Rathbun, J. M. (1982). Childhood depression. Developmental considerations. American Journal of Diseases of Children 136, 115-120.

Hindley, C. B., & Owen, C. F. (1978). The extent of individual changes in I.Q. for ages between 6 months and 17 years, in a British longitudinal sample. Journal of Child Psychology and Psychiatry and Allied Disciplines 19, 329-350.

Hixson, P. H. (1979). Guidelines for recognizing delayed language development. Ear, Nose, and Throat Journal 58, 310-315.

Hock, E., Kroll, B. C., Frantz, J., Janson, K. A., & Widaman, K. (1984). Infants in play groups: Time related changes in behavior toward mothers, peers, and toys. Journal of Genetic Psychology 144, 51-67.

Hoff-Ginsberg, E. (1983). Sound-based errors in early word use. Journal of Child Language 10, 459-464.

Hoff-Ginsberg, E., & Shatz, M. (1982). Linguistic input and the child's acquisition of language. Psychological Bulletin 92, 3-26.

Holaday, B. (1982). Maternal conceptual set development: Identifying patterns of maternal response to chronically ill infant crying. Maternal-Child Nursing Journal 11, 47-59.

Holaday, B. (1985). Sensorimotor development in the presence of atypical object manipulation during infancy. Maternal-Child Nursing Journal 14, 1-7.

Holt, K. S. (1985). A developmental approach to physical disability in childhood. International Rehabilitation Medicine 7, 18-26.

Honig, A. S. (1988). Secure attachment: Key to infant mental health [Review of Bretherton & Waters, Growing points of attachment theory and research]. Infant Mental Health Journal 9(2), 181-183.

Horgan, D. (1981). Learning to tell jokes: A case of study of metalinguistic abilities. Journal of Child Language 8, 217-224.

Horner, T. M. (1980). Test-retest and home-clinic characteristics of the Bayley scales of infant development in nine- and fifteen-month-old infants. Child Development 51, 751-758.

Horowitz, F. D. (1982). Child development for the pediatrician. Pediatric Clinics of North America 29, 359-375.

Hubatch, L. M., Johnson, C. J., Kistler, D. J., Burns, W. J., & Moneka, W. (1985). Early language abilities of high-risk infants. Journal of Speech and Hearing Disorders 50, 195-207.

Hudson, J., & Nelson, K. (1984). Play with language: Overextensions as analogies. Journal of Child Language 11, 337-346.

Hulse, A. (1983). Congenital hypothyroidism and neurological development. Journal of Child Psychology and Psychiatry and Allied Disciplines 24, 629-635.

Inoff, G. E., Halverson, C. F., Allen, M. G., & Cohen, D. J. (1980). Pathways between constitution and competence during the first five years of life. Developmental Psychobiology 13, 191-204.

Ireton, H., & Thwing, E. (1976). Appraising the development of a preschool child by means of a standardized report prepared by the mother. The Minnesota child development inventory. Clinical Pediatrics 15, 875-882.

Isay, R. A. (1987). Fathers and their homosexually inclined sons in childhood. In A. Solnit, et al. (Eds.), Psychoanalytic study of the child (Vol. 42, pp. 275-294). New Haven: Yale University Press.

Jenkins, S., Owen, C., Bax, M., & Hart, H. (1984). Continuities of common behaviour problems in preschool children. Journal of Child Psychology and Psychiatry and Allied Disciplines 25, 75-89.

Jolly, H. (1985). Helping parents achieve optimal development for their children. Journal of Psychosomatic Research 29, 593-595.

Joos, S. K., Pollitt, E., Mueller, W. H., & Albright, D. L. (1983). The Bacon Chow study: Maternal nutritional supplementation and infant behavior development. Child Development 54, 669-676.

Joseph, R. (1982). The neuropsychology of development hemispheric laterality, limbic language, and the origin of thought. Journal of Clinical Psychology 38, 4-33.

Jung, E., & Czajka-Narins, D. M. (1985). Birth weight doubling and tripling times: An updated look at the effects of birth weight, sex, race and type of feeding. American Journal of Clinical Nutrition 42, 182-189.

Junker, K. S., Barr, B., Maliniemi, S., & Wasz-Hockert, O. (1978). BOEL screening: A program for the early detection of communicative disorders. Preliminary reports from a study on 1,000 infants. Audiology 17, 51-61.

Kaga, M., Ohuchi, M., Kaga, K., & Tanaka, Y. (1984). Normalization of poor auditory brainstem response in infants and children. Brain Development 6, 458-466.

Kagan, J. (1976). Emergent themes in human development. American Scientist 64, 186-196.

Kagan, J. (1982). Canalization of early psychological development. Pediatrics 70, 474-483.

Kagan, J., Lapidus, D. R., & Moore, M. (1978). Infant antecedents of cognitive functioning: A longitudinal study. Child Development 49, 1005-1023.

Kamhi, A. G. (1986). The elusive first word: The importance of the naming insight for the development of referential speech. Journal of Child Language 13, 155-161.

Kastein, S., & Gillman, A. E. (1976). The interaction of emotional stress and language development: Case studies of three visually impaired children. Journal of Communication Disorders 9, 135-141.

Kavanaugh, R. D., Whittington, S., & Cerbone, M. J. (1983). Mothers' use of fantasy in speech to young children Journal of Child Language 10, 45-55.

Keane, S. P., & Conger, J. C. (1981). The implications of communication development for social skills training. Journal of Pediatric Psychology 6, 369-381.

Kent, R. D. (1984). Psychobiology of speech development: Coemergence of language and a movement system. American Journal of Physiology 246, 888-894.

Klein, R. P., & Durfee, J. T. (1979). Prediction of preschool social behavior from social-emotional development at one year. Child Psychiatry and Human Development 9, 145-151.

Klykylo, W. M. (1989). [Review of J. Bloom-Feshbach, S. Bloom-Feshbach & Associates, The psychology of separation and loss]. Journal of the American Academy of Child and Adolescent Psychiatry 28(3), 459-460.

Knobloch, H., & Pasamanick, B. (1976). Assessing development in the first three years. American Family Physician 13, 108-114.

Knobloch, H., Stevens, F., Malone, A., Ellison, P., & Risemberg, H. (1979). The validity of parental reporting of infant development. Pediatrics 63, 872-878.

Kramer, M. S., Rooks, Y., Washington, L. A., & Pearson, H. A. (1980). Pre- and postnatal growth and development in sickle cell anemia. Journal of Pediatrics 96, 857-860.

Krishnamoorthy, K. S., Kuehnle, K. J., Todres, I. D., & DeLong, G. R. (1984). Neurodevelopmental outcome of survivors with posthemorrhagic hydrocephalus following grade II neonatal intraventricular hemorrhage. Annals of Neurology 15, 201-204.

Krummel, T. M., Greenfield, L. J., Kirkpatrick, B. V., Mueller, D. G., Kerkering, K. W., Ormazabal, M., Myer, E. C., & Barnes, R. W. (1984). The early evaluation of survivors after extracorporeal membrane oxygenation for neonatal pulmonary failure. Journal of Pediatric Surgery 19, 585-590.

La Veck, B., & Hammond, M. A. (1982). Performance on the motor scale of the McCarthy scales of children's abilities as related to home environment and neonatal reflexes. Perceptual and Motor Skills 54, 1265-1266.

Lamb, M. E. (1976). Parent-infant interaction in 8-month-olds. Child Psychiatry and Human Development 7, 56-63.

Lamb, M. E. (1977). A re-examination of the infant social worlds. Human Development 20, 65-85.

Lamb, M. E. (1978). The development of sibling relationships in infancy: A short-term longitudinal study. Child Development 49, 1189-1192.

Lane, V. W., & Samples, J. M. (1984). Tuberous sclerosis: Case study of early seizure control and subsequent normal development. Journal of Autism and Developmental Disorders 14, 423-427.

Largo, R. H., & Howard, J. A. (1979). Developmental progression in play behavior of children between nine and thirty months. I: Spontaneous play and imitation. Developmental Medicine and Child Neurology 21, 299-310.

Largo, R. H., & Stutzle, W. (1977a). Longitudinal study of bowel and bladder control by day and at night in the first six years of life. I: Epidemiology and interrelations between bowel and bladder control. Developmental Medicine and Child Neurology 19, 598-606.

Largo, R. H., & Stutzle, W. (1977b). Longitudinal study of bowel and bladder control by day and at night in the first six years of life. II: The role of potty training and the child's initiative. Developmental Medicine and Child Neurology 19, 607-613.

Lasky, E. Z., & Klopp, K. (1982). Parent-child interactions in normal and language-disordered children. Journal of Speech and Hearing Disorders 47, 7-18.

Lasky, R. E., Klein, R. E., Yarbrough, C., Engle, P. L., Lechtig, A., & Martorell, R. (1981). The relationship between physical growth and infant behavioral development in rural Guatemala. Child Development 52, 219-226.

Lasky, R. E., Klein, R. E., Yarbrough, C., & Kallio, K. D. (1981). The predictive validity of infant assessments in rural Guatemala. Child Development 52, 847-856.

Lasky, R. E., Tyson, J. E., Rosenfeld, C. R., & Gant, N. F. (1984). Maternal-infant interactions at one-year adjusted age in infants at low- and high-risk as newborns. Early Human Development 9, 145-152.

Leonard, M. F., Sparrow, S., & Schowalter, J. E. (1982). A prospective study of development of children with sex chromosome anomalies. New Haven study III. The middle years. Birth Defects 18, 193-218.

Levinson, N. A., & Call, J. D. (1987). New developments in early language acquisition. [Introduction by J. D. Call]. In J. D. Noshpitz (Ed.), Basic handbook of child psychiatry (Vol. 5, pp. 51-61). New York: Basic Books.

Lewis, M., & Brooks-Gunn, J. (1984). Age and handicapped group differences in infants' visual attention. Child Development 55, 858-868.

Lewis, M., Feiring, C., McGuffog, C., & Jaskir, J. (1984). Predicting psychopathology in six-year-olds from early social relations. Child Development 55, 123-136.

Lindsay, J., Ounsted, C., & Richards, P. (1979). Long-term outcome in children with temporal lobe seizures. II: Marriage, parenthood and sexual indifference. Developmental Medicine and Child Neurology 21, 433-440.

Lipsitt, L. P. (1979). Critical conditions in infancy: A psychological perspective. American Psychologist 34, 973-980.

Loeffel, M. (1985). Developmental considerations of infants and children with congenital heart disease. Heart and Lung 14, 214-217.

Long, N. V., & Dalston, R. M. (1983). Comprehension abilities of one-year-old infants with cleft lip and palate. Cleft Plate Journal 20, 303-306.

Loria, C. (1980). Relationship of proximal and distal function in motor development. Physical Therapy 60, 167-172.

Lounsbury, M. L., & Bates, J. E. (1982). The cries of infants of differing levels of perceived temperamental difficultness: Acoustic properties and effects on listeners. Child Development 53, 677-686.

Luger, G. F., Wishart, J. G., & Bower, T. G. (1984). Modelling the stages of the identity theory of object-concept development in infancy. Perception 13, 97-115.

Mahalski, P. A. (1983). The incidence of attachment objects and oral habits at bedtime in two longitudinal samples of children aged 1.5-7 years. Journal of Child Psychology and Psychiatry and Allied Disciplines 24, 283-295.

Mahalski, P. A., Silva, P. A., & Spears, G. F. (1985). Children's attachment to soft objects at bedtime, child rearing, and child development. Journal of the American Academy of Child Psychiatry 24, 442-446.

Malerstein, A. J., & Ahern, M. M. (1979). Piaget's stages of cognitive development and adult character structure. American Journal of Psychotherapy 33, 107-118.

Marcus, J., Auerbach, J., Wilkinson, L., & Burack, C. M. (1981). Infants at risk for schizophrenia. The Jerusalem Infant Development Study. Archives of General Psychiatry 38, 703-713.

Marcus, J., & Hans, S. L. (1982). A methodological model to study the effects of toxins on child development. Neurobehavioral Toxicology and Teratology 4, 483-487.

Masur, E. F. (1982). Mothers' response to infants' object-related gestures: influences on lexical development. Journal of Child Language 9, 23-30.

McCormick, M. C., Shapiro, S., & Starfield, B. (1982). Factors associated with maternal opinion of infant development--clues to the vulnerable child? Pediatrics 69, 537-543.

McDevitt, J. B. (1987). Separation-individuation and the beginning emergence of the sense of self. [Introduction by J. D. Call]. In J. D. Noshpitz (Ed.), Basic handbook of child psychiatry (Vol. 5, pp. 38-51). New York: Basic Books.

McDevitt, S. C., & Carey, W. B. (1981). Stability of rating vs. perceptions of temperament from early infancy to 1-3 years. American Journal of Orthopsychiatry 51, 342-345.

McGee, R., Silva, P. A., & Williams, S. (1984). Perinatal, neurological, environmental and developmental characteristics of seven-year-old children with stable behaviour problems. Journal of Child Psychology and Psychiatry and Allied Disciplines 25, 573-586.

McGraw, M. E., & Haka-Ikse, K. (1985). Neurologic-developmental sequelae of chronic renal failure in infancy. Journal of Pediatrics 106, 579-583.

McLaughlin, B., White, D., McDevitt, T., & Raskin, R. (1983). Mothers' and fathers' speech to their young children: Similar or different? Journal of Child Language 10, 245-252.

Mehta, M. N., Munshi, N. N., & Krishnan, P. (1983). Adoptions: Follow-up from an orphanage in Bombay. Child Abuse and Neglect 7, 79-82.

Meier-Seethaler, C. (1982). The child: Erich Neumann's contribution to the psychopathology of child development. Journal of Analytic Psychology 27, 357-379.

Melnick, C. R., Michals, K. K., & Matalon, R. (1981). Linguistic development of children with phenylketonuria and normal intelligence. Journal of Pediatrics 98, 272-369.

Mercer, R. T., Hackley, K. C., & Bostrom, A. (1984). Adolescent motherhood. Comparison of outcome with older mothers. Journal of Adolescent Health Care 5, 7-13.

Messmer, B. J., Schallberger, U., Gattiker, R., & Senning, A. (1976). Psychomotor and intellectual development after deep hypothermia and circulatory arrest in early infancy. Journal of Thoracic and Cardiovascular Surgery 72, 495-502.

Miller, J. A., Jacobsen, R. B., & Bigner, J. J. (1981). The child's home environment for lesbian vs. heterosexual mothers: A neglected area of research. Journal of Homosexuality 7, 49-56.

Miller, J. F., Chapman, R. S., Branston, M. B., & Reichle, J. (1980). Language comprehension in sensorimotor stages V and VI. Journal of Speech and Hearing Research 23, 284-311.

Modarressi, T., & Kenny, T. (1977). Children's response to their true and distorted mirror images. Child Psychiatry and Human Development 8, 94-101.

Moller, M. A. (1983). The visually handicapped. Pediatric Clinics of North America 30, 1185-1193.

Mordock, J. B. (1979). The separation-individuation process and developmental disabilities. Exceptional Children 46, 176-184.

Morgan, S. B. (1979). Development and distribution of intellectual and adaptive skills in Down syndrome children: Implications for early intervention. Mental Retardation 17, 247-249.

Mutch, L. M., Moar, V. A., Ounsted, M. K., & Redman, C. W. (1977). Hypertension during pregnancy, with and without specific hypotensive treatment. II. The growth and development of the infant in the first year of life. Early Human Development 1, 49-67.

Nation, J. E., & Wetherbee, M. A. (1985). Cognitive-communicative development of identical triplets, one with unilateral cleft lip and palate. Cleft Palate Journal 22, 38-50.

Neilson, I. (1982). An alternative explanation of the infant's difficulty in the stage III, IV, and V object-concept tasks. Perception 11, 577-588.

Ninio, A. (1979). The naive theory of the infant and other maternal attitudes in two subgroups in Israel. Child Development 50, 976-980.

Noble-Jamieson, C. M., Lukeman, D., Silverman, M., & Davies, P. A. (1982). Low birth weight children at school age: Neurological, psychological, and pulmonary function. Seminars in Perinatology 6, 266-273.

Noller, K., & Ingrisano, D. (1984). Cross-sectional study of gross and fine motor development. Birth to six years of age. Physical Therapy 64, 308-316.

Nwuga, V. C. (1977). Effect of severe kwashiorkor in intellectual development among Nigerian children. American Journal of Clinical Nutrition 30, 1423-1430.

Oller, D. K., Eilers, R. E., Bull, D. H., & Carney, A. E. (1985). Prespeech vocalizations of a deaf infant: A comparison with normal metaphonological development. Journal of Speech and Hearing Research 28, 47-63.

Olsen-Fulero, L. (1983). Informational functions of mother-child discourse: Knowing them when we see them. Journal of Child Language 10, 223-229.

Oski, F. A., & Honig, A. S. (1978). The effects of therapy on the developmental scores of iron-deficient infants. Journal of Pediatrics 92, 21-25.

Ounsted, M., Moar, V. A., & Scott, A. (1984). Associations between size and development at four years among children who were small-for-dates and large-for-dates at birth. Early Human Development 9, 259-268.

Owens, M. E. (1986). Assessment of infant pain in clinical settings. Journal of Pain and Symptom Management 1, 29-31.

Paine, P. A., & Pasquali, L. (1983). Is motor development really more advanced in third world infants? Perceptual and Motor Skills 57, 729-730.

Palti, H., Pevsner, B., & Adler, B. (1983). Does anemia in infancy affect achievement on developmental and intelligence tests? Human Biology 55, 183-194.

Parmelee, A. H. (1986). Children's illnesses: Their beneficial effects on behavioral development. Child Development 57, 1-10.

Parmelee, A. H., Howard, J., & Beckwith, L. (1984). Infant mental health and biological risk. Child Abuse and Neglect 8, 219-226.

Pedersen, F. A., Rubenstein, J. L., & Yarrow, L. J. (1979). Infant development in father-absent families. Journal of Genetic Psychology 135, 51-61.

Penman, R., Cross, T., Milgrom-Friedman, J., & Meares, R. (1983). Mothers' speech to prelingual infants: A pragmatic analysis. Journal of Child Language 10, 17-34.

Perrin, E. C., & Gerrity, P. S. (1984). Development of children with a chronic illness. Pediatric Clinics of North America 31, 19-31.

Persson-Blennow, I., & McNeil, T. F. (1979). A questionnaire for measurement of temperament in six-month-old infants: Development and standardization. Journal of Child Psychology and Psychiatry and Allied Disciplines 20, 1-13.

Peters, T. J., Golding, J., Lawrence, C. J., Fryer, J. G., Chamberlain, G. V., & Butler, N. R. (1984). Delayed onset of regular respiration and subsequent development. Early Human Development 9, 225-239.

Pettit, G. S., & Bates, J. E. (1984). Continuity of individual differences in the mother-infant relationship from six to thirteen months. Child Development 55, 729-739.

Philipp, C. (1983). Parental perceptions of children who were hospitalized in neonatal intensive care units. Child Psychiatry and Human Development 14, 76-86.

Pine, F. (1979). On the expansion of the affect array. A developmental description. Bulletin of the Menninger Clinic 43, 79-95.

Priel, B., & de Schonen, S. (1986). Self-recognition: A study of a population without mirrors. Journal of Experimental Child Psychology 41, 237-250.

Development

Prizant, B. M., Audet, L.R., Burke, G.M., Hummel, L.S., Maher, S.R., & Theadore, G. (1990). Communication disorders and emotional/behavioral disorders in children. Journal of Speech and Hearing Disorders 55, 179-192.

Ramey, C. T., Yeates, K. O., & Short, E. J. (1984). The plasticity of intellectual development: Insights form preventive intervention. Child Development 55, 1913-1925.

Rice, T., Plomin, R., & De Fries, J. C. (1984). Development of hand preference in the Colorado Adoption Project. Perceptual and Motor Skills 58, 683-689.

Rieser, J. J., & Heiman, M. L. (1982). Spatial self-reference systems and shortest-route behavior in toddlers. Child Development 53, 524-533.

Robertson, S. S., & Suci, G. J. (1980). Event perception by children in the early stages of language production. Child Development 51, 89-96.

Robson, P. (1984). Prewalking locomotor movements and their use in predicting standing and walking. Child Care and Health Development 10, 317-330.

Rogers, G. L., Chazan, S., Fellows, R., & Tsou, B. H. (1982). Strabismus surgery and its effect upon infant development in congenital esotropia. Ophthalmology 89, 479-483.

Rogers, J. G., Perry, M. A., & Rosenberg, L. A. (1979). IQ measurement in children with skeletal dysplasia. Pediatrics 63, 894-897.

Rogow, S. M. (1980). Language development in blind multihandicapped children: A model of co-active intervention. Child Care and Health Development 6, 301-308.

Ross, G. (1985). Use of the Bayley scales to characterize abilities of premature infants. Child Development 56, 835-842.

Ross, G., Nelson, K., Wetstone, H., & Tanouye, E. (1986). Acquisition and generalization of novel object concepts by young language learners. Journal of Child Language 13, 67-83.

Ross, G. S. (1982). Language functioning and speech development of six children receiving tracheotomy in infancy. Journal of Communication Disorders 15, 95-111.

Rubenstein, J. L., Howes, C., & Boyle, P. (1981). A two-year follow-up of infants in community-based day care. Journal of Child Psychology and Psychiatry and Allied Disciplines 22, 209-218.

Rutter, M. (1979). Maternal deprivation, 1972-1978: New findings, new concepts, new approaches. Child Development 50, 283-305.

Rutter, M. (1980). The long-term effects of early experience. Developmental Medicine and Child Neurology 22, 800-815.

Rutter, M. (1981). Social-emotional consequence of day care for preschool children. American Journal of Orthopsychiatry 51, 4-28.

Rutter, M. L. (1986). Child psychiatry: The interface between clinical and developmental research. Psychological Medicine 16, 151-169.

Ryan, N. M. (1983). Body rocking, head banging, and head rolling: An Analysis of rhythmic motor activities in normal infants. Pediatric Nursing 9, 281-285, 296.

Sankey, C. G., Elmer, E., Halechko, A. D., & Schulberg, P. (1985). The development of abused and high-risk infants in different treatment modalities: Residential versus in-home care. Child Abuse and Neglect 9, 237-243.

Schaffer, H. R., Hepburn, A., & Collis, G. M. (1983). Verbal and nonverbal aspects of mothers' directives. Journal of Child Language 10, 337-355.

Schiff-Myers, N. B. (1982). Sign and oral language development of preschool hearing children of deaf parents in comparison with their mothers' communication system. American Annals of the Deaf 127, 322-330.

Schiff-Myers, N. B. (1983). From pronoun reversals to correct pronoun usage: A case study of a normally developing child. Journal of Speech and Hearing Disorders 48, 394-402.

Schneider-Rosen, K., & Cicchetti, D. (1984). The relationship between affect and cognition in maltreated infants: Quality of attachment and the development of visual self-recognition. Child Development 55, 648-658.

Schneiderman, M. H. (1983). 'Do what I mean, not what I say!' Changes in mothers' action-directives to young children. Journal of Child Language 10, 357-367.

Schnur, E., & Shatz, M. (1984). The role of maternal gesturing in conversations with one-year-olds. Journal of Child Language 11, 29-41.

10. Parental Influence on Infant Development

Ainsworth, M. D. (1985). Patterns of infant-mother attachments: Antecedents and effects on development. Bulletin of the New York Academy of Medicine 61, 771-791.

Bauman, P. S., & Dougherty, F. E. (1983). Drug-addicted mothers' parenting and their children's development. International Journal of the Addictions 18, 291-302.

Baumrind, D. (1975). The contributions of the family to the development of competence in children. Schizophrenia Bulletin 14, 12-37.

Bee, H. L., Hammond, M. A., Eyres, S. J., Barnard, K. E., & Snyder, C. (1986). The impact of parental life change on the early development of children. Research in Nursing and Health 9, 65-74.

Belsky, J. (1984). The determinants of parenting: A process model. Child Development 55, 83-96.

Belsky, J., Gilstrap, B., & Rovine, M. (1984). The Pennsylvania infant and family development project. I: Stability and change in mother-infant and father-infant interaction in a family setting at one, three, and nine months. Child Development 55, 692-705.

Berman, P. W., Smith, V. L., & Goodman, V. (1983). Development of sex differences in response to an infant and to the caretaker role. Journal of Genetic Psychology 143, 283-284.

Bernstein, V., Jeremy, R. J., Hans, S. L., & Marcus, J. (1984). A longitudinal study of offspring born to methadone-maintained women. II. Dyadic interaction and infant behavior at 4 months. American Journal of Drug and Alcohol Abuse 10, 161-193.

Boukydis, C. F., & Burgess, R. L. (1982). Adult physiological response to infant cries: Effects of temperament of infant, parental status, and gender. Child Development 53, 1291-1298.

Brewster, L. C. (1985). Interaction analysis of mother and hearing-impaired child. Ear and Hearing 6, 54-56.

Bruner, J. (1984). Interaction, communication, and self. Journal of the American Academy of Child Psychiatry 23, 1-7.

Buckhalt, J. A., Rutherford, R. B., & Goldberg, K. E. (1978). Verbal and nonverbal interaction of mothers with their Down's syndrome and nonretarded infants. American Journal of Mental Deficiency 82, 337-343.

Camp, B. W., Burgess, D., Morgan, L., & Malpiede, D. (1984). Infants of adolescent mothers. Maternal characteristics and developmental status at one year of age. American Journal of Diseases of Children 138, 243-246.

Cantwell, D. P., & Baker, L. (1978). The language environment of autistic and dysphasic children Journal of the American Academy of Child Psychiatry 17, 604-613.

Cassidy, J., & Main, M. (1985). The relationship between infant-parent attachment and the ability to tolerate brief separation at six years. In J. D. Call, E. Galenson, & R. L. Tyson (Eds.), Frontiers of infant psychiatry. New York: Basic Books.

Cravioto, J., & Arrieta, R. (1979). Stimulation and mental development of malnourished infants [Letter]. Lancet 2, 899.

Crnic, K. A., Greenberg, M. T., Robinson, N. M., & Ragozin, A. S. (1984). Maternal stress and social support: Effects on the mother-infant relationship from birth to eighteen months. American Journal of Orthopsychiatry 54, 224-235.

Cummings, E. M., Zahn-Waxler, C., & Radke-Yarrow, M. (1984). Developmental changes in children's reactions to anger in the home. Journal of Child Psychology and Psychiatry and Allied Disciplines 25, 63-74.

Donovan, W. L. (1981). Maternal learned helplessness and physiologic response to infant crying. Journal of Personality and Social Psychology 40, 919-926.

Easterbrooks, M. A., & Goldberg, W. A. (1984). Toddler development in the family: Impact of father involvement and parenting characteristics. Child Development 55, 740-752.

Egeland, B., Sroufe, L. A., & Erickson, M. (1983). The developmental consequence of different patterns of maltreatment. Child Abuse and Neglect 7, 459-469.

Eiduson, B. T. (1983). Conflict and stress in nontraditional families: Impact on children. American Journal of Orthopsychiatry 53, 426-435.

Elder, G. H., Jr., Nguyen, T. V., & Caspi, A. (1985). Linking family hardship to children's lives. Child Development 56, 361-375.

Ervin, C. S., Little, R. E., Streissguth, A. P., & Beck, D, E. (1984). Alcoholic fathering and its relation to child's intellectual development: A pilot investigation. Alcoholism 8, 362-365.

Field, T., Gewirtz, J. L., Cohen, D., Garcia, R., Greenberg, R., & Collins, K. (1984). Leave-takings and reunions of infants, toddlers, preschoolers, and their parents. Child Development 55, 628-635.

Field, T., Widmayer, S., Greenberg, R., & Stoller, S. (1982). Effects of parent training on teenage mothers and their infants. Pediatrics 69, 703-707.

Friedman, A. S., & Friedman, D. B. (1977). Parenting: A developmental process. Pediatric Annals 6, 564-572.

Friedman, R. (1975). The vicissitudes of adolescent development and what it activates in adults. Adolescence 10, 520-526.

Gaiter, J. L., & Johnson, A. A. S. (1985). Contact with intensive-care infants: Father's sex type, infant preference, and frequency of visits. In J. D. Call, E. Galenson, & R. L. Tyson (Eds.), Frontiers of infant psychiatry. New York: Basic Books.

Gamble, T. J., & Zigler, E. (1986). Effects of infant day care: Another look at the evidence. American Journal of Orthopsychiatry 56, 26-42.

Garbarino, J., Sebes, J., & Schellenbach, C. (1984). Families at risk for destructive parent-child relations in adolescence. Child Development 55, 174-183.

Gauthier, Y., Fortin, C., Drapeau, P., Breton, J. J., Gosselin, J., Quintal, L., Weisnagel, J., & Tetreault, L. (1977). The mother-child relationship and the development of autonomy and self-assertion in young (14-30 months) asthmatic children. Correlating allergic and psychological factors. Journal of the American Academy of Child Psychiatry 16, 109-131.

Goldin-Meadow, S., & Mylander, C. (1984). Gestural communication in deaf children: The effects and noneffects of parental input on early language development. Monographs of the Society for Research in Child Development (Vol. 49, pp. 1-151). Chicago: University of Chicago Press.

Goodnow, J. J. (1988). Parents' ideas, actions, and feelings: Models and methods from developmental and social psychology. Child Development 59, 286-320.

Gordon, A. H., & Jameson, J. C. (1979). Infant-mother attachment in patients with nonorganic failure to thrive syndrome. Journal of the American Academy of Child Psychiatry 18, 251-259.

Greenspan, S. I., & Greenspan, N. T. (1989). The essential partnership: How parents and children can meet the emotional challenges of infancy and childhood. New York: Viking/Penguin Press.

Gross, D. (1984). Relationships at risk: Issues and interventions with a disturbed mother-infant dyad. Perspectives in Psychiatric Care 22, 159-164.

Heinicke, C. M. (1984). The role of pre-birth parent characteristics in early family development. Child Abuse and Neglect 8, 169-181.

Hershorn, M., & Rosenbaum, A. (1985). Children of marital violence: A closer look at the unintended victims. American Journal of Orthopsychiatry 55, 260-266.

Hinde, R. A., & Stevenson-Hinde, J. (Eds.). (1988). Relations between relationships within families. Oxford: Oxford University Press.

Hock, E., Kroll, B. C., Frantz, J., Janson, K. A., & Widaman, K. (1984). Infants in play groups: Time related changes in behavior toward mothers, peers, and toys. Journal of Genetic Psychology 144, 51-67.

Jolly, H. (1985). Helping parents achieve optimal development for their children. Journal of Psychosomatic Research 29, 593-595.

Lamb, M. E. (1978). The development of sibling relationships in infancy: A short-term longitudinal study. Child Development 49, 1189-1192.

Lamb, M. E. (1985). Mothers, fathers, and child care in a changing world. In J. D. Call, E. Galenson, & R. L. Tyson (Eds.), Frontiers of infant psychiatry. New York: Basic Books.

Larsen, J. J., & Juhasz, A. M. (1985). The effects of knowledge of child development and social-emotional maturity on adolescent attitudes toward parenting. Adolescence 20, 823-839.

Laskey, R. E., Tyson, J. E., Rosenfeld, C. R., & Gant, N. F. (1984). Maternal-infant interactions at one-year adjusted age in infants at low- and high-risk as newborns. Early Human Development 9, 145-152.

Lerner, H., & Beagan, J., Sr. (1986). Promoting child development for hard-to-reach high-risk families. Issues in Comprehensive Pediatric Nursing 9, 97-106.

Lindsay, J., Ounsted, C., & Richards, P. (1979). Long-term outcome in children with temporal lobe seizures. II: Marriage, parenthood and sexual indifference. Developmental Medicine and Child Neurology 21, 433-440.

Liptak, G. S., Keller, B. B., Feldman, A. W., & Chamberlin, R. W. (1983). Enhancing infant development and parent-practitioner interaction with the Brazelton neonatal assessment scale. Pediatrics 72, 71-78.

McConkey, R., & O'Connor, M. (1982). A new approach to parental involvement in language intervention programmes. Child Care and Health Development 8, 163-176.

McCormick, M. C., Shapiro, S., & Starfield, B. (1982). Factors associated with maternal opinion of infant development--clues to the vulnerable child? Pediatrics 69, 537-543.

Murray, A. D. (1979). Infant crying as an elicitor of parental behavior: An examination of two models. Psychological Bulletin 86, 191-215.

Namerow, P. B., & Philliber, S. G. (1983). The value of children to children. Adolescence 18, 775-786.

Orvaschel, H., Mednick, S., Schulsinger, F., & Rock, D. (1979). The children of psychiatrically disturbed parents: Differences as a function of the sex of the sick parent. Archives of General Psychiatry 36, 691-695.

Orvaschel, H., Weissman, M. M., & Kidd, K. K. (1980). Children and depression--the children of depressed parents; the childhood of depressed patients; depression in children. Journal of Affective Disorders 2, 1-16.

Ounsted, M. K., & Hendrick, A. M. (1977). The first-born child: Patterns of development. Developmental Medicine and Child Neurology 19, 446-453.

Papousek, H., & Papousek, M. (1985). The evolution of parent-infant attachment: New psychobiological perspectives. In J. D. Call, E. Galenson, & R. L. Tyson (Eds.), Frontiers of infant psychiatry. New York: Basic Books.

Pedersen, F. A., Rubenstein, J. L., & Yarrow, L. J. (1979). Infant development in father-absent families. Journal of Genetic Psychology 135, 51-61.

Pollak, M. (1979). Housing and mothering: Their effects upon the developmental levels of 3-year-old children. Archives of Disease in Childhood 54, 54-58.

Popplewell, J. F., & Sheikh, A. A. (1979). The role of the father in child development: A review of the literature. International Journal of Social Psychiatry 25, 267-284.

Provence, S., & Solnit, A. J. (1983). Development-promoting aspects of the sibling experience. Vicarious mastery. In A. Solnit, et al. (Eds.), Psychoanalytic study of the child (Vol. 38, pp. 337-351). New Haven: Yale University Press.

Pruett, K. D. (1985). Children of the fathermothers: Infants of Primary nurturing fathers. In J. D. Call, E. Galenson, & R. L. Tyson (Eds.), Frontiers of infant psychiatry. New York: Basic Books.

Rosenfeld, A., Siegel-Gorelick, B., Haavik, D., Duryea, M., Wenegrat, A., Martin, J., & Bailey, R. (1984). Parental perceptions of children's modesty: A cross-sectional survey of ages tow to 10 year. Psychiatry 47, 351-365.

Sadler, L. S., & Catrone, C. (1983). The adolescent parent: A dual developmental crisis. Journal of Adolescent Health Care 4, 100-105.

Sameroff, A. J., & Emde, R. N. (Eds.). (1989). Relationship disturbances in early childhood: A developmental approach. New York: Basic Books.

Scharff, J. S. (1985). Understanding and satisfying the psychological needs of infants and toddlers. Journal of the American Medical Women's Association 40, 77-79.

Scherer, N. J., & Olswang, L. B. (1984). Role of mothers' expansions in stimulating children's language production. Journal of Speech and Hearing Research 27, 387-396.

Schneider-Rosen, K. & Cicchetti, D. (1984). The relationship between affect and cognition in maltreated infants: Quality of attachment and the development of visual self-recognition. Child Development 55, 648-658.

Schneiderman, M. H. (1983). 'Do what I mean, not what I say!' Changes in mothers' action-directives to young children. Journal of Child Language 10, 357-367.

Schnur, E., & Shatz, M. (1984). The role of maternal gesturing in conversations with one-year-olds. Journal of Child Language 11, 29-41.

Schwartz, P. (1983). Length of day-care attendance and attachment behavior in eighteen-month-old infants. Child Development 54, 1073-1078.

Sharav, T., Collins, R., & Shlomo, L. (1985). Effect of maternal education on prognosis of development in children with Down Syndrome. Pediatrics 76, 387-391.

Simkins, L. (1984). Consequences of teenage pregnancy and motherhood. Adolescence 19, 39-54.

Sroufe, L. A., & Fleeson, J. (1988). Relationships within families: Mutual influences. In R. A. Hinde & J. Stevenson-Hinde (Eds.), The coherence of family relationships (pp. 27-47). Oxford: Oxford University Press.

Steinglass, P., Bennett, L., Wolin, S., & Reiss, D. (1987). The alcoholic family. New York: Basic Books.

Stern, D. N., Jaffe, J., Beebe, B., & Bennett, S. L. (1975). Vocalizing in unison and in alternation: Two modes of communication within the mother-infant dyad. Annals of the New York Academy of Sciences 263, 89-100.

Stern, D. N., Spieker, S., Barnett, R. K., & MacKain, K. (1983). The prosody of maternal speech: Infant age and context related changes. Journal of Child Language 10, 1-15.

Wadsworth, J., Burnell, I., Taylor, B., & Butler, N. (1985). The influence of family type on children's behaviour and development at five years. Journal of Child Psychology and Psychiatry and Allied Disciplines 26, 245-254.

Wellen, C. J. (1985). Effects of older siblings on the language young children hear and produce. Journal of Speech and Hearing Disorders 50, 84-99.

Wheeler, M. P. (1983). Context-related age changes in mothers' speech: Joint book reading. Journal of Child Language 10, 259-263.

Yogman, M. W. (1985). The father's role with preterm and fullterm infants. In J. D. Call, E. Galenson, & R. L. Tyson (Eds.), Frontiers of infant psychiatry. New York: Basic Books.

Zahn-Waxler, C., Chapman, M., & Cummings, E. M. (1984). Cognitive and social development in infants and toddlers with a bipolar parent. Child Psychiatry and Human Development 15, 75-85.

11. Factors in Development and Developmental Disorders

Abel, E. L. (1980). Prenatal exposure to cannabis: A critical review of effects on growth, development, and behavior. Behavioral and Neural Biology 29, 137-156.

Anderson, R. C., & Anderson, K. E. (1984). Day care--social, emotional and intellectual effect. Occupational Health Nursing 32, 301-306.

Apolloni, T., & Cooke, T. P. (1975). Peer behavior conceptualized as a variable influencing infant and toddler development. American Journal of Orthopsychiatry 45, 4-17.

Baltes, P. B. (1984). Some constructive caveats on action psychology and the study of intention. Human Development 27, 135-138.

Beardslee, W. R., Wolff, P. H., Hurwitz, I., Parikh, B., & Schwachman, H. (1982). The effects of infantile malnutrition on behavioral development: A follow-up study. American Journal of Clinical Nutrition 35, 1437-1441.

Beratis, S., Rubin, M., Miller, R. T., Galenson, E., & Rothstein, A. (1979). Developmental aspects of an infant with transient moderate to severe hearing impairment. Pediatrics 63, 153-155.

Bock, J. K., & Hornsby, M. E. (1981). The development of directives: How children ask and tell. Journal of Child Language 8, 151-163.

Boesch, E. E. (1984). The development of affective schemata. Human Development 27, 173-183.

Brandtstadter, J. (1984). Action development and development through action. Human Development 27, 115-118.

Carey, W. B. (1982). Validity of parental assessments of development and behavior. American Journal of Diseases of Children 136, 97-99.

Chandler, L., & Roe, M. D. (1977). Behavioral and neurological comparisons of neonates born to mothers of differing social environments. Child Psychiatry and Human Development 8, 25-30.

Chapman, M. (1984). Action, intention, and intersubjectivity. Human Development 27, 139-144.

Chasnoff, I. J. (1985). Effects of maternal narcotic vs. non-narcotic addiction on neonatal neurobehavior and infant development. National Institute on Drug Abuse Research Monograph Series 59, 84-95.

Chisholm, J. S., Woodson, R. H., & da Costa Woodson, E. M. (1978). Maternal blood pressure in pregnancy and newborn irritability. Early Human Development 2, 171-178.

Dunn, J., & Munn, P. (1986). Siblings and the development of prosocial behavior. International Journal of Behavioral Development 9, 265-284.

Eckensberger, L. H., & Meacham, J. A. (1984a). Action theory, control and motivation: A symposium. Human Development 27, 163-165.

Eckensberger, L. H., & Meacham, J. A. (1984b). The essentials of action theory: A framework for discussion. Human Development 27, 166-172.

Ellwood, L. C. (1980). Effects of alcoholism as a family illness on child behavior and development. Military Medicine 145, 188-192.

Frese, M., & Stewart, J. (1984). Skill learning as a concept in life-span developmental psychology: An action theoretic analysis. Human Development 27, 145-162.

Harris, A. E. (1984). Action theory, language, and the unconscious. Human Development 27, 196-210.

Hunt, J. V., & Eichorn, D. H. (1972). Maternal and child behaviors: A review of data from the Berkeley growth study. Seminars in Psychiatry 4, 367-381.

Jacobvitz, D., & Sroufe, L. A. (1987). The early caregiver-child relationship and attention deficit disorder with hyperactivity in kindergarten: A prospective study. Child Development 58, 1488-1495.

Joos, S. K., Pollitt, E., Mueller, W. H., & Albright, D. L. (1983). The Bacon Chow study: Maternal nutritional supplementation and infant behavioral development. Child Development 54, 669-676.

Kagan, J. (1982). Canalization of early psychological development. Pediatrics 70, 182.

Klein, R. P., & Durfee, J. T. (1979). Prediction of preschool social behavior form social-emotional development at one year. Child Psychiatry and Human Development 9, 145-151.

Lasky, R. E., Klein, R. E., Yarbrough, C., Engle, P. L., Lechtig, A., & Martorell, R. (1981). The relationship between physical growth and infant behavioral development in rural Guatemala. Child Development 52, 219-226.

Liebert, R. M. (1986). Effects of television on children and adolescents. Journal of Developmental and Behavioral Pediatrics 7, 43-48.

Mischel, H. N. (1984). From intention to action: The role of rule knowledge in the development of self-regulation. Human Development 27, 124-129.

Mitchell, W. G., Gorrell, R. W., & Greenberg, R. A. (1980). Failure-to-thrive: A study in a primary care setting. Epidemiology and follow-up. Pediatrics 65, 971-977.

Paludetto, R., Rinaldi, P., Mansi, G., Andolfi, M., & Del Giudice, G. (1984). Early behavioural development of preterm infants. Developmental Medicine and Child Neurology 26, 347-352.

Parmelee, A. H., Jr. (1986). Children's illnesses: Their beneficial effects on behavioral development. Child Development 57, 1-10.

Ratcliffe, J. M. (1977). Developmental and behavioural functions in young children with elevated blood lead levels. British Journal of Preventive and Social Medicine 31, 258-264.

Rutter, M. (1980). School influences on children's behavior and development: The 1979 Kenneth Blackfan lecture, Children's Hospital Medical Center, Boston. Pediatrics 65, 208-220.

Skinner, E. A., & Chapman, M. (1984). Control beliefs in an action perspective. Human Development 27, 129-133.

Stott, D. H., & Latchford, S. A. (1976). Prenatal antecedents of child health, development, and behavior. An epidemiological report of incidence and association. Journal of the American Academy of Child Psychiatry 15, 161-191.

Vanderpool, N. A., & Parcel, G. S. (1979). Interacting with children in elementary schools: An effective approach to teaching child development. Journal of Medical Education 54, 418-420.

Wadsworth, J., Burnell, I., Taylor, B., & Butler, N. (1985). The influence of family type on children's behaviour and development at five years. Journal of Child Psychology and Psychiatry and Allied Disciplines 26, 245-254.

12. Biological Aspects of Infant Development

Anders, T. F., & Zeanah, C. H. (1985). Early infant development from a biological point of view. In J. D. Call, E. Galenson, & R. L. Tyson (Eds.), Frontiers of infant psychiatry. New York: Basic Books.

Coyle, J. T., & Harris, J. C. (1987). The development of neurotransmitters and neuropeptides. [Introduction by J. D. Call]. In J. D. Noshpitz (Ed.), Basic handbook of child psychiatry (Vol. 5, pp. 14-25). New York: Basic Books.

Diamond, M. C. (1987). Environmental influences on the young brain. [Introduction by J. D. Call]. In J. D. Noshpitz (Ed.), Basic handbook of child psychiatry (Vol. 5, pp. 6-13). New York: Basic Books.

Hamilton, J. A., & Conrad, C. D. (1986). Toward a developmental psychopharmacology: The physiological basis of age, gender, and hormonal effects on drug responsivity. In J. Noshpitz (Ed.), Basic handbook of child psychiatry (Vol. 5, pp. 66-81). New York: Basic Books.

Hinde, R. A. (1985). Biological bases of the mother-child relationship. In J. D. Call, E. Galenson, & R. L. Tyson (Eds.), Frontiers of infant psychiatry. New York: Basic Books.

Mosier, H. D., Jr. (1987). Endocrine factors in fetal development. [Introduction by J. D. Call]. In J. D. Noshpitz (Ed.), Basic handbook of child psychiatry (Vol. 5, pp. 26-36). New York: Basic Books.

Rangell, L. (1985). Structure, somatic and psychic: The biopsychological base of infancy. In J. D. Call, E. Galenson, & R. L. Tyson (Eds.), Frontiers of infant psychiatry. New York: Basic Books.

13. Physical Development of Infants and Children

Arshavskii, I. A. (1979). Physiological analysis of physical development with special reference to the new born infant. Human Physiology 5, 169-180.

Bailey, S. M., Gershoff, S. N., McGandy, R. B., Nondasuta, A., Tantiwongse, P., Suttapreyasri, D., Miller, J., & McCree, P. (1984). A longitudinal study of growth and maturation in rural Thailand. Human Biology 56, 530-557.

Bauman, P. S., & Dougherty, F. E. (1983). Drug-addicted mothers' parenting and their children's development. International Journal of the Addictions 18, 291-302.

Berkey, C. S., & Kent, R. L., Jr. (1983). Longitudinal principal components and non-linear regression models of early childhood growth. Annals of Human Biology 10, 523-536.

Branta, C., Haubenstricker, J., & Seefeldt, V. (1984). Age changes in motor skills during childhood and adolescence. Exercise and Sport Sciences Reviews 12, 467-520.

Bruch, H. (1981). Developmental considerations of anorexia nervosa and obesity. Canadian Journal of Psychiatry 26, 212-217.

Carey, W. B. (1985). Temperament and increased weight gain in infants. Journal of Developmental and Behavioral Pediatrics 6, 128-131.

Chang, P. N., Weisberg, S., & Fisch, R. O. (1984). Growth development and its relationship to intellectual functioning of children with phenylketonuria. Journal of Developmental and Behavioral Pediatrics 5, 127-131.

Drabman, R. S., Cordua, G. D., Hammer, D., Jarvie, G. J., & Horton, W. (1979). Developmental trends in eating rates of normal and overweight preschool children. Child Development 50, 211-216.

Elwood, P. C., Haley, T. J., Hughes, S. J., Sweetnam, P. M., Gray, O. P., & Davies, D. P. (1981). Child growth (0-5 years), and the effect of entitlement to a mild supplement. Archives of Disease in Childhood 56, 831-835.

Emde, R. N., & Walker, S. (1976). Longitudinal study of infant sleep: Results of 14 subjects studied at monthly intervals. Psychophysiology 13, 456-461.

Galler, J. R., Ramsey, F., & Solimano, G. (1985a). A follow-up study of the effects of early malnutrition on subsequent development. I. Physical growth and sexual maturation during adolescence. Pediatric Research 19, 518-523.

Galler, J. R., Ramsey, F., & Solimano, G. (1985b). A follow-up study of the effects of early malnutrition on subsequent development. II. Fine motor skills in adolescence. Pediatric Research 19, 524-527.

Gillberg, C., Rasmussen, P., & Wahlstrom, J. (1982). Long-term follow-up of children born after amniocentesis. Clinical Genetics 21, 69-73.

Grantham-McGregor, S. M., Powell, C., Stewart, M., & Schofield, W. N. (1982). Longitudinal study of growth and development of young Jamaican children recovering from severe protein-energy malnutrition. Developmental Medicine and Child Neurology 24, 321-331.

Hass, J. D., Moreno-Black, G., Frongillo, E. A., Jr., Pabon, J., Pareja, G., Ybarnegarary, J., & Hurtado, L. (1982). Altitude and infant growth in Bolivia: A longitudinal study. American Journal of Physical Anthropology 59, 251-262.

Development

Heiman, M. F. (1978). The management of obesity in the post-adolescent developmentally disabled client with Prader-Willi syndrome. Adolescence 13, 291-296.

Jansen, A. A., Thiuri, B., & 't Mannetje, W. (1985). The predictive and retrospective values of weight and height measurements of below fives. Journal of Tropical Pediatrics 31, 320-322.

Jordan, R. P. (1981). The neuromotor development of bipedal locomotion in the normal infant. Journal of the American Podiatry Association 71, 84-91.

Kramer, M. S., Rooks, Y., Washington, L. A., & Pearson, H. A. (1980). Pre- and postnatal growth and development in sickle cell anemia. Journal of Pediatrics 96, 857-860.

Lebenthal, E., & Lee, P. C. (1985). Gastrointestinal physiologic considerations in the feeding of the developing infant. Current Concepts in Nutrition 14, 125-145.

Lyon, A. J., Preece, M. A., & Grant, D. B. (1985). Growth curve for girls with Turner syndrome. Archives of Disease in Childhood 60, 932-935.

McCullough, J. M., & McCullough, C. S. (1984). Age-specific variation in the secular trend for stature: A comparison of samples from industrialized and nonindustrialized regions. American Journal of Physical Anthropology 65, 169-180.

Meisels, S. J., Plunkett, J. W., Roloff, D. W., Pasick, P. L., & Stiefel, G. S. (1986). Growth and development of preterm infants with respiratory distress syndrome and bronchopulmonary dysplasia. Pediatrics 77, 345-352.

Meredith, H. V. (1984). Body size of infants and children around the world in relation to socioeconomic status. Advances in Child Development and Behavior 18, 81-145.

Oates, R. K., Peacock, A., & Forrest, D. (1984). Development in children following abuse and nonorganic failure to thrive. American Journal of Diseases of Children 138, 764-767.

Ounsted, M., Moar, V., & Scott, A. (1982). Growth in the first four years: III. The Effects of maternal factors associated with small-for-dates and large-for-dates pregnancies. Early Human Development 7, 347-356.

Partington, M. W. (1984). The fragile X syndrome II: Preliminary data on growth and development in males. American Journal of Medical Genetics 17, 175-194.

Rantakallio, P., von Wendt, L., & Makinen, H. (1985). Influence of social background on psychomotor development in the first year of life and its correlation with later intellectual capacity: A prospective cohort study. Early Human Development 11, 141-148.

Satterfield, J. H., Cantwell, D. P., Schell, A., & Balschke, T. (1979). Growth of hyperactive children treated with methylphenidate. Archives of General Psychiatry 36, 212-217.

Sauve, R. S., & Singhal, N. (1985). Long-term morbidity of infants with bronchopulmonary dysplasia. Pediatrics 76, 725-733.

Teberg, A. J., Wu, P. Y., Hodgman, J. E., Mich, C., Garfinkle, J., Azen, S., & Wingert, W. A. (1982). Infants with birth weight under 1500 g: Physical, neurological, and developmental outcome. Critical Care in Medicine 10, 10-14.

Weeks, Z. R. (1979). Effects of the vestibular system on human development, Part I. Overview of functions and effects of stimulation. American Journal of Occupational Therapy 33, 376-381.

Weinstein, A. G. (1984). Crying-induced bronchospasm in childhood asthma. Journal of Asthma 21, 161-165.

Weston, A. J., & Mader, N. T. (1984). Infants' vocalizations as a diagnostic tool. Perceptual and Motor Skills 58, 787-796.

14. Development of Visual and Auditory Perception and Language

Atkinson, J. (1984). Human visual development over the first six months of life. A review and a hypothesis. Human Neurobiology 3, 61-74.

Banks, M. S., & Ginsburg, A. P. (1985). Infant visual preferences: A review and new theoretical treatment. Advances in Child Development and Behavior 19, 207-246.

Barnes, S., Gutfreund, M., Satterly, D., & Wells, G. (1983). Characteristics of adult speech which predict children's language development. Journal of Child Language 10, 65-84.

Bertenthal, B. I., Campos, J. J., & Haith, M. M. (1980). Development of visual organization: The perception of subjective contours. Child Development 51, 1072-1080.

Blom, J. L., Barth, P. G., & Visser, S. L. (1980). The visual evoked potential in the first six years of life. Electroencephalography and Clinical Neurophysiology 48, 395-405.

Brennan, M., & Kirkland, J. (1979). Discrimination of infants' cry-signals. Perceptual and Motor Skills 48, 683-686.

Brooks, J., & Lewis, M. (1976). Infants' responses to strangers: Midget, adult, and child. Child Development 47, 323-332.

Broussard, E. R. (1976). Neonatal prediction and outcome at 10/11 years. Child Psychiatry and Human Development 7, 85-93.

Chance, J. E., Turner, A. L., & Goldstein, A. G. (1982). Development of differential recognition for own- and other-race faces. Journal of Psychology 112, 29-37.

Cousino, M. E., & Rastatter, M. P. (1985). Reaction times of four year old children to monaurally presented verbal stimuli: Some evidence for right-hemisphere linguistic function. Cortex 21, 445-452.

Diamond, R., & Carey, S. (1977). Developmental changes in the representation of faces. Journal of Experimental Child Psychology 23, 1-22.

Dickie, J. R., & Strader, W. H. (1974). Development of mirror image responses in infancy. Journal of Psychology 88, 333-337.

Dixon, J. C., & Street, J. W. (1975). The distinction between self and not-self in children and adolescents. Journal of Genetic Psychology 127, 157-162.

Duncan, E. M., Whitney, P., & Kunen, S. (1982). Integration of visual and verbal information in children's memories. Child Development 53, 1215-1223.

Eimas, P. D. (1981). Infants, speech, and language: A look at some connections. Cognition 10, 79-84.

Etaugh, C., & Turton, W. J. (1977). Sex differences in discrimination of forms by elementary school children. Journal of Genetic Psychology 130, 49-55.

Fagan, J. F. (1978). Facilitation of infants' recognition memory. Child Development 49, 1066-1075.

Fennell, E. B., Satz, P., & Morris, R. (1983). The development of handedness and dichotic ear listening asymmetries in relation to school achievement: A longitudinal study. Journal of Experimental Child Psychology 35, 248-262.

Field, J. (1977). Coordination of vision and prehension in young infants. Child Development 48, 97-103.

Fiorentini, A. (1984). Visual development. Human Neurobiology 3, 59-60.

Fivush, R., & Mandler, J. M. (1985). Developmental changes in the understanding of temporal sequence. Child Development 57, 1437-1446.

Flavell, J. H. (1977). The development of knowledge about visual perception. Nebraska Symposium on Motivation 25, 43-76.

Flin, R. H. (1985). Development of face recognition: An encoding switch? British Journal of Psychology 76, 123-134.

Forrest, E. B. (1981). Visual imagery as an information processing strategy. Journal of Learning Disabilities 14, 584-586.

Franken, R. E., & Diamond, D. C. (1983). Picture recognition memory in children: Effects of homogeneous versus heterogeneous classes of pictures. Perceptual and Motor Skills 57, 749-750.

Freeburg, T. J., & Lippman, M. Z. (1986). Factors affecting discrimination of infant cries. Journal of Child Language 13, 3-13.

Freedman, D. A. (1981a). The effects of sensory and other deficits in children on their experience of people. Journal of the American Psychoanalytic Association 29, 831-867.

Freedman, D. A. (1981b). Speech, language, and the vocal-auditory connection. In A. Solnit, et al. (Eds.), Psychoanalytic study of the child (Vol. 36, pp. 105-127). New Haven: Yale University Press.

Fritz, J. J., & Suci, G. J. (1982). Facilitation of semantic comprehension at the one-word state of language development. Journal of Child Language 9, 31-39.

Gaines, R., & Powell, G. J. (1981). Children's color perception in relation to habitat and skin color. Child Development 52, 914-920.

Geffen, G. (1976). Development of hemispheric specialization for speech perception. Cortex 12, 337-346.

Gellert, E. (1975). Children's constructions of their self-image. Perceptual and Motor Skills 40, 307-324.

Giray, E. F., Altkin, W. M., Vaught, G. M., & Roodin, P. A. (1976). The incidence of eidetic imagery as a function of age. Child Development 47, 1207-1210.

Gladding, S. T. (1979). Effects of training versus non-training in identification of infant cry-signals: A longitudinal study. Perceptual and Motor Skills 48, 752-754.

Gopnik, A. (1984). The acquisition of "gone" and the development of the object concept. Journal of Child Language 11, 273-292.

Grusser, O. J., Selke, T., & Zynda, B. (1985). A developmental study of face recognition in children and adolescents. Human Neurobiology 4, 33-39.

Green, J. A., & Gustafson, G. E. (1983). Individual recognition of human infants on the basis of cries alone. Developmental Psychobiology 16, 485-493.

Gustafson, G. E., Green, J. A., & Tomic, T. (1984). Acoustic correlates of individuality in the cries of human infants. Developmental Psychobiology 17, 311-324.

Guttentag, R. E. (1985). A developmental study of attention to auditory and visual signals. Journal of Experimental Child Psychology 39, 546-561.

Harcherik, D. F., Carbonari, C. M., & Cohen, D. J. (1982). Attentional and perceptual measure: Developmental changes. Schizophrenia Bulletin 8, 349-355.

Highnam, C. L., & Beykirch, H. I. (1978). Effect of mothers' voices on auditory comprehension in children. Perceptual and Motor Skills 47, 435-439.

Huba, M. E., & Vellutino, F. R. (1980). The development of visual encoding and retention skills. Journal of Experimental Child Psychology 30, 88-97.

Jones-Molfese, V. (1975). Preferences of infants for regular and distorted facial stimuli. Child Development 46, 1005-1009.

Joseph, R., & Gallagher, R. E. (1985). Interhemispheric transfer and the completion of reversible operations in non-conserving children. Journal of Clinical Psychology 41, 796-800.

Kramer, M., Chamorro, I., Green, D., & Knudtson, F. (1975). Extra tactile stimulation of the premature infant. Nursing Research 24, 324-334.

Krumhansl, C. L., & Keil, F. C. (1982). Acquisition of the hierarchy of tonal functions in music. Memory and Cognition 10, 243-251.

Levin, I., Wilkening, F., & Dembo, Y. (1984). Development of time quantification: Integration and nonintegration of beginnings and endings in comparing durations. Child Development 55, 2160-2172.

Lewandowski, L. (1982). Hemispheric asymmetries in children. Perceptual and Motor Skills 54, 1011-1019.

Lindgren, S. D., & Benton, A. L. (1980). Developmental patterns of visuospatial judgment. Journal of Pediatric Psychology 5, 217-225.

Lounsbury, M. L., & Bates, J. E. (1982). The cries of infants of differing levels of perceived temperamental difficultness: Acoustic properties and effects on listeners. Child Development 53, 677-686.

Luger, G. F., Wishart, J. G., & Bower, T. G. (1984). Modelling the stages of identity theory of object-concept development in infancy. Perception 13, 97-115.

May, J. W., & May, J. G. (1981). Effects of age on color preference for black and white by infants and young children. Perceptual and Motor Skills 52, 255-261.

Modarressi, T., & Kenny, T. (1977). Children's response to their true and distorted mirror images. Child Psychiatry and Human Development 8, 94-101.

Montagu, A. (1984). The skin, touch, and human development. Clinics in Dermatology 2, 17-26.

Morrison, F. J., & Haith, M. M. (1976). Recognition versus recall of briefly presented visual information: A developmental study. Journal of Experimental Child Psychology 21, 191-200.

Myers, F. L., Myers, R. W., & Abromoski, M. (1981). Strategies in processing new versus old information by children. Journal of Psycholinguistic Research 10, 571-579.

Nelson, C. A., & Horowitz, F. D. (1983). The perception of facial expressions and stimulus motion by two- and five-month-old infants using holographic stimuli. Child Development 54, 868-877.

Owens, R. (1988). Language development: An introduction (2nd ed.). Columbus, Ohio: Merrill Publishing Co.

Perry, F. L., & Shwedel (1979). Interaction of visual information, verbal information, and linguistic competence in the preschool-aged child. Journal of Psycholinguistic Research 8, 559-566.

Pezdek, K., & Chen, H. C. (1982). Development differences in the role of detail in picture recognition memory. Journal of Experimental Child Psychology 33, 207-215.

Piazza Gordon, D. (1983). The influence of sex on the development of lateralization of speech. Neuropsychologia 21, 139-146.

Plante, M., Bernard, L., & Morais-Rochon, T. (1975). Drawing of a man: Development of the number of elements by age and school level. Union Medicale du Canada 104, 432-436.

Pomerleau, A., & Malcuit, G. (1980). Development of cardiac and behavioral responses to a three-dimensional toy stimulation in one- to six-month-old infants. Child Development 51, 1187-1196.

Powell, G. J., & Gaines, R. (1982). An in-progress research report of perceptual-cognitive development of young black children in three cultures. Journal of the National Medical Association 74, 115-123.

Priel, B., & de Schonen, S. (1986). Self-recognition: A study of a population without mirrors. Journal of Experimental Child Psychology 41, 237-250.

Prior, M. R., Frolley, M., & Sanson, A. (1983). Language lateralization in specific reading retarded children and backward readers. Cortex 19, 149-163.

Rose, S. A., & Wallace, I. F. (1985). Visual recognition memory: A predictor of later cognitive functioning in preterms. Child Development 56, 843-852.

Ruff, H. A. (1980). The development of perception and recognition of objects. Child Development 51, 981-992.

Schneider-Rosen, K., & Cicchetti, D. (1984). The relationship between affect and cognition in maltreated infants: Quality of attachment and the development of visual self-recognition. Child Development 55, 648-658.

Shucard, J. L., Shucard, D. W., Cummins, K. R., & Campos, J. J. (1981). Auditory evoked potentials and sex-related differences in brain development. Brain and Language 13, 91-102.

Streeter, L. A. (1976). Language perception of 2-month-old infants shows effects of both innate mechanism and experience. Nature 259, 39-41.

Young, A. W., & Bion, P. J. (1980). Absence of any developmental trend in right hemisphere superiority for face recognition. Cortex 16, 213-221.
Young, A. W., & Bion, P. J. (1981). Accuracy of naming laterally presented known faces by children and adults. Cortex 17, 97-106.
Yule, W., & Rutter, M. (Eds.). (1987). Language development and disorders. Oxford: Blackwell Scientific Publications Ltd.; Philadelphia: Lippincott.
Zeskind, P. S., & Huntington, L. (1984). The effects of within-group and between-group methodologies in the study of perception of infant crying. Child Development 55, 1658-1665.
Zeskind, P. S., Sale, J., Maio, M. L., Huntington, L., & Weiseman, J. R. (1985). Adult perceptions of pain and hunger cries: A synchrony of arousal. Child Development 56, 549-554.

15. Development of Memory

Achenbach, T. M., & Weisz, J. R. (1975). A longitudinal study of relations between outer-directedness and IQ changes in preschoolers. Child Development 46, 650-657.
Baker-Ward, L., Ornstein, P., & Holden, D. J. (1984). The expression of memorization in early childhood. Journal of Experimental Child Psychology 37, 555-575.
Baumeister, A. A. (1985). Age of acquisition and meaningfulness as predictors of word availability. Journal of Genetic Psychology 112, 109-112.
Cantor, D. S., Andreassen, C., & Waters, H. S. (1985). Organization in visual episodic memory: Relationships between verbalized knowledge, strategy use, and performance. Journal of Experimental Child Psychology 40, 218-232.
Cohen, M., & Grossberg, S. (1986). Neural dynamics of speech and language coding: Developmental programs, perceptual grouping, and competition for short-term memory. Human Neurobiology 5, 1-22.
Cramer, P. (1976). Changes from visual to verbal memory organization as a function of age. Journal of Experimental Child Psychology 22, 50-57.
DeLoache, J. S., & Brown, A. L. (1983). Very young children's memory for the location of objects in a large-scale environment. Child Development 54, 888-897.
DeLoache, J. S., Cassidy, D. J., & Brown, A. L. (1985). Precursors of mnemonic strategies in very young children's memory. Child Development 56, 125-137.
DeLoache, J. S., Sugarman, S., & Brown, A. L. (1985). The development of error correction strategies in young children's manipulative play. Child Development 56, 928-939.
Duncan, E. M., Whitney, P., & Kunen, S. (1982). Integration of visual and verbal information in children's memories. Child Development 53, 1215-1223.
Emmerich, H. J., & Ackerman, B. P. (1976). The effect of pictorial detail and elaboration on children's retention. Journal of Experimental Child Psychology 21, 241-248.
Fagan, J. F. (1978). 3d facilitation of infants' recognition memory. Child Development 49, 1066-1075.

Fagen, J. W., Ohr, P. S., Fleckenstein, L. K., & Ribner, D. R. (1985). The effect of crying on long-term memory in infancy. Child Development 56, 1584-1592.

Foellinger, D. B., & Trabasso, T. (1977). Seeing, hearing, and doing: A developmental study of memory for actions. Child Development 48, 1482-1489.

Foley, M. A., & Johnson, M. K. (1985). Confusions between memories for performed and imagined actions: A developmental comparison. Child Development 56, 1145-1155.

Foley, M. A., Johnson, M. K., & Raye, C. L. (1983). Age-related changes in confusion between memories for thoughts and memories for speech. Child Development 54, 51-60.

Fox, N., Kagan, J., & Weiskopf, S. (1979). The growth of memory during infancy. Genetic Psychology Monographs 99, 91-130.

Gladding, S. T. (1979). Effects of training versus non-training in identification of infant cry-signals: A longitudinal study. Perceptual and Motor Skills 48, 752-754.

Hirschman, R., & Katkin, E. S. (1974). Psychophysiological functioning, arousal, attention, and learning during the first year of life. Advances in Child Development and Behavior 9, 115-150.

Joseph, R., & Gallagher, R. E. (1985). Interhemispheric transfer and the completion of reversible operations in non-conserving children. Journal of Clinical Psychology 41, 796-800.

Lawson, A. E., & Shepherd, G. D. (1979). Written language maturity and formal reasoning in male and female adolescents. Language and Speech 22, 117-127.

Levin, I., Goldstein, R., & Zelniker, T. (1984). The role of memory and integration in early time concepts. Journal of Experimental Child Psychology 37, 262-270.

Lockman, J. J., Ashmead, D. H., & Bushnell, E. W. (1984). The development of anticipatory hand orientation during infancy. Journal of Experimental Child Psychology 37, 176-186.

Morgan, S.F. (1982). Measuring long-term memory storage and retrieval in children. Journal of Clinical Neuropsychology 4, 77-85.

Pinker, S. (1979). Formal models of language learning. Cognition 7, 217-283.

Ratner, H. H. (1984). Memory demands and the development of young children's memory. Child Development 55, 2173-2191.

Rees, K. (1978). The child's understanding of his past: Cognitive factors in reconstruction with children. In A. Solnit, et al. (Eds.), Psychoanalytic study of the child (Vol. 33, pp. 237-259). New Haven: Yale University Press.

Riseborough, M. G. (1982). Meaning in movement: An investigation into the interrelationship of physiographic gestures and speech in seven-year-olds. British Journal of Psychology 73, 497-503.

Rose, S. A. (1981). Developmental changes in infants' retention of visual stimuli. Child Development 52, 227-233.

Rose, S. A., & Wallace, I. F. (1985). Visual recognition memory: A predictor of later cognitive functioning in preterms. Child Development 56, 843-852.

Ross, B. M., & Kerst, S. M. (1978). Developmental memory theories: Baldwin and Piaget. Advances in Child Development and Behavior 12, 183-229.

Sak, R. J., & Ruben, R. J. (1981). Recurrent middle ear effusion in childhood: Implications of temporary auditory deprivation for language and learning. Annals of Otology, Rhinology and Laryngology 90, 546-551.

16. Development of Cognition

Baltaxe, C. A., & Simmons, J. Q. (1977). Bedtime soliloquies and linguistic competence in autism. Journal of Speech and Hearing Disorders 42, 376-393.

Bibace, R., & Walsh, M. E. (1980). Development of children's concepts of illness. Pediatrics 66, 912-917.

Fivush, R. (1984). Learning about school: The development of kindergarteners' school scripts. Child Development 55, 1697-1709.

Gopnik, A. (1982). Words and plans: Early language and the development of intelligent action. Journal of Child Language 9, 303-318.

Gopnik, A. (1984). The acquisition of gone and the development of the object concept. Journal of Child Language 11, 273-292.

Gottschalk, L. A. (1981). Psychoanalytic contributions to the generation of creativity in children. Psychiatry 44, 210-229.

Joseph, R. (1982). The neuropsychology of development hemispheric laterality, limbic language, and the origin of thought. Journal of Clinical Psychology 38, 4-33.

Kamhi, A. G. (1981). Nonlinguistic symbolic and conceptual abilities of language-impaired and normally developing children. Journal of Speech and Hearing Research 24, 446-453.

Kister, M. C., & Patterson, C. J. (1980). Children's conceptions of the causes of illness: Understanding of contagion and use of immanent justice. Child Development 51, 839-846.

Kohlberg, L., & Elfenbein, D. (1975). The development of moral judgments concerning capital punishment. American Journal of Orthopsychiatry 45, 614-640.

Kotchabhakdi, P., & Beardslee, C. (1985). School-age children's conceptions of the heart and its function: Part I: Review of Literature. Maternal-Child Nursing Journal 14, 139-152.

Lawson, A. E., & Shepherd, G. D. (1979). Written language maturity and formal reasoning in male and female adolescents. Language and Speech 22, 117-127.

Leeds, A., Dirlam, D., & Brannigan, G. G. (1983). The development of spatial representation in children from five to thirteen years of age. Genetic Psychology Monographs 108, 137-165.

Miller, P. H. (1985). Children's reasoning about the causes of human behavior. Journal of Experimental Child Psychology 39, 343-362.

Ross, R. J. (1974). The empirical status of the formal operations. Adolescence 9, 413-420.

Shorr, D. N., & Dale, P. S. (1984). Reflectivity bias in picture-pointing grammatical comprehension tasks. Journal of Speech and Hearing Research 27, 549-556.

Smolak, L. (1982). Cognitive precursors of receptive vs. expressive language. Journal of Child Language 9, 13-22.

Speece, M. W., & Brent, S. B. (1984). Children's understanding of death: A review of three components of a death concept. Child Development 55, 1671-1686.

17. Effects of Craniofacial Birth Defects on Development

Adams, G. (1980). The effects of physical attractiveness on the socialization process. In G. Lucker, K. Ribbens, & J. McNamara (Eds.), Psychological aspects of facial form. Ann Arbor: University of Michigan Press.

Affleck, G., McGrade, B., Allen, D., & McQueeney, M. (1985). Mother's beliefs about behavioral causes for their developmentally disabled infant's condition: What do they signify? Journal of Pediatric Psychology 10, 293-303.

Barden, C., Ford, M., Jensen, A., Rogers-Salyea, M., & Salyea, K. (1988). Effects of physical unattractiveness/craniofacial deformity in infancy on the quality of mother-infant interactions. Child Development 60, 819-824.

Barnard, K. E., Bee, H. L., & Hammond, M. A. (1984). Developmental changes in maternal interactions with term and preterm infants. Infant Behavior and Development 7, 101-113.

Barnard, K. E., Hammond, M., Booth, C., Bee, H., Mitchell, S., & Spieker, S. (1988). Measurement and meaning of parent-child interactions. In F. Morrison, C. Lord, & D. Keating (Eds.), Applied developmental psychology. New York: Academic Press.

Belsky, J. (1984). The determinants of parenting: A process model. Child Development 55, 83-96.

Brantley, H. J., & Clifford, E. (1979). Maternal and child locus of control and field-independence in cleft palate children. Cleft Palate Journal 16, 183-187.

Clifford, E. (1969). Parental ratings of cleft palate infants. Cleft Palate Journal 6, 235-244.

Combrinck-Graham, L. (1985). A developmental model for family systems. Family Process 24(21), 139-150.

Crnic, K. A., Greenberg, M. T., Ragozin, A. S., Robinson, N. M., & Basham, R. B. (1983). Social interaction and developmental competence of preterm and full-term infants during the first year of life. Child Development 52, 44-52.

Drotar, D., Baskiewicz, A., Irvin, N., Kennell, J., & Klaus, M. (1975). The adaptation of parents to the birth of an infant with a congenital malformation. A hypothetical model. Pediatrics 6, 710-717.

Field, T., & Vega-Lahr, N. (1984). Early interaction between infants with craniofacial anomalies and their mother. Infant Behavior and Development 7, 527-530.

Field, T. M. (1977). Effects of early separation, interactive deficits, and experimental manipulations on infant-mother face-to-face interactions. Child Development 48, 763-771.

Fox, D., Lynch, J., & Brookshire B. (1978). Selected developmental factors of cleft palate children between two and 33 months of age. Cleft Palate Journal 15, 239-245.

Goldberg, S., Brachfeld, S., & DeVito, B. (1980). Feeding, fussing, and playing: Parent-infant interaction in the first year as a function of prematurity and perinatal problems. In T. Field, S. Goldberg, D. Stern, & A. Sostek (Eds.), High risk infants and children: Adult and peer interactions. New York: Academic Press.

Greenberg, M., & Speltz, M. L. (1987). Contributions of attachment theory to the understanding of conduct problems during the preschool years. In J. Belsky & T. Nezowrski (Eds.), Clinical implications of attachment (pp. 177-218). Hillsdale, N.J.: Erlbaum.

Heller, A., Tidmarsh, W., & Pless, I. (1981). The psychosocial functioning of young adults born with cleft lip or palate. Clinical Pediatrics 20, 459-465.

Horan, M. (1982). Parental reaction to the birth of an infant with a defect: An attributional approach. Advances in Nursing Science 5, 57-68.

Kapp, K. (1979). Self-concept of the cleft lip or palate child. Cleft Palate Journal 16, 171-176.

McWilliams, B. J. (1982). Social and psychological problems associated with cleft palate. In F. C. Macgregor (Ed.), Clinics in plastic surgery. Philadelphia: W. B. Saunders.

Minde, K., Perrotta, M., & Hellman, J. (1988). Impact of delayed development in premature infants on mother-infant interaction. A prospective investigation. Journal of Pediatrics 116, 136-142.

Peter, J. P., & Chinsky, R. R. (1974). Sociological aspects of cleft palate adults: I. Marriage. Cleft Palate Journal 11, 295-309.

Richman, L. C. (1978). The effects of facial disfigurement on teachers' perception of ability in cleft palate children. Cleft Palate Journal 15, 155-160.

Richman, L. C., & Eliason, M. (1982). Psychological characteristics of children with cleft lip and palate: Intellectual, achievement, behavioral, and personality variables. Cleft Palate Journal 19, 251-257.

Richman, L. C., & Harper, D. C. (1978). Observable stigmata and perceived maternal behaviors. Cleft Palate Journal 15, 215-219.

Richman, L. C., & Harper, D. C. (1979). Self-identified personality patterns of children with facial or orthopedic disfigurement. Cleft Palate Journal 16, 257-261.

Sroufe, L. A. (1983). Infant caregiver attachment and patterns of adaptation in preschool: The roots of maladaptation and competence. In M. Perlmutter (Ed.), Minnesota symposium on child psychology (Vol. 16, pp. 41-81). Hillsdale, N.J.: Erlbaum.

Simonds, J. F., & Heimberger, R. E. (1978). Psychiatric evaluation of youth with cleft lip palate or matched with a control group. Cleft Palate Journal 15, 193-201.

Spriesterbach, D. C. (1973). Psychological aspects of the cleft palate problem (Vols. 1 and 2). Iowa City: University of Iowa Press.

Starr, P., Chinsky, R., Canter, H., & Meier, J. (1977). Mental, motor and social behavior of infants with cleft lip and/or palate. Cleft Palate Journal 14, 140-147.

Tobiason, J. (1984). Psychosocial correlates of congenital facial clefts: Conceptualization and model. Cleft Palate Journal 21, 131-139.

Tobiason, J., & Hiebert, J. (1984). Parents' tolerance for the conduct problems of the child with cleft lip and palate. Cleft Palate Journal 21, 140-147.

Wasserman, G. A., Allen, R., & Solomon, C. R. (1985). At risk toddlers and their mothers: The special case of physical handicap. Child Development 56, 73-83.

Wasserman, G. A., Lennon, M. L., Allen, R., & Shilansky, M. A. (1987). Contributors to attachment in normal and physically handicapped infants. Journal of the American Academy of Child and Adolescent Psychiatry 26, 9-15.

18. Neonatal Development

Aleksandrowicz, M. K., & Aleksandrowicz, D. R. (1975). The case history of a happy child. Child Psychiatry and Human Development 5, 174-181.

Als, H., & Brazelton, T. B. (1981). A new model of assessing the behavioral organization in preterm and full-term infants: Two case Studies. Journal of the American Academy of Child Psychiatry 20, 239-263.

Als, H., Tronick, E., Adamson, L., & Brazelton, T. B. (1976). The behavior of the full-term but underweight newborn infant. Developmental Medicine and Child Neurology 18, 590-602.

Amirhakimi, G. H. (1974). Growth from birth to two years of rich urban and poor rural Iranian children compared with Western norms. Annals of Human Biology 1, 427-441.

Anders, T. F. (1982). Biological rhythms in development. Psychosomatic Medicine 44, 61-72.

Arshavskii, I. A. (1979). Physiological analysis of physical development with special reference to the newborn infant. Human Physiology 5, 169-180.

Bakeman, R., & Brown, J. V. (1980). Early interaction: Consequences for social and mental development at three years. Child Development 51, 437-447.

Ball, R. S. (1977). The Gesell developmental schedules: Arnold Gesell (1880-1961). Journal of Abnormal Child Psychology 5, 233-239.

Barnard, K. E. (1983). Nursing research related to infants and young children. Annual Review of Nursing Research 1, 3-25.

Barnet, A. G. (1975). Auditory evoked potentials during sleep in normal children from ten days to three years of age. Electroencephalographic Clinical Neurophysiology 39, 29-41.

Beardslee, W. R., Wolff, P. H., Hurwitz, I., Parikh, B., & Shwachman, H. (1982). The effects of infantile malnutrition on behavioral development: A follow-up study. American Journal of Clinical Nutrition 35, 1427-1441.

Bee, H. L., Barnard, K. E., Eyres, S. J., Gray, C. A., Hammond, M. A., Spietz, A. L., Snyder, C., & Clark, B. (1982). Prediction of IQ and language skill from perinatal status, child performance, family characteristics, and mother-infant interaction. Child Development 53, 1134-1156.

Bennett, F. C., Robinson, N. M., & Sells, C. J. (1983). Growth and development of infants weighing less than 800 grams at birth. Pediatrics 71, 319-323.

Bertoncini, J., & Mehler, J. (1980). Language perception in the newborn infant: Some observations. Reproduction, Nutrition, Development 20, 859-869.

Bradley, R. H., & Caldwell, B. M. (1978). Screening the environment. American Journal of Orthopsychiatry 48, 114-130.

Brazelton, T. B. (1983). Developmental framework of infants and children: A future for pediatric responsibility. Journal of Pediatrics 102, 967-972.

Brazelton, T. B., & Als, H. (1979). Four early stages in the development of mother-infant interaction. In A. Solnit, et al. (Eds.), Psychoanalytic study of the child (Vol. 34, pp. 349-369). New Haven: Yale University Press.

Brazelton, T. B., Tronick, E., Lechtig, A., Lasky, R. E., & Klein, R. E. (1977). The behavior of nutritionally deprived Guaelmalan infants. Developmental Medicine and Child Neurology 19, 364-372.

Bromwich, R. M. (1976). Focus on maternal behavior in infant intervention. American Journal of Orthopsychiatry 46, 439-446.

Brooks-Gunn, J., & Hearn, R. P. (1982). Early intervention and developmental dysfunction: Implications for pediatrics. Advances in Pediatrics 29, 497-527.

Broussard, E. R. (1976). Neonatal prediction and outcome at 10/11 years. Child Psychiatry and Human Development 7, 85-93.

Call, J. D. (1980). Some prelinguistic aspects of language development. Journal of the American Psychoanalytic Association 28, 259-289.

Capute, A. J., & Accardo, P. J. (1978). Linguistic and auditory milestones during the first two years of life: A language inventory for the practitioner. Clinical Pediatrics 17, 847-853.

Caputo, D. V., Taub, H. B., Goldstein, K. M., Smith, N., Dalack, J. D., Pursner, J. P., & Silberstein, R. M. (1974). An evaluation of various parameters of maturity at birth as predictors of development at one year of life. Perceptual and Motor Skills 39, 631-652.

Chamberlin, R. W., & Szumowski, E. K. (1980). A follow-up study of parent education in pediatric office practices: Impact at age two and a half. American Journal of Public Health 70, 1180-1188.

Chandler, L., & Roe, M. D. (1977). Behavioral and neurological comparisons of neonates born to mothers of differing social environments. Child Psychiatry and Human Development 8, 25-30.

Chevrie-Muller, C. (1978). Early detection of deafness in young children. Developmental Medicine and Child Neurology 20, 814-822.

Chisholm, J. S., Woodson, R. H., & da Costa Woodson, E. M. (1978). Maternal blood pressure in pregnancy and newborn irritability. Early Human Development 2, 171-178.

Christoffel, K. K., Anzinger, N. K., & Amari, M. (1983). Homicide in childhood. Distinguishable patterns of risk related to developmental levels of victims. American Journal of Forensic Medicine and Pathology 4, 129-137.

Clarke, B. A. (1983). Improving adolescent parenting through participant modeling and self-evaluation. Nursing Clinics of North America 18, 303-311.

Development

Clore, E. R., & Newberry, Y. S. (1981). Nurse practitioner guidance for the adoptive family from birth to adolescence. Pediatric Nursing 7, 16-25, 52.

Cohen, S. E., & Beckwith, L. (1979). Preterm infant interaction with the caregiver in the first year of life and competence at age two. Child Development 50, 767-776.

Colombo, J. (1982). The critical period concept: Research, methodology, and theoretical issues. Psychological Bulletin 91, 260-275.

Cremer, H. D., Florez, A., de Navarro, L., Vuori, L., & Wagner, M. (1977). The influence of food supplementation and/or psychological stimulation on mental development. Nutrition and Metabolism 21, 358-371.

Crockenberg, S. B. (1981). Infant irritability, mother responsiveness, and social support influences on the security of infant-mother attachment. Child Development 52, 857-865.

Crosby, J. F. (1980). When does human life begin? American Journal of Orthopsychiatry 50, 356-364.

Czarniecki, L. (1978). Developmental nursing care: Infant stimulation for high risk children. Pediatric Nursing 4, 32-38.

Drotar, D. D., Stern, R. C., & Polmar, S. H. (1976). Intellectual and social development following prolonged isolation. Journal of Pediatrics 89, 675-678.

Dunn, J., & Kendrick, C. (1980). Studying temperament and parent-child interaction: Comparison of interview and direct observation. Developmental Medicine and Child Neurology 22, 484-496.

Dunn, J. F. (1976). Mother-infant relations: Continuities and discontinuities over the first 14 months. Journal of Psychosomatic Research 20, 273-277.

Earls, F. (1976). The fathers (not the mothers): Their importance and influence with infants and young children. Psychiatry 39, 209-226.

Egeland, B., & Sroufe, L. A. (1981). Attachment and early maltreatment. Child Development 42, 44-52.

Elwood, P. C., Haley, T. J., Hughes, S. J., Sweetnam, P. M., Gray, O. P., & Davies, D. P. (1981). Child growth (0-5 years), and the effect of entitlement to a mild supplement. Archives of Diseases in Childhood 56, 831-835.

Escalona, S. K. (1984). Social and other environmental influences on the cognitive and personality development of low birthweight infants. American Journal of Mental Deficiency 88, 508-512.

Fergusson, D. M., & Horwood, L. J. (1983). Childhood disadvantage and the planning of pregnancy. Social Science and Medicine 17, 1223-1227.

Ferrari, F., Grosoli, M. V., Fontana, G., & Cavazzuti, G. B. (1983). Neurobehavioural comparison of low-risk preterm and fullterm infants at term conceptional age. Developmental Medicine and Child Neurology 24, 450-458.

Ferry, P. C. (1981). On growing new neurons: Are early intervention programs effective. Pediatrics 67, 38-41.

Field, T., Hallock, N., Ting, G., Dempsey, J., Dabiri, C., & Shuman, H. H. (1978). A first-year follow-up of high-risk infants: Formulating a cumulative risk index. Child Development 49, 119-131.

Field, T., Widmayer, S., Greenberg, R., & Stoller, S. (1982). Effects of parent training on teenage mothers and their infants. Pediatrics 69, 703-707.

Fleshood, L. (1981). Public health report: Physical growth assessments of infants and children: Training aids. Journal of the Tennessee Medical Association 74, 199-200.

Freedman, D. A. (1981a). The effects of sensory and other deficits in children on their experience of people. Journal of the American Psychoanalytic Association 29, 831-867.

Freedman, D. A. (1981b). Speech, language, and the vocal-auditory connection. In A. Solnit, et al. (Eds.), Psychoanalytic study of the child (Vol. 36, pp. 105-127). New Haven: Yale University Press.

Freedman, D. A., Montgomery, J. R., Wilson, R., Bealmear, P. M., & South, M. A. (1976). Further observations on the effect of reverse isolation from birth on cognitive and affective development. Journal of the American Academy of Child Psychiatry 15, 593-603.

Fried, P. A. (1982). Marihuana use by pregnant women and effects on offspring: An update. Neurobehavioral Toxicology and Teratology 4, 451-454.

Fuller, P., Newcombe, F., & Ounsted, C. (1983). Late language development in a child unable to recognize or produce speech sounds. Archives of Neurology 40, 165-168.

Gaddini, R. (1984). On the origins of the battered child syndrome: Abuse as acting out of preverbal events. Childhood Abuse and Neglect 8, 41-45.

Gamer, E., Gallant, D., & Grunebaum, H. (1976). Children of psychotic mothers. An evaluation of 1-year-olds on a test of object permanence. Archives of General Psychiatry 33, 311-317.

Garbarino, J. (1980). Changing hospital childbirth practices: A developmental perspective on prevention of child maltreatment. American Journal of Orthopsychiatry 50, 588-597.

Gauthier, Y. (1982). The outcome of the premature infant. Union Medicale du Canada 111, 786-790, 817.

Golub, H. L., & Corwin, M. J. (1982). Infant cry: A clue to diagnosis. Pediatrics 69, 197-201.

Gorski, P. A. (1985). Experience following premature birth: Stresses and opportunities for infants, parents, and professionals. In J. D. Call, E. Galenson, & R. L. Tyson (Eds.), Frontiers of infant psychiatry. New York: Basic Books.

Gorski, P. A., Davison, M. F., & Brazelton, T. B. (1979). Stages of behavioral organization in the high-risk neonate: Theoretical and clinical considerations. Seminars in Perinatology 3, 61-72.

Green, J. A., & Gustafson, G. E. (1983). Individual recognition of human infants on the basis of cries alone. Developmental Psychobiology 16, 485-493.

Greenspan, S. I. (1982). Developmental morbidity in infants in multi-risk-factor families: Clinical perspective. Public Health Reports 97, 16-23.

Haas, J. D., Moreno-Black, G., Frongillo, E. A., Jr., Pabon, J., Pareja, G., Ybarnegaray, J., & Hurtado, L. (1982). Altitude and infant growth in Bolivia: A longitudinal study. American Journal of Physical Anthropology 59, 251-262.

Development

Harbin, R. E. (1975). Is there a place for a rocking chair in your newborn nursery? A review of studies on the effect of rocking the newborn. Pediatric Nursing 1, 16.

Harding, C. B. (1982). Development of the intention to communicate. Human Development 25, 140-151.

Harper, R. M., Leake, B., Hodgman, J. E., & Hoppenbrouwers, T. (1982). Developmental patterns of heart rate and heart rate variability during sleep and waking in normal infants and infants at risk for the sudden infant death syndrome. Sleep 5, 28-38.

Hartz, S. C., Heinonen, O. P., Shapiro, S., Siskind, V., & Slone, D. (1975). Antenatal exposure to meprobamate and chlordiazepoxide in relation to malformations, mental development, and childhood mortality. New England Journal of Medicine 292, 726-728.

Hines, R. B., Minde, K., Marton, P., & Trehub, S. (1980). Behavioral development of premature infants: An ethnological approach. Developmental Medicine and Childhood Neurology 22, 623-632.

Hunt, J. V., & Rhodes, L. (1977). Mental development of preterm infants during the first year. Child Development 48, 204-210.

The influence of early deficits on later development. (1985). Panel report. Journal of the American Psychoanalytic Association 33, 631-644.

Inoff, G. E., Halverson, C. F., Jr., Allen, M. G., & Cohen, D. J. (1980). Pathways between constitution and competence during the first five years of life. Developmental Psychobiology 13, 191-204.

Iosub, S., Fuchs, M., Bingol, N., Stone, R. K., & Gromisch, D. S. (1981). Long-term follow-up of three siblings with fetal alcohol syndrome. Alcoholism 5, 523-527.

Kierscht, M., & Meuwissen, J. (1979). Follow-up of preschool age survivors of neonatal intensive care. Journal of Psychology 101, 129-134.

Knobloch, H., Stevens, F., Malone, A., Ellison, P., & Risemberg, H. (1979). The validity of parental reporting of infant development. Pediatrics 63, 872-878.

Kornor, A. F., Kraemer, H. C., Haffner, M. E., & Cosper, L. M. (1975). Effects of waterbed flotation on premature infants: A pilot study. Pediatrics 56, 361-367.

Kornor, A. F., Schneider, P., & Forrest, T. (1983). Effects of vestibular-proprioceptive stimulation on the neurobehavioral development of preterm infants: A pilot study. Neuropediatrics 14, 170-175.

Kramer, M., Chamorro, I., Green, D., & Knudtson, F. (1975). Extra tactile stimulation of the premature infant. Nursing Research 24, 324-334.

LaVeck, B., Hammond, M. A., & LaVeck, G. D. (1980). Minor congenital anomalies and behavior in different homes environments. Journal of Pediatrics 96, 940-943.

Lawrence, R. A., & Merritt, T. A. (1981). Infants of adolescent mothers: Perinatal, neonatal, and infancy outcome. Seminars in Perinatology 5, 19-32.

Leib, S. A., Benfield, D. G., & Guidubaldi, J. (1980). Effects of early intervention and stimulation in the preterm infant. Pediatrics 66, 83-90.

Leijon, I., & Finnstrom, O. (1982). Correlation between neurological examination and behavioural assessment of the newborn infant. Early Human Development 7, 119-130.

Lewis, M. (1981). Child psychiatry perspectives. Child development research and child analysis. Journal of the American Academy of Child Psychiatry 20, 189-199.

Liakopoulou, M., Patterson, A., Samaraweera, S., & Finnegan, L. (1983). Developmental interventions in infancy during lengthy hospitalizations. Journal of Developmental and Behavioral Pediatrics 4, 213-217.

Liptak, G. S., Keller, B. B., Feldman, A. W., & Chamberlin R. W. (1983). Enhancing infant development and parent-practitioner interaction with the Brazelton neonatal assessment scale. Pediatrics 72, 71-78.

Litt, C. J. (1981). Children's attachment to transitional objects: A study of two pediatric populations. American Journal of Orthopsychiatry 51, 131-139.

Morikawa, Y., Goto, K., Kimura, K., Sai, H., Izumi, H., Miyoshi, K., & Mizuta, R. (1983). Development of responses by facial expressions and eye movements in neonates and young infants. Brain Development 5, 278-285.

Murray, A. D. (1979). Infant crying as an elicitor of parental behavior: An examination of two models. Psychological Bulletin 86, 191-215.

Ness, M. (1983). Encouraging early learning through play--an experiment in a deprived area. Health Visitor 56, 61-64.

Ounsted, M. K., & Hendrick, A. M. (1977). The first-born child: Patterns of development. Developmental Medicine and Childhood Neurology 19, 446-453.

Palti, H., Pevsner, B., & Adler, B. (1983). Does anemia in infancy affect achievement on developmental and intelligence tests? Human Biology 55, 183-194.

Palti, H., Zilber, N., & Kark, S. L. (1982). A community-orientated early intervention programme integrated in a primary preventive child health service--evaluation of activities and effectiveness. Community Medicine 4, 302-314.

Pechstein, J. (1978). Psychohygienic knowledge of child development and its application in the early care of handicapped children. International Journal of Rehabilitation Research 1, 149-166.

Philipp, C. (1983). Parental perceptions of children who were hospitalized in neonatal intensive care units. Child Psychiatry and Human Development 14, 76-86.

Pridham, K. F., & Chang, A. S. (1985). Parents' beliefs about themselves as parents of a new infant: Instrument development. Research in Nursing and Health 8, 19-29.

Pruett, K. D., & Leonard, M. F. (1978). The screaming baby: Treatment of a psychophysiological disorder of infancy. Journal of the American Academy of Child Psychiatry 17, 289-298

Ruddy, M. G., & Bornstein, M. H. (1982). Cognitive correlates of infant attention and maternal stimulation over the first year of life. Child Development 53, 183-188.

Sadler, L. S., & Catrone, C. (1983). The adolescent parent: A dual developmental crisis. Journal of Adolescent Health Care 4, 100-105.

Sardello, R. J. (1974). A phenomenological approach to development: The contributions of Maurice Merleau-Ponty. Human Development 17, 401-423.

Segal, H. (1982). Early infantile development as reflected in the psychoanalytic process: Steps in integration. International Journal of Psycho-Analysis 63, 15-22.

Siegel, L. S. (1982). Reproductive, perinatal, and environmental factors as predictors of the cognitive and language development of preterm and full-term infants. Child Development 53, 963-973.

Solomons, H. C. (1980). Standardization of the Bayley motor scales of infant development in Yucatan, Mexico. Developmental Medicine and Childhood Neurology 22, 580-587.

St. James-Roberts, I. (1979). Neurological plasticity, recovery from brain insult, and child development. Advances in Child Development and Behavior 14, 253-319.

Staisey, N. L., & Fried, P. A. (1983). Relationships between moderate maternal alcohol consumption during pregnancy and infant neurological development. Journal of Studies on Alcohol 44, 262-270.

Stillman, P. L., Ruggill, J. S., & Sabers, D. (1978). Improved student learning of infant growth and development. Pediatrics 62, 775-777.

Sugar, M. (1977a). Five early milestones in premature infants. Child Psychiatry and Human Development 8, 11-24.

Sugar, M. (1977b). Some milestones in premature infants at 6 to 24 months. Child Psychiatry and Human Development 8, 67-80.

Thoman, E. B., Acebo, C., & Becker, P. T. (1983). Infant crying and stability in the mother-infant relationship: A systems analysis. Child Development 54, 653-659.

Valentine, G. H. (1982). The growth and development of six XYY children: A continuative report. Birth Defects 18, 219-226.

Waber, D. P., Vuori-Christiansen, L., Ortiz, N., Clement, J. R., Christiansen, N. E., Mora, J. O., Reed, R. B., & Herrera, M. G. (1981). Nutritional supplementation, maternal education and cognitive development of infants at risk of malnutrition. American Journal of Clinical Nutrition 34, 807-813.

Walzer, S., Wolff, P. H., Bowen, D., Silbert, A. R., Bashir, A. S., Gerald, P. S., & Richmond, J. B. (1978). A method for the longitudinal study of behavioral development in infants and children: The early development of XXY children. Journal of Child Psychology and Psychiatry 19, 213-299.

Werner, E. E. (1986). Resilient offspring of alcoholics: A longitudinal study from birth to age 18. Journal of Studies on Alcohol 47, 34-40.

19. History of Studies in Infant Development

Ainsworth, M., Andry, R. G., Harlow, R. G., Lebovici, S., Mead, M., Prugh, D., & Wootton, B. (1962). Deprivation of maternal care: A reassessment of its effects. Monograph 14. Geneva: World Health Organization.

Ainsworth, M., Bell, S. M., & Stayton, D. (1974). Infant-mother attachment and social development: Socialization as a product of reciprocal responsiveness to signals. In M. Richards (Ed.), The integration of the child into a social world. Cambridge: Cambridge University Press.

Ainsworth, M., Blehar, M., Waters, E., & Wall, S. (1978). Patterns of attachment. Hillsdale, N.J.: Erlbaum.

Ainsworth, M., & Wittig, B. (1969). Attachment and exploratory behavior of one year olds in a strange situation. In B. M. Foss (Ed.), Determinants of infant behavior (Vol. 4). New York: Wiley.

Alpert, A. (1959). Reversibility of pathological fixations associated with maternal depression in infancy. In R. S. Eissler, et al. (Eds.), Psychoanalytic study of the child (Vol. 14, pp. 169-185). New York: International Universities Press.

Als, H., Tronick, E., & Brazelton, T. B. (1980). The achievement of affective reciprocity and the beginnings of the development of autonomy: The study of a blind infant. Journal of the American Academy of Child Psychiatry 19, 22-40.

Als, H., Tronick, E., Lester, B., & Brazelton, T. B. (1979). The Brazelton neonatal behavioral assessment scales (BNBAS). In J. Osofsky (Ed.), Handbook of infant development. New York: Wiley.

Barrera, M., & Maurer, D. (1981). The perception of facial expressions by the three month old. Child Development 52, 203-206.

Bayley, N. (1969). Bayley scales of infant development. New York: The Psychological Corporation.

Bayley, N., & Schaefer, E. S. (1964). Correlations of maternal and child behaviors with the development of mental abilities: Data from the Berkeley growth study. Chicago: Child Development Publications.

Bell, S. M. (1970). The development of the concept of the object as related to infant-mother attachment. Child Development 41, 291-311.

Benjamin, J. (1961). Some developmental observations relating to the theory of anxiety. Journal of the American Psychoanalytic Association 9, 652-668.

Bergman, P., & Escalona, S. K. (1949). Unusual sensitivities in very young children. In R. S. Eissler, et al. (Eds.), Psychoanalytic study of the child (Vol. 31, pp. 333-352). New York: International Universities Press.

Bowlby, J. (1969). Attachment and loss. Vol. 1: Attachment. New York: Basic Books.

Brazelton, T. B. (1962a). Crying in infancy. Pediatrics 29, 588-597.

Brazelton, T. B. (1962b). Observations of the neonate. Journal of the American Academy of Child Psychiatry 1, 38-47.

Brazelton, T. B. (1973). Neonatal assessment scale. London and Philadelphia: Spastics International Medical Publishers.

Brazelton, T. B. (1980). Neonatal assessment. In S. Greenspan & G. Pollock (Eds.), The course of life. Vol. 1. Infancy and early childhood (DHHS Publication No. ADM 80-999). Washington, D.C.: Government Printing Office.

Brazelton, T. B. (1983). Precursors for the development of emotions in early infancy. In R. Plutchik & H. Kellerman (Eds.), Emotions in early development. Vol. 2. The emotions. New York: Academic Press.

Brazelton, T. B., Scholl, M. L., & Robey, J. S. (1966). Visual responses in the newborn. Pediatrics 37, 284-290.

Development

Brazelton, T. B., Young, G. G., & Bullowa, M. (1982). Inception and resolution of early developmental pathology: A case history. Journal of the American Academy of Child Psychiatry 10, 124.

Brody, S. (1956). Patterns of mothering. New York: International Universities Press.

Brody, S., & Axelrad, S. (1966). Anxiety, socialization and ego formation in infancy. International Journal of Psycho-Analysis 47, 218-229.

Brody, S., & Axelrad, S. (1970). Anxiety and ego formation in infancy. New York: International Universities Press.

Bronson, G. W., & Pankey, W. (1977). On the distinction between fear and wariness. Child Development 48, 1167-1183.

Brown, A., Matheny, A., & Wilson, R. (1973). Baldwin's kindness concept measure as related to children's cognition and temperament: A twin study. Child Development 44, 193-195.

Burlingham, D. (1961). Some notes on the development of the blind. In R. S. Eissler, et al. (Eds.), Psychoanalytic study of the child (Vol. 16, pp. 121-145). New York: International Universities Press.

Burns, P., Sander, L., Stchler, G., & Julia, H. (1972). Distress in feeding, short-term effects of caretaker environment on the first 10 days. Journal of the American Academy of Child Psychiatry 11, 427-439.

Call, J. (1964). Newborn approach behavior and early ego development. International Journal of Psycho-Analysis 45, 286-294.

Caplan, G., Mason, E. A., & Kaplan, D. M. (1965). Four studies of crisis in parents of prematures. Community Mental Health Journal 1, 149-161.

Caplan, H., Bibace, R., & Rabinovitch, M. S. (1963). Paranatal stress, cognitive organization and ego function: A controlled follow-up study of children born prematurely. Journal of the American Academy of Child Psychiatry 2, 434-450.

Carmichael, L. (1970). The onset and early development of behavior. In L. Carmichael (Ed.), Manual of child psychology (3rd ed.) (pp. 447-563). New York: Wiley.

Chess, S. (1973). Temperament in the normal infant. In S. G. Sapir & A. C. Nitzburg (Eds.), Children with learning problems: Readings in a developmental-interaction approach (pp. 291-307). New York: Brunner/Mazel.

Cohen, D. J., Allen, M. G., Pollin, W., Inoff, G., Werner, M., & Dibble, E. (1972). Personality development in twins: Competence in the newborn and preschool periods. Journal of the American Academy of Child Psychiatry 11, 625-644.

Condon, W. S., & Sander, L. W. (1974). Neonate movement is synchronized with adult speech: Interactional participation and language acquisition. Science 183, 99-101.

Dudek, S. (1972). Longitudinal study of Piaget's developmental stages and the concept of regression. II. Journal of Personality Assessment 36, 468-478.

Dudek, S., & Dyer, S. (1972). A longitudinal study of Piaget's developmental stages and the concept of regression. Journal of Personality Assessment 36, 1025-1034.

Eisenberg, R. (1969). Auditory behavior in the human neonate: Functional properties of sound and their ontogenic implications. International Audiology 8, 34.

Elmer, E., & Gregg, G. (1967). Developmental characteristics of abused children. Pediatrics 40, 596-602.

Emde, R., Gaensbauser, T., & Harmon, R. (1976). Emotional expression in infancy: A biobehavioral study. Psychological Issues, Monograph 37 (Vol. 10). New York: International Universities Press.

Engel, G., Reichsman, F., & Monica, F. K. (1979). A 25 year longitudinal study of the consequences of trauma in infancy, reported by Milton Vederman. Journal of the American Psychoanalytic Association 27, 127-144.

Erikson, E. H. (1937). Configurations in play--clinical notes. Psychoanalytic Quarterly 6, 139-214.

Erikson, E. H. (Ed.). (1950). Childhood and society. New York: Norton.

Erikson, E. H. (1970). The theory of infantile sexuality. In E. H. Erikson (Ed.), Childhood and society (pp. 48-108). New York: Norton.

Erikson, E. H. (1980). Elements of a psychoanalytic theory of psychosocial development in infancy and early childhood. In S. Greenspan & G. Pollock (Eds.), The course of life. Vol. 1. Infancy and early childhood (DHHS Publication No. ADM 80-999). Washington, D.C.: Government Printing Office.

Escalona, S. K. (1968). The roots of individuality: Normal patterns of development in infancy. Chicago: Aldine.

Evans, J. (1961). Rocking at night. Journal of Child Psychology and Psychiatry and Allied Disciplines 2, 71-85.

Fish, B. (1963). The maturation of arousal and attention in the first months of life. Journal of the American Academy of Child Psychiatry 2, 253-270.

Fraiberg, S. (1959). The magic years: Understanding and handling the problems of early childhood. New York: Scribner's.

Fraiberg, S. (1974a). Blind infants and their mothers. An examination of the sign system. In M. Lewis & L. Rosenblum (Eds.), The effect of the infant on its caregiver. New York: Wiley.

Fraiberg, S. (1974b). The clinical dimension of baby games. Journal of the American Academy of Child Psychiatry 13, 202-220.

Fraiberg, S. H., & Freedman, D. A. (1964). Studies in ego development of the congenitally blind child. In R. S. Eissler, et al. (Eds.), Psychoanalytic study of the child (Vol. 19, pp. 113-169). New York: International Universities Press.

Freedman, D. A., Fox-Kolendal, B. J., Margileth, D. A., & Miller, D. H. (1969). The development of the use of sound as a guide to affective and cognitive behavior: A two phase process. Child Development 40, 1099-1105.

Freud, A. (1965). Normality and pathology in childhood. The writings of Anna Freud (Vol. 6). New York: International Universities Press.

Freud, A., & Burlingham, D. (1973). Infants without families. Reports on the Hampstead nurseries, 1939-1945. In A. Freud, The collected writings of Anna Freud (Vol. 3, pp. 543-664). New York: International Universities Press.

Fries, M. E. (1946). The child's ego development and the training of adults in his environment. In R. S. Eissler, et al. (Eds.), Psychoanalytic study of the child (Vol. 2, pp. 85-112). New York: International Universities Press.

Fries, M. E., & Woolf, P. J. (1953). Some hypotheses on the role of congenital activity type in personality development. In R. S. Eissler, et al. (Eds.), Psychoanalytic study of the child (Vol. 8, pp. 48-632). New York: International Universities Press.

Gaensbauer, T., & Emde, R. N. (1973). Wakefulness and feeding in human newborns. Archives of General Psychiatry 28, 894-987.

Gaensbauer, T., & Sands, S. (1979). Distorted affective communication in abused/neglected infants and their potential impact on caretakers. Journal of the American Academy of Child Psychiatry 18, 236-250.

Garmezy, N. (1974). The study of competence in children at risk for severe psychopathology. In E. J. Anthony & C. Koupernik (Eds.), The child in his family: Children at psychiatric risk (Vol. 3). New York: Wiley.

Geschwind, N. (1970). The organization of language and the brain. Science 170, 940-952.

Gesell, A. L., & Amatruda, C. (1945). The embryology of behavior: The beginnings of the human mind. New York: Harper.

Gewirtz, J. L. (1969). Levels of conceptual analysis in environment-infant interaction research. Merrill-Palmer Quarterly 15, 9.

Greenacre, P. C (1960). Considerations regarding the parent-infant relationship. International Journal of Psycho-Analysis 1, 571-584.

Greespan, S. I. (1979). Intelligence and adaptation: An integration of psychoanalytic and Piagetian developmental psychology. Psychological Issues, Monographs 47-48. New York: International Universities Press.

Greenspan, S. I., & Curry, J. (1989). An overview of the contributions of Piaget to understanding intellectual development. In H. Kaplan & B. Sadock (Eds.), Comprehensive textbook of psychiatry (5th ed.). Baltimore and London: Williams and Wilkins

Greenspan, S. I., & Pollock, G. H. (Eds.) (1980). The course of life: Psychoanalytic contributions toward understanding personality development. Vol. 1. Infancy and early childhood (DHHS Publication No. ADM 80-999). Washington, D.C.: Government Printing Office.

Harlow, H. F. (1958). The nature of love. American Psychologist 13, 673-685.

Hartmann, H., Kris, E., & Loewenstein, R. M. (1946). Comments on the formation of psychic structure. In R. S. Eissler, et al. (Eds.), Psychoanalytic study of the child (Vol. 2, pp. 11-38). New York: International Universities Press.

Hoffer, W. (1949). Mouth, hand, and ego integration. In R. S. Eissler, et al. (Eds.), Psychoanalytic study of the child (Vol. 3/4, pp. 49-56). New York: International Universities Press.

Hollos, M., & Cowan, P. (1973). Social isolation and cognitive development: Logical operations and role-taking abilities in three Norwegian social settings. Child Development 44, 630-641.

Hunt, J. M. (1941). Infants in an orphanage. Journal of Abnormal and Social Psychology 36, 338.

Inhelder, B., & Piaget, J. (1958). The growth of logical thinking from childhood to adolescence. New York: Basic Books.

Josselyn, I. M. (1962). Concepts related to child Development: 1. The oral stage. Journal of the American Academy of Child Psychiatry 1, 209-224.

Kanner, L. (1949). Autistic disturbance of affective contact. The Nervous Child 2, 217-250.

Katan, A. (1972). The infant's first reaction to strangers: Distress or anxiety? International Journal of Psycho-Analysis 53, 501-503.

Kennell, J. H., & Bergen, M. E. (1966). Early childhood separation. Pediatrics 37, 291-298.

Klaus, M. H., Jerauld, R., Kreger, N. C., McAlpine, W., Steffa, M., & Kennell, J. H. (1972). Maternal attachment, importance of the first postpartum days. New England Journal of Medicine 286, 460-463.

Korner, A. (1964). Some hypotheses regarding the significance of individual differences at birth for later development. In R. S. Eissler, et al. (Eds.), Psychoanalytic study of the child (Vol. 19, pp. 58-72). New York: International Universities Press.

Korner, A., & Thoman, E. (1970). Visual alertness in neonates as evoked by maternal care. Journal of Experimental Child Psychology 10, 67.

Lewis, M., & Rosenblum, L. A. (1974). The effect of the infant on its caregiver. New York: Wiley.

Lipsitt, L. (1966). Learning processes of newborns. Merrill-Palmer Quarterly 12, 45.

Lipton, E. L., Steinsschneider, A., & Richmond, J. D. (1960). Autonomic function in the neonate. Psychosomatic Medicine 22, 57-65.

Lourie, R. S. (1971). The first three years of life: An overview of a new frontier of psychiatry. American Journal of Psychiatry 127, 1457-1463.

Lowrey, L. G. (1940). Personality distortion and early institutional Care. American Journal of Orthopsychiatry 10, 546.

Mahler, M. S. (1958). On two crucial phases of integration of the sense of identity: Separation-individuation and bisexual identity. Abstract in panel on problems of identity. 1957, rep. D. L. R. Rubintine. Journal of the American Psychoanalytic Association 6, 131-142.

Mahler, M. S. (1965). On the significance of the normal separation-individuation phase. In M. Schur (Ed.), Drive, affects, behavior (Vol. 2, pp. 161-169). New York: International Universities Press.

Mahler, M. S. (1972). Rapprochement subphase of the separation-individuation process. Psychoanalytic Quarterly 41, 487-506.

Mahler, M., Pine, F., & Bergman, P. (1975). The psychological birth of the infant: Symbiosis and individuation. New York: Basic Books.

Matas, L., Arend, R., & Sroufe, L. A. (1978). Continuity of adaptation in the second year: The relationship between quality of attachment and later competent functioning. Child Development 489, 547-556.

McCall, R. B. (1972). Smiling and vocalization in infants as indices of perceptual-cognitive processes. Merrill-Palmer Quarterly 18, 341-347.

McCall, R. B., Hogarty, P. S., & Hurlburt, N. (1974). Transitions in infant sensorimotor development and the prediction of childhood IQ. In S. Chess & A.

Thomas (Eds.), Annual progress in child psychiatry and child development: 1973 (pp. 50-83). New York: Brunner/Mazel.

Meadow, K. (1975). The development of deaf children. In E. M. Heterington (Ed.), Review of child development research (Vol. 5). Chicago: University of Chicago Press.

Meltzoff, A., & Moore, K. (1977). Imitation of facial and manual gestures by human neonates. Science 198, 75-78.

Muir, D., & Field, J. (1979). Newborn infants orient to sound. Child Development 50, 431-436.

Murphy, L. B., & Moriarty, A. E. (1976). Vulnerability, coping and growth. New Haven: Yale University Press.

Osofsky, J., & Danzger, B. (1974). Relationships between neonatal characteristics and mother infant interaction. Developmental Psychology 16, 124.

Paine, R. S. (1965). The contribution of developmental neurology to child psychiatry. Journal of the American Academy of Child Psychiatry 4, 353-386.

Parmelee, A. H., Wenner, W. H., & Schulz, H. R. (1964). Infant sleep patterns: From birth to 16 weeks of age. Journal of Pediatrics 65, 576-582.

Pasamanick, B., & Knobloch, H. (1956). Pregnancy experience and the development of behavior disorder in children. American Journal of Psychiatry 112(8), 613-618.

Piaget, J. (1952). The origins of intelligence in children. New York: Norton.

Piaget, J. (1954). The construction of reality in the child New York: Basic Books.

Piaget, J. (1962a). Play, dreams and imitation in children. New York: Norton.

Piaget, J. (1962b). The stages in the intellectual development of the child. In S. Harrison & J. McDermott (Eds.), Childhood psychopathology. New York: International Universities Press.

Piaget, J. (1981). Intelligence and affectivity: Their relationship during child development [1954]. Palo Alto: Annual Reviews.

Piaget, J., & Inhelder, B. (1969). The psychology of the child. New York: Basic Books.

Provence, S., & Lipton, R. C. (1962). Infants in institutions. New York: International Universities Press.

Richmond, J. B., & Caldwell, B. M. (1963). Child-rearing practices and their consequences. In A. J. Solnit & S. A. Provence (Eds.), Modern perspectives in child development. (pp. 627-654). New York: International Universities Press.

Ritvo, S., McCollum, A. T., Omwake, E., Provence, S. A., & Solnit, A. J. (1963). Some relations of constitution, environment and personality as observed in a longitudinal study of child development. In A. J. Solnit & S. A. Provence (Eds.), Modern perspectives in child development. New York: International Universities Press.

Ritvo, S., & Solnit, A. J. (1958). Influence of early mother child interaction on identification processes. Discussion by R. Loewenstein, J. Arlow, and R. Knight. In R. S. Eissler, et al. (Eds.), Psychoanalytic study of the child (Vol. 13, pp. 64-91). New York: International Universities Press.

Robson, K. (1967). The role of eye-to-eye contact in maternal-infant attachment. Journal of Child Psychology and Psychiatry and Allied Disciplines 8, 13-25.

Rubin, K. (1973). Egocentrism in childhood: A unitary construct? Child Development 44, 102-110.

Rutter, M., Korn, S., & Birch, H. G. (1963). Genetic and environmental factors in the development of "primary reaction patterns." British Journal of Social and Clinical Psychology 2, 161-173.

Sander, L. (1962). Issues in early mother child interaction. Journal of the American Academy of Child Psychiatry 1, 141.

Sander, L. (1975). Infant and caretaking environment. In E. J. Anthony (Ed.), Explorations in child psychiatry (pp. 129-166). New York: Plenum Press.

Sander, L. (1976). Primary prevention and some aspects of temporal organization in early infant caretaker interaction. In E. Rexford, L. Sander, & T. Shapiro (Eds.), Infant psychiatry: A new syntheses (pp. 187-204). New Haven: Yale University Press.

Sander, L., Julia, H., Stechler, G., & Burns, P. (1972). Continuous 24 hour interactional monitoring in infants reared in two caretaking environments. Psychosomatic Medicine 34, 20-282.

Sandler, J., & Rosenblatt, B. (1962). The concept of the representational world. In R. S. Eissler, et al. (Eds.), Psychoanalytic study of the child (Vol. 1, pp. 128-145). New York: International Universities Press.

Scarr, S., & Salapatek, P. (1970). Patterns of fear development during infancy. Merrill-Palmer Quarterly 16, 53-90.

Schlesinger, H., & Meadow, J. (1972). Sound and sign: Childhood deafness and mental health. Berkeley: University of California Press.

Silberstein, R. M., Blackman, S., & Mandell, W. (1966). Auto-erotic head banging: A reflection on the opportunism of infants. Journal of the American Academy of Child Psychiatry 5, 235-242.

Spitz, R. (1946). Anaclitic depression. In R. S. Eissler, et al. (Eds.), Psychoanalytic study of the child (Vol. 11, pp. 313-342). New York: International Universities Press.

Spitz, R. A. (1946). Hospitalism: An inquiry into the genesis of psychiatric conditions in early childhood. In R. S. Eissler, et al. (Eds.), Psychoanalytic study of the child (Vol. 12, pp. 53-74). New York: International Universities Press.

Spitz, R. A. (1959). A genetic field theory of ego formation. New York: International Universities Press.

Spitz, R. A. (1965). The first year of life. New York: International Universities Press.

Spitz, R., & Wolf, M. (1946). The smiling response. Genetic Psychology Monographs 34, 57-125.

Spock, B. (1963). The striving for autonomy and regressive object relationship. In R. S. Eissler, et al. (Eds.), Psychoanalytic study of the child (Vol. 18, pp. 340-343). New York: International Universities Press.

Spock, B. (1965). Innate inhibition of aggressiveness in infancy. In R. S. Eissler, et al. (Eds.), Psychoanalytic study of the child (Vol. 20, pp. 340-343). New York: International Universities Press.

Sroufe, L., Waters, E., & Matas, L. (1977). Attachment as an organizational construct. Child Development 48, 1184.

Sroufe, L. A. (1979). The coherence of individual development: Early care, attachment, and subsequent developmental issues. American Psychologist 34, 834-841.

Sroufe, L. A., & Wunsch, J. (1977). The development of laughter in the first year of life. Child Development 43, 1326-1344.

Stechler, G., & Latz, E. (1966). Some observations on attention and arousal in the human infant. Journal of the Academy of Child Psychiatry 5, 517.

Stern, D. (1971). A micro-analysis of mother-infant interactions: Behavior regulating social contact between a mother and her 3 1/2 month old twins. Journal of the American Academy of Child Psychiatry 10, 501-517.

Stern, D. (1974). The goal and structure of mother-infant play. Journal of the American Academy of Child Psychiatry 13, 402-421.

Thomas, A., & Chess, S. (1977). Temperament and development. New York: Brunner/Mazel.

Thomas, A., Chess, S., & Birch, H. (1968). Temperament and behavior disorders in children. New York: New York University Press.

Tronick, E., Als, H., Adamson, L., Wise, S., & Brazelton, T. B. (1978). The infant's response to entrapment between contradictory messages in face-to-face interaction. Journal of the American Academy of Child Psychiatry 17, 1-13.

Vygotsky, L. (1962). Thought and language. Boston: MIT Press.

Waddington, C. H. (1966). Principles of development and differentiation. New York: Macmillan.

Werner, E. E., Bierman, J. M., French, F. E. (1971). The children of Kauai. Honolulu: University of Hawaii Press.

White, R. W. (1960). Competence and the psychosexual stages of development. Nebraska Symposium on Motivation 8, 97-141.

Winick, M. (1973). Effects of prenatal nutrition upon pregnancy risk. Clinical Obstetrics and Gynecology 16, 1.

Winnicott, D. W. (1953). Transitional objects and transitional phenomena: A study of the first not-me possession. International Journal of Psycho-Analysis 34, 89-97.

Winnicott, D. W. (1958). Collected works, through pediatrics to psychoanalysis. New York: Basic Books.

Winnicott, D. W. (1960). Transitional objects and transitional phenomena. International Journal of Psycho-Analysis. 1953. Reprinted in Collected papers: Through pediatrics to psychoanalysis (pp. 229-242). New York: Basic Books.

Winnicott, D. W. (1962). The maturational processes and the facilitating environment. New York: International Universities Press.

Wolf, K. M. (1952). Observations of individual tendencies in the first year of life. In M. Senn (Ed.), Problems of infancy and childhood. New York: Josiah Macy Foundation.

Wolff, P. H. (1966). The causes, controls, and organizations of behavior in the neonate. Psychological Issues, Monograph 17. New York: International Universities Press.

Wolff, P. H., & Feinbloom, R. L. (1969). Critical periods and cognitive development. Pediatrics 44, 999.

Wolff, P. H., & White, B. L. (1965). Visual pursuit and attention in young infants. Journal of the American Academy of Child Psychiatry 4, 437-484.

Yarrow, L. J. (1964). Separation from parents during early childhood. In M. Hoffman & L. Hoffman (Eds.), Review of child development research (Vol. 1). New York: Russell Sage Foundation.

Yarrow, L. J., Rubenstein, J. L., Pedersen, F. A., & Jankowski, J. J. (1974). Dimensions of early stimulation and their differential effects on infant development. In S. Chess & A. Thomas (Eds.), Annual progress in child psychiatry and child development: 1973 (pp. 3-17). New York: Brunner/Mazel.

Yorke, C., Kennedy, H., & Wiseberg, S. (1980). Some clinical and theoretical aspect of two development lines. In S. Greenspan & G. Pollock (Eds.), The course of life. Vol. 1. Infancy and early childhood (DHHS Publication No. ADM 80-999). Washington, D.C.: Government Printing Office.

Zahn-Waxler, C., Radke-Yarrow, M., & King, R. A. (1979). Childrearing and children's prosocial initiations towards victims of distress. Child Development 50, 319-330.

20. Emergence of Self

Ainsworth, M., Bell, S. M., & Stayton, D. (1974). Infant-mother attachment and social development: Socialization as a product of reciprocal responsiveness to signals. In M. Richards (Ed.), The integration of the child into a social world. Cambridge: Cambridge University Press.

Ainsworth, M., & Witting, B. (1969). Attachment and exploratory behavior of one year olds in a strange situation. In B. M. Foss (Ed.), Determinants of infant behavior (Vol. 4). New York: Wiley

Bell, S. M. (1970). The development of the concept of the object as related to infant-mother attachment. Child Development 41, 291-311.

Bronson, W. (1981). Toddler's behaviors with agemates: Issues of interaction, cognition and affect. In L. Lipsitt (Ed.), Monographs on infancy. Norwood, N.Y.: Ablex.

Brown, A., Matheny, A., & Wilson, R. (1973). Baldwin's kindness concept measure as related to children's cognition and temperament: A twin study. Child Development 44, 193-195.

Call, J. D. (1968). Lap and finger play in infancy, implications for ego development. International Journal of Psycho-Analysis 49, 373.

Call, J. D. (1975). The adaptive process in early infancy: A research odyssey. In E. J. Anthony (Ed.), Explorations in child psychiatry. New York: Plenum Press.

Call, J. D., & Marschak, M. (1966). Styles and games in infancy. Journal of the American Academy of Child Psychiatry 5(2), 193-210.

Erikson, E. H. (1937). Configurations in play--clinical notes. Psychoanalytic Quarterly 6, 139-214.

Feffer, M. (1959). The cognitive implications of role taking behavior. Journal of Personality 27, 152-168.

Feffer, M., & Gurevitch, V. (1960). Cognitive aspects of role-taking in children. Journal of Personality 28, 383-396.

Feinman, S., & Lewis, M. (1983). Social referencing and second order effects in 10 month old infants. Child Development 54, 878-887.

Ferenczi, S. (1916). States in the development of the sense of reality (1913). In S. Ferenczi, Sex in psychoanalysis (pp 213-239). Boston: Badger.

Flavell, J., Botkin, P., Fry, C., Wright, J., & Jarvis, P. (1968). The development of role-taking and communication skills in children. New York: Wiley.

Fraiberg, S. (1969). Libidinal object constancy and mental representation. In R. S. Eissler, et al. (Eds.), Psychoanalytic study of the child (Vol. 24, pp. 9-47). New York: International Universities Press.

Goldschmid, M. (1968). The relation of conservation to emotional and environmental aspects of development. Child Development 35, 579-589.

Greenspan, S. I. (1979). Intelligence and adaptation: An integration of psychoanalytic and Piagetian developmental psychology. Psychological Issues, Monographs 47-48. New York: International Universities Press.

Hoffman, M. L. (1982). Development of prosocial motivation: Empathy and guilt. In N. Eisenberg (Ed.), The development of prosocial behavior (pp. 281-313). New York: Academic Press.

Hollos, M., & Cowan, P. (1973). Social isolation and cognitive development: Logical operations and role-taking abilities in three Norwegian social settings. Child Development 44, 630-641.

Inhelder, B., & Piaget, J. (1958). The growth of logical thinking from childhood to adolescence. New York: Basic Books.

Kagan, J. (1981). The second year. Cambridge: Harvard University Press.

Kernberg, O. (1966). Structural derivatives of object relationships. International Journal of Psycho-Analysis 47, 236-253.

Kernberg, P. F. (1985). Reflections in the mirror: Mother-child interactions, self-awareness, and self-recognition. In J. D. Call, E. Galenson, & R. L. Tyson (Eds.), Frontiers of infant psychiatry. New York: Basic Books.

Klinnert, M. D., Campos, J., Sorce, J. F., Emde, R. N., & Svejda, M. J. (1983). Social referencing: Emotional expressions as behavior regulators. In R. Plutchik & H. Kellerman (Eds.), Emotions in early development. New York: Academic Press.

Korner, A. F. (1983). Individual differences in neonatal activity: Implications for the origins of different coping styles. In J. D. Call, E. Galenson, & R. L. Tyson (Eds.), Frontiers of infant psychiatry. New York: Basic Books.

Luger, G. F., Wishart, J. G., & Bower, T. G. (1984). Modeling the stages of the identity theory of object-concept development in infancy. Perception 13, 97-115.

Mahler, M., & McDevitt, J. (1980). The separation-individuation process and identity formation. In S. Greenspan & G. Pollock (Eds.), The course of life. Vol. 1.

Infancy and early childhood (DHHS Publication No. ADM 80-999). Washington, D.C.: Government Printing Office.

Mahler, M. S. (1958). On two crucial phases of integration of the sense of identity: Separation-individuation and bisexual identity. Abstract in E. L. R. Rubintine (Rep.): Panel on problems of identity, 1957. Journal of the American Psychoanalytic Association 6, 131-142.

Mahler, M. S. (1965). On the significance of the normal separation-individuation phase. In M. Schur (Ed.), Drive, affects, behavior (Vol. 2, pp. 161-169). New York: International Universities Press.

Mahler, M. S. (1972). Rapprochement subphase of the separation-individuation process. Psychoanalytic Quarterly 41, 487-506.

Matas, L., Arend, R., & Sroufe, L. A. (1978). Continuity of adaptation in the second year: The relationship between quality of attachment and later competent functioning. Child Development 49, 547-556.

McDevitt, J., & Mahler, M. (1980). Object constancy, individuality, and internalization. In S. Greenspan & G. Pollock (Eds.), The course of life. Vol. 1. Infancy and early childhood (DHHS Publication No. ADM 80-999). Washington, D.C.: Government Printing Office.

Modarressi, T., & Kenny, T. (1977). Children's response to their true and distorted mirror images. Child Psychiatry and Human Development 8, 94-101.

Nicholich, L. (1981). Towards symbolic functioning: Structure of early pretend games and potential parallels with language. Child Development 52, 386-388.

Novey, A. (1958). The meaning of the concept of mental representation of objects. Psychoanalytic Quarterly 27, 47-79.

Paret, I. (1983). Night waking and its relation to mother-infant interaction in nine-month-old infants. In J. D. Call, E. Galenson, & R. L. Tyson (Eds.), Frontiers of infant psychiatry. New York: Basic Books.

Peller, L. (1954). Libidinal phases, ego development and play. In R. S. Eissler, et al. (Eds.), Psychoanalytic study of the child (Vol. 9, pp. 178-198). New York: International Universities Press.

Provence, S. (1980). Direct observation and psychoanalytic developmental psychology, the child from one to three. In S. Greenspan & G. Pollock (Eds.), The course of life. Vol. 1. Infancy and early childhood (DHHS Publication No. ADM 80-999). Washington, D.C.: Government Printing Office.

Ramey, C. T., Yeates, K. O., & Short, E. J. (1984). The plasticity of intellectual development: Insights from preventive intervention. Child Development 55, 1913-1925.

Ritvo, S., & Solnit, A. J. (1958). Influence of early mother-child interaction on identification processes. Discussion by R. M. Loewenstein, J. Arlow, & R. Knight. In R. S. Eissler, et al. (Eds.), Psychoanalytic study of the child (Vol. 13, 64-91). New York: International Universities Press.

Rubin, K. (1973). Egocentrism in childhood: A unitary construct? Child Development 44, 102-110.

Sandler, J. & Rosenblatt, B. (1962). The concept of the representational world. In R. S. Eissler, et al. (Eds.), Psychoanalytic study of the child (Vol. 17, pp. 128-145). New York: International Universities Press.

Sroufe, L., & Wunsch, J. (1977). The development of laughter in the first year of life. Child Development 43, 1326-1344.

Sroufe, L. A. (1979). The coherence of individual development: Early care, attachment, and subsequent developmental issues. American Psychologist 34, 834-841.

Sroufe, L., Waters, E., & Matas, L. (1977). Attachment as an organizational construct. Child Development 48, 1184.

Stenberg, C., Campos, J., & Emde, R. (1983). The facial expressions of anger in seven month old infants. Child Development 54, 178-184.

Stern, D. (1974). The goal and structure of mother-infant play. Journal of the American Academy of Child Psychiatry 13, 402-421.

Stern, D. N. (1985). Affect attunement. In J. D. Call, E. Galenson, & R. L. Tyson (Eds.), Frontiers of infant psychiatry. New York: Basic Books.

Zahn-Waxler, C., Radke-Yarrow, M., & King, R. A. (1979). Childrearing and children's prosocial initiations towards victims of distress. Child Development 50, 319-330.

21. Evaluation and Assessment of Infant Functions

Call, J. D. (1981). Psychopathological development in infancy. In S. Arieti & H. K. H. Brodie (Eds.), American handbook of psychiatry (2d ed.). (Vol. 7). New York: Basic Books.

Call, J. D. (1985). Psychiatric evaluation of the infant, child and adolescent. In H. I. Kaplan, A. M. Freedman, & B. J. Sadock (Eds.), Comprehensive textbook of psychiatry (Vol. 4, pp. 1614-1625). New York: Williams and Wilkins.

Massie, H. N. & Campbell, B. K. (1983). The Massie-Campbell Scale of mother-infant attachment indicators during stress (AIDS scale). In J. D. Call, E. Galenson, & R. L. Tyson (Eds.), Frontiers of infant psychiatry. New York: Basic Books.

Rosenfield, A. G. (1983). Clinical use of the Bayley test of infant development for diagnosis of developmental dysfunction in very low birthweight infants. In J. D. Call, E. Galenson, & R. L. Tyson (Eds.), Frontiers of infant psychiatry. New York: Basic Books.

B. Development of the Preschool Child

Stanley Greenspan, M.D., Section Editor

1. History of Developmental Study of the Preschool Child

Anthony, E. J. (1970). The reactions of parents to the oedipal child. In E. J. Anthony & T. Benedek (Eds.), Parenthood (pp 275-288). Boston: Little, Brown.

Barnes, M. J. (1964). Reactions to the death of a mother. In R. S. Eissler, et al. (Eds.), Psychoanalytic study of the child (Vol. 19, pp. 334-357). New York: International Universities Press.

Biber, B., & Fanklin, M. B. (1967). The relevance of developmental and psychodynamic concepts to the education of the preschool child. Journal of the American Academy of Child Psychiatry 6, 5-24.

Briggs, J. L. (1974). The issues of autonomy and aggression in the three-year-old: The Utku Eskimo case. In S. Chess & A. Thomas (Eds.), Annual progress in child psychiatry and child development: 1973 (pp 139-155). New York: Brunner/Mazel.

Erikson, E. H. (1963a). The growth of the ego. In E. H. Erikson (Ed.), Childhood and society (pp. 187-274). New York: Norton.

Erikson, E. H. (1963b). The theory of infantile sexuality. In E. H. Erikson (Ed.), Childhood and society (pp. 48-108). New York: Norton.

Flavell, J. H. (1963). The developmental psychology of Jean Piaget. Princeton, N.J.: Van Nostrand.

Fraiberg, S. (1969). Libidinal object constancy and mental representation. Psychoanalytical Study of the Child 24, 9-47.

Freud, A. (1952). The role of bodily illness in the mental life of children. Psychoanalytical Study of the Child 7, 69-81.

Freud, A. (1963). The concept of developmental lines. Psychoanalytical Study of the Child 18, 245-265.

Furman, R. A. (1964). Death and the young child: Some preliminary considerations. Psychoanalytical Study of the Child 19, 321-333.

Graham, P., Rutter, M., & George, S. (1973). Temperamental characteristics as predictors of behavior disorders in children. American Journal of Orthopsychiatry 43, 328-339.

Hoffman, M. L. (1970). Moral development. In L. Carmichael (Ed.), Manual of child psychology (3rd ed.) (pp. 261-359). New York: Wiley.

Karnes, M. B., Teska, J. A., & Hodgins, A. S. (1970). The effects of four programs of classroom intervention on the intellectual and language development of 4-year-old disadvantaged children. American Journal of Orthopsychiatry 40, 58-76.

Katan, A. (1961). Some thoughts about the role of verbalization in early childhood. Psychoanalytical Study of the Child 16, 184-188.

Kleeman, J. A. (1966). Genital self-discovery during a boy's second year. A follow-up. Psychoanalytical Study of the Child 21, 358-392.

Kris, E. (1955). Neutralization and sublimation: Observations on young children. Psychoanalytical Study of the Child 10, 30-46.

Kris, E. (1962). Decline and recovery in the life of a three-year-old; Or, data in psychoanalytic perspective on the mother-child relationship. Psychoanalytical Study of the Child 17, 175-215.

Levenstein, P. (1970). Cognitive growth of preschoolers through verbal interaction with mothers. American Journal of Orthopsychiatry 40, 426-432.

Lewis, H. (1965). The psychiatric aspects of adoption. In J. G. Howells (Ed.), Modern perspectives in child psychiatry (pp. 428-451). London: Oliver and Boyd.

Lidz, T. F. (1970). The family as the developmental setting. In E. J. Anthony & C. Koupernik (Eds.), The child in his family (pp. 19-39). New York: Wiley.

Mahler, M. S. (1967). On human symbiosis and the vicissitudes of individuation. Journal of the American Psychoanalytic Association 15, 740-763.

Mahler, M. S., Pine, F., & Bergman, A. (1970). The mother's reaction to her toddler's drive for individuation. In E. J. Anthony & T. Benedek (Eds.), Parenthood (pp. 257-274). Boston: Little, Brown.

Moore, T., & Ucko, L. E. (1961). Four to six: Constructiveness and conflict in meeting doll play problems. Journal of Child Psychology and Psychiatry and Allied Disciplines 2, 21-47.

Murphy, L. B. (1962). The widening world of childhood, paths toward mastery (pp. 189-374). New York: Basic Books.

Nagera, H. (1966). Sleep and its disturbances approached developmentally. Psychoanalytical Study of the Child 21, 393-447.

Nagera, H. (1970). Children's reactions to the death of important objects: A developmental approach. Psychoanalytical Study of the Child 25, 260-400.

Neubauer, P. B. (1960). The one-parent child and his oedipal development. Psychoanalytical Study of the Child 15, 286-309.

Raph, J. B., et al. (1968). The influence of nursery school on social interactions. American Journal of Orthopsychiatry 38, 144-152.

Robertson, J. (1962). Mothering as an influence on early development: A study of well-baby clinic records. Psychoanalytical Study of the Child 17, 245-264.

Schwarz, J. C., Krolick, G., & Strickland, R. G. (1973). Effects of early day care experience on adjustment to a new environment. American Journal of Orthopsychiatry 43, 340-346.

Sears, R. R., Maccoby, E. E., & Levin, H. (1957). Patterns of child rearing (pp. 102-269, 362-393). Evanston, Ill.: Row, Peterson.

Shapiro, T., & Stine, J. (1965). The figure drawings of three-year-old children: A contribution to the early development of body image. Psychoanalytical Study of the Child 20, 298-309.

Sperling, O. E. (1954). An imaginary companion, representing a prestage of the superego. Psychoanalytical Study of the Child 9, 252-258.

van Leeuwen, K., & Tuma, J. M. (1972). Attachment and exploration: A systematic approach to the study of separation-adaptation phenomena in response to nursery school entry. Journal of the American Academy of Child Psychiatry 11, 314-340.

Waldrop, M. F., & Bell, R. Q. (1964). Relations of preschool dependency behavior to family size and density. Child Development 35, 1187-1195.

Wender, P. H., Pedersen, F. A., & Waldrop, M. F. (1967). A longitudinal study of early social behavior and cognitive development. American Journal of Orthopsychiatry 37, 691-696.

Westman, J. C., Rice, D. L., & Bermann, E. (1967). Nursery school behavior and later school adjustment. American Journal of Orthopsychiatry 37, 725-731.

Winnicott, D. W. (1965). The maturational process and the facilitating environment (pp. 56-93). London: Hogarth Press.

Wolins, M. (1970). Group care: Friends or foe? In S. Chess & A. Thomas (Eds.), Annual progress in child psychiatry and child development: 1973 (pp. 218-245). New York: Brunner/Mazel.

2. Development of the Preschool Child

Abelson, A. G. (1979). Development of psychosexual concepts in relation to expressive language performance. Psychiatry 42, 274-279.

Abrams, S. (1984). Fantasy and reality in the oedipal phase. A conceptual overview. Psychoanalytical Study of the Child 39, 83-100.

Achenbach, T. M., & Weisz, J. R. (1975). A longitudinal study to relations between outer-directedness and IQ changes in preschoolers. Child Development 46, 650-657.

Aggernaes, A., & Haugsted, R. (1976). Experienced reality in three to six year-old children: A study of direct reality testing. Journal of Child Psychology and Psychiatry and Allied Disciplines 17, 323-335.

Arend, R., Gove, F. L., & Sroufe, L. A. (1979). Continuity of individual adaptation from infancy to kindergarten: A predictive study of ego-resiliency and curiosity in preschoolers. Child Development 50, 950-959.

Bates, J. E., Bentler, P. M., & Thompson, S. K. (1979). Gender-deviant boys compared with normal and clinical control boys. Journal of Abnormal Child Psychology 7, 243-259.

Belsky, J., & Nezworski, T. (Eds.). (1988). Clinical implications of attachment. Hillsdale, N.J.: Erlbaum.

Beratis, S., Kolb, R., Sperling, E., & Stein, R. E. (1981). Development of a child with long-lasting deprivation of oral feeding. Journal of the American Academy of Child Psychiatry 20, 53-64.

Best, D. L., Williams, J. E., Cloud, J. M., Davis, S. W., Robertson, L. S., Edwards, J. R., Giles, H., & Folwes, J. (1977). Development of sex-trait stereotypes among young children in the United States, England, and Ireland. Child Development 48, 1375-1384.

Bloom-Feshbach, S., Bloom-Feshbach, J., & Gaughran, J. (1980). The child's tie to both parents: Separation patterns and nursery school adjustment. American Journal of Orthopsychiatry 50, 505-521.

Bower, E. M. (1978). Pathways upstream: Risks and realities of early screening efforts. American Journal of Orthopsychiatry 48, 131-139.

Bruneau, O. J. (1984). Comparison of behavioral characteristics and self-concepts of American Indian and Caucasian preschoolers. Psychological Reports 54, 571-574.

Capute, A. J., & Accardo, P. J. (1978). Linguistic and auditory milestones during the first two years of life: A language inventory for the practitioner. Clinical Pediatrics 17, 847-853.

Carey, W. B., & McDevitt, S. C. (1978). Stability and change in individual temperament diagnoses from infancy to early childhood. Journal of the American Academy of Child Psychiatry 17, 331-337.

Development

Chess, S. (1978). The plasticity of human development. Alternative pathways. Journal of the American Academy of Child Psychiatry 17, 80-91.

Cicchetti, D. (1989). How research on child maltreatment has informed the study of child development: Perspectives from developmental psychopathology. In D. Cicchetti & V. Carlson (Eds.), Child maltreatment: Theory and research on causes and consequences of child abuse and neglect. Cambridge: Cambridge University Press.

Clarke, A. D., & Clarke, A. M. (1984). Constancy and change in the growth of human characteristics. Journal of Child Psychology and Psychiatry and Allied Disciplines 25, 191-210.

Cobb, P. R., Chissom, B. S., & Davis, M. W. (1975). Relationships among perceptual-motor, self-concept, and academic measures for children in kindergarten, grades one and two. Perceptual and Motor Skills 41, 539-546.

Cohen, K. N., & Clark, J. A. (1984). Transitional object attachments in early childhood and personality characteristics in later life. Journal of Personality and Social Psychology 46, 106-111.

Condry, J. C., & Ross, D. F. (1985). Sex and aggression: The influence of gender label on the perception of aggression in children. Child Development 56, 225-233.

Cordua, G. D., McGraw, K. O., & Drabman, R. S. (1979). Doctor or nurse: Children's perception of sex typed occupations. Child Development 50, 590-593.

Cornoldi, C., & Fattori, L. C. (1976). Age spacing in firstborns and symbiotic dependence. Journal of Personality and Social Psychology 33, 431-434.

Corrigan, S. A., & Moskowitz, D. S. (1983). Type A behavior in preschool children: Construct validation evidence for the myth. Child Development 54, 1513-1521.

Craig, H. K., & Gallagher, T. M. (1979). The structural characteristics of monologues in the speech of normal children: Syntactic nonconversational aspects. Journal of Speech and Hearing Research 22, 46-62.

Dahl, E. K. (1983). First class or nothing at all? Aspects of early feminine development. In A. Solnit, et al. (Eds.), Psychoanalytic study of the child (Vol. 38, pp. 405-428). New Haven: Yale University Press.

Darwin, C. (1977). A biographical sketch of an infant. American Journal of Diseases of Children 131, 909-912.

DeGangi, G., & Greenspan, S. I. (1988). The development of sensory functioning in infants. Journal of Physical and Occupational Therapy in Pediatrics 8(3), 21-33.

Derevensky, J. L. (1979). Relative contributions of active and passive touch to a child's knowledge of physical objects. Perceptual and Motor Skills 48, 1331-1346.

Drabman, R. S., Cordua, G. D., Hammer, D., Jarvie, G. J., & Horton, W. (1979). Developmental trends in eating rates of normal and overweight preschool children. Child Development 50, 211-216.

Drucker, J., & Shapiro, C. B. (1979). First scribbles: The emergence of an ego function. Journal of the American Academy of Child Psychiatry 18, 628-646.

Dunn, J., Wooding, C., & Hermann, J. (1977). Mothers' speech to young children: Variation in context. Developmental Medicine and Child Neurology 19, 629-638.

Egeland, B., Sroufe, L. A., & Erickson, M. (1983). The developmental consequence of different patterns of maltreatment. Child Abuse and Neglect 7, 459-469.

Emde, R. N. (1983). The prerepresentational self and its affective core. In A. Solnit, et al. (Eds.), Psychoanalytic study of the child (Vo. 38, pp. 165-192). New Haven: Yale University Press.

Emmerich, H. J., & Ackerman, B. P. (1976). The effect of pictorial detail and elaboration on children's retention. Journal of Experimental Child Psychology 21, 241-248.

Fagot, B. I., & Leinbach, M. D. (1985). Gender identity: Some thoughts on an old concept. Journal of the American Academy of Child Psychiatry 24, 684-688.

Feilitzen, C. V., & Linne, O. (1975). The effects of television on children and adolescents: Identifying with television characters. Journal of Communication 25, 51-55.

Foellinger, D. B., & Trabasso, T. (1977). Seeing, hearing, and doing: A developmental study of memory for actions. Child Development 48, 1482-1489.

Frankel, S., & Sherick, I. (1977). Observations on the development of normal envy. In A. Solnit, et al. (Eds.), Psychoanalytic study of the child (Vol. 32, pp. 257-281). New Haven: Yale University Press.

Galenson, E., Miller, R., Kaplan, E., & Rothstein, A. (1979). Assessment of development in the deaf child. Journal of the American Academy of Child Psychiatry 18, 128-142.

Gauthier, Y., Fortin, C., Drapeau, P., Breton, J. J., Gosselin, J., Quintal, L., Weisnagel, J., & Tetreault, L. (1977). The mother-child relationship and the development of autonomy and self-assertion in young (14-30 months) asthmatic children. Correlating allergic and psychological factors. Journal of the American Academy of Child Psychiatry 16, 109-131.

Golombok, S., Spencer, A., & Rutter, M. (1983). Children in lesbian and single-parent households: Psychosexual and psychiatric appraisal. Journal of Child Psychology and Psychiatry and Allied Disciplines 24, 551-572.

Green, R. (1979). Childhood cross-gender behavior and subsequent sexual preference. American Journal of Psychiatry 136, 106-108.

Green, R., Williams, K., & Goodman, M. (1982). Ninety-nine "tomboys" and "non-tomboys": Behavioral contrasts and demographic similarities. Archives of Sexual Behavior 11, 247-266.

Greenspan, S. I. (1988). A clinical approach to normal child development. In H. Kaplan & B. Sadock (Eds.), Comprehensive textbook of psychiatry (5th ed.). Baltimore and London: Williams and Wilkins.

Greenspan, S. I. (1989a). The development of the ego: Implications for personality theory, psychopathology, and the psychotherapeutic process. Madison, Conn.: International Universities Press.

Greenspan, S. I. (1989b). The development of the ego: Insights from clinical work with infants and young children. Journal of the American Psychoanalytic Association 36, 3-55.

Greenspan, S. I., & Pollock, G. H. (Eds.). (1989a). The course of life (2nd ed.). Vol. 1: Infancy. Madison, Conn.: International Universities Press.

Greenspan, S. I., & Pollock, G. H. (Eds.). (1989b). The course of life (2nd ed.). Vol. 2: Early childhood. Madison, Conn.: International Universities Press.

Harter, S., & Pike, R. (1984). The pictorial scale of perceived competence and social acceptance for young children. Child Development 55, 1969-1982.

Himmelfarb, S., Hock, E., & Wenar, C. (1985). Infant temperament and noncompliant behavior at four years: A longitudinal study. Genetic, Social, and General Psychology Monographs 111, 7-21.

Kashani, J. H. (1986). Self-esteem of handicapped children and adolescents. Developmental Medicine and Child Neurology 28, 81-83.

Kennedy, J. H., & Bakeman, R. (1984). The early mother-infant relationship and social competence with peers and adults at three years. Journal of Psychology 116, 23-34.

Lotterman, A. (1981). Superman as a male latency stage myth. Bulletin of the Menninger Clinic 45, 491-498.

Mahon, E. (1985). Some aspects of separation and loss in therapy with disturbed children. American Journal of Psychoanalysis 45, 35-51.

Mauser, H. J., & Reynolds, R. P. (1977). Effects of a developmental physical activity program on children's body coordination and self-concept. Perceptual and Motor Skills 22, 1057-1058.

Meyer, J. K., & Dupkin, C. (1985). Gender disturbance in children. An interim clinical report. Bulletin of the Menninger Clinic 49, 236-269.

Money, J., & Lewis, V. (1982). Homosexual/heterosexual status in boys at puberty: Idiopathic adolescent gynecomastia and congenital virilizing adrenocorticism compared. Psychoneuroendocrinology 7, 339-346.

Oates, R. K., Forrest, D., & Peacock, A. (1985). Self-esteem of abused children. Child Abuse and Neglect 9, 159-163.

Papenfuss, R. L., Curtis, J. D., Beier, B. J., & Menze, J. D. (1983). Teaching positive self-concepts in the classroom. Journal of School Health 53, 618-620.

Scanlon, M. K. (1985). A chronically ill child's progression through the separation-individuation process. Maternal- Child Nursing Journal 14, 91-102.

Siegal, M. (1985). Mother-child relations and the development of empathy: A short-term longitudinal study. Child Psychiatry and Human Development 16, 77-86.

Skilbeck, W. M., Bates, J. E., & Bentler, P. M. (1975). Human figure drawing of gender-problem and school problem boys. Journal of Abnormal Child Psychology 3, 151-199.

Stingle, S. F., & Cook, H. (1985). Age and sex differences in the cooperative and noncooperative behavior of pairs of American children. Journal of Psychology 119, 335-345.

Story, M. D. (1979). Factors associated with more positive body self-concepts in preschool children. Journal of Social Psychology 108, 49-56.

Strauss, J. S., Harder, D. W., & Chandler, M. (1979). Egocentrism in children of parents with a history of psychotic disorders. Archives of General Psychiatry 36, 191-196.

Suter, B., Seegmiller, B. R., & Dunivant, N. (1980). Effects of age, sex, and income level on sex-role differentiation in preschoolers. Journal of Psychology 104, 217-220.

Taylor, M., & Flavell, J. H. (1984). Seeing and believing: Children's understanding of the distinction between appearance and reality. Child Development 55, 1710-1720.

Ullian, D. (1984). Why girls are good: A constructivist view. American Journal of Orthopsychiatry 54, 71-82.

Ullian, D. Z. (1981). Why boys will be boys: A structural perspective. American Journal of Orthopsychiatry 51, 493-501.

Zimet, S. G., & Farley, G. K. (1984). The self-concepts of children entering day psychiatric treatment. Child Psychiatry and Human Development 15, 142-150.

Zuger, B. (1978). Effeminate behavior present in boys from childhood: Ten additional years of follow-up. Comprehensive Psychiatry 19, 363-369.

Zuger, B. (1984). Early effeminate behavior in boys. Outcome and significance for homosexuality. Journal of Nervous and Mental Disease 172, 90-97.

C. Development of the Latency Age Child

Paul Adams, M.D., Section Editor

1. History of Studies on the Latency Age Child

Bayley, N., & Schaefer, E. S. (1964). Correlations of maternal and child behaviors with the development of mental abilities: Data from the Berkeley growth study. Chicago: Child Development Publications.

Blos, P. (1958). Preadolescent drive organization. Journal of the American Psychoanalytic Association 6, 47-56.

Bornstein, B. (1951). On latency. In R. S. Eissler, et al. (Eds.), Psychoanalytic study of the child (Vol. 6, 47-56). New York: International Universities Press.

Bornstein, B. (1953). Masturbation in the latency period. In R. S. Eissler, et al. (Eds.), Psychoanalytic study of the child (Vol. 8, pp. 65-78). New York: International Universities Press.

Buxbaum, E. (1950). A contribution to the psychoanalytic knowledge of the latency period. Workshop, 1950. American Journal of Orthopsychiatry 21, 132-198.

Erikson, E. H. (1963). Genital modes and spatial modalities. In E. H. Erikson (Ed.), Childhood and society (pp. 97-108). New York: Norton.

Flavell, J. H. (1963). Concrete operations. In J. H. Flavell (Ed.), The developmental psychology of Jean Piaget (pp. 165-201). Princeton, N.J.: Van Nostrand.

Freud, S. (1953). The period of sexual latency in childhood and its interruptions (1905). In E. Jones (Ed.), Collected papers. Standard edition (pp. 173-179). New York and London: Hogarth Press.

Freud, S. (1961). The dissolution of the Oedipus complex (1924). In E. Jones (Ed.), Collected papers. Standard edition (pp. 173-179). New York and London: Hogarth Press.

Fries, M. E. (1958). Review of the literature on the latency period, with special emphasis on the so-called "normal case." Journal of the Hillside Hospital 7, 3-16.
Grinder, R. E. (1964). Relations between behavioral and cognitive dimensions of conscience in middle childhood. Child Development 35, 881-891.
Kaplan, E. B. (1965). Reflections regarding psychomotor activities during the latency period. Psychoanalytical Study of the Child 20, 220-238.
Kestenberg, J. S. (1970). The effect on parents of the child's transition into and out of latency. In E. J. Anthony & T. Benedek (Eds.), Parenthood (pp. 289-306). Boston: Little, Brown.
Konopka, G. (1973). Formation of values in the developing person. American Journal of Orthopsychiatry 43, 86-96.
Lapouse, R., & Monk, M. A. (1959). Fears and worries in an representative sample of children. American Journal of Orthopsychiatry 29, 803-818.
Peller, L. (1958). Reading and daydreams in latency, boy-girl differences. Journal of the American Psychoanalytic Association 6, 57-70.
Sarnoff, C. A. (1971). Ego structure in latency. Psychoanalytic Quarterly 40, 387-414.
Stierlin, H. (1974). Shame and guilt in family relations. Archives of General Psychiatry 30, 381-389.
Thomas, A., & Chess, S. (1974). Development in middle childhood. In S. Chess & A. Thomas (Eds.), Annual progress in child psychiatry and child development: 1973 (pp. 172-186). New York: Brunner/Mazel.
Wolfenstein, M. (1954). Development of the joke facade. In M. Wolfenstein (Ed.), Children's humor: A psychological analysis (pp. 159-191). Glencoe, Ill.: The Free Press.

2. Latency as a Developmental Phase

Abrams, S. (1984). Fantasy and reality in the oedipal phase. A conceptual overview. Psychoanalytical Study of the Child 39, 83-100.
Aleksandrowicz, M. K. (1975). The biological strangers: An attempted suicide of a seven-and-a-half-year-old girl. Bulletin of the Menninger Clinic 39, 163-176.
Anderson, J. R. (1984). The development of self-recognition: A review. Developmental Psychobiology 17, 35-49.
Anthony, E. J. (1977). Nonverbal and verbal systems of communication. A study in complementarity. In A. Solnit, et al. (Eds.), Psychoanalytic study of the child (Vol. 32, pp. 307-325). New York: International Universities Press.
Archer, J. (1984). Gender roles as developmental pathways. British Journal of Social Psychology 23, 245-256.
Archer, J., & Westeman, K. (1981). Sex differences in the aggressive behaviour of schoolchildren. British Journal of Social Psychology 20, 31-36.
August, G. J., Rychlak, J. F., & Felker, D. W. (1975). Affective assessment, self-concept, and the verbal learning styles of fifth-grade children. Journal of Educational Psychology 67, 801-806.

Battle, J., & Blowers, T. (1982). A longitudinal comparative study of the self esteem of students in regular and special education classes. Journal of Learning Disabilities 15, 100-102.

Benedek, E. P., Poznanski, E., & Mason, S. (1979). A note on the female adolescent's psychological reactions to breast development. Journal of the American Academy of Child Psychiatry 18, 537-545.

Block, J. H. (1983). Differential premises arising from differential socialization of the sexes: Some conjectures. Child Development 54, 1335-1354.

Bowlby, J. (1977). The making and breaking of affectional bonds. I. Aetiology and psychopathology in the light of attachment theory. An expanded version of the Fiftieth Maudsley Lecture, delivered before the Royal College of Psychiatrists, 19 November 1976. British Journal of Psychiatry 130, 201-210.

Brim, O. G. (1976). Life-span development of the theory of oneself: Implications for child development. Advances in Child Development and Behavior 11, 241-251.

Brinich, P. M. (1980). Some potential effects of adoption on self and object representations. Psychoanalytical Study of the Child 35, 107-133.

Burka, A. A., & Glenwick, D. S. (1978). Egocentrism and classroom adjustment. Journal of Abnormal Child Psychology 6, 61-70.

Cath, S. H., & Cath, C. (1978). On the other side of Oz: Psychoanalytic aspects of fairy tales. In A. Solnit, et al. (Eds.), Psychoanalytic study of the child (Vol. 33, pp. 621-639). New York: International Universities Press.

Chandler, L. A., Million, M. E., & Shermis, M. D. (1985). The incidence of stressful life events of elemental school-aged children. American Journal of Community Psychology 13, 743-746.

Chiland, C. (1976). Social adaptation of the child in the latency period. Canadian Psychiatric Association Journal 21, 192-196.

Clingempeel, W. G., & Reppucci, N. D. (1982). Joint custody after divorce: Major issues and goals for research. Psychological Bulletin 91, 109-127.

Coates, S., & Person, E. S. (1985). Extreme boyhood femininity: Isolated behavior or pervasive disorder? Journal of the American Academy of Child Psychiatry 24, 702-709.

Cook, T. P., Goldman, J. A., & Olczak, P. V. (1978). The relationship between self-esteem and interpersonal attraction in children. Journal of Genetic Psychology 132, 149-150.

Coopersmith, S., Sakai, D., Beardslee, B., & Coopersmith, A. (1976). Figure drawing as an expression of self-esteem. Journal of Personality Assessment 40, 370-375.

Cropley, A. J., & Ahlers, K. H. (1975). Development of verbal skills in first-born and only boys. Journal of Biosocial Science 7, 297-306.

Dent, K. A. (1982). Two daughters of a deaf mute mother: Implications for ego and cognitive development. Journal of the American Academy of Psychoanalysis 10, 427-441.

Derevensky, J. L. (1979). Children's fears: A developmental comparison of normal and exceptional children. Journal of Genetic Psychology 135, 11-21.

Dienstbier, R. A., Hillman, D., Lehnhoff, J., Hillman, J., & Valkenaar, M. C. (1975). An emotion-attribution approach to moral behavior: Interfacing cognitive and avoidance theories of moral development. Psychological Review 82, 299-315.

DiVasto, P. V., Kaufman, A., Rosner, L., Jackson, R., Christy, J., Pearson, S., & Burgett, T. (1984). The prevalence of sexually stressful events among females in the general population. Archives of Sexual Behavior 13, 59-67.

Dixon, J. C., & Street, J. W. (1975). The distinction between self and not-self in children and adolescents. Journal of Genetic Psychology 127, 157-162.

Dodson, P. K., & Evans, E. D. (1985). A developmental study of school theft. Adolescence 20, 209-223.

Donnellan, G. J. (1980). Conceptual models and symbol formation during the latency period. Psychoanalytic Review 67, 291-312.

Duryea, E. J., & Glover, J. A. (1982). A review of the research on reflection and impulsivity in children. Genetic Psychology Monographs 106, 217-237.

Ebata, K. (1981). A comparative study of children's television programmes: American and Japanese. International Journal of Social Psychiatry 27, 301-306.

Egeland, B., Sroufe, L. A., & Erickson, M. (1983). The developmental consequence of different patterns of maltreatment. Child Abuse and Neglect 7, 459-469.

Eiduson, B. T. (1983). Conflict and stress in nontraditional families: Impact on children. American Journal of Orthopsychiatry 53, 426-435.

Eiser, C. (1986). Effects of chronic illness on the child's intellectual development [Editorial]. Journal of the Royal Society of Medicine 79, 2-4.

Elkind, D. (1976). Cognitive adaptation in latency. The construction of social reality. Canadian Psychiatric Association Journal 21, 186-191.

Elkisch, P. (1979). "Totem and Taboo" in a latency boy. Journal of the American Psychoanalytic Association 27, 65-77.

Ellwood, L. C. (1980). Effects of alcoholism as a family illness on child behavior and development. Military Medicine 145, 188-192.

Emde, R. N. (1983). The prerepresentational self and its affective core. In A. Solnit, et al. (Eds.), Psychoanalytic study of the child (Vol. 38, 165-192). New Haven: Yale University Press.

Eme, R., & Schmidt, D. (1978). The stability of children's fears. Child Development 49, 1277-1279.

Etaugh, C., & Turton, W. J. (1977). Sex differences in discrimination of forms by elementary school children. Journal of Genetic Psychology 130, 49-55.

Evans, P. D., & White, D. G. (1980). Sex differences in the development and projection of a simple fear. British Journal of Medical Psychology 53, 151-153.

Feagans, L., & Short, E. J. (1984). Developmental differences in the comprehension and production of narratives by reading-disabled and normally achieving children. Child Development 55, 1727-1736.

Fein, D., O'Neill, S., Frank, C., & Velit, K. M. (1975). Sex differences in preadolescent self-esteem. Journal of Psychology 90, 179-183.

Fennell, E. B., Satz, P., & Morris, R. (1983). The development of handedness and dichotic ear listening asymmetries in relation to school achievement: A longitudinal study. Journal of Experimental Child Psychology 35, 248-262.

Foley, M. A., & Johnson, M. K. (1985). Confusions between memories for performed and imagined actions: A developmental comparison. Child Development 56, 1145-1155.

Frey, K. S., & Ruble, D. N. (1985). What children say when the teacher is not around: Conflicting goals in social comparison and performance assessment in the classroom. Journal of Personality and Social Psychology 48, 550-562.

Friedrich, M. H. (1983). Partial brain dysfunctions. Their nature and their significance in child development. Munchener Medizinische Wochenschrift 125, 971-973.

Galler, J. R., Ramsey, F., & Solimano, G. (1985). A follow-up study of the effects of early malnutrition on subsequent development. I. Physical growth and sexual maturation during adolescence. Pediatric Research 19, 518-523.

Garber, J. (1984). Classification of childhood psychopathology: A developmental perspective. Child Development 55, 30-48.

Gilligan, C. (1982). New maps of development: New visions of maturity. American Journal of Orthopsychiatry 52, 199-212.

Goetz, R. R., Hanlon, C., Puig-Antich, J., & Weitzman, E. D. (1985). Signs of REM prior to the first REM period in prepubertal children. Sleep 8, 1-10.

Goldman, R., & Goldman, J. (1983). Children's perceptions of sex differences in babies and adolescents: A cross-national study. Archives of Sexual Behavior 12, 277-294.

Golombok, S., Spencer, A., & Rutter, M. (1983). Children in lesbian and single-parent households: Psychosexual and psychiatric appraisal. Journal of Child Psychology and Psychiatry and Allied Disciplines 24, 551-572.

Green, R. (1985). Gender identity in childhood and later sexual orientation: Follow-up of 78 males. American Journal of Psychiatry 142, 339-341.

Greenspan, S. I., Hatleberg, J. L., & Cullander, C. C. (1976). A systematic metapsychological assessment of the personality in childhood. Journal of the American Psychoanalytic Association 24, 875-903.

Hare, B. R. (1980). Self-perception and academic achievement: Variations in a desegregated setting. American Journal of Psychiatry 137, 683-689.

Harvey, D., & Greenway, P. (1982). How parent attitudes and emotional reactions affect their handicapped child's self-concept. Psychological Medicine 12, 357-370.

Hawkins, J. D., Lishner, D. M., & Catalano, R. F. (1985). Childhood predictors and the prevention of adolescent substance abuse. National Institute on Drug Abuse Research Monograph Series 56, 75-126.

Hershorn, M., & Rosenbaum, A. (1985). Children of marital violence: A closer look at the unintended victims. American Journal of Orthopsychiatry 55, 260-266.

Hoeffer, B. (1981). Children's acquisition of sex-role behavior in lesbian-mother families. American Journal of Orthopsychiatry 51, 536-544.

Holmes, C. S., Thompson, R. G., & Hayford, J. T. (1984). Factors related to grade retention in children with short stature. Child: Care, Health and Development 10, 199-210.

Hong, S. D., & Kim, S. P. (1981). Self-concept and body-image of children during physical illness. Psychosomatics 22, 128-130, 135.

James, J., & Meyerding, J. (1977). Early sexual experience and prostitution. American Journal of Psychiatry 134, 1381-1385.

Jarman, R. F. (1979). Matching of auditory-visual and temporal-spatial information by seven- and nine-year-old children. Child Development 50, 575-577.

Jensen, P. S., Lewis, R. L., & Xenakis, S. N. (1986). The military family in review: Context, risk, and prevention. Journal of the American Academy of Child Psychiatry 25, 225-234.

Johnson, D. S. (1981). Naturally acquired learned helplessness: The relationship of school failure to achievement behavior, attributions, and self-concept. Journal of Educational Psychology 73, 174-180.

Kagan, J., Klein, R. E., Finley, G. E., Rogoff, B., & Nolan, E. (1979). A cross-cultural study of cognitive development. Monographs of the Society for Research in Child Development (Vol. 44, pp. 1-77). Chicago: University of Chicago Press.

Kalter, N., Pickar, J., & Lesowitz, M. (1984). School-based developmental facilitation groups for children of divorce: A preventive intervention. American Journal of Orthopsychiatry 54, 613-623.

Kashani, J. H. (1986). Self-esteem of handicapped children and adolescents. Developmental Medicine and Child Neurology 28, 81-83.

Kay, P. (1980). The imaginary companion: Review of the literature. Maternal-Child Nursing Journal 9, 7-11.

Kerrins, K. M. (1983). Comparing the self-image of prepubescent girls before and after four sessions on body awareness. Journal of School Health 53, 541-543.

Khantzian, E. J., & Mack, J. E. (1983). Self-preservation and the care of the self. Ego instincts reconsidered. In A. Solnit, et al. (Eds.), Psychoanalytic study of the child (Vol. 38, pp. 209-232). New Haven: Yale University Press.

Kohlberg, L., & Elfenbein, D. (1975). the development of moral judgments concerning capital punishment. American Journal of Orthopsychiatry 45, 614-640.

Krell, R. (1985). Therapeutic value of documenting child survivors. Journal of the American Academy of Child Psychiatry 24, 397-400.

Kurdek, L. A. (1981). An integrative perspective on children's divorce adjustment. American Psychologist 36, 856-866. American Psychologist 36, 856-866.

Lazarus, P. J. (1982). Correlation of shyness and self-esteem for elementary school children. Perceptual and Motor Skills 55, 8-10.

Ledingham, J. E., Younger, A., Schwartzman, A., & Bergeron, G. (1982). Agreement among teacher, peer, and self-ratings of children's aggression, withdrawal, and likability. Journal of Abnormal Child Psychology 10, 363-372.

Lepper, M. R., Ross, L., & Lau, R. R. (1986). Persistence of inaccurate beliefs about the self: Perseverance effects in the classroom. Journal of Personality and Social Psychology 50, 482-491.

Lewis, M. (1985). Trends and directions in developmental research. Psychiatric Clinics of North America 8, 623-636.

Liebert, R. M. (1986). Effects of television on children and adolescents. Journal of Developmental and Behavioral Pediatrics 7, 43-48.

Livingood, A. B., & Cohen-Sandler, R. (1980). Failures of individuation and communication disorders in children. Journal of Pediatric Psychology 5, 179-187.

Loewald, H. W. (1985). Oedipus complex and development of self. Psychoanalytic Quarterly 54, 435-443.

Lyles, M. R., Yancey, A., Grace, C., & Carter, J. H. (1985). Racial identity and self-esteem: Problems peculiar to biracial children. Journal of the American Academy of Child Psychiatry 24, 150-153.

Maddux, J. E., Roberts, M. C., Sledden, E. A., & Wright, L. (1986). Developmental issues in child health psychology. American Psychologist 41, 25-34.

Masten, A. S. (1986). Humor and competence in school-aged children. Child Development 57, 461-473.

Masters, L., & Marsh, G. E. (1978). Middle ear pathology as a factor in learning disabilities. Journal of Learning Disabilities 11, 103-106.

Maziade, M., Cote, R., Boudreault, M., Thivierge, J., & Boutin, P. (1986). Family correlates of temperament continuity and change across middle childhood. American Journal of Orthopsychiatry 56, 195-203.

McCown, D. E. (1984). Moral development in children. Pediatric Nursing 10, 42-44.

McGuire, W. J., McGuire, C. V., Child, P., & Fujioka, T. (1978). Salience of ethnicity in the spontaneous self-concept as a function of one's ethnic distinctiveness in the social environment. Journal of Personality and Social Psychology 36, 511-520.

McLaughlin, B. E. (1975). Mental and emotional disturbances of school-age children: The exceptional and middle school-age child. Journal of School Health 45, 217-220.

McWhirter, L., Young, V., & Majury, J. (1983). Belfast children's awareness of violent death. British Journal of Social Psychology 22, 81-92.

Meacham, J. A. (1984). The social basis of intentional action. Human Development 27, 119-124.

Mehta, M. N., Munshi, N. N., & Krishnan, P. (1983). Adoptions: Follow-up from an orphanage in Bombay. Child Abuse and Neglect 7, 79-82.

Meyer, B. (1980). The development of girls' sex-role attitudes. Child Development 51, 508-514.

Meyer, N. (1985). Lost boys wandering around the Peter pantheon. In S. C. Feinstein, et al. (Eds.), Adolescent psychiatry: Developmental and clinical studies (Vol. 12, pp. 46-58). Chicago: University of Chicago Press.

Meyer-Bahlburg, H. F. (1985). Gender identity disorder of childhood. Introduction. Journal of the American Academy of Child Psychiatry 24, 681-683.

Milgram, R. M., Yitzhak, V., & Milgram, N. A. (1977). Creative activity and sex-role identity in elementary school children. Perceptual and Motor Skills 45, 371-376.

Milrod, D. (1982). The wished-for self image. In A. Solnit, et al. (Eds.), Psychoanalytic study of the child (Vol. 37, pp. 95-120). New Haven: Yale University Press.

Molla, P. M. (1981). Self-concept in children with and without physical disabilities. Journal of Psychiatric Nursing and Mental Health Services 19, 22-27.

Mondell, S., & Tyler, F. B. (1981). Child psychosocial competence and its measurement. Journal of Pediatric Psychology 6, 145-154.

Money, J. (1986). Longitudinal studies in clinical psychoendocrinology: Methodology. Journal of Developmental and Behavioral Pediatrics 7, 31-34.

Moses, R. (1978). Adult psychic trauma: The questions of early predisposition and some detailed mechanisms. International Journal of Psycho-Analysis 59, 353-363.

Moskowitz, D. S., Schwartzman, A. E., & Ledingham, J. E. (1985). Stability and change in aggression and withdrawal in middle childhood and early adolescence. Journal of Abnormal Psychology 94, 30-41.

Neubauer, P. B. (1980). The life cycle as indicated by the nature of the transference in the psychoanalysis of children. International Journal of Psycho-Analysis 61, 137-144.

Nippold, M. A., Leonard, L. B., & Kail, R. (1984). Syntactic and conceptual factors in children's understanding of metaphors. Journal of Speech and Hearing Research 27, 197-205.

Orbach, I., Gross, Y., Glaubman, H., & Berman, D. (1985). Children's perception of death in humans and animals as a function of age, anxiety and cognitive ability. Journal of Child Psychology and Psychiatry and Allied Disciplines 26, 453-463.

Orton, G. L. (1982). A comparative study of children's worries. Journal of Psychology 110, 153-162.

Orvaschel, H., Mednick, S., Schulsinger, F., & Rock, D. (1979). The children of psychiatrically disturbed parents: Differences as a function of the sex of the sick parent. Archives of General Psychiatry 36, 691-695.

Palmer, A. J. (1984). Tom Sawyer: Early parent loss. Bulletin of the Menninger Clinic 48, 155-169.

Papenfuss, R. L., Curtis, J. D., Beier, B. J., & Menze, J. D. (1983). Teaching positive self-concepts in the classroom. Journal of School Health 53, 618-620.

Parmelee, A. H. (1985). Comments on teaching developmental pediatrics and behavioral pediatrics. Journal of Developmental and Behavioral Pediatrics 6, 227-228.

Patten, M. D. (1983). Relationships between self-esteem, anxiety, and achievement in young learning disabled students. Journal of Learning Disabilities 16, 43-45.

Peckham, C. S., & Sheridan, M. D. (1976). Follow-up at 11 years of 46 children with severe unilateral hearing loss at 7 years. Child: Care, Health and Development 2, 107-111.

Penman, K. A., Christopher, J. R., & Wood, G. S. (1977). Using gross motor activity to improve language arts concepts by third grade students. Research Quarterly 48, 134-137.

Peterson, C. C., Peterson, J. L., & Seeto, D. (1983). Developmental changes in ideas about lying. Child Development 54, 1529-1535.

Pfeffer, C. R., Plutchik, R., & Mizruchi, M. S. (1983). Predictors of assaultiveness in latency age children. American Journal of Psychiatry 140, 31-35.

Phillips, D. (1984). The illusion of incompetence among academically competent children. Child Development 55, 2000-2016.

Pickar, D. B. (1986). Psychosocial aspects of learning disabilities. A review of research. Bulletin of the Menninger Clinic 50, 22-32.

Pihl, R. O., & McLarnon, L. D. (1984). Learning disabled children as adolescents. Journal of Learning Disabilities 17, 96-100.

Plank, E. N., & Plank, R. (1978). Children and death: As seen through art and autobiographies. In A. Solnit, et al. (Eds.), Psychoanalytic study of the child (Vol. 33, pp. 593-620). New Haven: Yale University Press.

Rae-Grant, Q. (1976). New family structure and the latency child. Canadian Psychiatric Association Journal 21, 197-198.

Richardson, S. A., Koller, H., & Katz, M. (1985). Continuities and change in behavior disturbance: A follow-up study of mildly retarded young children. American Journal of Orthopsychiatry 55, 220-229.

Richardson, S. A., Koller, H., & Katz, M. (1986). Factors leading to differences in the school performance of boys and girls. Journal of Developmental and Behavioral Pediatrics 7, 49-55.

Richmond, J. B. (1985). Coming of age: Developmental pediatrics in the late twentieth century. Journal of Developmental and Behavioral Pediatrics 6, 181-187.

Richter, H. E. (1976). The role of family life in child development. International Journal of Psycho-Analysis 57, 385-395.

Roe, K. V., McClure, A., & Roe, A. (1983). Infant Gesell scores vs. cognitive skills at age 12 years. Journal of Genetic Psychology 142, 143-147.

Rothman, G. R. (1976). The influence of moral reasoning on behavioral choices. Child Development 47, 397-406.

Rubin, J. A., Schachter, J., & Ragins, N. (1983). Intraindividual variability in human figure drawings: A developmental study. American Journal of Orthopsychiatry 53, 654-667.

Sandler, I. (1985). Children's environments and mental health: Opportunity and responsibility. American Journal of Community Psychology 13, 335-337.

Santrock, J. W. (1975). Father absence, perceived, maternal behavior, and moral development in boys. Child Development 46, 753-757.

Sarnoff, C. A. (1978-1979). Developmental considerations in the psychotherapy of latency-age children. International Journal of Psychoanalytic Psychotherapy 7, 283-304.

Satterfield, J. H., Cantwell, D. P., Schell, A., & Blaschke, T. (1979). Growth of hyperactive children treated with methylphenidate. Archives of General Psychiatry 36, 212-217.

Selman, R. L., & Demorest, A. P. (1984). Observing troubled children's interpersonal negotiation strategies: Implications of and for a developmental model. Child Development 55, 288-304.

Selman, R. L., Jaquette, D., & Lavin, D. R. (1977). Interpersonal awareness in children: Toward an integration of developmental and clinical child psychology. American Journal of Orthopsychiatry 47, 264-274.

Seymour, H. N., & Ralabate, P. K. (1985). The acquisition of a phonologic feature of Black English. Journal of Communication Disorders 18, 139-148.

Shapiro, T., & Perry, R. (1976). Latency revisited. The age 7 plus or minus 1. In R. S. Eissler, et al. (Eds.), Psychoanalytic study of the child (Vol. 31, pp. 79-105). New York: International Universities Press.

Shaw, L., Levine, M. D., & Belfer, M. (1982). Developmental double jeopardy: A study of clumsiness and self esteem in children with learning problems. Journal of Developmental and Behavioral Pediatrics 3, 191-196.

Shengold, L. (1981). Insight as metaphor. In A. Solnit, et al. (Eds.), Psychoanalytic study of the child (Vol. 36, pp. 289-306). New Haven: Yale University Press.

Siegal, M. (1985). Mother-child relations and the development of empathy: A short-term longitudinal study. Child Psychiatry and Human Development 16, 77-86.

Siegel, A. E. (1984). Working mothers and their children. Journal of the American Academy of Child Psychiatry 23, 486-488.

Silva, P. A., Justin, C., McGee, R., & Williams, S. M. (1984). Some developmental and behavioural characteristics of seven-year-old children with delayed speech development. British Journal of Disorders of Communication 19, 147-154.

Smith, W. P., & Rossman, B. B. (1986). Developmental changes in trait and situational denial under stress during childhood. Journal of Child Psychology and Psychiatry and Allied Disciplines 27, 227-235.

Solnit, A. J., & Newman, L. M. (1984). Anna Freud: The child expert. In A. Solnit, et al. (Eds.), Psychoanalytic study of the child (Vol. 39, pp. 45-63). New Haven: Yale University Press.

Solomon, S. B. (1986). Children with short stature. Journal of Pediatric Nursing 1, 80-89.

Sreenivasan, U. (1985). Effeminate boys in a child psychiatric clinic: Prevalence and associated factors. Journal of the American Academy of Child Psychiatry 24, 689-694.

Stainton, M. C. (1980). The effect of ordinal position or birth order on child development. Nursing Forum 19, 165-179.

Stilwell, B. M., & Galvin, M. (1985). Conceptualization of conscience in 11-12-year-olds. Journal of the American Academy of Child Psychiatry 24, 630-636.

Stingle, S. F., & Cook, H. (1985). Age and sex differences in the cooperative and noncooperative behavior of pairs of American children. Journal of Psychology 119, 335-345.

Stoller, R. J., & Herdt, G. H. (1982). The development of masculinity: A cross-cultural contribution. Journal of the American Psychoanalytic Association 30, 29-59.

Strunk, C. S., & Witkin, L. J. (1974). The transformation of a latency-age girls' group from unstructured play to problem-focused discussion. International Journal of Group Psychotherapy 24, 460-470.

Sunseri, A. J., Alberti, J. M., Kent, N. D., Schoenberger, J. A., Sunseri, J. K., Amuwo, S., & Vickers, P. (1983). Reading, demographic, social and psychological factors related to pre-adolescent smoking and non-smoking behaviors and attitudes. Journal of School Health 53, 257-263.

Taylor, J. J., & Achenbach, T. M. (1975). Moral and cognitive development in retarded and nonretarded children. American Journal of Mental Deficiency 80, 43-50.

Terry, G. E. (1975). The separation-individuation process in same-sex twins: A review of the literature. Maternal-Child Nursing Journal 4, 128-141.

Terry, R. L., Berg, A. J., & Phillips, P. E. (1983). The effect of eyeglasses on self-esteem. Journal of the American Optometry Association 54, 947-949.

Thomas, A., & Chess, S. (1972). Development in middle childhood. Seminars in Psychiatry 4, 331-341.

Ullian, D. (1984). Who girls are good: A constructivist view. American Journal of Orthopsychiatry 54, 71-82.

van der Velde, C. D. (1985). Body images of one's self and of others: Developmental and clinical significance. American Journal of Psychiatry 142, 527-537.

Wadden, T. A., Foster, G. D., Brownell, K. D., & Finley, E. (1984). Self-concept in obese and normal-weight children. Journal of Consulting and Clinical Psychology 52, 1104-1105.

Weiss, R. S. (1985). Men and the family. Family Process 24, 49-58.

Wolf, T. M., Hunter, S. M., & Webber, L. S. (1979). Psychosocial measures and cardiovascular risk factors in children and adolescents. Journal of Psychology 101, 139-146.

Yorke, C. (1983). Clinical notes on developmental pathology. In A. Solnit, et al. (Eds.), Psychoanalytic study of the child (Vol. 38, pp. 389-402). New Haven: Yale University Press.

Zuger, B. (1984). Early effeminate behavior in boys. Outcome and significance for homosexuality. Journal of Nervous and Mental Disease 172, 90-97.

D. Prevention and Early Intervention

Justin Call, M.D., Section Editor

1. Prevention and Early Intervention

Berlin, I. N. (1986). Prevention of psychiatric disorder in American Indian children and adolescents. In J. Noshpitz (Ed.), Basic handbook of child psychiatry (Vol. 5). New York: Basic Books.

Brazelton, T. B. (1985). Why early intervention. In J. D. Call, E. Galenson, & R. L. Tyson (Eds.), Frontiers of infant psychiatry. New York: Basic Books.

Greenspan, S. I., & White, K. R. (1986). Conducting research with preventive early intervention programs. In J. Noshpitz (Ed.), Basic handbook of child psychiatry (Vol. 5, pp. 554-564). New York: Basic Books.

Notman, M. T., Nadelson, C. C., Sauzier, M., & Gean, M. P. (1986). Preventive programs with pregnant teenagers and young mothers. In J. Noshpitz (Ed.), Basic handbook of child psychiatry (Vol. 5, pp. 590-599). New York: Basic Books.

Nurcombe, B., Rauh, V., Howell, D. C., Teti, D. M., Ruoff, P., Murphy, B., & Brennan, J. (1985). An intervention program for mothers of low-birthweight babies: Outcome at six and twelve months. In J. D. Call, E. Galenson, & R. L. Tyson (Eds.), Frontiers of infant psychiatry. New York: Basic Books.

Soule, M. (1985). Medical and nursing staff at risk: Very early prevention of psychosomatic illness in infancy. In J. D. Call, E. Galenson, & R. L. Tyson (Eds.), Frontiers of infant psychiatry. New York: Basic Books.

White, K. R., & Greenspan, S. I. (1986). An overview of the effectiveness of preventive early intervention programs. In J. Noshpitz (Ed.), Basic handbook of child psychiatry (Vol. 5, pp. 541-553). New York: Basic Books.

2. Psychiatric Factors in Development

Call, J. D. (1978). Differential vulnerability and coping in boys and girls at birth. In E. J. Anthony, C. Koupernik, & C. Chiland (Eds.), The child in his family: Vulnerable children. (Vol. 4, pp. 145-172). New York: Wiley.

Call, J. D. (1987). Psychiatric syndromes of infancy. In J. Noshpitz (Ed.), Basic handbook of child psychiatry (Vol. 5, pp. 242-262). New York: Basic Books.

Chatoor, I., & Egan, J. (1986). Etiology and diagnosis of failure to thrive and growth disorders in infants and children. In J. Noshpitz (Ed.), Basic handbook of child psychiatry (Vol. 5, pp. 272-279). New York: Basic Books.

Cytryn, L., & McKnew, D. H., Jr. (1986). Childhood depression: An update. In J. Noshpitz (Ed.), Basic handbook of child psychiatry (Vol. 5, pp. 286-293). New York: Basic Books.

Galdston, R. (1985). Teasing as an inducer of violence. In J. D. Call, E. Galenson, & R. L. Tyson (Eds.), Frontiers of infant psychiatry. New York: Basic Books.

Gislason, I. L., & Call, J. D. (1982). Dogbite in infancy: Trauma and personality development. A case report. Journal of the American Academy of Child Psychiatry 21, 203-207.

Goodwin, J. (1986). Developmental impacts of incest. In J. D. Call, E. Galenson, & R. L. Tyson (Eds.), Frontiers of infant psychiatry. New York: Basic Books.

Lourie, I. S., & Blick, L. C. (1986). Child sexual abuse. In J. Noshpitz (Ed.), Basic handbook of child psychiatry (Vol. 5, pp. 280-283). New York: Basic Books.

Solnit, A. J., & Call, J. D. (1979). Psychosexual development: Five to ten years. In J. D. Call, J. Noshpitz, & R. L. Cohen (Eds.), Basic handbook of child psychiatry (Vol. 1, pp. 184-190). New York: Basic Books.

Terr, L. C. (1986). Childhood psychic trauma. In J. Noshpitz (Ed.), Basic handbook of child psychiatry (Vol. 5, pp. 262-271). New York: Basic Books.

E. Early Treatment

Justin Call, M.D., Section Editor

1. Treatment of Disorders in Infancy

Fraiberg, S., Shapiro, V., & Cherniss, D. (1983). Treatment modalities. In J. D. Call, E. Galenson, & R. L. Tyson (Eds.), Frontiers of infant psychiatry. New York: Basic Books.

Gorski, P. A. (1983). Premature infant behavioral and physiological responses to caregiving interventions in the intensive care nursery. In J. D. Call, E. Galenson, & R. L. Tyson (Eds.), Frontiers of infant psychiatry. New York: Basic Books.

Herzog, J. M. (1983). A neonatal intensive care syndrome: A pain complex involving neuroplasticity and psychic trauma. In J. D. Call, E. Galenson, & R. L. Tyson (Eds.), Frontiers of infant psychiatry. New York: Basic Books.

Nachman, P. A., & Stern, D. N. (1985). Affect retrieval: A form of recall memory in prelinguistic infants. In J. D. Call, E. Galenson, & R. L. Tyson (Eds.), Frontiers of infant psychiatry. New York: Basic Books.

Parmelee, A. H., Beckwith, L., Cohen, S. E., & Sigman, M. (1983). Social influences on infants at medical risk for behavioral difficulties. In J. D. Call, E. Galenson, & R. L. Tyson (Eds.), Frontiers of infant psychiatry. New York: Basic Books.

Prugh, D. G., Jordan, K., Beresford, T. P., Marshall, P., Black, D., & Wood, D. (1983). Hypertrophic pyloric stenosis in infancy: Innate and experiential factors. In J. D. Call, E. Galenson, & R. L. Tyson (Eds.), Frontiers of infant psychiatry. New York: Basic Books.

Sander, L. W. (1983). A twenty-five-year follow-up of the Pavenstedt Longitudinal Research Project, its relation to early intervention. In J. D. Call, E. Galenson, & R. L. Tyson (Eds.), Frontiers of infant psychiatry. New York: Basic Books.

Sanders-Woudstra, J. A. R., Visser, H. K. A., De Raeymaecker, D. M. J., Skoda, I., & Uleman-Vleeschdrager, M. (1983). Low-birthweight children in their first two years of life and their difficulties. In J. D. Call, E. Galenson, & R. L. Tyson (Eds.), Frontiers of infant psychiatry. New York: Basic Books.

Seitz, V., Rosenbaum, L. K., & Apfel, N. H. (1985). Effects of family support intervention: A ten-year follow-up. Child Development 56, 387-391.

Stern, D. N., Barnett, R. K., & Spieker, S. (1983). Early transmission of affect: Some research issues. In J. D. Call, E. Galenson, & R. L. Tyson (Eds.), Frontiers of infant psychiatry. New York: Basic Books.

F. Books

Justin Call, M.D., Section Editor

1. Important Books and Papers on Development

Bowlby, J. (1982). Attachment and loss. Vols. 1, 2, 3 (2nd eds.). New York: Basic Books.

Bretherton, I., & Waters, E. (Eds.). (1985). Growing points in attachment theory and research. Monographs of the Society for Research in Child Development (Vol. 50). Chicago: University of Chicago Press.

Call, J., Galenson, E., & Tyson, R. L. (Eds.). (1983). Frontiers of infant psychiatry. Vol. 1. New York: Basic Books.

Call, J., Galenson, E., & Tyson, R. L. (Eds.). (1985). Frontiers of infant psychiatry. Vol. 2. New York: Basic Books.

Erikson, E. H. (1950). Childhood society. New York: Norton.

Freud, A. (1965a). Normality and pathology in childhood. New York: International Universities Press.

Freud, A. (1965b). The psychoanalytic view of childhood: Long distance and close up. Normality and pathology in childhood: Assessment of development. New York: International Universities Press.

Freud, S. (1926). Inhibitions, symptoms and anxiety. In E. Jones (Ed.), Collected papers. Standard edition. Vol. 20. New York and London: Hogarth Press.

Garmezy, N., & Rutter, M. (1983). Stress, coping and development in children. New York: McGraw-Hill.

Kagan, J. (1984). The nature of the child. New York: Basic Books.

Mahler, M. S. (1974). Symbiosis and individuation. In R. S. Eissler, et al. (Eds.), Psychoanalytic study of the child (Vol. 29, pp. 39-106). New York: International Universities Press.

Mahler, M., & Pine, F. (1975). The psychological birth of the human infant. New York: Basic Books.

Osofsky, J. D. (Ed.). (1987). Handbook of infant development. New York: Wiley.

Provence, S., & Lipton, R. (1962). Infants in institutions. New York: International Universities Press.

Spitz, R. A. (1946). Anaclitic depression. In R. S. Eissler, et al. (Eds.), Psychoanalytic study of the child (Vol. 2, pp. 313-342). New York: International Universities Press.

Spitz, R. A., & Wolf, K. M. (1949). Autoeroticism: Some empirical findings and hypothesis on three of its manifestations in the first year of life. In R. S. Eissler, et al. (Eds.), Psychoanalytic study of the child (Vol. 3, pp. 4, 85-120). New York: International Universities Press.

Stern, D. N. (1985). The interpersonal world of the infant. New York: Basic Books.

Winnicott, D. W. (1953). Transitional objects and transitional phenomena. International Journal of Psycho-Analysis 34, 89-97.

Woelder, R. (1933). The psychoanalytic theory of play. Psychoanalytic Quarterly 2, 208-224.

G. Adolescent Development

Brian McConville, M.D., Section Editor

1. Historical References

Anthony, E. J. (1969). The reactions of adults to adolescents and their behavior. In G. Caplan & S. Lebovici (Eds.), Adolescence: Psychosocial perspectives (pp. 54-78). New York: Basic Books.
Baittle, B., & Offer, D. (1971). On the nature of male adolescent rebellion. Annals of the American Society for Adolescent Psychiatry 1, 139-160.
Berman, S. (1970). Alienation: An essential process of the psychology of adolescence. Journal of the American Academy of Child Psychiatry 9, 233-250.
Blos, P. (1962). On adolescence: A psychoanalytic interpretation. New York: The Free Press.
Erikson, E. H. (1968). Identity, youth and crisis. New York: Norton.
Freeman, D. M. A. (1968). Adolescent crises of the Kiowa-Apache Indian male. In E. B. Brody (Ed.), Minority group adolescents in the United States (pp. 157-204). Baltimore: Williams and Wilkins.
Freud, A. (1969). Adolescence as a developmental disturbance. In G. Caplan & S. Lebovici (Eds.), Adolescence: Psychosocial perspective (pp. 5-10). New York: Basic Books.
Greenacre, P. (1970). Youth, growth, and violence. In R. S. Eissler, et al. (Eds.), Psychoanalytic study of the child (Vol. 25, pp. 340-359). New York: International Universities Press.
Hart, M., & Sarnoff, C. A. (1971). The impact of the menarche: A study of two stages of organization. Journal of the American Academy of Child Psychiatry 10, 257-271.
Hollingshead, A. B. (1961). Elmtown's youth. New York: Science Editions.
Keniston, K. (1971a). Youth and dissent. New York: Harcourt, Brace, Jovanovich.
Keniston, K. (1971b). Youth as a stage of life. Annals of the American Society for Adolescent Psychiatry 1, 161-175.
Laufer, M. (1966). Object loss and mourning during adolescence. In R. S. Eissler, et al. (Eds.), Psychoanalytic study of the child (Vol. 21, pp. 269-293). New York: International Universities Press.
Lidz, T. F. (1969). The adolescent and his family. In G. Caplan & S. Lebovici (Eds.), Adolescence: Psychosocial perspective (pp. 105-112). New York: Basic Books.
Marcus, I. M. (1969). From school to work: Certain aspects of psychosocial interaction. In G. Caplan & S. Lebovici (Eds.), Adolescence: Psychosocial perspective (pp. 157-164). New York: Basic Books.

Mays, J. B. (1971). The adolescent as a social being. In J. G. Howells (Ed.), Modern perspectives in adolescent psychiatry (pp. 126-151). Edinburgh: Oliver and Boyd.
Mead, M. (1939). From the South Seas: Studies of adolescence and sex in primitive societies. New York: Morrow.
Noshpitz, J. D. (1979). Certain cultural and familial factors contributing to adolescent alienation. Journal of the American Academy of Child Psychiatry 9, 216-223.
Offer, D., & Offer, J. (1971). Four issues in the developmental psychology of adolescent. In J. G. Howells (Ed.), Modern perspectives in adolescent psychiatry (pp. 28-44). Edinburgh: Oliver and Boyd.
Piaget, J. (1969). The intellectual development of the adolescent. In G. Caplan & S. Lebovici (Eds.), Adolescence: Psychosocial perspective (pp. 22-26). New York: Basic Books.
Pierce, C. M. (1968). Problems of the Negro adolescent in the next decade. In E. B. Brody (Ed.), Minority group adolescents in the United States (pp. 17-47). Baltimore: Williams and Wilkins.
Schonfeld, W. A. (1969). The body and the body-image in adolescents. In G. Caplan & S. Lebovici (Eds.), Adolescence: Psychosocial perspective (pp. 27-53). New York: Basic Books.
Shaffer, C. & Pine, F. (1972). Pregnancy, abortion, and the developmental tasks of adolescence. Journal of the American Academy of Child Psychiatry 11, 511-536.

2. Current Issues

Abramowitz, R. H., Petersen, A. C., & Schulenberg, J. E. (1984). Changes if self-image during early adolescence. New Directions for Mental Health Services 1, 19-28.
Adams, G. R. (1985). Family correlates of female adolescents ego-identity development. Journal of Adolescence 8, 69-82.
Adams, G. R., Ryan, J. H., Hoffman, J. J., Dobson, W. R., & Nielsen, E. C. (1984). Ego identity status, conformity behavior, and personality in late adolescence. Journal of Personalality and Social Psychology 47, 1091-1104.
Adler, I., & Kandel, D. B. (1981). Cross-cultural perspectives on developmental stages in adolescent drug use. Journal of Studies on Alcohol 42, 701-715.
Ahlgren, A., & Norem-Hebeisen, A. A. (1979). Self-esteem patterns distinctive of groups of drug abusing and other dysfunctional adolescents. International Journal of the Addictions 14, 759-777.
Andolina, C. (1980). Syntactic maturity and vocabulary richness of learning disabled children at four age levels. Journal of Learning Disabilities 13, 372-377.
Anthony, E. J. (1982). Normal adolescent development from a cognitive viewpoint. Journal of the American Academy of Child Psychiatry 21, 318-327.
Antonucci, T., Gillett, N., & Hoyer, F. W. (1979). Values and self-esteem in three generations of men and women. Journal of Gerontology 34, 415-422.
Arnstein, R. L. (1989). Overview of normal transition to young adulthood. In S. C. Feinstein, et al. (Eds.), Adolescent psychiatry: Developmental and clinical studies (Vol. 16, pp. 127-141). Chicago: University of Chicago Press.

Ashway, J. A. (1980). The changing needs of female adolescents. In S. C. Feinstein, et al. (Eds.), Adolescent psychiatry: Developmental and clinical studies (Vol. 8, pp. 482-498). Chicago: University of Chicago Press.

Bailey, G. W. (1989). Current perspectives of substance abuse in youth. Journal of the American Academy of Child and Adolescent Psychiatry 28, 151-162.

Bart, W. M. (1983). Adolescent thinking and the quality of life. Adolescence 18, 875-888.

Bassoff, B. Z., & Ortiz, E. T. (1984). Teen women: Disparity between cognitive values and anticipated life events. Child Welfare 63, 125-138.

Battista, J. R. (1982). Empirical test of Vaillant's hierarchy of ego function. American Journal of Psychiatry 139, 356-357.

Battle, J. (1980). Relationship between self-esteem and depression among high school students. Perceptual and Motor Skills 51, 157-158.

Baumeister, R. F., Shapiro, J. P., & Tice, D. M. (1985). Two kinds of identity crisis. Journal of Personality 53, 407-424.

Baumrind, D. (1985). Familial antecedents of adolescent drug use: A developmental perspective. National Institute on Drug Abuse Research Monograph Series 56, 13-44.

Baumrind, D., & Moselle, K. A. (1985). A development perspective on adolescent drug abuse. Advances in Alcohol and Substance Abuse 4, 41-67.

Becker, T. (1976). Self and social responsibility: A comparative view of American and Israeli youth. American Journal of Psychoanalysis 36, 155-162.

Beit-Hallahmi, B. (1977). Identity integration, self-image crisis and "superego victory" in postadolescent university students. Adolescence 12, 57-64.

Belsky, J. (1984). The determinants of parenting: A process model. Child Development 55, 83-96.

Benson, R. M. (1980). Narcissistic guardians: Developmental aspects of transitional objects, imaginary companions, and career fantasies. In S. C. Feinstein, et al. (Eds.), Adolescent psychiatry: Developmental and clinical studies (Vol. 8, pp. 253-264). Chicago: University of Chicago Press.

Berg, D. H. (1985). Reality construction at the family/society interface: The internalization of family themes and values. Adolescence 20, 605-618.

Berlin, I. N. (1978a). Developmental issues in the psychiatric hospitalization of children. American Journal of Psychiatry 135, 1044-1048.

Berlin, I. N. (1978b). Some implications of the development process for treatment of depression in adolescence. Journal of Adolescence 1, 135-145.

Berlin, I. N. (1978c). Anglo adoptions of Native Americans: Repercussions in adolescence. Journal of the American Academy of Child Psychiatry 17, 387-388.

Berlin, I. N. (1979). A developmental approach to work with disorganized families. Journal of the American Academy of Child Psychiatry 18, 354-365.

Berlin, I. N. (1980). Opportunities in adolescence to rectify developmental failures. In S. C. Feinstein, et al. (Eds.), Adolescent psychiatry: Developmental and clinical studies (Vol. 8, pp. 231-243). Chicago: University of Chicago

Development

Bird, H., Canino, G., Rubio-Stipec, M., et al. (1988). Estimates of the prevalence of childhood maladjustment in a community sample in Puerto Rico. Archives of General Psychiatry 45, 1120-1126.

Black, C., & DeBlassie, R. R. (1985). Adolescent pregnancy: Contributing factors, consequences, treatment, and plausible solutions. Adolescence 20, 281-290.

Blos, P. (1980). Modifications in the traditional psychoanalytic theory of female adolescent development. In S. C. Feinstein, et al. (Eds.), Adolescent psychiatry: Developmental and clinical studies (Vol. 8, pp. 8-25). Chicago: University of Chicago Press.

Blos, P. (1989). Masculinity: Developmental aspects of adolescence. In S. C. Feinstein, et al. (Eds.), Adolescent psychiatry: Developmental and clinical studies (Vol. 16, pp. 5-15). Chicago: University of Chicago Press.

Blotcky, A. D. (1984). A framework for assessing the psychologic functioning of adolescents. Journal of Developmental and Behavioral Pediatrics 5, 74-77.

Blotcky, M. J., & Looney, J. G. (1980). Normal female and male adolescent psychological development: An overview of theory and research. In S. C. Feinstein, et al. (Eds.), Adolescent psychiatry: Developmental and clinical studies (Vol. 8, pp. 184-199). Chicago: University of Chicago Press.

Botvin, G. J. (1983). Prevention of adolescent substance abuse through the development of personal and social competence. National Institute on Drug Abuse Research Monograph Series 47, 115-140.

Bowlby, J. (1988). Developmental psychiatry comes of age. American Journal of Psychiatry 145, 1-10.

Brent, D. A., Perper, J. A., Goldstein, C. E., et al. (1988). Risk factors for adolescent suicide. Archives of General Psychiatry 45, 581-588.

Brodzinsky, D. M., Singer, L. M., & Braff, A. M. (1984). Children's understanding of adoption. Child Development 55, 869-878.

Brooks, B. (1985). Sexually abused children and adolescent identity development. American Journal of Psychotherapy 39, 401-410.

Broughton, J. M. (1981). The divided self in adolescence. Human Development 24, 13-32.

Brown, T., Cash, T. F., & Lewis, R. J. (1989). Body-image disturbances in adolescent female binge-purgers: A brief report of the results of a national survey in the USA. Journal of Child Psychology and Psychiatry and Allied Disciplines 30, 605-613.

Burch, C. A. (1985). Identity foreclosure in early adolescence: A problem of narcissistic equilibrium. In S. C. Feinstein, et al. (Eds.), Adolescent psychiatry: Developmental and clinical studies (Vol. 12, pp. 145-161). Chicago: University of Chicago Press.

Burke, E. L., Zilberg, N. J., Amini, F., Salasnek, S., & Forkin, D. (1978). Some empirical evidence for Erikson's concept of negative identity in delinquent adolescent drug abusers. Comprehensive Psychiatry 19, 141-152.

Butcher, J. (1983). Socialization of adolescent girls into physical activity. Adolescence 18, 753-766.

Camp, B. W., Burgess, D., Morgan, L., & Malpiede, D. (1984). Infants of adolescent mothers. Maternal characteristics and developmental status at 1 year of age. American Journal of Diseases of Children 138, 243-246.
Campagna, A. F., & Harter, S. (1975). Moral judgment in sociopathic and normal children. Journal of Personality and Social Psychology 31, 199-205.
Carlson, G. A., & Kashani, J. H. (1988). Phenomenology of major depression from childhood through adulthood: Analysis of three studies. American Journal of Psychiatry 145, 1222-1225.
Carlson, H. M., & Steuer, J. (1985). Age, sex-role categorization, and psychological health in American homosexual and heterosexual men and women. Journal of Social Psychology 125, 203-211.
Chabassol, D. J. (1978). Fear of success in high school girls as related to family composition. Psychological Reports 42, 889-890.
Chambliss, J., Muller, D., Hulnick, R., & Wood, M. (1978). Relationships between self-concept, self-esteem, popularity, and social judgments of junior high school students. Journal of Psychology 98, 91-98.
Chance, J. E., Turner, A. L., & Goldstein, A. G. (1982). Development of differential recognition for own- and other-race faces. Journal of Psychology 112, 29-37.
Chassin, L., Tetzloff, C., & Hershey, M. (1985). Self-image and social-image factors in adolescent alcohol use. Journal of Studies on Alcohol 46, 39-47.
Clarke, A. D., & Clarke, A. M. (1984). Constancy and change in the growth of human characteristics. Journal of Child Psychology and Psychiatry and Allied Disciplines 25, 191-210.
Clifford, R. (1978). Development of masturbation in college women. Archives of Sexual Behavior 7, 559-573.
Clifford, R. E. (1978). Subjective sexual experience in college women. Archives of Sexual Behavior 7, 183-197.
Cohen, P., Velez, C. N., Brook, J., et al. (1989). Mechanisms of the relation between perinatal problems, early childhood illness, and psychopathology in late childhood and adolescence. Child Development 60, 701-709.
Colarusso, C. A. (1988). The development of time sense in adolescence. In A. Solnit, et al. (Eds.), Psychoanalytic study of the child (Vol. 43, pp. 179-197). New Haven: Yale University Press.
Coleman, E. (1981-1982). Developmental stages of the coming out process. Journal of Homosexuality 7, 31-43.
Conley, J. J. (1985). Longitudinal stability of personality traits: A multitrait-multimethod-multioccasion analysis. Journal of Personality and Social Psychology 49, 1266-1828.
Copeland, A. D. (1981). The impact of pregnancy on adolescent psychosocial development. In S. C. Feinstein, et al. (Eds.), Adolescent psychiatry: Developmental and clinical studies (Vol. 9, pp. 224-253). Chicago: University of Chicago Press.
Cvetkovich, G., Grote, B., Lieberman, E. J., & Miller, W. (1978). Sex role development and teenage fertility-related behavior. Adolescence 13, 231-236.

Development

D'Hondt, W., & Vandewiele, W. (1982). Retrospective considerations in training teachers regarding problems faced in adolescence. Adolescence 17, 855-861.

Daniels, D., Dunn, J., Furstenberg, F. F., & Plomin, R. (1985). Environmental differences within the family and adjustment differences within pairs of adolescent sibling. Child Development 56, 764-774.

Darling, C. A., & Hicks, M. W. (1983). Recycling parental sexual messages. Journal of Sex and Marital Therapy 9, 233-243.

Dashef, S. S. (1984). Aspects of identification and growth during late adolescence and young adulthood. American Journal of Psychotherapy 38, 239-247.

Dembo, R., Pilaro, L., Burgos, W., Des Jarlais, D. C., & Schmeidler, J. (1979). Self-concept and drug involvement among urban junior high school youths. International Journal of the Addictions 14, 1125-1144.

Dien, D. S. (1983). Big me and little me: A Chinese perspective on self. Psychiatry 46, 281-286.

Dixon, J. C., & Street, J. W. (1975). The distinction between self and not-self in children and adolescents. Journal of Genetic Psychology 127, 157-162.

Earls, F. (1989). Epidemiology and child psychiatry: Entering the second phase. American Journal of Orthopsychiatry 59, 279-283.

Egeland, B., Sroufe, L. A., & Erickson, M. (1983). The developmental consequence of different patterns of maltreatment. Child Development 55, 753-771.

Emans, S. J. (1983). The sexually active teenager. Journal of Developmental and Behavioral Pediatrics 4, 37-42.

Enright, R. D., Olson, L. M., Ganiere, D., Lapsley, D. K., & Buss, R. R. (1984). A clinical model for enhancing adolescent ego identity. Journal of Adolescence 7, 119-130.

Ensminger, M. E., Brown, C. H., & Kellam, S. G. (1984). Social control as an explanation of sex differences in substance use among adolescents. National Institute on Drug Abuse Research Monograph Series 49, 296-304.

Esman, A. H. (1985). A developmental approach to the psychotherapy of adolescent. In S. C. Feinstein, et al. (Eds.), Adolescent psychiatry: Developmental and clinical studies (Vol. 12, pp. 119-133). Chicago: University of Chicago Press.

Eyo, I. E. (1981). Relationship between social desirability and self-criticism in subgroups of male and female delinquents and non-delinquents. Psychological Reports 49, 711-716.

Farber, S. S., Felner, R. D., & Primavera, J. (1985). Parental separation/divorce and adolescents: An examination of factors mediating adaptation. American Journal of Community Psychology 13, 171-185.

Faust, M. S. (1977). Somatic development of adolescent girls. Monographs of the Society for Research in Child Development (Vol. 42, pp. 1-90). Chicago: University of Chicago Press.

Fischer, M., Rolf, J. E., Hasazi, J. E., & Commings, L. (1984). Follow-up of a preschool epidemiological sample: Cross-age continuities and predictions of later adjustment with internalizing and externalizing dimensions of behavior. Child Development 55, 137-150.

Flaherty, L. T. (1982). To love and/or to work: The ideological dilemma of young women. In S. C. Feinstein, et al. (Eds.), Adolescent psychiatry: Developmental and clinical studies (Vol. 10, pp. 41-51). Chicago: University of Chicago Press.

Flament, M. F., Whitaker, A., Rapoport, J. L., et al. (1988). Obsessive compulsive disorder in adolescence: An epidemiological study. Journal of the American Academy of Child and Adolescent Psychiatry 27, 764-771.

Fleck, J. R., Fuller, C. C., Malin, S. Z., Miller, D. H., & Acheson, K. R. (1980). Father psychological absence and heterosexual behavior, personal adjustment and sex-typing in adolescent girls. Adolescence 15, 847-860.

Fleming, M., & Feinbloom, D. (1984). Similarities in becoming transsexuals and adolescents. Adolescence 19, 729-748.

Flora, R. R. (1978). The effect of self concept upon adolescents; communication with parents. Journal of School Health 28, 100-102.

Foulds, G. A., & Bedford, A. (1977). Self-esteem and psychiatric syndromes. British Journal of Medical Psychology 50, 237-242.

Franzoi, S. (1985). Personality characteristics of the crosscountry hitchhiker. Adolescence 20, 655-668.

Friend, M. R. (1980). Vicissitudes of adolescent development and its relationship to young adulthood. Canadian Journal of Psychiatry 25, 377-380.

Friends and lovers in the college years. (1983). Public Group for the Advancement of Psychiatry 11, 1-120.

Frisancho, A. R., Matos, J., & Bollettino, L. A. (1984). Role of gynecological age and growth maturity status in fetal maturation and prenatal growth of infants born to young still-growing adolescent mothers. Human Biology 56, 583-593.

Frost, A. D. (1984). The use of rock music to assist adolescent sexual identity. Imprint 13, 36-42.

Furnham, A., & Kirris, R. (1983). Self-image disparity, ethnic identity and sex-role stereotypes in British and Cypriot adolescents. Journal of Adolescence 6, 275-292.

Gadpailler, W. J. (1983). Innate masculine/feminine traits: Their contributions to conflict. Journal of the American Academy of Psychoanalysis 11, 401-424.

Galler, J. R., Ramsey, F., & Solimano, G. (1985). A follow-up study of the effects of early malnutrition on subsequent development. II. Fine motor skills in adolescence. Pediatric Research 19, 524-527.

Garbarino, J., Sebes, J., & Schellenbach, C. (1984). Families at risk for destructive parent-child relations in adolescence. Child Development 55, 174-183.

Giovacchini, P. L. (1984). The psychoanalytic paradox: The self as a transitional object. Psychoanalytic Review 71, 881-894.

Goldberg, E. H. (1989). Severity of depression and developmental levels of psychological functioning in 8-16 year old girls. American Journal of Orthopsychiatry 59, 167-178.

Goldmeier, H. (1982). Children of the gilded ghetto in revolt: The early years, 1967-1974. Adolescence 17, 881-894.

Gooden, W., & Toye, R. (1984). Occupational dreams, relation to parents and depression in the early adult transition. Journal of Clinical Psychology 40, 945-954.

Gough, H. G. (1975). Personality factors related to reported severity of menstrual distress. Journal of Abnormal Psychology 84, 59-65.

Grossman, B., Wirt, R., & Davids, A. (1985). Self-esteem, ethnic identity, and behavioral adjustment among Anglo and Chicano adolescents in west Texas. Journal of Adolescence 8, 57-68.

Grotevant, H. D. (1979). Environmental influences on vocational interest development in adolescents from adoptive and biological families. Child Development 50, 854-860.

Grotevant, H. D., & Cooper, C. R. (1985). Patterns of interaction in family relationships and the development of identity exploration in adolescence. Child Development 56, 415-428.

Haber, C. H., Nitkin, R., & Shenker, I. R. (1979). Adverse reactions to hypnotherapy in obese adolescents: A developmental viewpoint. Psychiatric Quarterly 51, 55-63.

Hains, A. A., & Ryan, E. B. (1983). The development of social cognitive processes among juvenile delinquents and nondelinquent peers. Child Development 54, 1536-1544.

Hammen, C., Marks, T., deMayo, R., & Mayol, A. (1985). Self-schemas and risk for depression: A prospective study. Journal of Personality and Social Psychology 49, 1147-1159.

Hansen, S. L., & Darling, C. A. (1985). Attitudes of adolescents toward division of labor in the home. Adolescence 20, 61-72.

Harris, I. D., & Howard, K. I. (1984). On psychological resemblance: A questionnaire study of high school students. Psychiatry 47, 125-134.

Harris, P. L., Olthof, T., & Terwogt, M. M. (1981). Children's knowledge of emotion. Journal of Child Psychology and Psychiatry and Allied Disciplines 22, 247-261.

Hawkins, J. D., Lishner, D. M., & Catalano, R. F. (1985). Childhood predictors and the prevention of adolescent substance abuse. National Institute on Drug Abuse Research Monograph Series 56, 75-126.

Hawton, K. (1982). Attempted suicide in children and adolescents. Journal of Child Psychology and Psychiatry and Allied Disciplines 23, 297-503.

Hechtman, L. (1989). Teenage mothers and their children: Risks and problems--a review. Canadian Journal of Psychiatry 34, 569-575.

Held, L. (1981). Self-esteem and social network of the young pregnant teenager. Adolescence 16, 905-912.

Henderson, A. F. (1984). Homosexuality in the college years: Developmental differences between men and women. Journal of American College Health 32, 216-219.

Herold, E. S., Goodwin, M. S., & Lero, D. S. (1979). Self-esteem, locus of control, and adolescent contraception. Journal of Psychology 101, 83-88.

Hertsgaard, D., & Light, H. (1984). Adolescent females' perceived parental sex-role attributes. Psychological Reports 55, 253-254.

Hetherington, E. M. (1989). Coping with family transitions: Winners, losers and survivors. Child Development 60, 1-14.

Hodges, J., & Tizard, B. (1989). IQ and behavioral adjustment of institutional adolescents. Journal of Child Psychology and Psychiatry and Allied Disciplines 30, 53-75.

Hoover, M. L. (1984). The self-image of overweight adolescent females: A review of the literature. Maternal-Child Nursing Journal 13, 125-137.

Howe, C. L. (1986). Developmental theory and adolescent sexual behavior. Nurse Practitioner 11, 65, 68, 71.

Hummel, R., & Roselli, L. L. (1983). Identity status and academic achievement in female adolescents. Adolescence 18, 17-27.

Humphrey, M., & Lenham, C. (1984). Adolescent fantasy and self-fulfillment: The problem of female passivity. Journal of Adolescence 7, 295-304.

Jacobs, S. B., & Wagner, M. K. (1984). Obese and nonobese individuals: Behavioral and personality characteristics. Addictive Behaviors 9, 223-226.

Jessor, R. (1976). Predicting time of onset of marijuana use: A developmental study of high school youth. Journal of Consulting and Clinical Psychology 44, 125-134.

Jessor, R., & Jessor, S. L. (1975). Adolescent development and the onset of drinking. A longitudinal study. Journal of Studies on Alcohol 36, 27-51.

Joffe, R. T., Offord, D. R., & Boyle, M. H. (1988). Ontario Child Health Study: Suicidal behavior in youth age 12-16 years. American Journal of Psychiatry 145, 1420-1423.

Johnson, C. F., Loxterkamp, D., & Albanese, M. (1982). Effect of high school students' knowledge of child development and child health on approaches to child discipline. Pediatrics 69, 558-563.

Johnson, R. L. (1985). Black adolescents: Issues critical to their survival. Journal of the National Medical Association 77, 447-448.

Johnson, R. T., Johnson, D. W., & Rynders, J. (1981). Effect of cooperative, competitive, and individualistic experiences on self-esteem of handicapped and nonhandicapped students. Journal of Psychology 108, 31-34.

Kahle, L. R., Kulka, R. A., & Klingel, D. M. (1980). Low adolescent self-esteem leads to multiple interpersonal problems: A test of social adaptation theory. Journal of Personality and Social Psychology 39, 496-502.

Kandel, D. B. (1980). Developmental stages in adolescent drug involvement. National Institute on Drug Abuse Research Monograph Series 30, 120-127.

Kandel, D. B. (1985). On processes of peer influences in adolescent drug use: A developmental perspective. Advances in Alcohol and Substance Abuse 4, 139-163.

Kaplan, H. B., Martin, S. S., & Robbins, C. (1982). Application of a general theory of deviant behavior: Self-derogation and adolescent drug use. Journal of Health and Social Behavior 23, 274-294.

Kashani, J. H., Orvaschel, H., Rosenberg, T. K., et al. (1989). Psychopathology in a community sample of children and adolescents: A developmental perspective.

Journal of the American Academy of Child and Adolescent Psychiatry 28, 701-706.

Kauffman, C., Grunebaum, H., Cohler, B., & Gamer, E. (1979). Superkids: Competent children of psychotic mothers. American Journal of Psychiatry 136, 1398-1402.

Keil, T. J. (1980). Social correlates of female abstinence from marijuana: Results of a household survey. International Journal of the Addictions 15, 957-967.

Kellerman, J., Zeltzer, L., Ellenberg, L., Dash, J., & Rigler, D. (1980). Psychological effects of illness in adolescence. I. Anxiety, self-esteem, and perception of control. Journal of Pediatrics 97, 126-131.

Kestenbaum, G. I., & Weinstein, L. (1985). Personality, psychopathology, and developmental issues in male adolescent video game use. Journal of the American Academy of Child Psychiatry 24, 329-333.

Kester, P. A. (1984). Effects of prenatally administered 17 alpha-hydroxyprogesterone caproate on adolescent males. Archives of Sexual Behavior 13, 441-455.

Kipper, D. A., & Jaffe, Y. (1978). Dimensions of assertiveness: Factors underlying the college self-expression scale. Perceptual and Motor Skills 46, 47-52.

Kistner, J., White, K., Haskett, M., & Robbins, F. (1985). Development of learning-disabled and normally achieving children's causal attributions. Journal of Abnormal Child Psychology 13, 639-647.

Kitahara, M. (1983). Female puberty rites: Reconsideration and speculation. Adolescence 18, 957-964.

Klein, R. G., & Mannuzza, S. (1988). Hyperactive boys almost grown up. Archives of General Psychiatry 45, 1131-1134.

Kroger, J. (1985). Relationships during adolescence: A cross-national comparison of New Zealand and United States teenagers. Journal of Adolescence 8, 47-56.

Krueger, D. W. (1983). Childhood parent loss: Developmental impact and adult psychopathology. American Journal of Psychotherapy 37, 582-592.

La Gaipa, J. J. (1979). A developmental study of the meaning of friendship in adolescence. Journal of Adolescence 2, 201-213.

Laufer, M. E. (1982). Female masturbation in adolescence and the development of the relationship to the body. International Journal of Psycho-Analysis 63, 295-302.

Lawler, K. A., & Schmied, L. A. (1986). Cardiovascular responsivity, type A behavior, and parental history of heart disease in young women. Psychophysiology 23, 28-32.

Lawson, A. E., & Shepherd, G. D. (1979). Written language maturity and formal reasoning in male and female adolescents. Language and Speech 22, 117-127.

Lechner, C. R., & Rosenthal, D. A. (1984). Adolescent self-consciousness and the imaginary audience. Genetic Psychology Monographs 110, 289-305.

Leonardson, G. R. (1977). Relationship between self-concept and perceived physical fitness. Perceptual and Motor Skills 44, 62.

Lerner, R. M., Orlos, J. B., & Knapp, J. R. (1976). Physical attractiveness, physical effectiveness, and self-concept in late adolescents. Adolescence 11, 313-326.

Lewin, B. (1982). The adolescent boy and girl: First and other early experiences with intercourse from a representative sample of Swedish school adolescents. Archives of Sexual Behavior 11, 417-428.

Lewis, D. O., Lovely, R., Yeager, C., et al. (1989). Toward a theory of the genesis of violence: A follow-up study of delinquents. Journal of the American Academy of Child and Adolescent Psychiatry 28, 431-437.

Libow, J. A., & Doty, D. W. (1979). An exploratory approach to self-blame and self-derogation by rape victims. American Journal of Orthopsychiatry 49, 670-679.

Liebert, R. M. (1986). Effects of television on children and adolescents. Journal of Developmental and Behavioral Pediatrics 7, 43-48.

Litt, I. F. (1985). Know thyself--adolescents' self-assessment of compliance behavior. Pediatrics 75, 693-696.

Logan, R. D. (1983). A re-conceptualization of Erikson's identity stage. Adolescence 18, 943-946.

Lorr, M., & Manning, T. T. (1978). Personality correlates of the sex role types. Journal of Clinical Psychology 34, 884-888.

Louden, D. M. (1980). A comparative study of self-esteem among minority group adolescents in Britain. Journal of Adolescence 3, 17-23.

Magen, Z. (1983). Re-forming the boundaries: A trans-cultural comparison of positive experiences among adolescent males and females. Adolescence 18, 851-858.

Magrab, P. R., Shearin, R. B., Bronheim, S. M., Jones, R. L., & Ahmed, S. W. (1984). Georgetown adolescent psychosocial rating scale. Journal of Adolescent Health Care 5, 14-20.

Marschark, M., & Nall, L. (1985). Metaphoric competence in cognitive and language development. Advances in Child Development and Behavior 19, 49-81.

McBride, A. B. (1982). Obesity of women during the childbearing years: Psychosocial and physiologic aspects. Nursing Clinics of North America 17, 217-225.

McCabe, M. P., & Collins, J. K. (1983). The sexual and affectional attitudes and experiences of Australian adolescents during dating: The effects of age, church attendance, type of school, and socioeconomic class. Archives of Sexual Behavior 12, 525-539.

McClary, S. A., & Lubin, B. (1985). Effects of type of examiner, sex, and year in school on self report of drug use by high school students. Journal of Drug Education 15, 49-55.

McDermott, J. F., Robillard, A. B., Char, W. F., Hsu, J., Tseng, W. S., & Ashton, G. C. (1983). Reexamining the concept of adolescence: Difference between adolescent boys and girls in the context of their families. American Journal of Psychiatry 140, 1318-1322.

Mednick, R. A. (1977). Gender-specific variances in sexual fantasy. Journal of Personality Assessment 41, 248-254.

Mercer, R. T. (1986). The relationship of developmental variables to maternal behavior. Research in Nursing and Health 9, 25-33.

Merola, J. L., & Liederman, J. (1985). Developmental changes in hemispheric independence. Child Development 56, 1184-1194.

Miller, T. W. (1984). Paternal absence and its effect on adolescent self-esteem. International Journal of Social Psychiatry 30, 293-296.

Morris, L. W., Finkelstein, C. S., & Fisher, W. R. (1976). Components of school anxiety: Developmental trends and sex differences. Journal of Genetic Psychology 128, 49-57.

Moskowitz, D. S., Schwartzman, A. E., & Ledingham, J. E. (1985). Stability and change in aggression and withdrawal in middle childhood and early adolescence. Journal of Abnormal Psychology 94, 30-41.

Murray, D. M., & Perry, C. L. (1985). The prevention of adolescent drug abuse: Implications of etiological, developmental, behavioral, and environmental models. National Institute on Drug Abuse Research Monograph Series 56, 236-256.

Musser, J. M., & Fleck, J. R. (1983). The relationship of paternal acceptance and control to college females' personality adjustment. Adolescence 18, 907-916.

Newcomb, M. D., Huba, G. J., & Bentler, P. M. (1986). Determinants of sexual and dating behaviors among adolescents. Journal of Personality and Social Psychology 50, 428-438.

Newman, J. (1985). Adolescents: Why they can be so obnoxious. Adolescence 20, 635-646.

Nichtern, S. (1980). The missing adolescent. In S. C. Feinstein, et al. (Eds.), Adolescent psychiatry: Developmental and clinical studies (Vol. 8, pp. 54-64). Chicago: University of Chicago Press.

Norem-Hebeisen, A. A. (1976). A multidimensional construct of self-esteem. Journal of Educational Psychology 68, 559-565.

Norris, J., & Kunes-Connell, M. (1985). Self-esteem disturbance. Nursing Clinics of North America 20, 745-761.

Norvell, M., & Guy, R. F. (1977). A comparison of self-concept in adopted and non-adopted adolescents. Adolescence 12, 443-448.

Offer, D., Ostrov, E., & Howard, K. I. (1984). The self-image of normal adolescents. New Directions for Mental Health Services 1, 5-17.

Offer, D., Ostrov, E., & Howard, K. I. (1987). Epidemiology of mental health and mental illness among adolescents. [Introduction by J. D. Call]. In J. D. Noshpitz (Ed.), Basic handbook of child psychiatry (Vol. 5, pp. 82-88). New York: Basic Books.

Offord, D. R., Boyle, M. H., Fleming, J. E., et al. (1989). Ontario Child Health Study: Summary of selected results. Canadian Journal of Psychiatry 34, 483-491.

Olowu, A. A. (1983). A cross-cultural study of adolescent self-concept. Journal of Adolescence 6, 263-274.

Onyehalu, A. S. (1981). Identity crisis in adolescence. Adolescence 16, 629-632.

Otto, M. W., & Dougher, M. J. (1985). Sex differences and personality factors in responsivity to pain. Perceptual and Motor Skills 61, 383-390.

Overton, W. F., & Meehan, A. M. (1982). Individual differences in formal operational thought: Sex role and learned helplessness. Child Development 53, 1536-1543.

Parish, T. S., Baker, S. K., Arheart, K. L., & Adamchak, P. G. (1980). Normal and exceptional children's attitudes toward themselves and one another. Journal of Psychology 104, 249-253.

Parish, T. S., & Wigle, S. E. (1985). A longitudinal study of the impact of parental divorce on adolescents' evaluations of self and parents. Adolescence 20, 239-244.

Patten, M. A. (1981). Self concept and self esteem: Factors in adolescent pregnancy. Adolescence 16, 765-778.

Peck, D. G. (1981). Adolescent self-esteem, emotional learning disabilities, and significant others. In S. C. Feinstein, et al. (Eds.), Adolescent psychiatry: Developmental and clinical studies (Vol. 16, pp. 443-451). Chicago: University of Chicago Press.

Peterson, C. C., Peterson, J. L., & Seeto, D. (1983). Developmental changes in ideas about lying. Child Development 54, 1529-1535.

Pfeffer, C. R. (1988). Clinical dilemmas in the prevention of adolescent suicide behavior. In S. C. Feinstein, et al. (Eds.), Adolescent psychiatry: Developmental and clinical studies (Vol. 15, pp. 407-421). Chicago: University of Chicago Press.

Pontius, A. A. (1974). Basis for a neurological test of frontal lobe system functioning up to adolescence--a form analysis of action expressed in narratives. Adolescence 9, 221-232.

Power and authority in adolescence: The origins and resolutions of intergenerational conflict. (1978). Formulated by the committee on adolescence. Public Group for the Advancement of Psychiatry 10, 49-274.

Prawat, R. S. (1976). Mapping the affective domain in young adolescents. Journal of Educational Psychology 68, 566-572.

Prerost, F. J. (1982). The development of the mood-inhibiting effects of crowding during adolescence. Journal of Psychology 110, 197-202.

Ra, J. B. (1983). An analysis of the interpersonal perceptions of adolescents. Adolescence 18, 859-873.

Radelet, M. L. (1980). The effect of female social position on geographic variations in the sex ration of arrests. Bulletin of the American Academy of Psychiatry and the Law 8, 465-476.

Rae-Grant, N., Thomas, B. H., Offord, D., et al. (1989). Risk, protective factors, and the prevalence of behavioral and emotional disorders in children and adolescents. Journal of the American Academy of Child and Adolescent Psychiatry 28, 262-268.

Rahim, S. I., & Cederblad, M. (1984). Effects of rapid urbanisation on child behaviour and health in a part of Khartoum, Sudan. Journal of Child Psychology and Psychiatry and Allied Disciplines 25, 629-641.

Robson, B. E. (1983). And they lived happily ever after: Marriage concepts of olde adolescents. Canadian Journal of Psychiatry 28, 646-649.

Rosenheim, E., & Gaoni, B. (1977). Defensive passivity in adolescence. Adolescence 12, 449-459.

Ross, C. E., & Huber, J. (1985). Hardship and depression. Journal of Health and Social Behavior 26, 312-327.

Ross, R. J. (1974). The empirical status of the formal operations. Adolescence 9, 413-420.

Rubenstein, J. L., Heeren, T., Housman, D., et al. (1989). Suicidal behavior in "normal" adolescents: Risk and protective factors. American Journal of Orthopsychiatry 59, 59-71.

Rutter, M. (1980). School influences on children's behavior and development: The 1979 Kenneth Blackfan Lecture, Children's Hospital Medical Center, Boston. Pediatrics 65, 208-220.

Rutter, M. (1989). Isle of Wight revisited: Twenty-five years of child psychiatric epidemiology. Journal of the American Academy of Child and Adolescent Psychiatry 28, 633-653.

Rutter, M. (1989). Pathways from childhood to adult life. Journal of Child Psychology and Psychiatry and Allied Disciplines 30, 23-51.

Sabatelli, R. M., & Mazor, A. (1985). Differentiation, individuation, and identity formation: The integration of family system and individual developmental perspectives. Adolescence 20, 619-633.

Sadler, L. S., & Catrone, C. (1983). The adolescent parent: A dual developmental crisis. Journal of Adolescent Health Care 4, 100-105.

Scheibach, M. (1985). Transition to manhood: Effects of the Great Depression on male youth. Adolescence 20, 725-744.

Shaffer, D., Garland, A., Gould, M., et al. (1988). Preventing teenage suicide: A critical review. Journal of the American Academy of Child and Adolescent Psychiatry 27, 675-687.

Schowalter, J. E. (1983). Psyche and soma of physical illness during adolescence. Psychosomatics 24, 453-461.

Shane, P. G. (1989). Changing patterns among homeless and runaway youth. American Journal of Orthopsychiatry 59, 208-214.

Shaner, J. M., Peterson, K. L., & Roscoe, B. (1985). Older adolescent females' knowledge of child development norms. Adolescence 20, 53-59.

Shestowsky, B. J. (1983). Ego identity development and obesity in adolescent girls. Adolescence 18, 551-559.

Simkins, L. (1984). Consequences of teenage pregnancy and motherhood. Adolescence 19, 39-54.

Simmons, C. H., & Parsons, R. J. (1983). Empowerment for role alternatives in adolescence. Adolescence 18, 193-200.

Siomopoulos, G., & Inamdar, S. C. (1979). Developmental aspects of hopelessness. Adolescence 14, 233-239.

Slater, E. J., Stewart, K. J., & Linn, M. W. (1983). The effects of family disruption on adolescent males and females. Adolescence 18, 931-942.

Slavin, M. O. (1985-1986). A developmental disorder of late adolescence. International Journal of Psychoanalytic Psychotherapy 11, 219-241.

Smith, R. H., & Smith, A. R. (1976). Attachment and educational investment of adolescence. Adolescence 11, 349-357.

Snarey, J. R., & Vaillant, G. E. (1985). How lower- and working-class youth become middle-class adults: The association between ego defence mechanism and upward social mobility. Child Development 56, 899-910.

Steffenhagen, R. A. (1980). Self-esteem theory of drug abuse. National Institute on Drug Abuse Research Monograph Series 30, 157-163.

Steiner-Adair, C. (1986). The body politic: Normal female adolescent development and the development of eating disorders. Journal of the American Academy of Psychoanalysis 14, 95-114.

Streissguth, A. P., Clarren, S. K., & Jones, K. L. (1985). Natural history of the fetal alcohol syndrome: A 10-year follow-up of eleven patients. Lancet 2, 85-91.

Sunseri, A. J., Alberti, J. M., Kent, N. D., Schoenberger, J. A., Sunseri, J. K., Amuwo, S., & Vickers, P. (1983). Reading, demographic, social and psychological factors related to pre-adolescent smoking and non-smoking behaviors and attitudes. Journal of School Health 53, 257-263.

Svendsen, D. (1983). Factors related to changes in IQ: A follow-up study of former slow learners. Journal of Child Psychology and Psychiatry and Allied Disciplines 24, 405-413.

Svobodny, L. A. (1982). Biographical, self-concept and educational factors among chemically dependent adolescents. Adolescence 17, 847-853.

Swanson, H. L. (1983). A developmental study of vigilance in learning-disabled and nondisabled children. Journal of Abnormal Child Psychology 11, 415-429.

Thornton, W. E. (1982). Gender traits and delinquency involvement of boys and girls. Adolescence 17, 749-768.

Tyson, R. L. (1983). Some narcissistic consequences of object loss: A developmental view. Psychoanalytic Quarterly 52, 205-224.

Vaillant, G. E., & Drake, R. E. (1985). Maturity of ego defenses in relation to DSM-III axis II personality disorder. Archives of Genetic Psychiatry 42, 597-601.

Verhulst, F. C., Achenbach, T. M. & Akverhus, G. W. (1989). Problems reported for clinically referred American and Dutch children. Journal of the American Academy of Child and Adolescent Psychiatry 28, 516-524.

Wallerstein, J. B. & Corbin, S. B. (1989). Daughters of divorce: Report from a ten year follow-up. American Journal of Orthopsychiatry 59, 593-604.

Werner, E. E. (1989). High-risk children in young adulthood: A longitudinal study from birth to 32 years. American Journal of Orthopsychiatry 59, 72-81.

Zuravin, S. J. (1988). Child maltreatment and teenage first births: A relationship mediated by chronic sociodemographic stress? American Journal of Orthopsychiatry 58, 91-103.

3. Gender and Sex Role Development

Bates, J. E., Bentler, P. M., & Thompson, S. K. (1979). Gender-deviant boys compared with normal and clinical control boys. Journal of Abnormal Child Psychology 7, 243-259.

Bates, J. E., Skilbeck, W. M., Smith, K. V. R., & Bentler, P. M. (1974). Gender role abnormalities in boys: An analysis of clinical ratings. Journal of Abnormal Child Psychology 2, 1-16.

Bleiberg, E., Jackson, L., & Ross, J. L. (1986). Gender identity disorder and object loss. Journal of the American Academy of Child Psychiatry 25, 58-67.

Coates, S., & Person, E. S. (1985). Extreme boyhood femininity: Isolated behavior or pervasive disorder? Journal of the American Academy of Child Psychiatry 24, 702-709.

Davenport, C. W., & Harrison, S. I. (1977). Gender identity change in a female adolescent transsexual. Archives of Sexual Behavior 6, 327-340.

Dulcan, M. K., & Lee, P. A. (1984). Transsexualism in the adolescent girl. Journal of the American Academy of Child Psychiatry 23, 354-361.

Ehrhardt, A. A., & Meyer-Bahlburg, H. F. (1981). Effects of prenatal sex hormones on gender-related behavior. Science 211, 1312-1318.

Ehrhardt, A. A., Meyer-Bahlburg, H. F., Feldman, J. F., & Ince, S. E. (1984). Sex-dimorphic behavior in childhood subsequent to prenatal exposure to exogenous progestogens and estrogens. Archives of Sexual Behavior 13, 457-477.

Ehrhardt, A. A., Meyer-Bahlburg, H. F., Rosen, L. R., Feldman, J. F., Veridiano, N. P., Zimmerman, I., & McEwen, B. S. (1985). Sexual orientation after prenatal exposure to exogenous estrogen. Archives of Sexual Behavior 14, 57-77.

Eme, R. F. (1979). Sex differences in childhood psychopathology. Psychological Bulletin 86, 574-595.

Finegan, J. K., Zucker, K. J., Bradley, S. J., & Doering, R. W. (1982). Patterns of intellectual functioning and spatial ability in boys and gender identity disorder. Canadian Journal of Psychiatry 27, 135-139.

Gadpaille, W. J. (1975). Homosexuality in adolescent males. American Academy of Psychoanalysis 3, 361-371.

Golombok, S., Spencer, A., & Rutter, M. (1983). Children in lesbian and single-parent households: Psychosexual and psychiatric appraisal. Journal of Child Psychology and Psychiatry and Allied Disciplines 24, 551-572.

Green, R. (1976). One-hundred-ten feminine and masculine boys: Behavior contrasts and demographic similarities. Archives of Sexual Behavior 5, 425-446.

Green, R. (1978). Sexual identity of 37 children raised by homosexual or transsexual parents. American Journal of Psychiatry 135, 692-697.

Green, R. (1985). Gender identity in childhood and later sexual orientation: Follow-up of 78 males. American Journal of Psychiatry 142, 339-341.

Green, R. (1987). The sissy-boy syndrome and the development of homosexuality. New Haven: Yale University Press.

Green, R., Mandel, J. B., Hotvedt, M. E., Gray, J., & Smith, L. (1986). Lesbian mothers and their children: A comparison with solo parent heterosexual mothers and their children. Archives of Sexual Behavior 15, 167-184.

Green, R., & Money, J. (1960). Incongruous gender role: Nongenital manifestations in prepubertal boys. Journal of Nervous and Mental Disease 131, 160-168.

Green, R., Williams, K., & Goodman, M. (1985). Masculine or feminine gender identity in boys: Developmental differences between two diverse family groups. Sex Roles 12, 1155-1162.

Hoeffer, B. (1981). Children's acquisition of sex-role behavior in lesbian-mother families. American Journal of Orthopsychiatry 51, 536-544.

Imperato-McGinley, J., Peterson, R. E., Gautier, T., & Sturla, E. (1979). Androgens and the evolution of male-gender identity among male pseudohermaphrodites with 5 alpha-reductase deficiency. New England Journal of Medicine 300, 1233-1237.

Kirkpatrick, M., Smith, C., & Roy, R. (1981). Lesbian mothers and their children: A comparative survey. American Journal of Orthopsychiatry 51, 545-551.

Lothstein, L. M. (1980). The adolescent gender dysphoric patient: An approach to treatment and management. Journal of Pediatric Psychology 5, 93-109.

Martin, A. D. (1982). Learning to hide: The socialization of the gay adolescent. In S. C. Feinstein, et al. (Eds.), Adolescent psychiatry: Developmental and clinical studies (pp. 52-65). Chicago: University of Chicago Press.

McCauley, E., & Ehrhardt, A. A. (1984). Follow-up of females with gender identity disorders. Journal of Nervous and Mental Disease 172, 353-358.

Meyer, J. K., & Dupkin, C. (1985). Gender disturbance in children. An interim clinical report. Bulletin of the Menninger Clinic 49, 236-269.

Meyer-Bahlburg, H. F., Feldman, J. F., & Ehrhardt, A. A. (1985). Questionnaires for the assessment of atypical gender role behavior: A methodological study. Journal of the American Academy of Child Psychiatry 24, 695-701.

Money, J. (1985a). The conceptual neutering of gender and the criminalization of sex. Archives of Sexual Behavior 14, 279-290.

Money, J. (1985b). Pediatric sexology and hermaphroditism. Journal of Sex and Marital Therapy 11, 139-156.

Money, J., Devore, H., & Normal, B. F. (1986). Gender identity and gender transposition: Longitudinal outcome study of 32 male hermaphrodites assigned as girls. Journal of Sex and Marital Therapy 12, 165-181.

Money, J., Hampson, J. G., & Hampson, J. L. (1955). Hermaphroditism: Recommendations concerning assignment of sex, change of sex, and psychologic management. Bulletin of Johns Hopkins Hospital 97, 284-300.

Money, J., & Lewis, V. (1982). Homosexual/heterosexual status in boys at puberty: Idiopathic adolescent gynecomastia and congenital virilizing adrenocorticism compared. Psychoneuroendocrinology 7, 339-346.

Money, J., & Russo, A. J. (1979). Homosexual outcome of discordant gender identity/role: Longitudinal follow-up. Journal of Pediatric Psychology 4, 29-41.

Money, J., Schwartz, J., & Lewis, V. G. (1984). Adult erotosexual status and fetal hormonal masculinization and demasculinization: 46, XX congenital virilizing adrenal hyper-plasia and 46, XX androgen-insensitivity syndrome compared. Psychoneuroendocrinology 9, 405-414.

Myers, M. F. (1982). Counseling the parents of young homosexual male patients. Journal of Homosexuality 8, 131-143.

Newman, L. E. (1976). Treatment for the parents of feminine boys. American Journal of Psychiatry 133, 683-687.

Rekers, G. A. (1975). Stimulus control over sex-typed play in cross-gender identified boys. Journal of Experimental Child Psychology 20, 136-148.

Rekers, G. A. (1977a). Assessment and treatment of childhood gender problems. In B. B. Lahey & A. E. Kazdin (Eds.), Advances in clinical child psychology (pp. 267-306). New York: Plenum Press.

Rekers, G. A. (1977b). Atypical gender development and psychosocial adjustment. Journal of Applied Behavior Analysis 10, 559-571.

Rekers, G. A., & Yates, C. E. (1976). Sex-typed play in feminoid boys versus normal boys and girls. Journal of Abnormal Child Psychology 4, 1-8.

Roiphe, H., & Galenson, E. (1981). Infantile origins of sexual identity. New York: International Universities Press.

Ross, J. M. (1975). The development of paternal identity: A critical review of the literature on nurturance and generativity in boys and men. Journal of the American Psychoanalytic Association 23, 783-817.

Sreenivasan, U. (1985). Effeminate boys in a child psychiatric clinic: Prevalence and associated factors. Journal of the American Academy of Child Psychiatry 24, 689-694.

Stoller, R. J. (1985). Presentations of gender. New Haven: Yale University Press.

Tuber, S., & Coates, S. (1985). Interpersonal phenomena in the Rorschachs of extremely feminine boys. Psychoanalysis and Psychology 2, 251-265.

Weinrich, J. D. (1985). Transsexuals, homosexuals, and sissy boys: On the mathematics of follow-up studies. Journal of Sex Research 21, 322-328.

Williams, K., Goodman, M., & Green, R. (1985). Parent-child factors in gender role socialization in girls. Journal of the American Academy of Child Psychiatry 24, 720-731.

Wolfe, B. E. (1979). Behavioral treatment of childhood gender disorders: A conceptual and empirical critique. Behavior Modification 3, 550-575.

Zucker, K. J. (1982). Childhood gender disturbance: Diagnostic issues. Journal of the American Academy of Child Psychiatry 21, 274-280.

Zucker, K. J. (1985). Cross-gender-identified children. In B. W. Steiner (Ed.), Gender dysphoria: Development, research, management. (pp. 74-175). New York: Plenum Press.

Zucker, K. J., Bradley, S. J., Doering, R. W., & Lozinski, J. A. (1985). Sex-typed behavior in cross-gender-identified children: Stability and change at a one-year follow-up. Journal of the American Academy of Child Psychiatry 24, 710-719.

Zucker, K. J., Doering, R. W., Bradley, S. J., & Finegan, J. K. (1982). Sex-typed play in gender-disturbed children: A comparison to sibling and psychiatric controls. Archives of Sexual Behavior 11, 309-321.

Zucker, K. J., Finegan, J. K., Doering, R. W., & Bradley, S. J. (1983). Human figure drawings of gender-problem children: A comparison to sibling, psychiatric, and normal controls. Journal of Abnormal Child Psychology 11, 287-298.

4. Psychophysiologic Disorders

Abramson, H. A., & Krinsky, L. W. (1975). The first dream as the chief complaint of the unconscious, and its utilization by the primary physician. Journal of Asthma Research 12, 221-236.

Adams, J. A., & Weaver, S. J. (1986). Self-esteem and perceived stress in young adolescents with chronic disease. Unexpected findings. Journal of Adolescent Health Care 7, 173-177.

Bibliography of developmental medicine and child neurology: Selected books and articles received in 1985. (1986). Developmental Medicine and Child Neurology [Suppl.] 52, 1-154.

Bromfield, R., Weisz, J. R., & Messer, T. (1986). Children's judgments and attributions in response to the "mentally retarded" label: A developmental approach. Journal of Abnormal Psychology 95, 81-87.

Call, J. D., Christianson, M. D., Penrose, F. R., & Backlar, M. (1963). Psychogenic megacolon in three preschool boys: A study of etiology through collaborative treatment of child and parents. American Journal of Orthopsychiatry 33, 923-928.

Campbell, J. D. (1986). Similarity and uniqueness: The effects of attribute type, relevance, and individual differences in self-esteem and depression. Journal of Personality and Social Psychology 50, 281-294.

Eaves, L. J., Long, J., & Heath, A. C. (1986). A theory of developmental change in quantitative phenotypes applied to cognitive development. Behavior Genetics 16, 143-162.

Heilbrun, A. B., & Renert, D. (1986). Type A behavior, cognitive defense, and stress. Psychological Reports 58, 447-456.

Jurich, A. P., & Polson, C. J. (1986). Effect of a marriage and family therapy practicum upon students' self-perceived strengths and weaknesses. Psychological Reports 58, 527-533.

Larsen, R. J., & Seidman, E. (1986). Gender schema theory and sex role inventories: Some conceptual and psychometric considerations. Journal of Personality and Social Psychology 50, 205-211.

Notman, M. T., Zilbach, J. J., Baker-Miller, J., & Nadelson, C. C. (1986). Themes in psychoanalytic understanding of women: Some reconsiderations of autonomy and affiliation. Journal of the American Academy of Psychoanalysis 14, 241-253.

Severino, S. K. (1986). Use of a Holocaust fantasy for the consolidation of identity. Journal of the American Academy of Psychoanalysis 14, 227-239.

Sweda, M. G., Sines, J. O., Lauer, R. M., & Clarke, W. R. (1986). Familial aggregation of type A behavior. Journal of Behavioral Medicine 9, 23-32.

Weston, D. (1986). The superego: A revised developmental model. Journal of the American Academy of Psychoanalysis 14, 181-202.

White, K. M., Speisman, J. C., Jackson, D., Bartis, S., & Costos, D. (1986). Intimacy maturity and its correlates in young married couples. Journal of Personality and Social Psychology 50, 152-162.

Wilson, R. S. (1986). Continuity and change in cognitive ability profile. Behavioral Genetics 16, 45-60.

Wood, W., & Karten, S. J. (1986). Sex differences in interaction style as a product of perceived sex differences in competence. Journal of Personality and Social Psychology 50, 341-347.

PART III

PSYCHOPATHOLOGY: DISEASE AND DISORDER

Psychopathology: Disease and Disorder

Section Editor (Psychopathology):

Saul I. Harrison, M.D.
Professor and Director
Child and Adolescent Psychiatry
Harbor-UCLA Medical Center
Torrance, California
and
Professor Emeritus
University of Michigan

Subsection Editors:

Thomas Anders, M.D.
Professor of Psychiatry and Human Behavior
Director, Child and Adolescent Psychiatry
Brown University
Providence, Rhode Island

Irving N. Berlin, M.D.
Professor of Psychiatry and Pediatrics
University of New Mexico
Albuquerque, New Mexico

Dennis Cantwell, M.D.
Professor of Psychiatry
Director, Child and Adolescent Psychiatry
University of California at Los Angeles Medical Center
Los Angeles, California

Spencer Eth, M.D.
Associate Chief of Psychiatry
Assistant Professor of Psychiatry
University of California at Los Angeles
Associate Clinical Professor of Psychiatry
University of Southern California School of Medicine
Los Angeles, California

Lois T. Flaherty, M.D.
Director, Child and Adolescent Psychiatry
Associate Professor
University of Maryland School of Medicine
Baltimore, Maryland

Arthur Green, M.D.
Associate Clinical Professor of Psychiatry
Columbia University College of Physicians and Surgeons
New York, New York
and
Director, Child and Family Center
Columbia Presbyterian Medical Center
New York, New York
and
Clinical Director of Therapeutic Nurseries
Babies Hospital
New York, New York

Lionel Hersov, M.D., F.R.C.P., D.P.M.
Professor of Psychiatry and Pediatrics
Medical Center, University of Massachusetts
Worcester, Massachusetts

Charles Keith, M.D.
Professor of Psychiatry
Division of Child and Adolescent Psychiatry
Duke University Medical Center
Durham, North Carolina

Paulina K. Kernberg, M.D.
Professor of Psychiatry
Chief, Child and Adolescent Psychiatry
Cornell Medical Center, Westchester Division
White Plains, New York

Paul Laybourne, M.D.
Professor of Psychiatry
Director, Child and Adolescent Psychiatry
University of Kansas
Kansas City, Kansas

Alexander P. Lucas, M.D.
Consultant, Section of Child and Adolescent Psychiatry
Professor in Psychiatry, Mayo Medical School
Mayo Clinic
Rochester, Minnesota

Joseph D. Noshpitz, M.D.
Professor of Child Psychiatry
Children's Hospital and George Washington School of Medicine
Washington, D.C.

Theodore Petti, M.D.
Professor of Psychiatry
University of Pittsburgh School of Medicine
Pittsburgh, Pennsylvania

Cynthia Pfeffer, M.D.
Associate Professor
Division of Child Psychiatry
New York Hospital, Cornell School of Medicine
Westchester Division
White Plains, New York

Andrew Russell, M.D.
Associate Professor
Mental Retardation and Child Psychiatry Division
Neuropsychiatric Institute, Center for Health Sciences
University of California at Los Angeles
Los Angeles, California

John E. Schowalter, M.D.
Professor of Psychiatry and Pediatrics
Chief, Child and Adolescent Psychiatry
Child Study Center, Yale University
New Haven, Connecticut

Larry Silver, M.D.
Director of Training
Division of Child Psychiatry
Department of Psychiatry
Georgetown University School of Medicine
Washington, D.C.
and
Clinical Professor of Psychiatry
Georgetown University School of Medicine
Washington, D.C.

Peter E. Tanguay, M.D.
Professor of Child Psychiatry
Mental Retardation and Child Psychiatry Division
Neuropsychiatric Institute, School of Medicine
University of California at Los Angeles
Los Angeles, California

Jay Tarnow, M.D.
Professor of Psychiatry
University of Texas School of Medicine
and
Director, Houston Child Guidance Clinic
Houston, Texas

Harry H. Wright, M.D., M.B.A.
Associate Professor of Psychiatry
Division of Youth Services
Medical University of South Carolina
Columbia, South Carolina

Associate Section Editors:

Paul Adams, M.D.
Professor of Psychiatry
University of Texas School of Medicine
Galveston, Texas

Marc Amaya, M.D.
Professor of Psychiatry
Division of Child-Adolescent Psychiatry
Duke University Medical Center
Durham, North Carolina

William Arroyo, M.D.
Clinical Assistant Professor of Psychiatry
University of Southern California School of Medicine
Los Angeles, California

George Awad, M.D.
Family Court Clinic
Toronto, Ontario
Canada

Psychopathology: Disease and Disorder

Sidney Berman, M.D.
Professor Emeritus of Psychiatry
Georgetown University School of Medicine
Washington, D.C.

Efrain Bleiberg, M.D.
Director, Child and Adolescent Service
Menninger Clinic and Hospital
Topeka, Kansas

Eli M. Bower, Ph.D.
Professor of Education
College of Education
University of California
Berkeley, California

Donald J. Cohen, M.D.
Professor
Yale Child Study Center
Yale University School of Medicine
New Haven, Connecticut

Ken Farley, M.D.
Assistant Professor of Psychiatry
University of Massachusetts
Worcester, Massachusetts

Carl Feinstein, M.D.
Assistant Professor of Psychiatry
Brown University
Providence, Rhode Island

Jo Ann B. Fineman, M.D.
Visiting Assistant Professor of Psychiatry
Child and Adolescent Psychiatry
Harbor-UCLA Medical Center
Torrance, California

Steven Forness, Ed.D.
Professor
Department of Psychiatry
Mental Retardation and Child Psychiatry Division
The U.C.L.A. Neuropsychiatric Institute
Los Angeles, California

Fred Frankel, Ph.D.
Associate Professor
Department of Psychiatry
Mental Retardation and Child Psychiatry Division
The U.C.L.A. Neuropsychiatric Institute
Los Angeles, California

Thomas Haslip, M.D.
Professor of Psychiatry
Division of Child-Adolescent Psychiatry
Duke University Medical Center
Durham, North Carolina

Michael G. Kalogerakis, M.D.
Clinical Professor of Psychiatry
New York University School of Medicine
New York, New York

Connie Kasasi
Post Graduate Research Psychologist
Department of Psychiatry
Mental Retardation and Child Psychiatry Division
The U.C.L.A. Neuropsychiatric Institute
Los Angeles, California

William Klykylo, M.D.
Cincinnati, Ohio

James F. Leckman, M.D.
Associate Professor
Yale Child Study Center
Yale University School of Medicine
New Haven, Connecticut

John Looney, M.D.
Professor of Psychiatry
Director, Division of Child and Adolescent Psychiatry
University of North Carolina School of Medicine
Chapel Hill, North Carolina

Richard C. Marohn, M.D.
Clinical Professor of Psychiatry
Northwestern University School of Medicine
Chicago, Illinois

Psychopathology: Disease and Disorder

John McDermott, Jr., M.D.
Professor and Chairman
Department of Psychiatry
University of Hawaii School of Medicine at Manoa
Honolulu, Hawaii

John Meeks, M.D.
Clinical Professor of Psychiatry
University of Maryland School of Medicine
and
Medical Director
Psychiatric Institute of Montgomery County
Rockville, Maryland

Spyros J. Monopolis, M.D.
Assistant Professor
Division of Child and Adolescent Psychiatry
University of Maryland School of Medicine
Baltimore, Maryland

Cynthia Pfeffer, M.D.
Associate Professor of Psychiatry
Division of Child-Adolescent Psychiatry
New York Hospital Medical Center
Westchester Division
White Plains, New York

Andres Pumariega, M.D.
Houston Child Guidance Clinic
Houston, Texas

Richard M. Sarles, M.D.
Clinical Professor
University of Maryland School of Medicine
Baltimore, Maryland
and
Director of Child and Adolescent Psychiatry
Sheppard Enoch Pratt Hospital
Towson, Maryland

Marian Sigman, Ph.D.
Professor, Department of Psychiatry
Mental Retardation and Child Psychiatry Division
The U.C.L.A. Neuropsychiatric Institute
Los Angeles, California

Peter Toscano, M.D.
Assistant Professor of Psychiatry
University of Massachusetts
Worcester, Massachusetts

Alexander Tymchuck, Ph.D.
Associate Professor
Department of Psychiatry
Mental Retardation and Child Psychiatry Division
The U.C.L.A. Neuropsychiatric Institute
Los Angeles, California

Mario Valente, M.D.
Adjunct Associate Professor
Department of Psychiatry
Mental Retardation and Child Psychiatry Division
The U.C.L.A. Neuropsychiatric Institute
Los Angeles, California

Kenneth J. Zucker, Ph.D.
Assistant Professor
Department of Psychology and Psychiatry
University of Toronto
Toronto, Ontario
Canada

A. Classification of Psychopathology with Reference to DSM III and III-R

Dennis Cantwell, M.D., Section Editor

Achenbach, T. M. (1980). DSM-III in light of empirical research on the classification of child psychopathy. Journal of the American Academy of Child Psychiatry 19, 395-412.

Beitchman, J. H., Dielman, T. E., Landis, J. R., Benson, R. M., & Kemp, P. L. (1978). Reliability of the Group for Advancement of Psychiatry Diagnostic Categories in Child Psychiatry. Archives of General Psychiatry 35, 1461-1466.

Cantwell, D. P. (1983). Diagnostic validity of the hyperactive child (attention deficit disorder with hyperactivity) syndrome. Psychiatric Developments 1, 277-300.

Cantwell, D. P., Baker, L., & Mattison, R. E. (1979). The prevalence of psychiatric disorder in children with speech and language disorder: An epidemiologic study. Journal of the American Academy of Child Psychiatry 18, 450-461.

Cantwell, D. P., Baker, L., & Mattison, R. E. (1980). Psychiatric disorders in children with speech and language retardation. Archives of General Psychiatry 37, 423-426.

Cantwell, D. P., Mattison, R., Russell, A. T., & Will, L. (1979). A comparison of DSM-II and DSM-III in the diagnosis of childhood psychiatric disorders. IV. Difficulties in use, global comparison, and conclusions. Archives of General Psychiatry 36, 1227-1228.

Cantwell, D. P., Russell, A. T., Mattison, R., & Will, L. (1979). A comparison of DSM-II and DSM-III in the diagnosis of childhood psychiatric disorders. I. Agreement with expected diagnosis. Archives of General Psychiatry 36, 1208-1213.

Carlson, G. A., & Cantwell, D. P. (1982). Diagnosis of childhood depression: A comparison of the Weinberg and DSM-III criteria. Journal of the American Academy of Child Psychiatry 21, 247-250.

Cohen, D. J., Paul R., & Volkmar, F. R. (1986). Issues in the classification of pervasive and other developmental disorders: Toward DSM-IV. Journal of the American Academy of Child Psychiatry 25, 213-220.

Cohen, D. J., Volkmar, F. R. & Paul, R. (1986). Issues in the classification of pervasive and other developmental disorders and assoicated conditions: History and current status of nosology. Journal of the American Academy of Child Psychiatry 25, 158-161.

Forness, S. R., & Cantwell, D. P. (1982). DSM-III psychiatric diagnoses and special education categories. Journal of Special Education 16, 49-63.

Geller, B., Chestnut, E. C., Miller, M. D., Price, D. T., & Yates, E. (1985). Preliminary data on DSM-III associated features of major depressive disorder in children and adolescents. American Journal of Psychiatry 142, 643-644.

Harris, S. L. (1979). DSM-III: Its implications for children. Child Behavior Therapy 1, 37-46.

Lobovits, D. A., & Handal, P. J. (1985). Childhood depression: Prevalence using DSM-III criteria and validity of parent and child depression scales. Journal of Pediatric Psychology 10, 45-54.

Mezzich, A. C., & Mezzich, J. E. (1985). Perceived suitability and usefulness of DSM-III vs. DSM-II in child psychopathology. Journal of the American Academy of Child Psychiatry 24, 281-285.

Mezzich, A. C., Mezzich, J. E., & Coffman, G. A. (1985). Reliability of DSM-III vs. DSM-II in child psychopathology. Journal of the American Academy of Child Psychiatry 24, 273-280.

Quay, H. C. (1986). A crucial analysis of DSM-III as a taxonomy of psychopathology in childhood and adolescence. In T. Mullon & G. Klerman (Eds.), Contemporary directions in psychopathology: Toward the DSM-IV. New York: Guilford Press.

Russell, A. T., Cantwell, D. P., Mattison, R., & Will, L. (1979). A comparison of DSM-II and DSM-III in the diagnosis of childhood psychiatric disorders. III. Multiaxial features. Archives of General Psychiatry 36, 1223-1226.

Rutter, M., & Shaffer, D. (1980). DSM-III. A step forward or back in terms of the classification of child psychiatric disorders? Journal of the American Academy of Child Psychiatry 19, 371-394.

Spitzer, R. L., & Cantwell, D. P. (1980). The DSM-III classification of the psychiatric disorders of infancy, childhood, and adolescence. Journal of the American Academy of Child Psychiatry 9, 356-370.

Werry, J. S. (1985). ICD 9 & DSM III classification for the clinician. Journal of Child Psychology and Psychiatry and Allied Disciplines 26, 1-6.

Werry, J. S., Methven, R. J., Fitzpatrick, J., & Dixon, H. (1983). The interrater reliability of DSM-III in children. Journal of Abnormal Child Psychology 11, 341-354.

B. Psychopathology

Saul I. Harrison, M.D., Section Editor

1. Developmental Disorders Including Language Disorders

Larry Silver, M.D., Subsection Editor

Abuelo, D., Pueschel, S., & Stern, L. (1982). Screening the neonate for development and genetic disorders. Paediatrician 11, 45-71.

Allen, R., & Wasserman, G. A. (1985). Origins of language delay in abused infants. Child Abuse and Neglect 9, 335-340.

Aram, D. M., Ekelman, B. L., & Nation, J. E. (1984). Preschoolers with language disorders: 10 years later. Journal of Speech and Hearing Research 27, 232-244.

August, G. J., & Garfinkel, B. D. (1989). Behavioral and cognitive subtypes of ADHD. Journal of the American Academy of Child and Adolescent Psychiatry 28, 739-748.

Banus, B. J. (1983). The Miller assessment for preschoolers (MAP): An introduction and review. American Journal of Occupational Therapy 27, 232-244.

Beiser, H. R. (1979). Formal games in diagnosis and therapy. Journal of the American Academy of Child Psychiatry 18, 480-491.

Beitchman, J. H. (1985). Speech and language impairment and psychiatric risk. Psychiatric Clinics of North America 8, 721-735.

Beratis, S., Kolk, R., Sperling, E., & Stein, R. E. (1981). Development of a child with long-lasting deprivation of oral feeding. Journal of the American Academy of Child Psychiatry 20, 53-64.

Brier, N. M., & Demb, H. B. (1980). Psychotherapy with the developmentally disabled adolescent. Journal of Developmental and Behavioral Pediatrics 1, 19-23.

Buxbaum, E., & Sodergren, S. S. (1977). A disturbance of elimination and motor development. In A. Solnit, et al. (Eds.), Psychoanalytic study of the child (Vol. 32, pp. 195-214). New Haven: Yale University Press.

Cantwell, D. P., Baker, L., & Mattison, R. E. (1979). The prevalence of psychiatric disorder in children with speech and language disorder: An epidemiologic study. Journal of the American Academy of Child Psychiatry 18, 450-461.

Casey, P. H. (1983). Failure to thrive: A reconceptualization. Journal of Developmental and Behavioral Pediatrics 4, 63-66.

Cohen, D. J., Caparulo, B., & Shaywitz, B. (1976). Primary childhood aphasia and childhood autism: Clinical, biological and conceptual observations. Journal of the American Academy of Child Psychiatry 15, 604-645.

Cohen, D. J., Caparulo, B. K., & Wetstone, H. (1981). The emergence of meaning and intentions. Mother's dialogue with normal and language-impaired children. Psychiatric Clinics of North America 4, 489-508.

Doherty, M. B., & Rosenfeld, A. A. (1984). Play assessment in the differential diagnosis of autism and other cases of severe language disorder. Journal of Developmental and Behavioral Pediatrics 5, 26-29.

Emde, R. (1983). The prerepresentational self and its affective core. In A. Solnit, et al. (Eds.), Psychoanalytic study of the child (Vol. 38, pp. 169-192). New Haven: Yale University Press.

Fineman, J. B., & Smith, M. (1984). Object ties and interaction of infant and adolescent mother. In M. Sugar (Ed.), Adolescent parenthood. New York: Spectrum Publications.

Fischler, R. S., & Fleshman, C. (1985). Comprehensive health services for developmentally disabled Navajo children. Journal of Developmental and Behavioral Pediatrics 6. 9-14.

Fischler, R. S., & Tancer, M. (1984). The primary physician's role in care for developmentally handicapped children. Journal of Family Practice 18, 85-88.

Fish, B. (1976). An approach to prevention in infants at risk for schizophrenia developmental deviations from birth to 10 years. Journal of the American Academy of Child Psychiatry 15, 62-82.

Freud, A., & Burlingham, D. (1944). Infants without families. New York: International Universities Press.

Friedlander, K. (1945). Formation of the antisocial character. In R. S. Eissler, et al. (Eds.), Psychoanalytic study of the child (Vol. 1, pp. 189-203). New York: International Universities Press.

Gaensbauer, T. J., & Sands, K. (1979). Distorted affective communications in abused/neglected infants and their potential impact on caretaker. Journal of the American Academy of Child Psychiatry 18, 236-250.

Galenson, E., Miller, R., Kaplan, E., & Rothstein, A. (1979). Assessment of the development in the deaf child. Journal of the American Academy of Child Psychiatry 18, 128-142.

Gordan, A. H., & Jameson, J. C. (1979). Infant-mother attachment in patients with nonorganic failure to thrive. Journal of the American Academy of Child Psychiatry 18, 251-259.

Greenspan, S., & Lourie, R. S. (1981). Developmental structuralist approach to the classification of adaptive and pathologic personality organizations: Infancy and early childhood. American Journal of Psychiatry 138, 725-735.

Hansen, D. (1985). The influence of early deficits on later development. Panel report. Journal of the American Psychoanalytic Association 33, 631-644.

Lawrence, M.M. (1976). The appraisal of ego strength in evaluation, treatment and consultation. Journal of the American Academy of Child Psychiatry 15, 1-14.

Levinson, L. (1984). Witches--good and bad: Maternal psychopathology as a developmental interference. In A. Solnit, et al. (Eds.), Psychoanalytic study of the child (Vol. 39, p. 371). New Haven: Yale University Press.

Ornitz, E., & Ritvo, E. R. (1976). The syndrome of autism: A critical review. American Journal of Psychiatry 133, 609-621.

Ornitz, E. M., Guthrie, D., & Farley, A. H. (1977). The early development of autistic children. Journal of Autism and Childhood Schizophrenia 7, 207-229.

Paul, R., Cohen, D. J., & Caparulo, B. K. (1983). A longitudinal study of patients with severe developmental disorders of language learning. Journal of the American Academy of Child Psychiatry 22, 525-534.

Rescorla, L. A. (1986). Preschool psychiatric disorders: Diagnostic classification and symptom patterns. Journal of the American Academy of Child Psychiatry 25, 162-169.

Rubin, S. S. (1982). Expressive language deficits in preschool children and faulty development of the self: Description and case study. American Journal of Orthopsychiatry 52, 58-64.

Shengold, L. (1979). Child abuse and deprivation: Soul murder. Journal of the American Psychoanalytic Association 27, 533-559.

Sherman, M., & Hertzig, M. (1983). Treasured object use: A cognitive and developmental marker. Journal of the American Academy of Child Psychiatry 22, 541-544.

Sherman, M., Shapiro, T., & Glassman, M. (1983). Play and language in developmentally disordered preschoolers: A new approach to classification. Journal of the American Academy of Child Psychiatry 22, 511-524.

Special issue: Recent advances in infant psychiatry. (1981). Journal of the American Academy of Child Psychiatry 20, 215-337.

Stavrakaki, C. (1985). Developmental disabilities. Recent trends in prevention and treatment. Psychiatric Clinics of North America 8, 685-701.

Waelder, R. (1933). Psychoanalytic theory of play. Psychoanalytic Quarterly 2, 208-244.

2. Anxiety and Phobias

Achenbach, R. M., & Edelbrock, C. S. (1979). The child behavior profile: Boys aged 12-16 and girls aged 6-11 and 12-16. Journal of Consulting and Clinical Psychology 47, 2.

Atkinson, L., Quarrington, B., & Cyr, J. J. (1985). School refusal: The heterogeneity of a concept. American Journal of Orthopsychiatry 55, 83-101.

Baideme, S. M., Kern, R. M., & Taffel-Cohen, S. (1979). The use of Adlerian family therapy in a case of school phobia. Journal of Individual Psychology 35, 58-69.

Berecz, J. M. (1968). Phobias of childhood: Etiology and treatment. Psychological Bulletin 70, 694-720.

Berg, C. J., Rapoport, J. L., & Flament, M. (1986). The Leyton obsessional inventory--child version. Journal of the American Academy of Child Psychiatry 25, 84-91.

Berg, I. (1984). School refusal. British Journal of Hospital Medicine 31, 59-62.

Berg, I., Marks, I., McGuire, R., & Lipsedge, M. (1974). School phobia and agoraphobia. Psychological Medicine 4, 428-434.

Blagg, N. R., & Yule, W. (1984). The behavioural treatment of school refusal--a comparative study. Behavior Reserach and Therapy 22, 119-127.

Bloom-Feshbach, S., & Blatt, S. J. (1982). Separation response and nursery school adaptation. Journal of the American Academy of Child Psychiatry 21, 58-64.

Bornstein, B. (1949). The analysis of a phobic child: Some problems of theory and technique in a child analysis. In R. S. Eissler, et al. (Eds.), Psychoanalytic study of the child (Vol. 3/4, pp. 181-226). New York: International Universities Press.

Bowlby, J. (1960). Separation anxiety. International Journal of Psycho-Analysis 41, 89-113.

Bowlby, J. (1961). Separation anxiety: A critical review of the literature. Journal of Child Psychology and Psychiatry and Allied Disciplines 1, 251-269.

Bowlby, J. (1973). Attachment and loss (separation, anxiety, and anger). London: Hogarth Press.

Bowlby, J., Ainsworth, M., Boston, M., & Rosenbluth, D. (1956). The effects of mother-child separation: A follow-up study. British Journal of Medical Psychology 29, 211-247.

Briet, M. (1982). Separation anxiety in mothers of latency-age fearful children. Journal of Abnormal Child Psychology 10, 135-144.

Brogden, R. N., Heel, R. C., Speight, T. M., & Avery, G. S. (1980). Clobazam: A review of its pharmacological properties and therapeutic use in anxiety. Drugs 20, 161-178.

Burns, L. E., & Thorpe, G. L. (1977). Fears and clinical phobias: Epidemiological aspects and the national survey of agoraphobics. Journal of International Medical Research 5, 132-139.

Butcher, P. (1983). The treatment of childhood-rooted separation anxiety in an adult. Journal of Behavior Therapy and Experimental Psychiatry 14, 61-65.

Charney, D. S., & Redmond, D. E. (1983). Neurobiological mechanisms in human anxiety. Neuropharmacology 22, 1531-1536.

Coffey, B., Shader, R. I., & Greenblatt, D. J. (1983). Pharmacokinetics of benzodiazepines and psychostimulants in children. Journal of Clinical Psychopharmacology 3, 217-225.

Conners, C. K. (1969). A teacher rating scale for use in drug studies with children. American Journal of Psychiatry 126, 884-888.

Creak, M. (1969). Hysteria in childhood. Acta Paedopsychiatrica 36, 269-274.

Cretekos, C. J. (1977). Some techniques in rehabilitating the school phobic adolescent. Adolescence 12, 237-246.

Crowe, R. C., Pauls, D. L., Slymen, D. J., & Noyes, R. (1980). A family study of anxiety neurosis. Morbidity risk in families of patients with and without mitral valve prolapse. Archives of General Psychiatry 37, 77-79.

Crumley, F. E. (1974). A school phobia in a three-generational family conflict. Journal of the American Academy of Child Psychiatry 13, 536-550.

Dash, J. (1981). Rapid hypno-behavioral treatment of a needle phobia in a five-year-old cardiac patient. Journal of Pediatric Psychology 6, 37-42.

DuPont, R. L. (1983). Phobias in culture. Journal of Pediatrics 102, 999-1002.

Eisenberg, L. (1958). School phobia: A study in the communication of anxiety. American Journal of Psychiatry 114, 712-718.

Field, T., & Reite, M. (1984). Children's responses to separation from mother during the birth of another child. Child Development 55, 1308-1316.

Finch, A. J., Montgomery, L. E., & Deardorf, P. A. (1974). Reliability of state-trait anxiety with emotionally disturbed children. Journal of the American Academy of Child Psychiatry 2, 67-69.

Fond, K., & Brosnan, J. (1980). School phobia: The school anxiety symptom. Pediatric Nursing 6, 9-13.

Frances, A., & Petti, T. A. (1984). Boy with seriously ill mother manifests somatic complaints, withdrawal, disabling fears. Hospital and Community Psychiatry 35, 439-440.

Garrison, M. (1978). A new look at Little Hans. Psychoanalytic Review 65, 523-532.

Gittleman, R. (1985). Ratings for anxiety disorders. Psychopharmacology Bulletin 21, 931-948.

Gittelman, R., & Klein, D. F. (1985). Childhood separation anxiety and adult agoraphobia. In A. H. Tuma & J. D. Maser (Eds.), Anxiety and the anxiety disorders. Hillsdale, N.J.: Erlbaum

Gittelman-Klein, R. (1978). Psychopharmacological treatment of anxiety disorders, mood disorders, and Tourette's disorder in children. In M. A. Lipton, A. MiMascio, & K. F. Killam (Eds.), Psychopharmacology: A generation of progress. New York: Raven Press.

Gittelman-Klein, R., & Klein, D. F. (1973). School phobia: Diagnostic considerations in the light of the imipramine effects. Journal of Nervous and Mental Disease 150, 199-215.

Graziano, A. M., & De Giovanni, I. S. (1979). The clinical significance of childhood phobias: A note on the proportion of child-clinical referrals for the treatment of children's fears. Behavior Research and Therapy 17, 161-162.

Greenacre, P. (1941). The predisposition to anxiety. Psychoanalytic Quarterly 10, 66-94.

Gromska, J., Domoslawska, B., & Koczurowska, J. (1975). Music therapy in the treatment of hyperkinesis and anxiety neuroses in children. Psychiatria Polska 9, 605-612.

Haefely, W. E. (1979). Biological basis of the therapeutic effects of benzodiazepines. In R. G. Priest, U. V. Filho, R. Amrein, & M. Skreta (Eds.), Benzodiazepines today and tomorrow: Proceedings of the First International Symposium on Benzodiazepine in Rio de Janeiro. Baltimore: University Park Press.

Harris, E. (1981). Antidepressants: Old drugs, new uses. American Journal of Nursing 81, 1308-1309.

Henry, R. M. (1981). Validation of a projective measure of aggression-anxiety for five-year-old boys. Journal of Personality Assessment 45, 359-369.
Hershberg, S. G., Carlson, G. A., Cantwell, D. P., & Strober, M. (1982). Anxiety and depressive disorders in psychiatrically disturbed children. Journal of Clinical Psychiatry 43, 358-361.
Hoehn-Saric, R. (1982). Neurotransmitters in anxiety. Archives of General Psychiatry 39, 635-642.
Insel, T. R., Ninan, P. T., Aloi, J., et al. (1984). A benzodiazepine receptor mediated model of anxiety. Archives of General Psychiatry 41, 741-750.
Johnson, S. B., & Melamed, B. G. (1979). The assessment and treatment of children's fears. In B. B. Lahey & A. E. Kazdin (Eds.), Advances in clinical child psychology. New York: Plenum Press.
Kotsopoulos, S., & Mellor, C. (1986). Extralinguistic speech characteristics of children with conduct and anxiety disorders. Journal of Child Psychology and Psychiatry and Allied Disciplines 27, 99-108.
Lamb, M. E. (1979). Separation and reunion behaviors as criteria of attachment to mothers and fathers. Early Human Development 3, 329-339.
Lang, P. J. (1984). In state of the art conference reviews: New developments in characterizing, treatment anxiety. Hospital and Community Psychiatry 35, 9-10.
Lansky, S., & Gendel, M. (1978). Symbiotic regressive behavior patterns in childhood malignancy. A pattern characterized by a severe separation anxiety in the sick child and a parent, and extreme social withdrawal of the pair. Clinical Pediatrics 17, 133-138.
Lansky, S. B., Lowman, J. T., Vats, T., & Gyulay, J. E. (1975). School phobia in children with malignant neoplasms. American Journal of Diseases of Children 129, 42-46.
Lawlor, E. D. (1976). Hypnotic intervention with "school phobic" children. International Journal of Clinical and Experimental Hypnosis 24, 74-86.
Linet, L. S. (1985). Tourette syndrome, pimozide, and school phobia: The neuroleptic separation anxiety syndrome. American Journal of Psychiatry 142, 613-615.
Livingston, R., Nugent, H., Rader, L., & Smith, G. R. (1985). Family histories of depressed and severely anxious children. American Journal of Psychiatry 142, 1497-1499.
Mahler, M. S., Pine, F., & Bergman, A. (1975). The psychological birth of the human infant: Symbiosis and individuation. New York: Basic Books.
Mahon, E. (1985). Some aspects of separation and loss in therapy with disturbed children. American Journal of Psychoanalysis 45, 35-51.
Malmquist, C. P. (1965). School phobia. A problem in family neurosis. Journal of the American Academy of Child Psychiatry 4, 293-319.
Mansdorf, I. J. (1981). Eliminating somatic complaints in separation anxiety through contingency management. Journal of Behavior Therapy and Experimental Psychiatry 12, 73-75.
Mathai, J. (1983). An acute anxiety state in an adolescent precipitated by viewing a horror movie. Journal of Adolescence 6, 197-200.

Matson, J. L. (1983). Exploration of phobic behavior in a small child. Journal of Behavior Therapy and Experimental Psychiatry 14, 257-259.

Mavissakalian, M., Perel, J. M., & Michelson, L. (1984). The relationship of plasma imipramine and N-desmethylimipramine to improvement in agoraphobia. Journal of Clinical Psychopharmacology 4, 36-40.

McDermott, J. F. (1985a). Anxiety disorders in children. In R. Michels, et al. (Eds.), Psychiatry. Philadelphia: Lippincott.

McDermott, J. F. (1985b). Treatment of anxiety disorders in children and adolescents. In R. Michels, et al. (Eds.), Psychiatry. Philadelphia: Lippincott.

Menahem, S. & Cebon, A. (1984). Treat mother too--"failed" psychotherapy of an adolescent with school refusal. Child Psychiatry and Human Development 14, 170-177.

Nader, P. R., Bullock, D., & Caldwell, B. (1975). School phobia. Pediatric Clinics of North America 22, 605-617.

Norvell, N., Brophy, C., & Finch, A. J. (1985). The relationship of anxiety to childhood depression. Journal of Personality Assessment 49, 150-153.

Ost, L. G., & Hugdahl, K. (1983). Acquisition of agoraphobia, mode of onset and anxiety response patterns. Behavior Research and Therapy 21, 623-631.

Parenteau, P., & Lamontagne, Y. (1981). The thought-stopping technique: A treatment for different types of rumination? Canadian Journal of Psychiatry 26, 192-195.

Petti, T. A., & Sallee, F. R. (1986). Issues in childhood and adolescent psychopharmacology. In K. D. Gadow & A. D. Poling (Eds.), Advances in learning and behavioral disabilities. Greenwich, Conn.: JAI Press.

Phillips, D., & Wolpe, S. (1981). Multiple behavioral techniques in severe separation anxiety of a twelve-year-old. Journal of Behavior Therapy and Experimental Psychiatry 12, 329-332.

Poznanski, E. O. (1973). Children with excessive fears. American Journal of Orthopsychiatry 43, 428-438.

Preskorn, S. H., Weller, E. B., Weller, R. A., & Glotzbach, E. (1983). Plasma levels of imipramine and adverse effects in children. American Journal of Psychiatry 140, 1332-1335.

Puig-Antich, J., Perel, J., Luptakin, W., et al. (1987). Imipramine in prepubertal major depression Archives of General Psychiatry 44, 81-89.

Raskin, M., Peeke, H. V., Dickman, W., & Pinsker, H. (1982). Panic and generalized anxiety disorders. Developmental antecedents and precipitants. Archives of General Psychiatry 39, 687-689.

Reinhart, J. B., & Pisula, D. (1977). Phobic symptoms in a toddler. Early intervention can forestall serious developments. Clinical Pediatrics 16, 1100-1104.

Remschmidt, H. (1973). Observations on the role of anxiety in neurotic and psychotic disorders at an early age. Journal of Autism and Childhood Schizophrenia 3, 106-114.

Renik, O., Spielman, P., & Afterman, J. (1978). Bamboo phobia in an eighteen-month-old boy. Journal of the American Psychoanalytic Association 26, 255-282.

Reynolds, C. R., & Paget, K. D. (1981). Factor analysis of the revised children's manifest anxiety scale for blacks, whites, males, and females with a national normative sample. Journal of Consulting and Clinical Psychology 49, 352-359.
Richter, N. C. (1984). Efficacy of relaxation training with children. Journal of Abnormal Child Psychology 12, 319-344.
Roth, M. (1984). Agoraphobia, panic disorder and generalized anxiety disorder: Some implications of recent advances. Psychiatric Developments 2, 31-52.
Rutter, M. (1979). Separation experiences: A new look at an old topic. Journal of Pediatrics 95, 147-154.
Sandler, A. M. (1977). Beyond eight-month anxiety. International Journal of Psycho-Analysis 58, 195-207.
Saraf, K. R., Klein, D. F., Gittelman-Klein, R., Gootman, N., & Greenhill, P. (1978). EKG effects of imipramine treatment in children. Journal of the American Academy of Child Psychiatry 17, 60-69.
Schmeltz, K. (1977). An early latency child's use of obsessional ritual to master separation anxiety. Maternal-Child Nursing Journal 6, 117-134.
Sheehan, D. V., Davidson, J., Manschreck, T., et al. (1983). Lack of efficacy of a new antidepressant (bupropion) in the treatment of panic disorders with phobias. Journal of Clinical Psychopharmacology 3, 28-31.
Sheehan, D. V., Sheehan, K. E., & Minichiello, W. E. (1981). Age of onset of phobic disorders: A reevaluation. Comprehensive Psychiatry 22, 544-553.
Shill, M. (1981). TAT measures of gender identity (castration anxiety) in father-absent males. Journal of Personality Assessment 45, 136-146.
Shrand, H. (1982). Agoraphobia and imipramine withdrawal? [Letter]. Pediatrics 70, 825.
Simeon, J. G., & Ferguson, H. B. (1985). Recent developments in the use of antidepressant and anxiolytic medications. Psychiatric Clinics of North America 8, 893-907.
Sperling, M. (1952). Animal phobias in a two-year-old child. In R. S. Eissler, et al. (Eds.), Psychoanalytic study of the child (Vol. 7, pp. 115-125). New York: International Universities Press.
Spitz, R. (1965). The first year of life. New York: International Universities Press.
Sreenivasan, U., Manocha, S. N., & Jain, V. K. (1979). Treatment of severe dog phobia in childhood by flooding: A case report. Journal of Child Psychology and Psychiatry and Allied Disciplines 20, 255-260.
Stein, L., Beluzzi, J. D., & Wise, D. (1977). Benzodianepines: Behavioral or neurochemical mechanisms. American Journal of Psychiatry 134, 665-669.
Terr, L. C. (1981). "Forbidden games": Post-traumatic child's play. Journal of the American Academy of Child Psychiatry 20, 741-760.
Thyer, B. A., Parrish, R. T., Curtis, G. C., Nesse, R. M., & Cameron, O. G. (1985). Ages of onset of DSM-III anxiety disorders. Comprehensive Psychiatry 26, 113-122.
Trueman, D. (1984). What are the characteristics of school phobic children? Psychological Reports 54, 191-202.

Ultee, C. A., Griffisen, D., & Schellenkens, J. (1982). The reduction of anxiety in children: A comparison of the effects of systematic desensitization in vitro and systematic desensitization in vivo. Behavior Research and Therapy 20, 61-67.

Van Winter, J. T., & Stickler, G. B. (1984). Panic attack syndrome. Journal of Pediatrics 105, 661-665.

Waldron, S., Shrier, D. K., Stone, B., & Tobin, F. (1975). School phobia and other childhood neuroses: A systematic study of the children and their families. American Journal of Psychiatry 132, 802-808.

Wallick, M. M. (1979). Desensitization therapy with a fearful two-year-old. American Journal of Psychiatry 136, 1325-1326.

Weissman, M. M., Leckman, J. F., Merikangas, K. R., Gammon, G. D., & Prusoff, B. A. (1984). Depression and anxiety disorders in parents and children: Results from the Yale family study. Archives of General Psychiatry 41, 845-852.

Werry, J. S. (1979). Family therapy: Behavioral approaches. Journal of the American Academy of Child Psychiatry 18, 91-102.

White, W. C., & Davis, M. T. (1974). Vicarious extinction of phobic behavior in early childhood. Journal of Abnormal Child Psychology 2, 25-32.

Williams, D. T., Mehl, R., Yudofsky, S., et al. (1982). The effect of proporanolol on uncontrolled rage outbursts in children and adolescents with organic brain dysfunction. Journal of the American Academy of Child Psychiatry 2, 129-135.

Wolpe, J. (1981). The dichotomy between classical conditioned and cognitively learned anxiety. Journal of Behavior Therapy and Experimental Psychiatry 12, 35-42.

3. Conversion Hysteria

Adams, P. L., & Horovitz, J. H. (1980). Coping patterns of mothers of poor boys. Child Psychiatry and Human Development 10, 144-155.

Brooksbank, D. J. (1984). Management of conversion reaction in five adolescent girls. Journal of Adolescence 7, 359-376.

Carek, D. J., & Santos, A. B. (1984). Atypical somtoform disorder following infection in children--a depressive equivalent? Journal of Clinical Psychiatry 45, 108-111.

Chilcote, R. R., & Baehner, R. L. (1980). Atypical bleeding in hemophilia: Application of the conversion model to the case study of a child. Psychosomatic Medicine 42, 221-230.

Delamater, A. M., Rosenbloom, N., Conners, C. K., & Hertwick, L. (1983). The behavioral treatment of hysterical paralysis in a ten-year-old boy. A case study. Journal of the American Academy of Child Psychiatry 22, 73-79.

Dubowitz, V., & Hersov, L. (1976). Management of children with non-organic (hysterical) disorders of motor function. Developmental Medicine and Child Neurology 18, 358-368.

Ernst, A. R., Routh, D. K., & Harper, D. C. (1984). Abdominal pain in children and symptoms of somatization disorder. Journal of Pediatric Psychology 9, 77-86.

Goodyer, I. (1981). Hysterical conversion reactions in childhood. Journal of Child Psychology and Psychiatry and Allied Disciplines 22, 179-188.

Goodyer, I., & Taylor, D. C. (1985). Hysteria. Archives of Disease in Childhood 60, 680-681.

Greene, J. W., Walker, L. S., Hickson, G., & Thompson, J. (1985). Stressful life events and somatic complaints in adolescents. Pediatrics 75, 19-22.

Hryhorczuk, L. L. (1981). Conversion disorder: A developmental response to stress in adolescence? Psychosomatics 22, 636-638.

Kaufman, I. (1962). Conversion hysteria in latency. Journal of the American Academy of Child Psychiatry 1, 385-396.

Kenyon, F. E. (1965). Hypochondriasis: A survey of some historical, clinical and social aspects. British Journal of Medical Psychology 38, 117-138.

Krumholz, A., & Niedermeyer, E. (1983). Psychogenic seizures: A clinical study with follow-up data. Neurology 33, 498-502.

Lesse, S. (1981). Hypochondriacal and psychosomatic disorders masking depression in adolescents. American Journal of Psychotherapy 35, 356-367.

Livingson, R., & Martin-Cannici, C. (1985). Multiple somatic complaints and possible somatization disorder in prepubertal children. Journal of the American Academy of Child Psychiatry 24, 603-607.

Mai, F. M., & Merskey, H. (1980). Briquet's treatise on hysteria. A synopsis and commentary. Archives of General Psychiatry 37, 1401-1405.

Maloney, M. J. (1980). Diagnosing hysterical conversion reactions in children. Journal of Pediatrics 97, 1016-1020.

Nishiura, K., & Yamada, M. (1984). Therapeutic function of diagnostic label 'hysteria.' British Journal of Medical Psychology 57, 91-96.

Parker, G., & Lipscombe, P. (1980). The relevance of early parental experiences to adult dependency, hypochondriases and utilization of primary physicians. British Journal of Medical Psychology 53, 355-363.

Routh, D. K., & Ernst, A. R. (1984). Somatization disorder in relatives of children and adolescents with functional abdominal pain. Journal of Pediatric Psychology 9, 427-437.

Silber, G. W., & Borus, J. F. (1983). Outbreak of illness in a school chorus. Toxic poisoning or mass hysteria? New England Journal of Medicine 308, 632-635.

Small, G. W., & Nicholi, A. M. (1982). Mass hysteria among schoolchildren. Early loss as a predisposing factor. Archives of General Psychiatry 39, 721-724.

Volkmar, F. R., Poll, J., & Lewis, M. (1984). Conversion reactions in childhood and adolescence. Journal of the American Academy of Child Psychiatry 23, 424-430.

Weller, E. B., & Weller, R. A. (1983). Case report of conversion symptom associated with major depressive disorder in a child. American Journal of Psychiatry 140, 1079-1080.

Williams, D. T., Gold, A. P., Shrout, P., Shaffer, D., & Adams, D. (1979). The impact of psychiatric intervention on patients with uncontrolled seizures. Journal of Nervous and Mental Disease 167, 626-631.

Williams, D. T., Spiegel, H., & Mostofsky, D. I. (1978). Neurogenic and hysterical seizures in children and adolescents: Differential diagnostic and therapeutic considerations. American Journal of Psychiatry 135, 82-86.

Winnicott, D. W. (1958). The antisocial tendency. In D. W. Winnicott (Ed.), Collected papers. New York: Basic Books.

Winnicott, D. W. (1961). Delinquency as a sign of hope. Journal of Child Psychology and Psychiatry and Allied Disciplines 2, 269-276.

Wolff, S. (1984). The concept of personality disorder in childhood. Journal of Child Psychology and Psychiatry and Allied Disciplines 25, 5-13.

Woodside, M., Harrow, A., Basson, J. V., & Affleck, J. W. (1976). Experiment in managing sociopathic behavior disorders. British Medical Journal 2, 1056-1059.

Zander, K. (1984). "The fragile princess." Midway on the borderline-narcissistic personality continuum. Perspectives in Psychiatric Care 22, 77-84.

4. Obsessive Compulsive Disorders

Adams, P. L. (1985). The obsessive child: A therapy update. American Journal of Psychotherapy 39, 301-313.

Akhtar, S. (1978). Obsessional neurosis, marriage, sex and fertility: Some transcultural comparison. International Journal of Social Psychiatry 24, 164-166.

Apter, A., Bernhout, E., & Tyano, S. (1984). Severe obsessive compulsive disorder in adolescence: A report of eight cases. Journal of Adolescence 7, 347-358.

Behar, D., Rapoport, J. L., Berg, C. J., Denckla, M. B., Mann, L., Cox, C., Fedio, P., & Zahn, T. (1984). Computerized tomography and neuropsychological test measures in adolescents with obsessive-compulsive disorder. American Journal of Psychiatry 141, 363-368.

Berg, C. J., Rapoport, J. L., & Flament, M. (1986). The Leyton obsessional inventory--child version. Journal of the American Academy of Child Psychiatry 25, 84-91.

Berg, C. Z., Rapoport, J. L., Whitaker, A., Davies, M., Leonard, H., Swedo, S. E., Braiman, S., & Lenane (1989). Childhood obsessive compulsive disorder: A two-year prospective follow-up of a community sample. Journal of the American Academy of Child and Adolescent Psychiatry 28, 528-533.

Berg, C. Z., Whitaker, A., Davies, M., Flament, M. F., & Rapoport, J. L. (1988). The survey form of the Leyton Obsessional Inventory-Child Version: Norms from and epidemiological study. Journal of the American Academy of Child and Adolescent Psychiatry 27, 759-763.

Bolton, D., Collins, S., & Steinberg, D. (1983). The treatment of obsessive-compulsive disorder in adolescence: A report of fifteen cases. British Journal of Psychiatry 142, 456-464.

Bolton, D., & Turner, T. (1984). Obsessive-compulsive neurosis with conduct disorder in adolescence: A report of two cases. Journal of Child Psychology and Psychiatry and Allied Disciplines 25, 133-139.

Braconi, L. (1976). Gene interaction in the phenotypic expression of mental disease. Acta Geneticae Medicae et Gemellologiae (Roma) 25, 240-243.

Braconnier, A., & Ferrari, P. (1976). Moments depreeifs chez les adolescents presentant une organisation nevrotique, phobique ou obsessionnelle. [Periods of deprivation of adolescents presenting neurotic organization of phobias and obsessions]. Revue de Neuropsychiatrie Infantile 24, 329-339.

Brandrup, E., & Vanggaard, R. (1977). LSD treatment in a severe case of compulsive neurosis. Acta Psychiatrica Scandinavica 55, 127-141.

Burke, P., Meyer, V., Kocoshis, S., Orenstein, D., Chandra, R., & Sauer, J. (1989). Obsessive-compulsive symptoms in childhood inflammatory bowel disease and cystic fibrosis. Journal of the American Academy of Child and Adolescent Psychiatry 28, 525-527.

Cechakova, A., Tumova, S., & Vojtik, V. (1977). Obsessional syndrome as a result of minimal brain dysfunction in an adolescent. Ceskoslovenska Psychiatrie 73, 329-335.

Clark, D. A., & Bolton, D. (1985a). An investigation of two self-report measures of obsessional phenomena in obsessive-compulsive adolescents: Research note. Journal of Child Psychology and Psychiatry and Allied Disciplines 26, 429-437.

Clark, D. A., & Bolton, D. (1985b). Obsessive-compulsive adolescents and their parents: A psychometric study. Journal of Child Psychology and Psychiatry and Allied Disciplines 26, 267-276.

Collins, G. H. (1973). The use of parenteral and oral chlorimipramine (Anafranil) in the treatment of depressive state. British Journal of Psychiatry 122, 189-190.

Cooper, J. (1970). The Leyton obsessional inventory. Psychological Medicine 1, 48-64.

Coryell, W. (1981). Obsessive-compulsive disorder and primary unipolar depression: Comparison of background, family history, course and mortality. Journal of Nervous and Mental Disease 169, 220-224.

Dalton, P. (1983). Family treatment of an obsessive-compulsive child: A case report. Family Process 22, 99-108.

Elkins, R., Rapoport, J. L., & Lipsky, A. (1980). Obsessive-compulsive disorder of childhood and adolescence. Journal of the American Academy of Child Psychiatry 19, 511-524.

Fine, S. (1973). Family therapy and a behavioral approach to childhood obsessive-compulsive neurosis. Archives of General Psychiatry 28, 695-697.

Flament, M. F., Rapoport, J. L., Berg, C. J., Sceery, W., Kilts, C., Mellstrom, B., & Linnoila, M. (1985). Clomipramine treatment of childhood obsessive-compulsive disorder: A double-blind study. Archives of General Psychiatry 42, 977-983.

Flament, M. F., Whitaker, A., Rapoport, J. L., Davies, M., Berg, C. Z., Kalikow, K., Sceery, W., & Shaffer, D. (1988). Obsessive compulsive disorder in adolescence: An epidemiological study. Journal of the American Academy of Child and Adolescent Psychiatry 27, 764-771.

Fontana, D. (1980). Some standardization date for the Sandler-Hazari Obsessionality Inventory. British Journal of Medical Psychology 53, 267-275.

Friedmann, C. T., & Silvers, F. M. (1977). A multimodality approach to inpatient treatment of obsessive-compulsive disorder. American Journal of Psychotherapy 31, 456-465.

Gaines, T. (1978). A technique for reducing parental obsessions in family therapy. Family Therapy 5, 91-94.

Goodman, W. K., Price, L. H., Rasmussen, S. A., Mazure, C., Delgado, P., Heninger, G. R., & Charney, D. S. (1989). The Yale-Brown Obsessive Compulsive Scale. II. Validity. Archives of General Psychiatry 46, 1012-1016.

Goodman, W. K., Price, L. H., Rasmussen, S. A., Mazure, C., Fleischmann, R. L., Hill, C. L., Heninger, G. R., & Charney, D. S. (1989). The Yale-Brown Obsessive Compulsive Scale. I. Development, use, and reliability. Archives of General Psychiatry 46, 1006-1011.

Gylling, H. (1982). Treatment of the pediatric obsessions and compulsions with behavior modification: Two case studies. Scandinavian Journal of Behavior Therapy 11, 195-212.

Hafner, R. J., Gilchrist, P., Bowling, J., & Kalucy, R. (1981). The treatment of obsessional neurosis in a family setting. Australian and New Zealand Journal of Psychiatry 15, 145-151.

Harbin, H. T. (1979). Cure by ordeal: Treatment of an obsessive-compulsive neurotic. International Journal of Family Therapy 1, 324-332.

Hare, E. H., Price, J. S., & Slater, E. T. (1972). Fertility in obsessional neurosis. British Journal of Psychiatry 121, 197-205.

Hollinsworth, C. E., Tanguay, P. E., Grossman, L., & Pabst, P. (1980). Long-term outcome of obsessive-compulsive disorder in childhood. American Academy of Child Psychiatry 19, 134-144.

Holmes, J. (1982). Obsessional phenomena and the development of imaginative competence. British Journal of Medical Psychology 55, 147-158.

Hoover, C. F., & Insel, R. I. (1984). Families of origin in obsessive-compulsive disorder. Journal of Nervous and Mental Disease 172, 207-215.

Insel, T. R. (1982). Obsessive compulsive disorder--five clinical questions and a suggested approach. Comprehensive Psychiatry 23, 241-251.

Insel, T. R., Kalin, N. H., Guttmacher, L. B., Cohen, R. M., & Murphy, D. L. (1982). The dexamethasone suppression test in patients with primary obsessive-compulsive disorder. Psychiatric Research 6, 153-160.

Insel, T. R., Mueller, E. A., Gillin, J. C., Siever, L. J., & Murphy, D. L. (1985). Tricyclic response in obsessive compulsive disorder. Progress in Neuro-Psychopharmacology and Biological Psychiatry 9, 25-31.

Jenike, M. A. (1983). Obsessive compulsive disorder. Comprehensive Psychiatry 24, 99-115.

Jenike, M. A. (1984). Obsessive-compulsive disorder: A question of neurologic lesion. Comprehensive Psychiatry 25, 298-304.

Kellerman, J. (1981). Hypnosis as an adjunct to thought-stopping and covert reinforcement in the treatment of homicidal obsessions in a twelve-year-old boy. International Journal of Clinical and Experimental Hypnosis 29, 128-135.

Kendall, R. E., & Discipio, W. J. (1970). Obsessional symptoms and obsessional personality traits in patients with depressive illnesses. Psychological Medicine 1, 65-72.

Kettl, P. A., & Marks, I. M. (1986). Neurological factors in obsessive compulsive disorder: Two case reports and a review of the literature. British Journal of Psychiatry 149, 315-319.

Khanna, S., & Channabasavanna, S. M. (1986). Sociodemographic variables in obsessive compulsive neurosis in India. International Journal of Social Psychiatry 32, 47-52.

Klein, D. N., & Depue, R. A. (1985). Obsessional personality traits and risk for bipolar affective disorder: An offspring study. Journal of Abnormal Psychology 94, 291-297.

Kringlen, E. (1970). Natural history of obsessional neuroses. Seminars in Psychiatry 2, 403-419.

Leonard, H. L., Swedo, S. E., Rapoport, J. L., Koby, E. V., Lenane, M. C., Cheslow, D. L., & Hamburger, S. D. (1989). Treatment of obsessive-compulsive disorder with clomipramine and desipramine in children and adolescents: A double-blind crossover comparison. Archives of General Psychiatry 46, 1088-1092.

Lieberman, J. (1984). Evidence for a biological hypotheses of obsessive-compulsive disorder. Neuropsychobiology 11, 14-21.

Lieberman, J. A., Kane, J. M., Sarantakos, S., Cole, K., Howard, A., Borenstein, H., Novacenko, H., & Puig-Antich, J. (1985). Dexamethasone suppression tests in patients with obsessive-compulsive disorder. American Journal of Psychiatry 142, 747-751.

Lindley, P., Marks, I., Philpott, R., & Snowden, J. (1977). Treatment of obsessive-compulsive neurosis with history of childhood autism. British Journal of Psychiatry 130, 592-597.

Loeb, L. R. (1986). Traumatic contributions in the development of an obsessional neurosis in an adolescent. In S. C. Feinstein, et al. (Eds.), Adolescent psychiatry: Developmental and clinical studies (Vol. 13, pp. 201-217). Chicago: University of Chicago Press.

Luxenberg, J. S., Swedo, S. E., Flament, M. F., Friedland, R. P., Rapoport, J., & Rapoport, S. I. (1988). Neuroanatomical abnormalities in obsessive-compulsive disorder detected with quantitative X-ray computed tomography. American Journal of Psychiatry 145, 1089-1093.

Mallinger, A. E. (1984). The obsessive's myth of control. Journal of the American Academy of Psychoanalysis 12, 147-165.

Marks, I. (1983). Are there anticompulsive or antiphobic drugs? British Journal of Psychiatry 143, 338-347.

Marks, I. M., Crowe, M., Drewe, E., Young, J., & Dewhurst, W. G. (1969). Obsessive compulsive neuroses in identical twins. British Journal of Psychiatry 115, 991-998.

Marks, I. M., Stern, R. S., Mawson, D., Cobb, J., & McDonald, R. (1980). Clomipramine and exposure for obsessive-compulsive rituals. British Journal of Psychiatry 136, 1-25.

Mavissakalian, M., & Michelson, L. (1982). Tricyclic antidepressants in obsessive-compulsive disorder. Journal of Nervous and Mental Disease 171, 301-306.

McKean, J., McGuffin, P., & Robinson, P. (1984). Obsessive-compulsive neurosis following head injury: A report of four cases. British Journal of Psychiatry 144, 190-192.

Morelli, G. (1983). Adolescent compulsion: A case study involving cognitive-behavioral treatment. Psychological Reports 53, 519-522.

O'Connor, J. J. (1983). Why can't I get hives? Brief strategic therapy with an obsessional child. Family Process 22, 201-209.

Ong, S. B., & Leng, Y. K. (1979). The treatment of an obsessive-compulsive girl in the context of Malaysian Chinese culture. Australian and New Zealand Journal of Psychiatry 13, 255-259.

Ownby, R. L. (1983). A cognitive behavioral intervention for compulsive handwashing with a thirteen-year-old boy. Psychology in the Schools 20, 219-222.

Parnas, J., Teasdale, T. W., & Schulsinger, H. (1982). Continuity of character neurosis from childhood to adulthood: A prospective longitudinal study. Acta Psychiatrica Scandinavica 66, 491-498.

Pascalis, G., Igert, C. L., Berne, C. H., & Theret-Bacart, F. (1976). Death, psychosis and obsession: Statistical survey. Annales Medico-Psychologique 2, 453-458.

Pauls, D. L., Towbin, K. E., Leckman, J. F., Zahner, G. E., & Cohen, D. J. (1986). Gilles de la Tourette's syndrome and obsessive-compulsive disorder. Archives of General Psychiatry 43, 1180-1182.

Pivetta, R. (1973). Obsessional neurosis: Etiology and biopsychological presuppositions. A comparative study involving Freudian and Piagetian theory. Genetic Psychology Monographs 88, 287-304.

Pollak, J. M. (1979). Obsessive-compulsive personality: A review. Psychological Bulletin 86, 225-241.

Quality assurance project. (1985). Treatment outlines for the treatment of obsessive-compulsive disorders. Australian and New Zealand Journal of Psychiatry 19, 240-253.

Rachman, S., & DeSilva, P. (1978). Abnormal and normal obsessions. Behavior Research and Therapy 16, 233-238.

Rachman, S., & Hodgson, R. (1980). Obsessions and compulsions. Englewood Cliffs, N.J.: Prentice-Hall.

Ramos Brieva, J. A., & Irala San Jose, M. V. (1983). Mini-inventory of anankastic personality traits. Actas Luso-Espanolas de Neurologia y Psiquiatria 11, 219-230.

Rapoport, J. (1988). The neurobiology of obsessive-compulsive disorder. Journal of the American Medical Association 260, 2888-2890.

Rapoport, J. L. (1986). Annotations: Childhood obsessive compulsive disorder. Journal of Child Psychology and Psychiatry and Allied Disciplines 27, 289-295.

Rapoport, J. L., Elkins, R., Langer, D. H., Sceery, W., Buchsbaum, M. S., Gillin, C., Murphy, D. L., & Zahn, T. P. (1981). Childhood obsessive compulsive disorder. American Journal of Psychiatry 138, 1545-1554.

Rapoport, J. L., Elkins, R., & Mikkelsen, E. (1980). Clinical controlled trial of chlorimipramine in adolescents with obsessive-compulsive disorder. Psychopharmacology Bulletin 16, 61-63.

Rasmussen, S. A., & Tsuang, M. T. (1984). The epidemiology of obsessive-compulsive disorder. Journal of Clinical Psychiatry 45, 450-457.

Rasmussen, S. A., & Tsuang, M. T. (1986). Clinical characteristics and family history in DSM-III obsessive-compulsive disorder. American Journal of psychiatry 143, 317-322.

Rincover, A., & Newsom, C. D. (1979). Using sensory extinction procedures in the treatment of compulsive-like behavior of developmentally disabled children. Journal of Consulting and Clinical Psychology 47, 695-701.

Rinieris, P., Stefanis, C., & Rabaviles, A. (1981). Relationships between obsessional personality traits, neuroticism and extraversion in normal subjects. Comprehensive Psychiatry 22, 488-489.

Rosen, M. (1975). A dual model of obsessional neurosis. Journal of Consulting and Clinical Psychology 43, 453-459.

Salzman, L., & Thaler, F. H. (1981). Obsessive-compulsive disorders: A review of the literature. American Journal of Psychiatry 138, 286-296.

Sanavio, E., & Vidotto, G. (1985). The components of the Maudsley Obsessional-Compulsive Questionnaire. Behavior Research and Therapy 23, 659-662.

Schmeltz, K. (1977). An early latency child's use of obsessional ritual to master separation anxiety. Maternal-Child Nursing Journal 34, 117-134.

Shaw, B. A. (1978). Obsessional defenses and reading disabilities in adolescence as seen through art therapy. Art Psychotherapy 5, 61-69.

Silverman, J. S. (1972). Obsessional disorders in childhood and adolescence: Developmental, therapeutic and nosologic aspects. American Journal of Psychotherapy 26, 362-377.

Simons, J. M. (1974). Observations on compulsive behavior in autism. Journal of Autism and Childhood Schizophrenia 4, 1-10.

Solyom, L. (1982). A comparative psychometric study of anorexia nervosa and obsessive neurosis. Canadian Journal of Psychiatry 27, 282-286.

Solyom, L., Ledwidge, B., & Solyom, C. (1986). Obsessiveness and adjustment. Comprehensive Psychiatry 27, 234-240.

Stanley, L. (1980). Treatment of ritualistic behavior in an eight-year-old girl by response prevention: A case report. Journal of Child Psychology and Psychiatry and Allied Disciplines 21, 85-90.

Steketee, G., & Dopelt, H. (1986). Measurement of obsessive-compulsive symptomatology: Utility of the Hopkins symptom checklist. Psychiatry Research 19, 135-145.

Stroebel, C. F, Szarek, B. L., & Glueck, B. C. (1984). Use of clomipramine in treatment of obsessive-compulsive symptomatology. Journal of Clinical Psychopharmacology 4, 98-100.

Sugiyama, T. (1974). Clinico-electroencephalographic study on obsessive-compulsive neurosis. Bulletin of the Osaka Medical School 20, 95-114.

Taylor, R. E. (1984). Imagery for the treatment of obsessional behavior: A case study. American Journal of Clinical Hypnosis 27, 178-179.

Turner, S. M., Hersen, M., Bellack, A. S., Andrasik, F., & Capparell, H. V. (1980). Behavioral pharmacological treatment of obsessive-compulsive disorders. Journal of Nervous and Mental Disease 168, 651-657.

Warneke, L. B. (1985). Intravenous chlorimipramine in the treatment of obsessional disorder in adolescence: Case report. Journal of Clinical Psychiatry 46, 100-103.

Waxman, D. (1975). An investigation into the use of Anafranil in phobic and obsessional disorders. Scottish Medical Journal 20, 61-66.

Waxman, D. (1977). A clinical trial of clompipramine and diazepam in the treatment of phobic and obsessional illness. Journal of International Medical Research (Suppl.) 5, 99-110.

Weizman, A., Carmi, M., Hermesh, H., Shahar, A., Apter, A., Tyano, S., & Rehavi, M. (1986). High-affinity imipramine binding and serotonin uptake in platelets of eight adolescents and ten adult obsessive-compulsive patients. American Journal of Psychiatry 143, 335-339.

Willmuth, M. E. (1988). Cognitive-behavioral and insight-oriented psychotherapy of an eleven-year-old boy with obsessive-compulsive disorder. American Journal of Psychotherapy 42, 472-478.

Yaryura-Tobias, J. A., & Bhagavan, H. M. (1977). L-Tryptophan in obsessive-compulsive disorders. American Journal of Psychiatry 134, 1298-1299.

Young, J. G., & Solnit, A. L. (1981). Research on repetitive behaviors in childhood. American Journal of Psychiatry 138, 1598-1600.

Zikis, P. (1983). Treatment of an 11-year-old obsessive-compulsive ritualizer and tiqueur girl with in vivo exposure and response prevention. Behavior and Psychotherapy 11, 75-81.

5. Sleep Disorders

Thomas Anders, M.D., Subsection Editor

Abe, K., Amatomi, M., & Oda, N. (1984). Sleepwalking and recurrent sleeptalking in children of childhood sleepwalkers. American Journal of Psychiatry 141, 800-801.

Amir, N., Navon, P., & Silverberg-Shalev, R. (1985). Interictal electroencephalography in night terrors and somnambulism. Israel Journal of Medical Sciences 21, 22-26.

Baker, T. L. (1985). Sleep apnea disorders. Introduction to sleep and sleep disorders. Medical Clinics of North America 69, 1123-1152.

Barabas, G., Ferrari, M., & Matthews, W. S. (1983). Childhood migraine and somnambulism. Neurology 33, 948-949.

Barabas, G., Matthews, W. S., & Ferrari, M. (1984). Somnambulism in children with Tourette syndrome. Developmental Medicine and Child Neurology 26, 457-460.

Bax, M. C. (1980). Sleep disturbance in the young child. British Medical Journal 280, 1177-1179.

Berlin, R. M., Litovitz, G. L., Diaz, M. A., & Ahmed, S. W. (1984). Sleep disorders on a psychiatric consultation service. American Journal of Psychiatry 141, 582-584.

Bertelson, A. D., & Monroe, L. J. (1979). Personality patterns of adolescent poor and good sleepers. Journal of Abnormal Child Psychology 7, 191-197.

Bhatia, V. P., Katiyar, G. P., Agarwal, K. N., Das, T. K., & Dey, P. K. (1980). Sleep cycle studies in babies of undernourished mothers. Archives of Disease in Childhood 55, 134-138.

Billiard, M. (1985). Narcolepsy. Clinical features and aetiology. Annals of Clinical Research 17, 220-226.

Broughton, R. (1982). Pathophysiology of enuresis nocturna, sleep terrors and sleepwalking: Current status and the Marseilles contribution. Electroencephalography and Clinical Neurophysiology [Supplement] 35, 401-410.

Campbell, K. (1981). Association of the domestic set-up with sleeping difficulties in children under three years of age. Medical Journal of Australia 2, 254-255.

Carskadon, M. A., Harvey, K., & Dement, W. C. (1981). Multiple sleep latency tests during the development of narcolepsy. Western Journal of Medicine 135, 414-418.

Conner, A. E. (1977). Sleep disturbance in hyperkinetic children. Virginia Medical 104, 316-318.

Davies, S. M. (1982). Nocturnal epilepsy masquerading as a behavioral problem in children. Journal of Family Practice 15, 267-269.

Dement, W. C., Carskadon, M. A., Guilleminault, C., & Zarcone, V. P. (1976). Narcolepsy. Diagnosis and treatment. Primary Care 3, 609-623.

Dixon, K. N., Monroe, L. J., & Jakim, S. (1981). Insomniac children. Sleep 4, 313-318.

Felman, A. H., Loughlin, G. M., Leftridge, C. A., & Cassisi, N. J. (1979). Upper airway obstruction during sleep in children. American Journal of Roentgenology 133, 213-216

Ferber, R. (1985). Sleep, sleeplessness, and sleep disruptions in infants and young children. Annals of Clinical Research 17, 227-234.

Freidin, M. R., Jankowski, J. J., & Singer, W. D. (1979). Nocturnal head banging as a sleep disorder: A case report. American Journal of Psychiatry 136, 1469-1470.

Glaze, D. G., Frost, J. D., & Jankovic, J. (1983). Sleep in Gilles de la Tourette's syndrome: Disorder of arousal. Neurology 33, 586-592.

Graziano, A. M., & Mooney, K. C. (1982). Behavioral treatment of "nightfears" in children: Maintenance of improvement at 2 1/2- to 3-year follow-up. Journal of Consulting and Clinical Psychology 50, 598-599.

Greenhill, L., Puig-Antich, J., Goetz, R., Hanlon, C., & Davies, M. (1983). Sleep architecture and REM sleep measures in prepubertal children with attention deficit disorder with hyperactivity. Sleep 6, 91-101.

Guilleminault, C. (1978). Advances in the pathology of sleep. Electroencephalography and Clinical Neurophysiology [Supplement] 34, 67-70.

Guilleminault, C., & Dement, W. C. (1977). 235 cases of excessive daytime sleepiness. Diagnosis and tentative classification. Journal of Neurological Science 31, 13-27.

Guilleminault, C., Eldridge, F. L., Simmons, F. B., & Dement, W. C. (1976). Sleep apnea in eight children. Pediatrics 58, 23-30.

Guilleminault, C., Liebhaber, M., Navelet, Y., & Dement, W. C. (1975). Proceedings: Sleep-induced apnea syndrome in 6 children. Electroencephalography and Clinical Neurophysiology 39, 432.

Hauri, P., & Olmstead, E. (1980). Childhood-onset insomnia. Sleep 3, 59-65.

Hoshino, Y., Watanabe, H., Yashima, Y., Kaneko, M., & Kumashiro, H. (1984). An investigation on sleep disturbance of autistic children. Folia Psychiatrica et Neurologica Japonica 38, 45-51.

Hunter, J. (1983). Sleep disorders in childhood. Australian Family Physician 12, 503-505.

Jackson, H., & Rawlins, M. D. (1977). The sleepless child. British Medical Journal 2, 509.

Jones, D. P., & Verduyn, C. M. (1983). Behavioural management of sleep problems. Archives of Disease in Childhood 58, 442-444.

Kales, J. D., Kales, A., Bixler, E. O., & Soldatos, C. R. (1980). Sleep disorders: What the primary care physician needs to know. Postgraduate Medicine 67, 213-217, 220.

Kales, J. D., Kales, A., Soldatos, C. R., Chamberlin, K., & Martin, E. D. (1979). Sleepwalking and night terrors related to febrile illness. American Journal of Psychiatry 136, 1214-1215.

Kales, J. D., Soldatos, C. R., & Vela-Bueno, A. (1983). Treatment of sleep disorders III: Enuresis, sleepwalking, night terrors and nightmares. Rational Drug Therapy 17, 1-6.

Kane, J., Coble, P., Conners, K., & Kupfer, D. J. (1977). EEG sleep in a child with severe depression. American Journal of Psychiatry 134, 813-814.

Klackenberg, G. (1982a). Sleep behaviour studied longitudinally. Data from 4-16 years on duration, might-awakening and bed-sharing. Acta Paediatrica Scandinavica 71, 501-506.

Klackenberg, G. (1982b). Somnambulism in childhood --prevalence, course and behavioral correlations. A prospective longitudinal study (6-16 years). Acta Paediatrica Scandinavica 71, 495-499.

Kuo, P. C., West, R. A., Bloomquist, D. S., & McNeil, R. W. (1979). The effect of mandibular osteotomy in three patients with hypersomnia sleep apnea. Oral Surgery, Oral Medicine, Oral Pathololog̲y 48, 385-392.

Kupfer, D. J., & Reynolds, C. F. (1983). A critical review of sleep and its disorders from a developmental perspective. Psychiatric Developments 1, 367-386.

Langdon, N., Welsh, K. I., Van, D. M., Vaughan, R. W., & Parkes, D. (1984). Genetic markers in narcolepsy. Lancet 2, 1178-1180.

Largo, R. H., & Hunziker, U. A. (1984). A developmental approach to the management of children with sleep disturbances in the first three year of life. European Journal of Pediatrics 142, 170-173.

Lavie, P. (1983). Nasal obstructions, sleep, and mental function. Sleep 6, 244-246.

Lozoff, B., Wolf, A. W., & Davis, N. S. (1985). Sleep problems seen in pediatric practice. Pediatrics 75, 477-483.

Lugaresi, E., & Cirignotta, F. (1981). Hypnogenic paroxysmal dystonia: Epileptic seizure or a new syndrome? Sleep 4, 129-138.

Mangat, D., Orr, W. C., & Smith, R. O. (1977). Sleep apnea, hypersomnolence, and upper airway obstruction secondary to adenotonsillar enlargement. Archives of Otolaryngology 103, 383-386.

Mark, J. D., & Brooks, J. G. (1984). Sleep-associated airway problems in children. Pediatric Clinics of North America 31, 907-918.

Monroe, L. J., & Marks, P. A. (1977). MMPI differences between adolescent poor and good sleepers. Journal of Consulting and Clinical Psychology 45, 151-152.

Orr, W. C. (1985). Utilization of polysomnography in the assessment of sleep disorders. Medical Clinics of North America 69, 1153-1167.

Parkes, J. D. (1977). The sleepy patient. Lancet 1, 990-993.

Reimiao, R. N., & Lefievre, A. B. (1980). Prevalence of sleep-talking in childhood. Brain and Development 2, 353-357.

Richman, N. (1981a). A community survey of characteristics of one- to two-year-olds with sleep disruptions. Journal of the American Academy of Child Psychiatry 20, 281-291.

Richman, N. (1981b). Sleep problems in young children. Archives of Disease in Childhood 56, 491-493.

Richman, N. (1985). A double-blind drug trial of treatment in young children with waking problems. Journal of Child Psychology and Psychiatry and Allied Disciplines 26, 591-598.

Richman, N., Douglas, J., Hunt, H., Lansdown, R., & Levere, R. (1985). Behavioural methods in the treatment of sleep disorders--a pilot study. Journal of Child Psychology and Psychiatry and Allied Disciplines 26, 581-590.

Rogozea, R., & Florea-Ciocoiu, V. (1985). Orienting reaction in patients with night terrors. Biological Psychiatry 20, 894-905.

Salzarulo, P., & Chevalier, A. (1983). Sleep problems in children and their relationship with early disturbances of the waking-sleeping rhythms. Sleep 6, 47-51.

Salzarulo, P., Fagioli, I., Salomon, F., & Ricour, C. (1982). Developmental trend of quiet sleep is altered by early human malnutrition and recovered by nutritional rehabilitation. Early Human Development 7, 257-264.

Schmitt, B. D. (1981). Infants who do not sleep through the night. Journal of Developmental and Behavioral Pediatrics 2, 20-23.

Schmitt, B. D. (1985). The prevention of sleep problems. Clinics in Perinatology 12, 453-457.

Shows, W. D. (1974). A sleeping epidemic among first-grade children: Crisis intervention. Community Mental Health Journal 10, 332-336.

Simonds, J. F., & Parraga, H. (1982). Prevalence of sleep disorders and sleep behaviors in children and adolescents. Journal of the American Academy of Child Psychiatry 21, 383-388.

Simonds, J. F., & Parraga, H. (1984). Sleep behaviors and disorders in children and adolescents evaluated at psychiatric clinics. Journal of Developmental and Behavioral Pediatrics 5, 6-10.

Van, T. (1985). The relative influence of child and environmental characteristics on sleep disturbances in the first and second years of life. Journal of Developmental and Behavioral Pediatrics 6, 81-86.

Vela-Bueno, A., Kales, A., Soldatos, C. R., Dobladez-Blanco, B., Campos-Castello, J., Espino-Hurtado, P., & Olivan-Palacios, J. (1984). Sleep in the Prader-Willi syndrome. Clinical and polygraphic findings. Archives of Neurology 41, 294-296.

Walsh, J. K., Kramer, M., Skinner, J. E. (1981). A case report of jactatio capitis nocturna. American Journal of Psychiatry 138, 524-526.

Weissbluth, M. (1982). Modification of sleep schedule with reduction of night walking: A case report. Sleep 5, 262-266.

Younger, J. B. (1982). The management of night waking in older infants. Pediatric Nursing 8, 155-158.

6. Fire Setting

Awad, G. A., & Harrison, S. I. (1976). A female fire-setter: A case report. Journal of Nervous and Mental Disease 163, 432-437.

Bumpass, E. R., Fagelman, F. D., & Brix, R. J. (1983). Intervention with children who set fires. American Journal of Psychotherapy 37, 328-345.

Fineman, K. R. (1980). Firesetting in childhood and adolescence. Psychiatric Clinics of North America 3, 483-500.

Heath, G. A., Hardesty, V. A., Goldfine, P. E., & Walker, A. M. (1983). Childhood firesetting: An empirical study. Journal of the American Academy of Child Psychiatry 22, 370-374.

Jacobson, R. R. (1985). Child firesetters: A clinical investigation. Journal of Child Psychology and Psychiatry and Allied Disciplines 26, 759-768.

Kaufman, I., Heims, L. W., & Reiser, D. E. (1961). A reevaluation of the psychodynamics of firesetting. American Journal of Orthopsychiatry 31, 123-137.

Koles, M. R., & Jenson, W. R. (1985). Comprehensive treatment of chronic fire setting in a severely disordered boy. Journal of Behavior Therapy and Experimental Psychiatry 16, 81-85.

Kolko, D. J., & Kazdin, A. (1988). Prevalence of firesetting and related behaviours among child psychiatric patients. Journal of Consulting and Clinical Psychology 56, 628-630.

Kuhnley, E. J., Hendren, R. L., & Quinlan, D. M. (1982). Fire-setting by children. Journal of the American Academy of Child Psychiatry 21, 560-563.

Lewis, N., & Yarnell, H. (1951). Pathological firesetting. Nervous and Mental Disease Monographs 82, 8-26.
Macht, L. B., & Mack, J. E. (1968). The firesetter syndrome. Psychiatry 31, 277-288.
Sakheim, G. A., Vigdor, M. G., Gordon, M., & Helprin, L. M. (1985). A psychological profile of juvenile firesetters in residential treatment. Child Welfare 64, 453-476.

7. Elective Mutism

Paul Laybourne, M.D., Subsection Editor

Ambrosino, S. V., & Allesi, M. (1979). Elective mutism: Fixation and the double bind. American Journal of Psychoanalysis 39, 251-256.
Bradley, S., & Sloman, L. (1975). Elective mutism in immigrant families. Journal of the American Academy of Child Psychiatry 14, 510-514.
Browne, E., Wilson, V., & Laybourne, P. C. (1963). Diagnosis and treatment of elective mutism in children. Journal of the American Academy of Child Psychiatry 2, 605-617.
Chetnick, M. (1980). Amy: The intensive treatment of an elective mute. Journal of the American Academy of Child Psychiatry 12, 482-498.
Conrad, R. D., Delp, J. L., & Williams, C. (1974). Uses stimulus feeding procedures in the treatment of situation specific mutism. Journal of Behavior Therapy and Experimental Psychiatry 5, 99-100.
Croghan, L. M., & Craven, T. (1982). Elective mutism: Learning from the analysis of a successful case history. Journal of Pediatric Psychology 7, 85-93.
Goll, K. (1979). Role structure and subculture in families of elective mutists. Family Process 18, 55-68.
Hayden, T. L. (1980). Classification of elective mutism. Journal of the American Academy of Child Psychiatry 19, 118-133.
Heimlich, E. P. (1981). Patient as assistant therapist in paraverbal therapy with children. American Journal of Psychotherapy 35, 262-267.
Kolvin, I., & Fundudis, T. (1981). Elective mute children: Psychological development and background factors. Journal of Child Psychology and Psychiatry and Allied Disciplines 22, 219-232.
Labbe, E. E., & Williamson, D. A. (1984). Behavioral treatment of elective mutism: A review of the literature. Clinical Psychology Review 4, 273-292.
Pustrom, E., & Speers, R. W. (1964). Elective mutism in children. Journal of the American Academy of Child Psychiatry 3, 287-297.
Reed, G. F. (1963). Elective mutism in children: A re-appraisal. Journal of Child Psychology and Psychiatry and Allied Disciplines 4, 99-107.
Rosenberg, J. B., & Lindblad, M. B. (1978). Behavior therapy in a family context: Treating elective mutism. Family Process 17, 77-82.

Ruzicka, B. B., & Sackin, H. D. (1974). Elective autism. The impact of the patient's silent detachment upon the therapist. Journal of the American Academy of Child Psychiatry 13, 551-561.

Shaw, W. H. (1971). Aversive control in the treatment of elective mutism. Journal of the American Academy of Child Psychiatry 10, 572-581.

Wergeland, H. (1979). Elective mutism. Acta Psychiatrica Scandinavica 59, 218-228.

Wright, H. H., Miller, M. D., Cook, M. A., & Littmann, J. R. (1985). Early identification and intervention with children who refuse to speak. Journal of the American Academy of Child Psychiatry 24, 739-746.

8. Tics, Tourette's Syndrome

Barabas, G., Matthews, W. S., & Ferrare, M. (1984). Tourette syndrome and migraine. Archives of Neurology 41, 871-872.

Burd, L., Kerbeshian, J., Wikenheiser, M., & Fisher, W. (1986). Prevalence of Gilles de la Tourette's syndrome in North Dakota adults. American Journal of Psychiatry 14., 787-788.

Cohen, D. J., Brunn, R., & Leckman, J. F. (Eds.). (1987). Tourette syndrome and tic disorders: Clinical understanding and treatment. New York: Wiley.

Cohen, D. J., Leckman, J. F., & Shaywitz, B. A. (1984). The Tourette syndrome and other tics. In D. Shaffer, A. A. Ehrhart, & L. Greenhill (Eds.), A clinical guide to child psychiatry (pp. 2-28). New York: Macmillan Free Press.

Comings, D. E., & Comings, B. G. (1984). Tourette syndrome and attention deficit with hyperactivity: Are they genetically related? Journal of the American Academy of Child Psychiatry 23, 138-146.

Harcherik, D. J., Leckman, J. F., Deltor, J., & Cohen, D. G. (1984). A new instrument for clinical studies of Tourette's syndrome. Journal of the American Academy of Child Psychiatry 23, 152-160.

Leckman, J. F., Deltor, J., Harcherik, D., Ort, S., Shaywitz, B. A., & Cohen, D. J. (1985). Short and long term treatment of Tourette's disorder with clonidine: A clinical perspective. Neurology 35, 343-351.

Pauls, D. L., Hurst, C., Kruger, S. D., Leckman, J. F., Kidd, K. K., & Cohen, D. J. (1986). Evidence against a genetic relationship between Tourette syndrome and attention deficit disorder. Archives of General Psychiatry 43, 1177-1179.

Pauls, D. L., Kruger, S. D., Leckman, J. F., Cohen, D. J., & Kidd, K. K. (1984). The risk of TS/CMT among relatives of TS patients obtained by direct interview. Journal of the American Academy of Child Psychiatry 23, 134-137.

Pauls, D. L., & Leckman, J. F. (1986). The inheritance of Gilles de la Tourette syndrome and associated behaviors: Evidence for autosomal dominant transmission. New England Journal of Medicine 315, 993-997.

Pauls, D. L., Towbin, D. K., Leckman, J. F., Zahner, G. E., & Cohen, D. J. (1986). Gilles de la Tourette's syndrome and obsessive-compulsive disorder: Evidence supporting a genetic relationship. Archives of General Psychiatry 43, 1180-1183.

Price, R. A., Kidd, K. K., Cohen, D. J., Pauls, D. L., & Leckman, J. F. (1985). A twin study of Tourette syndrome. Archives of General Psychiatry 42, 815-820.

Price, R. A., Leckman, J. F., Pauls, D. L., Cohen, D. J., & Kidd, K. K. (1986). Tics and central nervous stimulants in twins and non-twins with Tourette syndrome. Neurology 36, 232-237.

Shapiro, A. K., & Shapiro, E. (1984). Controlled study of pimozide vs. placebo in Tourette syndrome. Journal of the American Academy of Child Psychiatry 23, 161-173.

Shapiro, A. K., Shapiro, E., & Eisenkraft, G. J. (1983). Treatment of Gilles de la Tourette's syndrome with clonidine and neuroleptics. Archives of General Psychiatry 40, 1235-1240.

9. Personality Disorders, Gender-Identity Problems, and Borderline Conditions

Ackerly, W. C. (1967). Latency-age children who threaten or attempt to kill themselves. Journal of the American Academy of Child Psychiatry 6, 242-261.

Adams, P. L. (1972). Family characteristics of obsessive children. American Journal of Psychiatry 128, 1414-1417.

Adams, P. L., Schwab, J. J., & Aponte, J. (1965). Authoritarian parents and disturbed children. American Journal of Psychiatry 121, 1162-1167.

Aichhorn, A. (1935). Wayward youth. New York: Viking Press.

Amado, H., & Lustman, P. J. (1982). Attention deficit disorders persisting in adulthood: A review. Comprehensive Psychiatry 23, 300-314.

Andrulonis, P. A., Glueck, B. C., Stroebel, C. F., Vogel, N. G., Shapiro, A. L., & Aldridge, D. M. (1981). Organic brain dysfunction and the borderline syndrome. Psychiatric Clinics of North America 4, 47-66.

Anthony, E. J. (1970). The mutative impact of serious mental and physical illness in a parent on family life. In E. J. Anthony & C. Koupernik (Eds.), The child in his family (pp. 131-163). New York: Wiley.

Archer, R. P., Ball, J. D., & Hunter, J. A. (1985). MMPI characteristics of borderline psychopathology in adolescent inpatients. Journal of Personality Assessment 49, 47-55.

Bandura, A. (1958). Dependency conflict in aggressive delinquents. Journal of Social Issues 143, 52-65.

Bemporad, J. R., Smith, H. F., Hanson, G., & Cicchetti, D. (1982). Borderline syndromes in childhood: Criteria for diagnosis. American Journal of Psychiatry 139, 596-602.

Bender, L. (1959). Children and adolescents who have killed. American Journal of Psychiatry 116, 510.

Blumberg, M. L. (1979). Character disorders in traumatized and handicapped children. American Journal of Psychotherapy 33, 201-203.

Bowlby, J. (1944). Forty-four juvenile thieves: Their characters and home life. International Journal of Psycho-Analysis 25, 19-52.

Bowlby, J. (1961). Separation anxiety: A critical review of the literature. Journal of Child Psychology and Psychiatry and Allied Disciplines 1, 251-269.

Bowlby, J., Ainsworth, M., Boston, M., & Rosenbluth, D. (1956). The effects of mother-child separation: A follow-up study. British Journal of Medical Psychology 29, 211-247.

Bradley, S. J. (1979). The relationship of early maternal separation to borderline personality in children and adolescents: A pilot study. American Journal of Psychiatry 136, 424-426.

Bradley, S. J. (1981). The borderline diagnosis in children and adolescents. Child Psychiatry and Human Development 12, 121-127.

Brazelton, T. B., Young, G. G., & Bullowa, M. (1971). Inception and resolution of early developmental pathology: A case history. Journal of the American Academy of Child Psychiatry 10, 124-135.

Broucek, F. J. (1982). Shame and its relationship to early narcissistic development. International Journal of Psycho-Analysis 63, 369-378.

Brunswick, R. M. (1943). The accepted lie. Psychiatric Quarterly 12, 458-464.

Bullard, M. D., et al. (1967). Failure to thrive in the "neglected" child. American Journal of Orthopsychiatry 37, 680-690.

Burks, H. L., & Harrison, S. I. (1962). Aggressive behavior as a means of avoiding depression. American Journal of Orthopsychiatry 32, 416-422.

Carlson, G. A., & Cantwell, D. P. (1980). Unmasking masked depression in children and adolescents. American Journal of Psychiatry 137, 445-449.

Chess, S. (1967). Healthy responses, developmental disturbances and stress or reactive disorders. I. Infancy and childhood. In A. M. Freedman & H. I. Kaplan (Eds.), Comprehensive textbook of psychiatry (pp. 1358-1366). Baltimore: Williams and Wilkins.

Chess, S., Thomas, A., Birch, H. G., & Hertzig, M. (1960). Implications of a longitudinal study of child development for child psychiatry. American Journal of Psychiatry 117, 434-441.

Chethik, M. (1986). Levels of borderline functioning in children: Etiological and treatment considerations. American Journal of Orthopsychiatry 56, 109-119.

Chethik, M., & Fast, I. (1970). A function of fantasy in the borderline child. American Journal of Orthopsychiatry 40, 756-765.

Chiland, C. (1988). Enfance et transsexualisme. [Infancy and transexuality]. Psychiatrie de l'Enfant 31, 313-373.

Coates, S., & Zucker, K. J. (1988). Gender identity disorders in children. In C. J. Kestenbaum & D. T. Williams (Eds.), Handbook of clinical assessment of children and adolescents (Vol. 2, pp. 893-914). New York: New York University Press.

Cohen, D. J., & Johnson, W. T. (1977). Cardiovascular correlates of attention in normal and psychiatrically disturbed children. Blood pressure, peripheral blood flow, and peripheral vascular resistance. Archives of General Psychiatry 34, 561-567.

Coles, R. (1967). Violence in ghetto children. Children 14, 101-104.

Deprivation of maternal care: A reassessment of its effects. (1962). Geneva: World Health Organization.

Easson, W. M., & Steinhilber, R. M. (1961). Murderous aggression by children and adolescents. Archives of General Psychiatry 4, 1.

Eaton, L. F., & Menolascino, F. J. (1982). Psychiatric disorders in the mentally retarded: Types, problems, and challenger. American Journal of Psychiatry 139, 1297-1303.

Erikson, E. H. (1959). Growth and crises of the healthy personality. Psychological Issues 1, 50-100.

Feldman, R. B., & Guttman, H. A. (1984). Families of borderline patients: Literal-minded parents, borderline parents, and parental protectiveness. American Journal of Psychiatry 141, 1392-1396.

Freud, A. (1965). Dissociality, delinquency, criminality. In A. Freud (Ed.), Normality and pathology in childhood: Assessment of development. New York: International Universities Press.

Freud, S. (1959). Inhibitions, symptoms and anxiety (1926). In E. Jones (Ed.), Collected papers. Standard edition (pp. 87-174). New York and London: Hogarth Press.

Friedman, R. C. (1988). Male homosexuality: A contemporary psychoanalytic perspective. New Haven: Yale University Press.

Friedman, R. M. (1982). Therapeutic techniques for the treatment of certain infantile personality disorders in ego-disturbed children. Psychoanalytic Review 69, 191-206.

Fries, M. E., Nelson, M. C., & Woolf, P. J. (1980). Developmental and etiological factors in the treatment of character disorders with archaic ego function. Psychoanalytic Review 67, 337-352.

Frijling-Schreuder, E. C. M. (1969). Borderline states in children. In R. S. Eissler, et al. (Eds.), Psychoanalytic study of the child (Vol. 24, pp. 307-327). New York: International Universities Press.

Frosch, J. (1971). Technique in regard to some specific ego defects in treatment of borderline patients. Psychiatric Quarterly 45, 216-220.

Gilpin, D. C., & Maltz, P. (1980). The oppositional personality in childhood. Child Psychiatry and Human Development 11, 79-86.

Golomeier, H. (1974). Vandalism: The effects of unmanageable confrontations. Adolescence 9, 49.

Green, R., & Green, J. (Eds.). (1969). Money, transsexualism, and sex reassignment. Baltimore: Johns Hopkins University Press.

Green, R., Roberts, C., Williams, K., & Mixon, A. (1987). Specific cross-gender behaviors in boyhood and later sexual orientation. British Journal of Psychiatry 151, 84-88.

Greenson, R. R. (1966). A transvestite boy and a hypothesis. International Journal of Psycho-Analysis 47, 396-403.

Greenspan, S., & Lourie, R. S. (1981). Developmental structuralist approach to the classification of adaptive and pathologic personality organizations: Infancy and early childhood. American Journal of Psychiatry 138, 725-735.

Groves, J. E. (1981). Current concepts in psychiatry: Borderline personality disorder. New England Journal of Medicine 305, 259-262.

Gunderson, J. G., & Englund, D. W. (1981). Characterizing the families of borderlines. A review of the literature. Psychiatric Clinics of North America 4, 159-168.

Harrison, S. I. (1970). Reared in the wrong sex. Journal of the American Academy of Child Psychiatry 9, 44-102.

Harrison, S. I., Cain, A. C., & Benedek, E. (1968). the childhood of a transsexual. Archives of General Psychiatry 19, 28-37.

Holman, S. L. (1985). A group program for borderline mothers and their toddlers. International Journal of Group Psychotherapy 35, 79-93.

Johnson, A. M., & Szurek, S. A. (1952). The genesis of antisocial acting out in children and adults. Psychoanalytic Quarterly 21, 323.

Kaufman, I., Heims, L. W., & Reiser, D. E. (1961). A re-evaluation of the psychodynamics of firesetting. American Journal of Orthopsychiatry 31, 123-136.

Kaufman, I., Makkay, E. S., & Zilbach, J. (1959). The impact of adolescence on girls with delinquent character formation. American Journal of Orthopsychiatry 29, 130-143.

Kirk, H. D., Jonassohn, K., & Fish, A. D. (1966). Are adopted children especially vulnerable to stress? Archives of General Psychiatry 14, 291-298.

Knight, R. P. (1942). Intimidation of others as a defense against anxiety. Bulletin of the Menninger Clinic 6, 4-14.

Kosky, R. J. (1987). Gender-disordered children: Does inpatient treatment help? Medical Journal of Australia 146, 565-569.

Lapouse, R., & Monk, M. A. (1964). Behavior deviations in a representative sample of children: Variation by sex, age, race, social class and family size. American Journal of Orthopsychiatry 34, 436-446.

Lax, R. F. (1958). Infantile deprivation and arrested ego development. Psychoanalytic Quarterly 27, 501-517.

Leicester, J. (1982). Temper tantrums, epilepsy and episodic dyscontrol. British Journal of Psychiatry 141, 262-266.

Levy, E. (1934). Psychoanalytic treatment of a child with a stealing compulsion. American Journal of Orthopsychiatry 4, 1-23.

Lewis, M., & Sarrel, P. M. (1969). Some psychological aspect of seduction, incest, and rape in childhood. Journal of the American Academy of Child Psychiatry 8, 606-619.

Lewis, N. D. C., & Yarnell, H. (1951). Pathological firesetting (pyromania). Nervous and Mental Disease Monographs 82.

Makkay, E. S., & Schwaab, E. H. (1962). Some problems in the differential diagnosis of antisocial character disorders in early latency. Journal of the American Academy of Child Psychiatry 1, 414-430.

Marohn, R. C. (1974). Trauma and the delinquent.In S. C. Feinstein, et al. (Eds.), Adolescent psychiatry: Developmental and clinical studies (Vol. 3, pp. 354-361). Chicago: University of Chicago Press.

Marohn, R. C. (1977). The juvenile imposter: Some thoughts on narcissism and the delinquent. In S. C. Feinstein, et al. (Eds.), Adolescent psychiatry:

Developmental and clinical studies (Vol. 5, pp. 186-212). Chicago: University of Chicago Press.

Marohn, R. C. (1979). A psychiatric overview of juvenile delinquency. In S. C. Feinstein, et al. (Eds.), Adolescent psychiatry: Developmental and clinical studies (Vol. 7, pp. 425-432). Chicago: University of Chicago Press.

Marohn, R. C. (1981). The negative transference in the treatment of juvenile delinquents. Annaul Psychoanalysis 9, 21-42.

Marohn, R. C., Locke, E., Rosenthal, R., & Curtiss, G. (1982). Juvenile delinquents and violent death. In S. C. Feinstein, et al. (Eds.), Adolescent psychiatry: Developmental and clinical studies (Vol. 10, pp. 147-170). Chicago: University of Chicago Press.

Marohn, R. C., Offer, D., Ostrov, E., & Trujillo, J. (1979). Psychodynamic types of hospitalized juvenile delinquents. In S. C. Feinstein, et al. (Eds.), Adolescent psychiatry: Developmental and clinical studies (Vol. 7, pp. 466-483). Chicago: University of Chicago Press.

Meeks, J. E. (1979). Behavioral and antisocial disorders. In J. D. Noshpitz (Ed.), Basic handbook of child psychiatry (pp. 482-533). New York: Basic Books.

Meissner, W. W. (1978). Theoretical assumptions of concepts of the borderline personality. Journal of the American Psychoanalytic Association 26, 559-598.

Meissner, W. W. (1985). A case of phallic-narcissistic personality. Journal of the American Psychoanalytic Association 33, 437-469.

Michaels, J. J. (1941). Parallels between persistent enuresis and delinquency in the psychopathic personality. American Journal of Orthopsychiatry 11, 260.

Millican, F. K., & Lourie, R. S. (1970). The child with pica and his family. In E. J. Anthony & C. Koupernik (Eds.), The child in his family (pp. 333-348). New York: Wiley.

Money, J. (1987). Sin, sickness, or status? Homosexual gender identity and psychoneuroendocrinology. American Psychologist 42, 384-399.

Money, J. (1988). Gay, straight, and in between: The sexology of erotic orientation. New York: Oxford University Press.

Monopolis, S., & Lion, J. R. (1983). Problems in the diagnosis of the intermittent explosive disorder. American Journal of Psychiatry 140, 1200-1202.

Morris, H. H., Jr., Escoll, P. J., & Wekler, R. (1956). Aggressive behavior disorders of childhood: A follow-up study. American Journal of Psychiatry 112, 991-997.

Morrison, J. (1980). Adult psychiatric disorders in parents of hyperactive children. American Journal of Psychiatry 137, 825-827.

Morrison, J. R., & Minkoff, K. (1975). Explosive personality as a sequel to the hyperactive-child syndrome. Comprehensive Psychiatry 16, 343-348.

Neubauer, P. B. (1960). The one-parent child and his oedipal development. In R. S. Eissler, et al. (Eds.), Psychoanalytic study of the child (Vol. 15, pp. 286-309). New York: International Universities Press.

Newman, M. B., & San Martino, M. R. (1971). The child and the seriously disturbed parent: Patterns of adaptation to parental psychosis. Journal of the American Academy of Child Psychiatry 10, 358-374.

Ornstein, A., Gropper, C., & Bogner, J. Z. (1983). Shoplifting: An expression of revenge and restitution. Annual Psychoanalysis 11, 311-331.

Perry, J. C. (1985). Depression in borderline personality disorder: Lifetime prevalence at interview and longitudinal course of symptoms. American Journal of Psychiatry 142, 15-21.

Petti, T. A., & Law, W. (1982). Borderline psychotic behavior in hospitalized children: Approaches to assessment and treatment. Journal of the American Academy of Child Psychiatry 21, 197-202.

Petti, T. A., & Unis, A. (1981). Imipramine treatment of borderline children: Case reports with a controlled study. American Journal of Psychiatry 138, 515-518.

Pleak, R. R., Meyer-Bahlburg, H. F. L., O'Brien, J. D., Bowen, H. A., & Morganstein, A. (1989). Cross-gender behavior and psychopathology in boy psychiatric out-patients. Journal of the American Academy of Child and Adolescent Psychiatry 28, 385-393.

Poznanski, E. O. (1973). Children with excessive fears. American Journal of Orthopsychiatry 43, 428-438.

Rainer, J. D. (1979). Heredity and character disorders. American Journal of Psychotherapy 33, 6-16.

Rekers, G. A. (1988). Psychosexual assessment of gender identity disorders. In R. J. Prinz (Ed.), Advances in behavioral assessment of children and families (Vol. 4, pp. 33-71). Greenwood, Conn.: JAI Press.

Rexford, E. N., & van Amerongen, S. T. (1957). The influence of unsolved maternal oral conflicts upon impulsive acting out in young children. American Journal of Orthopsychiatry 27, 75-87.

Rinsley, D. B. (1981a). Borderline psychopathology: The concepts of Masterson and Rinsley and beyond. In S. C. Feinstein, et al. (Eds.), Adolescent psychiatry: Developmental and clinical studies (Vol. 9, pp. 259-274). Chicago: University of Chicago Press.

Rinsley, D. B. (1981b). Dynamic and developmental issues in borderline and related "spectrum" disorders. Psychiatric Clinics of North America 4, 117-132.

Robbins, M. (1983). Toward a new mind model for the primitive personalities. International Journal of Psycho-Analysis 64, 127-148.

Robbins, M. D. (1976). Borderline personality organization: The need for a new theory. Journal of the American Psychoanalytic Association 24, 831-853.

Roberts, C. W., Green, R., Williams, K., & Goodman, M. (1987). Boyhood gender identity development: A statistical contrast of two family groups. Developmental Psychology 23, 554-557.

Sandler, A., Daunton, E., & Schnurmann, A. (1957). Inconsistency in the mother as a factor in character development: A comparative study of three cases. In R. S. Eissler, et al. (Eds.), Psychoanalytic study of the child (Vol. 12, pp. 209-225). New York: International Universities Press.

Scharer, K. M. (1979). Helping disturbed children change their passive-aggressive behavior through milieu therapy. American Nurses' Association Publication, No. 59: 275-292.

Sedman, A. B., Wilkening, G. N., Warady, B. A., Lum, G. M., & Alfrey, A. C. (1984). Encephalopathy in childhood secondary to aluminum toxicity. Journal of Pediatrics 105, 836-838.

Sendi, I. B., & Blombren, P. G. (1975). A comparative study of predictive criteria in the predisposition of homicidal adolescents. American Journal of Psychiatry 132, 423.

Settlage, C. F. (1977). The psychoanalytic understanding of narcissistic and borderline personality disorders: Advances in developmental theory. Journal of the American Psychoanalytic Association 25, 805-833.

Singer, M. (1974). Family structure, disciplinary configurations and adolescent psychopathology. In S. C. Feinstein, et al. (Eds.), Adolescent psychiatry: Developmental and clinical studies (Vol. 3, p. 372). Chicago: University of Chicago Press.

Smith, H. F., Bemporad, J. R., & Hanson, G. (1982). Aspects of the treatment of borderline children. American Journal of Psychotherapy 36, 181-197.

Spitz, R. A. (1951). The psychogenic diseases in infancy. An attempt at their etiologic classification. In R. S. Eissler, et al. (Eds.), Psychoanalytic study of the child (Vol. 6, pp. 255-275). New York: International Universities Press.

Spitz, R. A., & Wolf, K. M. (1946). Anaclitic depression. An inquiry into the genesis of psychiatric conditions in early childhood. II. In R. S. Eissler, et al. (Eds.), Psychoanalytic study of the child (Vol. 2, pp. 313-342). New York: International Universities Press.

Stierlin, H. (1973). A family perspective on adolescent runaways. Archives of General Psychiatry 29, 56.

Stoller, R. J. (1974). Symbiosis anxiety and the development of masculinity. Archives of General Psychiatry 30, 164-172.

Szurek, S. A. (1942). Notes of the genesis of psychopathic personality traits. Psychiatry 5, 1-6.

Thomas, A., Chess, S., & Birch, H. G. (1968). Temperament and behavior disorders in children. New York: New York University Press.

Tuber, S., & Coates, S. (1989). Indices of psychopathology in the Rorschachs of boys with severe gender identity disorder: A comparison with normal control subjects. Journal of Personality Assessment 53, 100-112.

Westman, J. C., Rice, D. L., & Bermann, E. (1967). Nursery school behavior and later school adjustment. American Journal of Orthopsychiatry 37, 725-731.

Winnicott, D. W. (1958). The antisocial tendency. In D. W. Winnicott (Ed.), Collected papers. New York: Basic Books.

Winnicott, D. W. (1973). Delinquency as a sign of hope. In S. C. Feinstein, et al. (Eds.), Adolescent psychiatry: Developmental and clinical studies (Vol. 2, pp. 364-371). Chicago: University of Chicago Press.

Wolff, S. (1961). Symptomatology and outcome of pre-school children with behaviour disorders attending a child guidance clinic. Journal of Child Psychology and Psychiatry and Allied Disciplines 2, 269-276.

Wolff, S. (1967). The contribution of obstetric complications to the etiology of behaviour disorders in childhood. Journal of Child Psychology and Psychiatry and Allied Disciplines 8, 57-66.
Wolff, S. (1984). The concept of personality disorder in childhood. Journal of Child Psychology and Psychiatry and Allied Disciplines 25, 5-13.
Woodside, M., Harrow, A., Basson, J. V., & Affleck, J. W. (1976). Experiment in managing sociopathic behaviour disorders. British Medical Journal 2, 1056-1059.
Woolley, L. F. (1937). Studies in obsessive ruminative tension states: III. The effect of erratic discipline in childhood on emotional tensions. Psychiatric Quarterly 11, 237-352.
Yates, A. (1981). Narcissistic traits in certain abused children. American Journal of Orthopsychiatry 51, 55-62.
Zander, K. (1984). "The fragile princess." Midway on the borderline-narcissistic personality continuum. Perspectives in Psychiatric Care 22, 77-84.
Zatolokina, E. I., & Ushakov, G. K. (1981). Types of personality reactions in children and adolescents with hysterical disorders. Zhurnal Nevropatologii i Psikhiatrii Imeni S. S. Korsakova 81, 1676-1681.
Zucker, K. J. (1988). Toward a developmental sexology [Review of The "sissy boy syndrome" and the development of homosexuality]. Contemporary Psychology 33, 197-199.
Zucker, K. J. (1989). Gender identity disorders. In C. G. Last & M. Hersen (Eds.), Handbook of child psychiatric diagnosis (pp. 388-406). New York: Wiley.
Zucker, K. J., Bradley, S. J., & Hughes, H. E. (1987). Gender dysphoria in a child with true hermaphroditism. Canadian Journal of Psychiatry 32, 602-609.
Zucker, K. J., & Green, R. (1989). Gender identity disorder of childhood. In T. B. Karasu (Ed.), Treatments of psychiatric disorders: A task force report of the American Psychiatric Association (Vol. 1, pp. 661-670). Washington, D.C.: American Psychiatric Association.
Zuger, B. (1974). Effeminate behavior in boys. Archives of General Psychiatry 30, 173-177.
Zuger, B. (1988). Is early effeminate behavior in boys early homosexuality? Comprehensive Psychiatry 29, 509-519.

10. Problems of Sexual Identification

Bates, J. E., Bentler, P. M., & Thompson, S. K. (1979). Gender-deviant boys compared with normal and clinical control boys. Journal of Abnormal Child Psychology 7, 243-259.
Bates, J. E., Skilbeck, W. M., Smith, K. V. R., & Bentler, P. M. (1974). Gender role abnormalities in boys: An analysis of clinical ratings. Journal of Abnormal Child Psychology 2, 1-16.
Bleiberg, E., Jackson, L., & Ross, J. L. (1986). Gender identity disorder and object loss. Journal of the American Academy of Child Psychiatry 25, 58-67.

Coates, S., & Person, E. S. (1985). Extreme boyhood femininity: Isolated behavior or pervasive disorder? Journal of the American Academy of Child Psychiatry 24, 702-709.

Davenport, C. W., & Harrison, S. I. (1977). Gender identity change in a female adolescent transsexual. Archives of Sexual Behavior 6, 327-340.

Dulcan, M. K., & Lee, P. A. (1984). Transsexualism in the adolescent girl. Journal of the American Academy of Child Psychiatry 23, 354-361.

Ehrhardt, A. A., & Meyer-Bahlburg, H. F. (1981). Effects of prenatal sex hormones on gender-related behavior. Science 211, 1312-1318.

Ehrhardt, A. A., Meyer-Bahlburg, H. F., Feldman, J. F., & Ince, S. E. (1984). Sex-dimorphic behavior in childhood subsequent to prenatal exposure to exogenous progestogens and estrogens. Archives of Sexual Behavior 13, 457-477.

Ehrhardt, A. A., Meyer-Bahlburg, H. F. L., Rosen, L. R., Feldman, J. F., Veridiano, N. P., Zimmerman, I., & McEwen, B. S. (1985). Sexual orientation after prenatal exposure to exogenous estrogen. Archives of Sexual Behavior 14, 57-77.

Eme, R. F. (1979). Sex differences in childhood psychopathology. Psychological Bulletin 86, 574-595.

Finegan, J. K., Zucker, K. J., Bradley, S. J., & Doering, R. W. (1982). Patterns of intellectual functioning and spatial ability in boys and gender identity disorder. Canadian Journal of Psychiatry 27, 135-139.

Gadpaille, W. J. (1975). Homosexuality in adolescent males. American Academy of Psychoanalysis 3, 361-371.

Glasser, M. (1977). Homosexuality in adolescence. British Journal of Medical Psychology 50, 217-225.

Golombok, S., Spencer, A., & Rutter, M. (1983). Children in lesbian and single-parent households: Psychosexual and psychiatric appraisal. Journal of Child Psychology and Psychiatry and Allied Disciplines 24, 551-572.

Green, R. (1976). One-hundred ten feminine and masculine boys: Behavioral contrasts and demographic similarities. Archives of Sexual Behavior 5, 425-446.

Green, R. (1985). Gender identity in childhood and later sexual orientation: Follow-up of 78 males. American Journal of Psychiatry 142, 339-341.

Green, R. (1987). The sissy-boy syndrome and the development of homosexuality. New Haven: Yale University Press.

Green, R., Mandel, J. B., Hotvedt, M. E., Gray, J., & Smith, L. (1986). Lesbian mothers and their children: A comparison with solo parent heterosexual mothers and their children. Archives of Sexual Behavior 15, 167-184.

Green, R., Williams, K., & Goodman, M. (1982). Ninety-nine "tomboys" and "non-tomboys": Behavioral contrasts and demographic similarities. Archives of Sexual Behavior 11, 247-266.

Green, R., Williams, K., & Goodman, M. (1985). Masculine or feminine gender identity in boys: Developmental differences between two diverse family groups. Sex Roles 12, 1155-1162.

Hoeffer, B. (1981). Children's acquisition of sex-role behavior in lesbian-mother families. American Journal of Orthopsychiatry 51, 536-544.

Kirkpatrick, M., Smith, C., & Roy, R. (1981). Lesbian mothers and their children: A comparative survey. American Journal of Orthopsychiatry 51, 545-551.

Lothstein, L. M. (1980). The adolescent gender dysphoric patient: An approach to treatment and management. Journal of Pediatric Psychology 5, 93-109.

Martin, A. D. (1982). Learning to hide: The socialization of the gay adolescent. In S. C. Feinstein, J. G. Looney, A. Z. Schwartzberg, & A. D. Sorosky (Eds.), Adolescent psychiatry: Developmental and clinical studies (pp. 52-65). Chicago: University of Chicago Press.

McCauley, E., & Ehrhardt, A. A. (1984). Follow-up of females with gender identity disorders. Journal of Nervous and Mental Disease 172, 353-358.

Meyer, J. K., & Dupkin, C. (1985). Gender disturbance in children. An interim clinical report. Bulletin of the Menninger Clinic 49, 236-269.

Meyer-Bahlburg, H. F., Feldman, J. F., & Ehrhardt, A. A. (1985). Questionnaires for the assessment of atypical gender role behavior: A methodological study. Journal of the American Academy of Child Psychiatry 24, 695-701.

Money, J. (1985a). The conceptual neutering of gender and the criminalization of sex. Archives of Sexual Behavior 14, 279-290.

Money, J. (1985b). Pediatric sexology and hermaphroditism. Journal of Sex and Marital Therapy 11, 139-156.

Money, J., Devore, H., & Normal, B. F. (1986). Gender identity and gender transposition: Longitudinal outcome study of 32 male hermaphrodites assigned as girls. Journal of Sex and Marital Therapy 12, 165-181.

Money, J., Hampson, J. G., & Hampson, J. L. (1955). Hermaphroditism: Recommendations concerning assignment of sex, change of sex, and psychologic management. Bulletin of the Johns Hopkins Hospital 97, 284-300.

Money, J., & Russo, A. J. (1979). Homosexual outcome of discordant gender identity/role: Longitudinal follow-up. Journal of Pediatric Psychology 4, 29-41.

Myers, M. F. (1982). Counseling the parents of young homosexual male patients. Journal of Homosexuality 8, 131-143.

Newman, L. E. (1976). Treatment for the parents of feminine boys. American Journal of Psychiatry 133, 683-687.

Rekers, G. A. (1975). Stimulus control over sex-typed play in cross-gender identified boys. Journal of Experimental Child Psychology 20, 136-148.

Rekers, G. A. (1977a). Assessment and treatment of childhood gender problems. In B. B. Lahey & A. E. Kazdin (Eds.), Advances in clinical child psychology (pp. 267-306). New York: Plenum Press.

Rekers, G. A. (1977b). Atypical gender development and psychosocial adjustment. Journal of Applied Behavior Analysis 10, 559-571.

Rekers, G. A., & Yates, C. E. (1976). Sex-typed play in feminoid boys versus normal boys and girls. Journal of Abnormal Child Psychology 4, 1-8.

Ross, J. M. (1975). The development of paternal identity: A critical review of the literature on nurturance and generactivity in boys and men. Journal of the American Psychoanalytic Association 23, 783-817.

Skilbeck, W. M., Bates, J. E., & Bentler, P. M. (1975). Human figure drawings of gender-problem and school-problem boys. Journal of Abnormal Child Psychology 3, 191-199.

Sreenivasan, U. (1985). Effeminate boys in a child psychiatric clinic: Prevalence and associated factors. Journal of the American Academy of Child Psychiatry 24, 689-694.

Stoller, R. J. (1974). Symbiosis, anxiety and the development of masculinity. Archives of General Psychiatry 30, 164-172.

Tuber, S., & Coates, S. (1985). Interpersonal phenomena in the Rorschachs of extremely feminine boys. Psychoanalytic Psychology 2, 251-265.

Weinrich, J. D. (1985). Transsexuals, homosexuals, and sissy boys: On the mathematics of follow-up studies. Journal of Sex Research 21, 322-328.

Williams, K., Goodman, M., & Green, R. (1985). Parent-child factors in gender role socialization in girls Journal of the American Academy of Child Psychiatry 24, 720-731.

Wolfe, B. E. (1979). Behavioral treatment of childhood gender disorders: A conceptual and empirical critique. Behavior Modification 3, 550-575.

Zucker, K. J. (1982). Childhood gender disturbance: Diagnostic issues. Journal of the American Academy of Child Psychiatry 21, 274-280.

Zucker, K. J., Bradley, S. J., Doering, R. W., & Lozinski, J. A. (1985). Sex-typed behavior in cross-gender-identified children: Stability and change at a one-year follow-up. Journal of the American Academy of Child Psychiatry 24, 710-719.

Zucker, K. J., Doering, R. W., Bradley, S. J., & Finegan, J. K. (1982). Sex-typed play in gender-disturbed children: A comparison to sibling and psychiatric controls. Archives of Sexual Behavior 11, 309-321.

Zucker, K. J., Finegan, J. K., Doering, R. W., & Bradley, S. J. (1984). Two subgroups of gender-problem children. Archives of Sexual Behavior 13, 27-39.

Zuger, B. (1984). Early effeminate behavior in boys. Outcome and significance for homosexuality. Journal of Nervous and Mental Disease 172, 90-97.

11. Affective Disorders

Theodore Petti, M.D., Subsection Editor

a. Assessment

Angold, A. (1988). Childhood and adolescent depression. I. Epidemiological and aetiological aspects. British Journal of Psychiatry 152, 601-617.

Annell, A. L. (1972). Depressive states in childhood and adolescence. New York: Halstead Press.

Anthony, E. J. (1983). Depression in adolescents. A psychodynamic approach to nosology. In H. Golombek & B. D. Garfinkel (Eds.), The adolescent and mood disturbances (pp. 151-165). New York: International Universities Press.

Brumback, R. A., Dietz-Schmidt, S. G., & Weinberg, W. A. (1977). Depression in children referred to an educational diagnostic center: Diagnostic and treatment and analysis of criteria and literature review. Diseases of the Nervous System 38, 529-535.

Brumback, R. A., Staton, R. D., & Wilson, H. (1980). Neuropsychological study of children during and after remission of endogenous depressive episodes. Perceptual and Motor Skills 50, 1163-1167.

Burke, P., Meyer, V., Kocoshis, S., Orenstein, D., Chandra, R., Nord, D., Sauer, J., & Cohen, E. (1989). Depression and anxiety in pediatric inflammatory bowel disease and cystic fibrosis. Journal of the American Academy of Child and Adolescent Psychiatry 28, 948-951.

Cantwell, D. P. (1985). Depressive disorders in children. Validation of clinical syndromes. Psychiatric Clinics of North America 8, 779-792.

Cantwell, D. P., & Carlson, G. A. (Eds.). (1983). Affective disorders in childhood and adolescents: An update. New York: Spectrum Publications.

Cicchetti, D., & Schneider Rosen, K., (Eds.), Childhood depression: New directions for child development. San Francisco: Jossey-Bass.

Cohen, D. J. (1980). Constructive and reconstructive activities in the analysis of a depressed child. In A. Solnit, et al. (Eds.), Psychoanalytic study of the child (Vol. 35, pp. 237-266). New Haven: Yale University Press.

Costello, E. J., & Angold, A. (1988). Scales to assess child and adolescent depression: Checklists, screens, and nets. Journal of the American Academy of Child and Adolescent Psychiatry 27, 726-737.

Cytryn, L., McKnew, D. H., & Bunney, W. E. (1980). Diagnosis of depression in children: A reassessment. American Journal of Psychiatry 137, 22-25.

Eastgate, J., & Gilmour, L. (1984). Long-term outcome of depressed children: A follow-up study. Developmental Medicine and Child Neurology 26, 68-72.

Emery, G., Bedrosian, R., & Garber, J. (1983). Cognitive therapy with depressed children and adolescent. In D. P. Cantwell & G. A. Carlson (Eds.), Affective disorders in childhood and adolescents: An update. New York: Spectrum Publications.

Fleming, J. E., Offord, D. R., & Boyle, M. H. (1989). Prevalence of childhood and adolescent depression in the community. Ontario child health study. British Journal of Psychiatry 155, 647-654.

French, A., & Berlin, I. (Eds.). (1979). Depression in childhood and adolescents. New York: Human Sciences Press.

Garber, J., Kriss, M. R., Koch, M., & Lindholm, L. (1988). Recurrent depression in adolescents: A follow-up study. Journal of the American Academy of Child and Adolescent Psychiatry 27, 49-54.

Glaser, K. (1978). The treatment of depressed and suicidal adolescents. American Journal of Psychotherapy 32, 252-269.

Glaser, K. (1981). Psychopathic patterns in depressed adolescents. American Journal of Psychotherapy 35, 368-382.

Golombek, H., & Garfinkel, B. D. (Eds.). (1983). The adolescent and mood disturbance. New York: International Universities Press.

Guttman, H. A. (1983). Family therapy in the treatment of mood disturbance in adolescents. In H. Golombek & B. D. Garfinkel (Eds.), The adolescent and mood disturbances (pp. 263-272). New York: International Universities Press.

Harmon, R. J., Wagonfeld, S., & Emde, R. N. (1982). Anaclitic depression. A follow-up from infancy to puberty. In A. Solnit, et al. (Eds.), Psychoanalytic study of the child (Vol. 37, pp. 67-94). New Haven: Yale University Press.

Hsu, L. K., Molcan, K., Cashman, M. A., Lee, S., Lohr, J. & Hindmarsh, D. (1983). The dexamethasone suppression test in adolescent depression. Journal of the American Academy of Child Psychiatry 22, 470-473.

Kandel, D. B., & Davies, M. (1982). Epidemiology of depressive mood in adolescents. Archives of General Psychiatry 39, 1205-1216.

Kaplan, S. L., Hong, G. K., & Weinhold, C. (1984). Epidemiology of depressive symptomatology in adolescents. Journal of the American Academy of Child Psychiatry 23, 91-98.

Kashani, J. H., Holcomb, W. R., & Orvadschel, H. (1986). Depression and depressive symptoms in preschool children from the general population. American Journal of Psychiatry 143, 1138-1143.

Kashani, J. H., & Priesmeyer, M. (1983). Differences in depressive symptoms and depression among college students. American Journal of Psychiatry 140, 1081-1082.

Kashani, J. H., Strober, M., Rosenberg, T. K., & Reid, J. C. (1988). Correlates of psychopathology in adolescents. Psychiatry Research 26, 141-148.

Kazdin, A. E. (1981). Assessment techniques for childhood depression: A critical appraisal. Journal of the American Academy of Child Psychiatry 20, 358-375.

Kazdin, A. E., & Petti, T. A. (1982). Self-report and interview measures of childhood and adolescent depression. Journal of Child Psychology and Psychiatry and Allied Disciplines 23, 437-457.

Kovacs, M. (1986). A developmental perspective on methods and measures in the assessment of depressive disorders: The clinical interview. In M. Rutter, C. Izard, & P. Read (Eds.), Depression in young people: Developmental and clinical perspectives. New York: Guilford Press.

Kovacs, M., Feinberg, T. L., Crouse-Novak, M. A., Paulauskas, S. L., & Finkelstein, R. (1984). Depressive disorders in childhood. I. A longitudinal prospective study of characteristics and recovery. Archives of General Psychiatry 41, 229-237.

Kovacs, M., Feinberg, T. L., Crouse-Novak, M., Paulauskas, S. L., Pollock, M., & Finkelstein, R. (1984). Depressive disorders in childhood. II. A longitudinal study of the risk for a subsequent major depression. Archives of General Psychiatry 41, 643-649.

Kovacs, M., Gatsonis, C., Paulauskas, S. L., & Richards, C. (1989). Depressive disorders in childhood. IV. A longitudinal study of comorbidity with and risk for anxiety disorders. Archives of General Psychiatry 46, 776-782.

Kovacs, M., Paulauskas, S., Gatsonis, C., & Richards, C. (1988). Depressive disorders in childhood. III. A longitudinal study of comorbidity with and risk for conduct disorders. Journal of Affective Disorders 15, 205-217.

Kramer, A. D., & Feiguine, R. J. (1984). Clinical effects of amitriptyline an adolescent depression: A pilot study. Journal of the American Academy of Child Psychiatry 20, 636-644.

Leahy, R. L. (1988). Cognitive therapy of childhood depression: Developmental considerations. In S. R. Shirk (Ed.), Cognitive development and child psychotherapy (pp. 187-204). New York: Plenum Press.

Lefkowitz, M. M., & Tesiny, E. P. (1980). Assessment of childhood depression. Journal of Consulting and Clinical Psychology 48, 43-50.

McConville, B. J., & Bruce, R. T. (1985). Depressive illnesses in children and adolescents: A review of current concepts. Canadian Journal of Psychiatry 30, 119-129.

Merikangas, K. R., Prusoff, B. A., & Weissman, M. M. (1988). Parental concordance for affective disorders: Psychopathology in offspring. Journal of Affective Disorders 15, 279-290.

Merikangas, K. R., Weissman, M. M., Prusoff, B. A., & John, K. (1988). Assortative mating and affective disorders: Psychopathology in offspring. Psychiatry 51, 48-57.

Pearce, J. B. (1978). The recognition of depressive disorder in children. Journal of the Royal Society of Medicine 71, 494-500.

Petti, T. A. (1983). Behavioral approaches in the treatment of depressed children. In D. Cantwell & G. Carlson (Eds.), Affective disorders of childhood and adolescence (pp. 417-443). New York: Spectrum Publications.

Petti, T. A. (Ed.) (1983). Childhood depression. New York: Hawthorne Press.

Petti, T. A. (1985). Scales of potential use in the psychopharmacologic treatment of depressed children and adolescents. Psychopharmacology Bulletin 21, 951-977.

Philips, I. (1979). Childhood depression: Interpersonal interactions and depressive phenomena. American Journal of Psychiatry 136, 511-555.

Poznanski, E., Mokros, H. B., Grossman, J., & Freeman, L. N. (1985). Diagnostic criteria in childhood depression. American Journal of Psychiatry 142, 1168-1173.

Poznanski, E. O. (1982). The clinical phenomenology of childhood depression. American Journal of Orthopsychiatry 52, 308-313.

Poznanski, E. O., Krahenbuhl, V., & Zrull J. P. (1976). Childhood depression: A longitudinal perspective. Journal of the American Academy of Child Psychiatry 15, 491-501.

Puig-Antich, J. (1987). Sleep and neuroendocrine correlates of affective illness in childhood and adolescence. Journal of Adolescent Health Care 8, 505-529.

Reynolds, W. M., Anderson, G., & Bartell, N. (1985). Measuring depression in children: A multimethod assessment investigation. Journal of Abnormal Child Psychology 13, 513-526.

Reynolds, W. M., & Coats, K. I. (1986). A comparison of cognitive-behavioral therapy and relaxation training in the treatment of depression in adolescents. Journal of Consulting and Clinical Psychology 54, 653-660.

Robbins, D. R., Alessi, N. E., Yanchyshyn, G. W., & Colfer, M. (1983). Psychodynamic and characterological heterogeneity among adolescents with major depressive disorders. Journal of the American Academy of Child Psychiatry 22, 487-491.

Rossman, G. P. (1982). Psychotherapeutic approaches with depressed acting-out adolescents: Interpretive tactics and their rationale. In S. C. Feinstein, et al. (Eds.), Adolescent psychiatry: Developmental and clinical studies (Vol. 10, pp. 455-468). Chicago: University of Chicago Press.

Rutter, M., Izard, C. E., & Read, P. B. (Eds.), Depression in young people: Developmental and clinical perspectives. New York: Guilford Press.

Ryan, N., & Puig-Antich, J. (1986). Affective illness in adolescents. In (Ed.), Annual review (pp. 420-450). Washington, D.C.: American Psychiatric Association.

Schoenbach, V. J., Kaplan, B. H., Wagner, E. H., Grimson, R. C., & Miller, F. T. (1983). Prevalence of self-reported depressive symptoms in young adolescents. American Journal of Public Health 73, 1281-1287.

Seligman, M. E., Peterson, C., Kaslow, N. J., Tanenbaum, R. L., Alloy, L. B., & Abramson, L. Y. (1984). Attributional style and depressive symptoms among children. Journal of Abnormal Psychology 93, 235-238.

Shaffer, D. (1985). Depression, mania, and suicidal acts. In M. Rutter & L. Hersov (Eds.), Child and adolescent psychiatry (pp. 698-719). Oxford: Blackwell Scientific Publication.

Spitz, R. A., & Wolf, K. M. (1946). Anaclitic depression. An inquiry into the genesis of psychiatric conditions in early childhood, II. In R. S. Eissler, et al. (Eds.), Psychoanalytic study of the child (Vol. 2, pp. 313-342). New York: International Universities Press.

Stark, K., Reynolds, W. M., & Kaslow, N. J. (1987). A comparison of the relative efficacy of self-control and behavior therapy for the reduction of depression in children. Journal of Consulting and Clinical Psychology 15, 91-113.

Strober, M. (1984). Familial aspects of depressive disorders in early adolescence. In E. B. Weller & R. A. Weller (Eds.), Current perspectives on major depressive disorders in children (pp. 38-48). Washington, D.C.: American Psychiatric Press.

Toolan, J. M. (1978). Therapy of depressed and suicidal children. American Journal of Psychotherapy 32, 243-251.

Trad, P. V. (1987). Infant and childhood depression: Developmental factors. New York: Wiley.

Waller, D. A., & Rush, A. J. (1983). Differentiating primary affective disease, organic affective syndromes, and situational depression on a pediatric service. Journal of the American Academy of Child Psychiatry 22, 52-58.

Waters, B. G., & Storm, V. (1985). Depression in prepubertal children. Australian and New Zealand Journal of Psychiatry 19, 6-17.

Weissman, M. M., Leckman, J. F., Merikangas, K. R., Gammon, G. D., & Prusoff, B. A. (1984). Depression and anxiety disorders in parents and children. Results from the Yale family study. Archives of General Psychiatry 41, 845-852.

Wilkes, T. C. R., & Rush, A. J. (1988). Adaptations of cognitive therapy for depressed adolescents. Journal of the American Academy of and Adolescent Child Psychiatry 27, 381-386.

Yanchyshyn, G. W., & Robbins, D. R. (1983). The assessment of depression in normal adolescents--a comparison study. Canadian Journal of Psychiatry 28, 522-526.

b. Unipolar Disorder

Beardslee, W. R., Bemporad, J., Keller, M. B., & Klerman, G. L. (1983). Children of parents with major affective disorder: A review. American Journal of Psychiatry 140, 825-832.

Beardslee, W. R., Klerman, G. L., Keller, M. B., Lavori, P. W., & Podorefsky, D. L. (1985). But are they cases? Validity of DSM-III major depression in children identified in a family study. American Journal of Psychiatry 142, 687-691.

Chambers, W. J., Puig-Antich, J., Hirsch, M., Paez, P., Ambrosini, P. J., Tabrizi, M. A., & Davies, M. (1985). The assessment of affective disorders in children and adolescents by semistructured interview. Archives of General Psychiatry 42, 696-702.

Geller, B., Chestnut, E. C., Miller, M. D., Price, D. T., & Yates, E. (1985). Preliminary data on DSM-III associated features of major depressive disorder in children and adolescents. American Journal of Psychiatry 142, 643-644.

Geller, B., Cooper, T. B., & Chestnut, E. C. (1985). Serial monitoring and achievement of steady state nortriptyline plasma levels in depressed children and adolescents: Preliminary data. Journal of Clinical Psychopharmacology 5, 213-216.

Geller, B., Cooper, T. B., McCombs, H. G., Graham, D., & Wells, J. (1989). Double-blind, placebo-controlled study of nortriptyline in depressed children using a "fixed plasma level" design. Psychopharmacology Bulletin 25, 101-108.

Hughes, M. C. (1984). Recurrent abdominal pain and childhood depression: Clinical observations of 23 children and their families. American Journal of Orthopsychiatry 54, 146-155.

Kashani, J. H. (1982). Epidemiology of childhood depression. In L. Grinspoon (Ed.), Psychiatry 1982: The American Psychiatric Association's annual review of psychiatry (pp. 281-288). Washington, D.C.: American Psychiatric Association.

Kashani, J. H., McGee, R. O., Clarkson, S. E., Anderson, J. C., Walton, L. A., Williams, S., Silva, P. A., & Robins, A. J. (1983). Depression in a sample of 9-year-old children, prevalence and associated characteristics. Archives of General Psychiatry 40, 1217-1223.

Kashani, J. H., Shekim, W. O., & Reid, J. C. (1984). Amitriptyline in children with major depressive disorder: A double-blind crossover pilot study. Journal of the American Academy of Child Psychiatry 23, 348-351.

Kasdin, A. E., French, N. H., & Unis, A. S. (1983). Child, mother, and father evaluation of depression in psychiatric inpatient children. Journal of Abnormal Child Psychology 11, 167-179.

Keller, M. B., Beardslee, W., Lavori, P. W., Wunder, J., Drs, D. L., & Samuelson, H. (1988). Course of major depression in non-referred adolescents: A retrospective study. Journal of Affective Disorders 15, 235-243.

Klerman, G. L., & Weissman, M. M. (1989). Increasing rates of depression. Journal of the American Medical Association 261, 2229-2235.

Orvaschel, H., Puig-Antich, J., Chambers, W., Tabrizi, M. A., & Johnson, R. (1982). Retrospective assessment of prepubertal major depression with the Kiddie-SADS-E. American Journal of Child Psychiatry 21, 392-397.

Puig-Antich, J., Goetz, D., Davies, M., Kaplan, T., Davies, S., Ostrow, L., Asnis, L., Twomey, J., Iyengar, S., & Ryan, N. D. (1989). A controlled family history study of prepubertal major depressive disorder. Archives of General Psychiatry 46, 406-418.

Puig-Antich, J., Perel, J. M., Lupatkin, W., Chambers, W. J., Tabrizi, M. A., King, J., Goetz, R., Davies, M., & Stiller, R. L. (1987). Imipramine in prepubertal major depressive disorders. Archives of General Psychiatry 44, 81-89.

Poznanski, E. O., Grossman, J. A., Buchsbaum, Y., Banegas, M., Freeman, L., & Gibbons, R. (1984). Preliminary studies of the reliability and validity of the children's depression rating scale. Journal of the American Academy of Child Psychiatry, 23 191-197.

Preskorn, S. H., Weller, E. B., & Weller, R. A. (1982). Depression in children: Relationship between plasma imipramine levels and response. Journal of Clinical Psychiatry 43, 450-453.

Preskorn, S. H., Weller, E. B., Weller, R. A., & Glotzbach, E. (1983). Plasma levels of imipramine and adverse effects in children. American Journal of Psychiatry 140, 1332-1335.

Puig-Antich, J. (1982). Major depression and conduct disorder in prepuberty. Journal of the American Academy of Child Psychiatry 21, 118-128.

Puig-Antich, J. (1986). Effects of age and puberty in psychobiological markers of depressive illness. In M. Rutter, C. Izard, & P. B. Read (Eds.), Depression in young people: Developmental and clinical perspectives (pp. 341-381). New York: Guilford Press.

Puig-Antich, J., Goetz, R., Davies, M., Tabrizi, M. A., Novacenko, H., Hanlon, C., Sachar, E. J., & Weitzman, E. D. (1984). Growth hormone secretion in prepubertal children with major depression. IV. Sleep-related plasma concentrations in a drug-free, fully recovered clinical state. Archives of General Psychiatry 41, 479-483.

Puig-Antich, J., Lukens, E., Davies, M., Goetz, D., Brennan-Quattrock, J., & Todak, G. (1985). Psychosocial functioning in prepubertal major depressive disorders. II. Interpersonal relationships after sustained recovery from affective episode. Archives of General Psychiatry 42, 511-517.

Robins, D. R., Alessi, N. E., Yanchyshyn, G. W., & Colfer, M. (1983). Psychodynamic and characterological heterogeneity among adolescents with major depressive disorders. Journal of the American Academy of Child Psychiatry 22, 487-491.

Ryan, N. D., Meyer, V., Dachille, S., Mazzie, D., & Puig-Antich, J. (1988). Lithium antidepressant augmentation in TCA-refractory depression in adolescents.

Journal of the American Academy of Child and Adolescent Psychiatry 27, 371-376.
Ryan, N. D., Puig-Antich, J., Cooper, T., Rabinovich, H., Ambrosini, P., Davies, M., King, J., & Torres, D. (1986). Imipramine in adolescent major depression: Plasma level and clinical response. Acta Psychiatrica Scandinavica 73, 275-288.
Ryan, N. D., Puig-Antich, J., Rabinovich, H., Ambrosini, P., Robinson, D., Nelson, B., & Novacenko, H. (1988). Growth hormone response to desmethylimipramine in depressed and suicidal adolescents. Journal of Affective Disorders 15, 323-337.
Ryan, N. D., Puig-Antich, J., Rabinovich, H., Fried, J., Ambrosini, P., Meyer, V., Torres, D., Dachille, S., & Mazzie, D. (1988). MAOIs in adolescent major depression unresponsive to tricyclic antidepressants. Journal of the American Academy of Child and Adolescent Psychiatry 27, 755-758.
Ryan, N. D., Puig-Antich, J., Ambrosini, P., Rabinovich, H., Robinson, D., Nelson, B., Iyengar, S., & Twomey, J. (1987). The clinical picture of major depression in children and adolescents. Archives of General Psychiatry 44, 854-861.
Strober, M., & Carlson, G. (1982). Bipolar illness in adolescents with major depression: Clinical, genetic, and psychopharmacological predictors in a 3-4 prospective follow-up investigation. Archives of General Psychiatry 39, 549-555.
Weissman, M. M., Warner, V., Wickramaratne, P., & Prusoff, B. A. (1988). Early-onset major depression in parents and their children. Journal of Affective Disorders 15, 269-277.

c. Bipolar Illness

Akiskal, H. S., Downs, J., Jordan, P., Watson, S., Daugherty, D., & Pruitt, D. B. (1985). Affective disorders in referred children and younger siblings of manic-depressives. Mode of onset and prospective course. Archives of General Psychiatry 42, 996-1003.
Anthony, E. J., & Scott, P. (1960). Manic-depressive psychosis in childhood. Journal of Child Psychology and Psychiatry and Allied Disciplines 1, 53-72.
Ballenger, J. C., Reus, V. I., & Post, R. M. (1982). The "atypical" clinical picture of adolescent mania. American Journal of Psychiatry 139, 602-606.
Carlson, G. A. (1984). Classification issues of bipolar disorders in childhood. Psychiatric Developments 2, 273-285.
Davis, R. E. (1979). Manic-depressive variant syndrome of childhood: A preliminary report. American Journal of Psychiatry 136, 702-706.
DeLong, G. R., & Nieman, G. W. (1983). Lithium-induced behavior changes in children with symptoms suggesting manic-depressive illness. Psychopharmacology Bulletin 19, 258-265.
Feinstein, S. C. (1982). Manic-depressive disorder in children and adolescents. In S. C. Feinstein, et al. (Eds.), Adolescent psychiatry: Developmental and clinical studies (Vol. 10, pp. 256-272). Chicago: University of Chicago Press.

Fine, S., Moretti, M., Haley, G., & Marriage, K. (1985). Affective disorders in children and adolescents: The dysthymic disorder dilemma. Canadian Journal of Psychiatry 30, 173-177.

Gammon, G. D., John, K., Rothblum, E. D., Mullen, K., Tischler, G. L., & Weissman, M. M. (1983). Use of a structured diagnostic interview to identify bipolar disorder in adolescent inpatients: Frequency and manifestations of the disorder. American Journal of Psychiatry 140, 543-547.

Strober, M., Morrell, W., Burroughs, J., Lampert, C., Danforth, H., & Freeman, R. (1988). A family study of bipolar 1 disorder in adolescence. Early onset of symptoms linked to increased familial loading and lithium resistance. Journal of Affective Disorders 15, 255-268.

Weissman, M. M., Warner, V., John, K., Prusoff, B. A., Merikangas, K. R., Wickramaratne, P., & Gammon, G. D. (1988). Delusional depression and bipolar spectrum: Evidence for a possible association from a family study of children. Neuropsychopharmacology 1, 257-264.

12. Suicide

Cynthia Pfeffer, M.D., Subsection Editor

Ackerly, W. C. (1967). Latency-age children who threaten or attempt to kill themselves. Journal of the American Academy of Child Psychiatry 6, 242-261.

Adam, K. S., Lohrenz, J. G., Harper, D., & Streiner, D. (1982). Early parental loss and suicidal ideation in university students. Canadian Journal of Psychiatry 27, 275-281.

Ahlburg, D. A., & Schapiro, M. O. (1984). Socioeconomic ramifications of changing cohort size: An analysis of U.S. postwar suicide rates by age and sex. Demography 21, 97-108.

Alcohol, drug abuse and mental health administration (1989). Report of the Secretary's Task Force on youth suicide. Washington, D.C.: U.S. Government Printing Office. Department of Health and Human Services Publication Number (ADM) 89-1624.

Aleksandrowicz, M. K. (1975). The biological strangers: An attempted suicide of a seven-and-a-half-year-old girl. Bulletin of the Menninger Clinic 39, 163-176.

Alessi, N. E., McManus, M., Brickman, A., & Grapentine, L. (1984). Suicidal behavior among serious juvenile offenders. American Journal of Psychiatry 141, 286-287.

Andress, V. R., & Corey, D. M. (1977). Suicide motives: Comparison of assignment of motives by coroners and psychologists. Psychological Reports 40, 11-14.

Apter, A., Bleich, A., Plutchik, R., Mendelsohn, S., & Tyano, S. (1988). Suicidal behavior, depression and conduct disorder in hospitalized adolescents. Journal of the American Academy of Child and Adolescent Psychiatry 27, 696-699.

Araki, S., & Murata, K. (1986). Factors affecting suicide in young, middle-aged and elderly men. Journal of Biosocial Science 18, 103-108.

Arffa, S. (1982). Predicting adolescent suicidal behavior and the order of Rorschach measurement. Journal of Personality Assessment 46, 563-568.

Asarnow, J. R., Carlson, G. A., & Guthrie, D. (1987). Coping strategies, self-perceptions, hopelessness, and perceived family environments in depressed and suicidal children. Journal of Counselling and Clinical Psychology 55, 361-366.

Baker, F. M. (1984). Black suicide attempters in 1980: A preventive focus. General Hospital Psychiatry 6, 131-137.

Barber, J. H., Hodgkin, G. K., Patel, A. R., & Wilson, G. M. (1975). Effect of teaching on students' attitudes to self-poisoning. British Medical Journal 2, 431-434.

Belfer, M. L. (1983). Suicide in children and adolescents. Emergency Medicine Clinics of North America 1, 201-206.

Berlin, I. N. (1985). Prevention of adolescent suicide among some Native American tribes. In S. C. Feinstein, et al. (Eds.), Adolescent psychiatry: Developmental and clinical studies (Vol. 12, pp. 77-93). Chicago: University of Chicago Press.

Bourque, L. B., Kraus, J. F., & Cosand, B. J. (1983). Attributes of suicide in females. Suicide and Life-Threatening Behavior 13, 123-138.

Boyd, J. H. (1983). The increasing rate of suicide by firearms. New England Journal of Medicine 308, 872-874.

Boyd, J. H., & Moscicki, E. E. (1986). Firearms and youth suicide. American Journal of Public Health 76, 1240-1242.

Brent, D. A., Kalas, R., Edelbrock, C., Costello, A. J., Dulcan, M., & Conover, N. (1986). Psychopathology and its relationship to suicidal ideation in childhood and adolescents. Journal of the American Academy of Child Psychiatry 25, 666-673.

Brent, D. A., Perper, J. A., & Allman, C. J. (1987). Alcohol, firearms, and suicide among youth: Temporal trends in Allegheny County, Pennsylvania 1960-1983. Journal of the American Medical Association 257, 3369-3372.

Brent, D. A., Perper, J. A., Goldstein, C. E., Kolko, D. J., Allman, M. S., Allman, C. J., & Zelenak, J. P. (1988). Risk factors for adolescent suicide: A comparison of adolescent suicide victims with suicidal inpatients. Archives of General Psychiatry 45, 581-586.

Burke, A. W. (1974). Socio-cultural aspects of attempted suicide among women in Trinidad and Tobago. British Journal of Psychiatry 125, 374-377.

Burke, A. W. (1985). Suicide in Jamaica. West Indian Medical Journal 34, 48-53.

Calhoun, L. G., Selby, J. W., & Faulstich, M. E. (1980). Reactions to the parents of the child suicide: A study of social impressions. Journal of Consulting and Clinical Psychology 48, 535-536.

Carlson, G. A., & Cantwell, D. P. (1982). Suicidal behavior and depression in children and adolescents. Journal of the American Academy of Child Psychiatry 21, 361-368.

Charnov, J. H., & Sturner, W. Q. (1985). Psychotropic drug-related suicides. American Journal of Forensic Medicine and Pathology 6, 312-318.

Clarkin, J. F., Friedman, R. C., Hurt, S. W., Corn, R., & Aronoff, M. (1984). Affective and character pathology of suicidal adolescent and young adult inpatients. Journal of Clinical Psychology 45, 19-22.

Cline, F. W. (1978). Adolescent suicide. Nursing Practice 3, 44-45, 53.
Cohen-Sandler, R., Berman, A. L., & King, R. A. (1982). Life stress and symptomatology: Determinants of suicidal behavior in children. Journal of the American Academy of Child Psychiatry 21, 178-186.
Combrinck-Graham, L. (1980). Suicidal children. Clinical Pediatrics 19, 447-448.
Copeland, A. R. (1985a). Childhood suicide: A report of four cases. Journal of Forensic Sciences 30, 965-967.
Copeland, A. R. (1985b). Teenage suicide--the five-year Metro Dade County experience from 1979 until 1983. Journal of Forensic Science International 28, 27-33.
Corder, B. F., & Haizlip, T. M. (1984). Environmental and personality similarities in case histories of suicide and self-poisoning by children under ten. Suicide and Life- Threatening Behavior 14, 59-66.
Cormier, H. J., & Klerman, G. L. (1985). Unemployment and male-female labor force participation as determinants of changing suicide rates of males and females in Quebec. Social Psychiatry 20, 109-114.
Cosand, B. J., Bourque, L. B., & Kraus, J. F. (1982). Suicide among adolescents in Sacramento County, California 1950-1979. Adolescence 17, 917-930.
Critical health problems in school-aged youth. (1984). Communique 3, 161-167.
Crompton, M. R. (1985). Alcohol and violent accidental and suicidal death. Medicine, Science and the Law 25, 59-62.
Crumley, F. E. (1982). The adolescent suicide attempt: A cardinal symptom of a serious psychiatric disorder. American Journal of Psychotherapy 36, 158-165.
Dashef, S. S. (1984). Active suicide intervention by a campus mental health service: Operation and rationale. Journal of American College Health 33, 118-122.
Davis, R. (1979). Black suicide in the seventies: Current trends. Suicide and Life-Threatening Behavior 9, 131-140.
DeMaio-Esteves, M., & Shuzman, E. (1983). Adolescent suicide in a technological society. Topics in Clinical Nursing 5, 59-65.
DenHouter, K. V. (1981). To silence one's self: A brief analysis of the literature on adolescent suicide. Child Welfare 60, 2-10.
Deykin, E. Y., Hsieh, C. C., Joshi, N., & McNamarra, J. J. (1986). Adolescent suicidal and self-destructive behavior. Journal of Adolescent Health Care 7, 88-95.
Diekstra, R. F. (1985). Suicide and suicide attempts in the European economic community: An analysis of trends, with special emphasis upon trends among the young. Suicide and Life-Threatening Behavior 15, 27-42.
Eisenberg, L. (1980). Adolescent suicide: On taking arms against a sea of troubles. Pediatrics 66, 315-320.
Eisenberg, L. (1984). The epidemiology of suicide in adolescents. Pediatric Annals 13, 47-54.
Emery, P. E. (1983). Adolescent depression and suicide. Adolescence 18, 245-258.
Ennis, J., Barnes, R. A., & Kennedy, S. (1985). The dexamethasone suppression test and suicidal patients. British Journal of Psychiatry 147, 419-423.

Eth, S., Pynoos, R. S., & Carlson, G. A. (1984). An unusual case of self-inflicted death in childhood. Suicide and Life-Threatening Behavior 14, 157-165.

Evans, D. L. (1982). Explaining suicide among the young: An analytical review of the literature. Journal of Psychosocial Nursing and Mental Health Services 20, 9-16.

Farber, M. L. (1977). Factors determining the incidence of suicide within families. Suicide and Life-Threatening Behavior 7, 3-6.

Fine, P., McIntire, M. S., & Fain, P. R. (1986). Early indicators of self-destruction in childhood and adolescence: A survey of pediatricians and psychiatrists. Pediatrics 77, 557-568.

Flaherty, M. G. (1983). The national incidence of juvenile suicide in adult jails and juvenile detention centers. Suicide and Life-Threatening Behavior 13, 85-94.

Fowler, R. C., Rich, C. L., & Young, D. (1986). San Diego suicide study: II. Substance abuse in young cases. Archives of General Psychiatry 43, 962-968.

Fox, J., Manitowabi, D., & Ward, J. A. (1984). An Indian community with a high suicide rate--5 years after. Canadian Journal of Psychiatry 29, 425-427.

Frances, A., & Clarkin, J. F. (1985). Considering family versus other therapies after a teenager's suicide attempt. Hospital and Community Psychiatry 36, 1041-1042, 1046.

Frazer, M. (1985). The female suicide victim. Trends in a metropolitan county (1963-1983). American Journal of Forensic Medicine and Pathology 6, 305-311.

Freese, A. S. (1985). Teenage suicides: Is there a preventive role for the dentist? Tic 44, 7, 13, 16.

French, A. P., & Steward, M. S. (1975). Family dynamics, childhood depression, and attempted suicide in a 7-year-old boy: A case study. Suicide 5, 29-37.

Friedman, J. M., Asnis, G. M., Boeck, M., & diFiore, J. (1987). Prevalence of specific suicidal behaviors in a high school sample. American Journal of Psychiatry 144, 1203-1206.

Friedman, R. C., Aronoff, M. S., Clarkin, J. F., Corn, R., & Hurt, S. W. (1983). History of suicidal behavior in depressed borderline inpatients. American Journal of Psychiatry 140, 1023-1026.

Friedman, R. C., Corn, R., Hurt, S. W., Fibel, B., Schulick, J., & Swirsky, S. (1984). Family history of illness in the seriously suicidal adolescent: A life-cycle approach. American Journal of Orthopsychiatry 54, 390-397.

Gardner, D. L, & Cowdry, R. W. (1985). Suicidal and parasuicidal behavior in borderline personality disorder. Psychiatric Clinics of North America 8, 389-403.

Garvey, M. J., & Spoden, F. (1980). Suicide attempts in antisocial personality disorder. Comprehensive Psychiatry 21, 146-149.

Gehlot, P. S., & Nathawat, S. S. (1983). Suicide and family constellation in India. American Journal of Psychotherapy, 37, 273-278.

Gilead, M. P., & Mulaik, J. S. (1983). Adolescent suicide: A response to developmental crisis. Perspectives in Psychiatric Care 21, 94-101.

Gillis, A. (1984). Early detection of the suicidal adolescent. Canadian Journal of Psychiatric Nursing 25, 6-8.

Glaser, K. (1978). The treatment of depressed and suicidal adolescents. American Journal of Psychotherapy 32, 252-269.

Goldacre, M., & Hawton, K. (1986). Repetition of self-poisoning and subsequent death in adolescents who take overdoses. British Journal of Psychiatry 146, 395-398.

Golombek, H., & Garfinkel, B. D. (1983). The adolescent and mood disturbance. New York: International Universities Press.

Gould, M. S., & Shaffer, D. (1986). The impact of suicide in television stories: Evidence for imitation. New England Journal of Medicine 135, 690-694.

Gould, R. E. (1965). Suicide problems in children and adolescent. American Journal of Psychotherapy 19, 228-246.

Green, A. H. (1978). Self-destructive behavior in battered children. American Journal of Psychiatry 135, 579-582.

Hafen, B. Q., & Peterson, B. (1983). Preventing adolescent suicide. Nursing 13, 47-48.

Hankoff, L. D. (1984). Poetry, adolescent, and suicide. Pharos of Alpha Omega Alpha Honor Medical Society 47, 7-12.

Hasekura, H., Fukushima, H., Yonemura, I., & Ota, M. (1985). A rare suicidal case of a ten-year-old child stabbing himself in the throat. Journal of Forensic Sciences 30, 1269-1271.

Hawton, K. (1986). Suicide in adolescents. In A. Roy (Ed.), Suicide (pp. 135-150). Baltimore: Williams & Wilkins.

Hawton, K., O'Grady, J., Osborn, M., & Cole, D. (1982). Adolescents who take overdoes: Their characteristics, problems and contacts with helping agencies. British Journal of Psychiatry 140, 118-123.

Headlam, H. K., Goldsmith, J., Hanenson, I. B., & Rauh, J. L. (1979). Demographic characteristics of adolescents with self-poisoning. A survey of 235 instances in Cincinnati, Ohio. Clinical Pediatrics 18, 147, 151, 154.

Heming, J. (1986). Saving teenage suicides. Journal of Psychosomatic Research 21, 291-296.

Hersh, S. P. (1975). Suicide: Youth's high vulnerability to it/signs to look for/how you can help. MH 59, 23-25.

Hickman, L. C. (1984). Descriptive differences between black and white suicide attempters. Issues of Mental Health Nursing 5, 293-310.

Hingson, R., Merrigan, D., & Heeren, T. (1985). Effects of Massachusetts raising its legal drinking age from 18 to 20 on deaths from teenage homicide, suicide, and nontraffic accidents. Pediatric Clinics of North America 32, 221-232.

Hodgman, C. H. (1985). Recent findings in adolescent depression and suicide. Journal of Developmental and Behavioral Pediatrics 6, 162-170.

Holden, C. (1986). Youth suicide: New research focus on a growing social problem. Science 233, 829-841.

Holinger, P. C. (1979). Violent deaths among the young: Recent trends in suicide, homicide, and accidents. American Journal of Psychiatry 136, 1144-1147.

Holinger, P. C., & Offer, D. (1982). Prediction of adolescent suicide: A population model. American Journal of Psychiatry 139, 302-307.

Holinger, P. C., & Offer, D. (1987). Suicide and homicide in the United States: An epidemiologic study of violent death, population changes, and potential for prediction. American Journal of Psychiatry 144, 215-219.

Iga, M. (1981). Suicide of Japanese youth. Suicide and Life-Threatening Behavior 11, 17-30.

Iga, M., Yamamota, J., & Noguchi, T. (1975). The vulnerability of young Japanese women and suicide. Suicide 5, 207-222.

Inamdar, S. C., Oberfield, R. A., & Darrell, E. B. (1983). A suicide by self-immolation--psychosocial perspectives. International Journal of Social Psychiatry 29, 130-133.

Joffe, R. T., & Offord, D. R. (1983). Suicidal behaviour in childhood. Canadian Journal of Psychiatry 28, 57-63.

Kahan, J., & Pattison, E. M. (1984). Proposal for a distinctive diagnosis: The deliberate self-harm syndrome (DSH). Suicide and Life-Threatening Behavior 14, 17-35.

Kazdin, A. E., French, N. H., Unis, A. S., Esveldt-Dawson, K., & Sherick, R. B. (1983). Hopelessness, depression, and suicidal intent among psychiatrically disturbed inpatient children. Journal of Consulting and Clinical Psychology 51, 504-510.

Keidel, G. C. (1983). Adolescent suicide. Nursing Clinics of North America 18, 323-332.

Kerfoot, M. (1980). The family context of adolescent suicidal behavior. Journal of Adolescence 3, 335-346.

Kessler, R. C., Downey, G., Milavsky, J. R., & Stipp, H. (1988). Clustering of teenage suicides after television news stories about suicides: A reconsideration. American Journal of Psychiatry 145, 1379-1383.

Klerman, G. L. (Ed.). (1986). Suicide and depression among adolescents and young adults. Washington, D.C.: American Psychiatric Press.

Konopka, G. (1983). Adolescent suicide. Exceptional Children 49, 390-394.

Kosky. R. (1983). Childhood suicidal behaviour. Journal of Child Psychology and Psychiatry and Allied Disciplines 24, 457-468.

Kuperman, S., Black, D. W., & Burns, T. L. (1988). Excess mortality among formerly hospitalized child psychiatric patients. Archives of General Psychiatry 45, 277-282.

Lampert, D. I., Bourque, L. B., & Kraus, J. F. (1984). Occupational status and suicide. Suicide and Life-Threatening Behavior 14, 254-269.

Leads from the MMWR. (1983). Violent deaths among persons 15 to 24 years of age--United States. Journal of the American Medical Association 250, 3147-3148.

Lester, D. (1982). The distribution of sex and age among completed suicides: A cross-national study. International Journal of Social Psychiatry 28, 256-260.

Lester, D. (1984). Suicide risk by birth cohort. Suicide and Life-Threatening Behavior 14, 132-136.,

Lester, D., & Beck, A. T. (1976). Early loss as a possible "sensitizer" to later loss in attempted suicides. Psychological Reports 39, 121-122.

Lester, D., Beck, A. T., & Trexler, L. (1975). Extrapolation from attempted suicides to completed suicides. Journal of Abnormal Psychology 84, 563-566.

Liberman, R. P., & Eckman, T. (1981). Behaviour therapy vs. insight-oriented therapy for repeated suicide attempters. Archives of General Psychiatry 38, 1126-1130.

Mann, J. J., & Stanley, M. (Eds.). (1986). Psychobiology of suicidal behavior. Annals of the New York Academy of Sciences 487, 1-82.

Maris, R. (1985). The adolescent suicide problem. Suicide and Life-Threatening Behavior 15, 91-109.

Marks, A. (1979). Management of the suicidal adolescent on a nonpsychiatric adolescent unit. Journal of Pediatrics 95, 305-308.

Markush, R. E., & Bartolucci, A. A. (1984). Firearms and suicide in the United States. American Journal of Public Health 74, 123-127.

Mattsson, A., Seese, L. R., & Hawkins, J. W. (1969). Suicidal behavior as a child psychiatric emergency: Clinical characteristics and follow-up results. Archives of General Psychiatry 20, 100-109.

McAnarney, E. R. (1975). Suicidal behavior of children and youth. Pediatric Clinics of North America 22, 595-604.

McClure, G. M. (1984). Recent trends in suicide amongst the young. British Journal of Psychiatry 144, 134-138.

McGoldrick, K. E. (1985). Adolescent suicide: The tragic end of childhood. Journal of the American Medical Women's Association 40, 99-100.

McGuire, D. J., & Ely, M. (1984). Childhood suicide. Child Welfare 63, 17-26.

McIntire, M. S., Angle, C. R., & Schlicht, M. L. (1977). Suicide and self-poisoning in pediatrics. Advances in Pediatrics 24, 291-309.

Miller, D. (1981). Adolescent suicide: Etiology and treatment. In S. C. Feinstein, et al. (Eds.), Adolescent psychiatry: Developmental and clinical studies (Vol. 9, pp. 327-342). Chicago: University of Chicago Press.

Miller, H. L., Coombs, D. W., Leeper, J. D., & Barton, S. N. (1984). An analysis of the effects of suicide prevention facilities on the suicide rates in the United States. American Journal of Public Health 74, 340-343.

Mitchell, K. (1985). Suicide: A preventable tragedy. Pediatric Nursing 11, 165.

Monahan, R. T. (1983). Suicidal children's and adolescents' responses to early memories test. Journal of Personality Assessment 47, 258-264.

Morrison, J. (1984). Suicide in psychiatric patients: Age distribution. Suicide and Life-Threatening Behavior 14, 52-58.

Motto, J. A., Heilbron, D. C., & Juster, R. P. (1985). Development of a clinical instrument to estimate suicide risk. American Journal of Psychiatry 142, 680-686.

Nuttall, E. A., Evenson, R. C., & Cho, D. W. (1980). A comparison of suicide and undetermined deaths in psychiatric patients. Suicide and Life-Threatening Behavior 10, 167-174.

Orbach, I., Feshbach, S., Carlson, G., Glaubman, H., & Gross, Y. (1983). Attraction and repulsion by life and death in suicidal and in normal children. Journal of Consulting and Clinical Psychology 51, 661-670.

Orbach, I., & Glaubman, H. (1978). Suicidal, aggressive, and normal children's perception of personal and impersonal death. Journal of Clinical Psychology 34, 850-856.

Paerregaard, G. (1980). Suicide in Denmark: A statistical review for the past 150 years. Suicide and Life-Threatening Behavior 10, 150-156.

Pallis, D. J., Gibbons, J. S., & Pierce, D. W. (1984). Estimating suicide risk among attempted suicides. II. Efficiency of predictive scales after the attempt. British Journal of Psychiatry 144, 139-148.

Peck, D. L. (1981). The loner: An exploration of a suicidal subtype in adolescence. In S. C. Feinstein, et al. (Eds.), Adolescent psychiatry: Developmental and clinical studies (Vol. 9, pp. 461-466). Chicago: University of Chicago Press.

Peck, D. L. (1984). Lethality of method of suicide among a youthful sample of committers: An examination of the intent hypotheses. Psychological Reports 55, 861-862.

Pepitone-Arreola-Rockwell, F., Rockwell, D., & Core, N. (1981). Fifty-two medical student suicides. American Journal of Psychiatry 138, 198-201.

Perrot, L. J., Froede, R. C., & Jones, A. M. (1985). Asphyxiation by hanging in two young Hispanic children--homicide, suicide, or accidental deaths? A review of pediatric hangings. American Journal of Forensic Medicine and Pathology 6, 284-288.

Pfeffer, C. R. (1978). Psychiatric hospital treatment of suicidal children. Suicide and Life-Threatening Behavior 8, 150-160.

Pfeffer, C. R. (1979). Clinical observations of play of hospitalized suicidal children. Suicide and Life-Threatening Behavior 9, 235-244.

Pfeffer, C. R. (1980). Unanswered questions about childhood suicidal behavior: Perspectives for the practicing physician. Journal of Developmental and Behavioral Pediatrics 1, 11-14.

Pfeffer, C. R. (1981a). The family system of suicidal children. American Journal of Psychotherapy 35, 330-341.

Pfeffer, C. R. (1981b.) Parental suicide: An organizing event in the development of latency age children. Suicide and Life-Threatening Behavior 11, 43-50.

Pfeffer, C. R. (1981c). Suicidal behavior of children: A review with implications for research and practice. American Journal of Psychiatry 138, 154-159.

Pfeffer, C. R. (1984). Modalities of treatment for suicidal children: An overview of the literature on current practice. American Journal of Psychotherapy 38, 364-372.

Pfeffer, C. R. (1985a). Death preoccupations and suicidal behavior in children. Issues in Comprehensive Pediatric Nursing 8, 261-278.

Pfeffer, C. R. (1985b). Self-destructive behavior in children and adolescents. Psychiatric Clinics of North America 8, 215-226.

Pfeffer, C. R. (1985c). Suicidal fantasies in normal children. Journal of Nervous and Mental Disease 173, 78-84.

Pfeffer, C. R. (1986a). Suicidal behavior in child psychiatric inpatients and outpatients and in nonpatients. American Journal of Psychiatry 143, 733-738.

Pfeffer, C. R. (1986b). The suicidal child. New York: Guilford Press.

Pfeffer, C. R. (1987a). Elements of treatment of suicidal children. American Journal of Psychotherapy 41, 172-184.

Pfeffer, C. R. (1987b). Reducing environmental stress for a suicidal ten-year-old. Hospital and Community Psychiatry 38, 22-24.

Pfeffer, C. R. (1988). Suicidal behavior among children and adolescents: Risk identification and intervention. A. J. Frances & R. E. Hales (Eds.), American Psychiatric Press review of psychiatry (Vol. 7, pp. 386-402). Washington, D.C.: American Psychiatric Press

Pfeffer, C. R. (1989a). Preoccupations with death in "normal" children: The relationship to suicidal behavior. Omega 20 (3), 205-212.

Pfeffer, C. R. (1989b). Risk factors associated with youth suicide: A clinical perspective. Psychiatric Annals 18 (11), 652-656.

Pfeffer, C. R. (1989c). Spotting the red flags for adolescent suicide. Contemporary Pediatrics 6, 59-70.

Pfeffer, C. R. (1989d). Studies of suicidal preadolescent and adolescent inpatients: A critique of research methods. Suicide and Life-Threatening Behavior 19, (1), 58-77.

Pfeffer, C. R. (1989e). Suicide among youth: Perspectives on risk and prevention. Washington, D.C.: American Psychiatric Press.

Pfeffer, C. R., Adams, D., Weiner, A., & Rosenberg, J. (1989). Stresses on parents of suicidal children. International Journal of Family Psychiatry 9 (4), 341-358.

Pfeffer, C. R., Lipkins, R., Plutchik, R., & Mizruchi, M. S. (1988). Normal children at risk for suicidal behavior: A two-year follow-up study. Journal of the American Academy of Child and Adolescent Psychiatry 27, 34-41. Reprinted in S. Chess, A. Thomas, & M. E. Hertzig (Eds.), Annual progress in child psychiatry and child development (Vol. 22) (in press).

Pfeffer, C. R., Newcorn, J., Kaplan, G., Plutchik, R., & Mizruchi, M. S. (1988). Suicidal behavior in adolescent psychiatric inpatients. Journal of the American Academy of Child and Adolescent Psychiatry 26, 256-261.

Pfeffer, C. R., Newcorn, J., Kaplan, G., Plutchik, R., & Mizruchi, M. S. (1989). Subtypes of suicidal and assaultive behavior in adolescent psychiatric inpatients. Journal of Child Psychology and Psychiatry and Allied Disciplines 30 (1), 151-161.

Pfeffer, C. R., Plutchik, R., Mizruchi, M. S., Faughnan, L., Mintz, M., & Shindledecker, R. (1989). Changes in suicidal behavior in child psychiatric inpatients. Acta Psychiatrica Scandinavica 79, 431-435.

Pfeffer, C. R., Plutchik, R., Mizruchi, M. S., & Lipkins, R. (1986). Suicidal behavior in child psychiatric inpatients and outpatients and in nonpatients. American Journal of Psychiatry 143 (6), 733-738.

Pfeffer, C. R., Solomon, G., Plutchik, R., Mizruchi, M. S., & Weiner, A. (1982). Suicidal behavior in latency-age psychiatric inpatients: A replication and cross validation. Journal of the American Academy of Child Psychiatry 21, 564-569.

Pfeffer, C. R., & Trad, P. V. (1988). Suicidality and sadness in pre-school children. Journal of Developmental and Behavioral Pediatrics 9, 86-88.

Pfeffer, C. R., Zuckerman, S., Plutchik, R., & Mizruchi, M. S. (1984). Suicidal behavior in normal school children: A comparison with child psychiatric inpatients. Journal of the American Academy of Child Psychiatry 23, 416-423.

Phillips, D. P., & Carstensen, M. S. (1986). Clustering of teenage suicide after television news stories about suicide. New England Journal of Medicine 135, 685-689.

Phillips, D. P., & Paight, D. J. (1987). The impact of televised movies about suicide: A replicative study. New England Journal of Medicine 317, 809-811.

Pless, I. B., & Stulginskas, J. (1982). Accidents and violence as a cause of morbidity and mortality in childhood. Advances in Pediatrics 29, 471-495.

Rachlin, S., Milton, J., & Pam, A. (1977). Countersymbiotic suicide. Archives of General Psychiatry 34, 965-967.

Renshaw, D. C. (1981). Suicide in children. American Family Physician 24, 123-127.

Rich, C. L., Young, D., & Fowler, R. C. (1986). San Diego suicide study: I. Young versus old subjects. Archives of General Psychiatry 43, 577-582.

Robbins, D. R., & Alessi, N. E. (1985a). Depressive symptoms and suicidal behavior in adolescents. American Journal of Psychiatry 142, 588-592.

Robbins, D. R., & Alessi, N. E. (1985b). Suicide and the dexamethasone suppression test in adolescence. Biological Psychiatry 20, 107-110.

Robinson, L. H. (1984). Outpatient management of the suicidal child. American Journal of Psychotherapy 38, 399-412.

Rosenblaum, S., & Faber, M. M. (1979). The adolescent sexual asphyxia syndrome. Journal of the American Academy of Child Psychiatry 18, 546-558.

Ross, C. A., & Davis, B. (1986). Suicide and parasuicide in an Northern Canadian native community. Canadian Journal of Psychiatry 31, 331-334.

Ross, C. P. (1980). Mobilizing schools for suicide prevention. Suicide prevention. Suicide and Life- Threatening Behavior 10, 239-243.

Rotherman-Borus, M. J., & Trautman,P. D. (1988). Hopelessness, depression, and suicidal intent among adolescent suicide attempters. Journal of the American Academy of Child and Adolescent Psychiatry 27, 700-704.

Rubinstein, D. H. (1983). Epidemic suicide among Micronesian adolescents. Social Science and Medicine 17, 657-665.

Rudestam, K. E., & Imbroll, D. (1983). Societal reactions to a child's death by suicide. Journal of Consulting and Clinical Psychology 51, 461-462.

Salk, L., Lipsitt, L. P., Sturner, W. Q., Reilly, B. M., & Levat, R. H. (1985). Relationship of maternal and perinatal conditions to eventual adolescent suicide. Lancet 1, 624-627.

Santostefano, S., Rieder, C., & Berk, S. A. (1984). The structure of fantasied movement in suicidal children and adolescents. Suicide and Life-Threatening Behavior 14, 3-16.

Schneer, H. I., Perlstein, A., & Brozovsky, M. (1975). Hospitalized suicidal adolescents. Two generations. Journal of the American Academy of Child Psychiatry 14, 268-280.

Schwartz, R. S., & Eisen, S. V. (1984). The risk of suicide in young psychiatric patients hospitalized out-of-state. Psychiatry 47, 342-350.

Scully, J. H., & Hutcherson, R. (1983). Suicide by burning. American Journal of Psychiatry 140, 905-906.

Seiden, R. H. (1984). Death in the West--a regional analysis of the youthful suicide rate. Western Journal of Medicine 140, 969-973.

Shaffer, D. (1982). Diagnostic consideration in suicidal behavior in children and adolescents. Journal of the American Academy of Child Psychiatry 21, 414-415.

Shaffer, D. (1988). The epidemiology of teen suicide: An examination of risk factors. Journal of Clinical Psychiatry 49, 36-41.

Shaffer, D., & Fisher, P. (1981). The epidemiology of suicide in children and young adolescents. Journal of the American Academy of Child Psychiatry 20, 545-565.

Shafii, M., Carrigan, S., Whittinghill, J. R., & Derrick A. (1985). Psychological autopsy of completed suicide in children and adolescents. American Journal of Psychiatry 142, 1061-1064.

Shulman, S., & Margalit, M. (1985). Suicidal behavior at school: A systemic perspective. Journal of Adolescence 8, 263-269.

Sickel, R. Z. (1979). Children who experience parental suicide. Pediatric Nursing 5, 37-39.

Smith, J. C., Mercy, J. A., & Warren, C. W. (1985). Comparison of suicides among Anglos and Hispanics in five southwestern states. Suicide and Life-Threatening Behavior 15, 14-26.

Smith, K., & Crawford, S. (1986). Suicidal behavior among "normal" high school students. Suicide and Life-Threatening Behavior 16, 313-325.

Sommer, B. (1984). The troubled teen: Suicide, drug use, and running away. Women and Health 9, 117-141.

Spalt, L. (1980). Suicide behavior and depression in university student psychiatric referrals. Psychiatry 52, 235-239.

Stack, S. (1983). The effect of religious commitment on suicide: A cross-national analysis. Journal of Health and Social Behavior 24, 362-374.

Stanley, M. (1984). Cholinergic receptor binding in the frontal cortex of suicide victims. American Journal of Psychiatry 141, 1432-1436.

Stoddard, F. J., Pahlavan, K., & Cahners, S. S. (1985). Suicide attempted by self-immolation during adolescence. I. Literature review, case reports, and personality precursors. In S. C. Feinstein, et al. (Eds.), Adolescent psychiatry: Developmental and clinical studies (Vol. 12, pp. 251-265). Chicago: University of Chicago Press.

Sudak, H. S., Ford, A. B., & Rushforth, N. B. (1984). Adolescent suicide: An overview. American Journal of Psychotherapy 38, 350-363.

Tabachnick, N. (1981). The interlocking psychologies of suicide and adolescence. In S. C. Feinstein, et al. (Eds.), Adolescent psychiatry: Developmental and clinical studies (Vol. 9, pp. 399-410). Chicago: University of Chicago Press.

Tardiff, K., & Sweillam, A. (1980). Assault, suicide, and mental illness. Archives of General Psychiatry 37, 164-169.

Topol, P., & Reznikoff, M. (1982). Perceived peer and family relationship, hopelessness and locus of control as factors in adolescent suicide attempts. Suicide and Life-Threatening Behavior 12, 141-150.

Toolan, J. M. (1962). Suicide and suicidal attempts in children and adolescents. American Journal of Psychiatry 118, 719-724.
Toolan, J. M. (1975). Suicide in children and adolescents. American Journal of Psychotherapy 29, 339-344.
Toolan, J. M. (1978). Therapy of depressed and suicidal children. American Journal of Psychotherapy 32, 243-251.
Toolan, J. M. (1981). Depression and suicide in children: An overview. American Journal of Psychotherapy 35, 311-322.
Trout, D. L. (1980). The role of social isolation in suicide. Suicide and Life-Threatening Behavior 10, 10-23.
Tsuang, M. T. (1983). Risk of suicide in the relatives of schizophrenics, manics, depressives, and controls. Journal of Clinical Psychiatry 44, 396-397, 398-400.
Valente, S. (1983). Suicide in school aged children: Theory and assessment. Pediatric Nursing 9, 25-29.
Violent deaths among persons 15-24 years of age--United States, 1970-1978. (1983). Morbidity and Mortality Weekly Report 32, 453-457.
Walker, B. A., & Mehr, M. (1983). Adolescent suicide--a family crisis: A model for effective intervention by family therapists. Adolescence 18, 285-292.
Weiner, A. S., & Pfeffer, C. R. (1986). Suicidal status, depression and cognitive functioning in child psychiatric inpatients. Comprehensive Psychiatry 27 (4), 372-380.
Wenz, F. V. (1978). Economic status, family anomie, and adolescent suicide potential. Journal of Psychology 98, 45-47.
Wright, L. S. (1985). Suicidal thoughts and their relationship to family stress and personal problems among high school seniors and college undergraduates. Adolescence 20, 575-580.

C. Psychophysiologic Disorders

Alexander P. Lucas, M.D., Section Editor

Eric K. Milliner, M.D., S. Wendell Obetz, M.D., and Lloyd A. Wells, Ph.D., M.D., Associate Editors

1. Theories of Psychosomatic Disorders

Alexander, F. (1943). Fundamental concepts of psychosomatic research: Psychogenesis, conversion, specificity. Psychosomatic Medicine 5, 205-210.
Becker, H. (1984). Significance of the patient's theory of disease for the physician-patient relation. Psychotherapie, Psychosomatik, Medizinische Psychologie 34, 313-321.
Benedek, T. (1949). The psychosomatic implications of the primary unit: Mother-child. American Journal of Orthopsychiatry 19, 642-654.
Demers-Desrosiers, L. (1982). Influence of alexithymia on symbolic function. Psychotherapy and Psychosomatics 38, 103-120.

Deutsch, F. (1953). The psychosomatic concept in psychoanalysis. New York: International Universities Press.

Engel, G. L. (1960). A unified concept of health and disease. Perspectives in Biology and Medicine 3, 459.

Engel, G. L. (1967). Training in psychosomatic research. Advances in Psychosomatic Medicine 5, 16.

Flannery, J., & Taylor, G. (1981). Toward integrating psyche and soma: Psychoanalysis and neurobiology. Canadian Journal of Psychiatry 26, 15-23.

Friedman, H. S., Hall, J. A., & Harris, M. J. (1985). Type A behavior, nonverbal expressive style, and health. Journal of Personality and Social Psychology 48, 1299-1315.

Gadlin, W. (1985). Psychiatric consultation to the medical ward: A group analytic and general systems theory point of view. International Journal of Group Psychotherapy 35, 263-278.

Gottschalk, L. A. (1982). Shortcomings in specificity research and remedial suggestions, including the involvement of language markers. Psychotherapy and Psychosomatics 38, 46-53.

Groen, J. J. (1979). The psychosomatic theory of bronchial asthma. Psychotherapy and Psychosomatics 31, 38-48.

Latimer, P. (1979). Psychophysiologic disorders: A critical appraisal of concept and theory illustrated with reference to the irritable bowel syndrome (IBS). Psychological Medicine 9, 71-80.

Lolas, F. (1985). The psychosomatic approach and the problem of diagnosis. Social Science and Medicine 21, 1355-1361.

McMahon, C. E., & Hastrup, J. L. (1980). The role of imagination in the disease process: Post-Cartesian history. Journal of Behavioral Medicine 3, 205-217.

Minuchin, S., et al. (1975). A conceptual model of psychosomatic illness in children: Family organization and family therapy. Archives of General Psychiatry 32, 1031-1038.

Mirsky, I. A. (1957). The psychosomatic approach to the etiology of clinical disorders. Psychosomatic Medicine 19, 424.

Mohl, P. C., & Burstein, A. G. (1982). The application of Kohutian self psychology to consultation--liaison psychiatry. General Hospital Psychiatry 4, 113-119.

Schmale, A. H. (1958). Relationship of separation and depression to disease. Psychosomatic Medicine 20, 259-277.

Schur, M. (1955). Comments on the metapsychology of somatization. In R. S. Eissler, et al. (Eds.), Psychoanalytic study of the child (Vol. 10, pp. 119-164). New York: International Universities Press.

Schwartz, G. E. (1981). A systems analysis of psychobiology and behavior therapy. Implications for behavioral medicine. Psychotherapy and Psychosomatics 36, 159-184.

Selye, H. (1946). The general adaptation syndrome and the diseases of adaptation. Journal of Clinical Endocrinology 6, 117.

Shipko, S. (1982). Further reflections on psychosomatic theory. Alexithymia and interhemispheric specialization. Psychotherapy and Psychosomatics 37, 83-86.

Speciani, A., & Milani, L. (1983). Acupuncture treatment of painful and dysfunctional syndromes in subjects exposed to severe stress. Psychosomatic interpretation in the light of the dermatoneuromeric theory. Minerva Medica 74, 953-960.

Sperling, M. (1950). Indirect treatment of psychoneurotic and psychosomatic disorders in children. Quarterly Journal of Child Behavior 2, 250-266.

Sperling, M. (1970). The clinical effects of parental neurosis on the child. In E. Anthony & T. Benedek (Eds.), Parenthood (pp. 539-569). New York: Little, Brown.

Spitz, R. (1951). The psychogenic diseases in infancy, an attempt at their etiologic classification. In R. S. Eissler, et al. (Eds.), Psychoanalytic study of the child (Vol. 6, pp. 255-278). New York: International Universities Press.

Stoudemire, A. (1985). Psychosomatic theory and pulmonary disease. Asthma as a paradigm for the biopsychosocial approach. Advances in Psychosomatic Medicine 14, 1-15.

Winnicott, D. W. (1966). Psycho-somatic illness in its positive and negative aspects. International Journal of Psycho-Analysis 47, 510-516.

Wolff, H. G. (1950). Life stress and bodily disease-formulation. Proceedings of the Association for Research in Nervous and Mental Disease 29, 1059.

Wooley, S. C., Blackwell, B., & Winget, C. (1978). A learning theory model of chronic illness behavior: Theory, treatment, and research. Psychosomatic Medicine 40, 379-401.

2. Effects of Psychological and Physical Trauma on Psychophysiologic Disorders

Bernstein, D. M. (1971). After transplantation: The child's emotional reactions. American Journal of Psychiatry 127, 1189-1193.

Freyberg, J. T. (1980). Difficulties in separation-individuation as experienced by offspring of Nazi holocaust survivors. American Journal of Orthopsychiatry 50, 87-95.

Green, M. (1967). Care of the child with a long-term, life-threatening illness: Some principles of management. Pediatrics 39, 441-445.

Heiligenstein, E., & Jacobsen, P. B. (1988). Differentiating depression in medically ill children and adolescents. Journal of the American Academy of Child and Adolescent Psychiatry 27(6), 719-719.

Korsch, B. M., Fine, R. N., Grushkin, C. M., & Negrete, V. F. (1971). Experiences with children and their families during extended hemodialysis and kidney transplantation. Pediatric Clinics of North America 18, 625-637.

Kriechman, A. V. (1987). Siblings with somatoform disorders in childhood and adolescence. Journal of the American Academy of Child and Adolescent Psychiatry 26(2), 226-231.

Leon, G. R., Butcher, J. N., Kleinman, M., Goldberg, A., & Almagor, M. (1981). Survivors of the holocaust and their children: Current status and adjustment. Journal of Personality and Social Psychology 41, 503-516.

Levy, S. (1959). Post-encephalitic behavior disorder--a forgotten entity: A report of 100 cases. American Journal of Psychiatry 115, 1062-1067.
Plionis, E. M. (1977). Family functioning and childhood accident occurrence. American Journal of Orthopsychiatry 47, 250-263.
Ravenscroft, K. (1982). Psychiatric consultation to the child with acute physical trauma. American Journal of Orthopsychiatry 52, 298-307.
Rosenheck, R., & Nathan, P. (1985). Secondary traumatization in children of Vietnam veterans. Hospital and Community Psychiatry 36, 538-539.
Terr, L. C. (1985). Psychic trauma in children and adolescents. Psychiatric Clinics of North America 8, 815-835.
Watson, E. J., & Johnson, A. M. (1958). The emotional significance of acquired physical disfigurement in children. American Journal of Orthopsychiatry 28, 85-97.

3. Psychiatric Disorders and Psychophysiologic Disease

Aronsson, G., & Koivunen, E. (1985). Differences in personality between parents of asthmatic children and parents of non-asthmatic children. Journal of Psychosomatic Research 29, 177-182.
Asnes, R. S. (1983). Depression and chest pain [Letter]. Journal of the American Academy of Child Psychiatry 22, 412.
Barclay, G. N. (1982). Functional complaints and the pediatric gastroenterologist. Pediatric Annals 11, 159-173.
Belmaker, E. (1984). Nonspecific somatic symptoms in early adolescent girls. Journal of Adolescent Health Care 5, 30-33.
Bentovim, A. (1985). Less orthodox psychological interventions. Archives of Disease in Childhood 60, 1198-1201.
Blackwell, B. (1981). Biofeedback in a comprehensive behavioral medicine program. Biofeedback and Self Regulation 6, 445-472.
Cadoret, R. J., Widmer, R. B., & Troughton, E. P. (1980). Somatic complaints--harbinger of depression in primary care. Journal of Affective Disorders 2, 61-70.
Conte, H. R., & Karasu, T. B. (1981). Psychotherapy for medically ill patients: Review and critique of controlled studies. Psychosomatics 22, 285-290, 297-300, 312, 315.
Edgecumbe, R. M. (1984). Modes of communication. The differentiation of somatic and verbal expression. In A. Solnit, et al. (Eds.), Psychoanalytic study of the child (Vol. 39, pp. 137-154). New Haven: Yale University Press.
Esman, A., Hertzig, M. E., Lewis, N. B., Sherman, M., Snow, M., & Spiegel, L. (1985). A case of psychogenic pain [Clinical Conference] Journal of the American Academy of Child Psychiatry 24, 781-787.
Ferholt, J. B., Rotnem, D. L., Genel, M., Leonard, M., Carey, M., & Hunter, D. E. (1985). A psychodynamic study of psychosomatic dwarfism: A syndrome of depression, personality disorder, and impaired growth. Journal of the American Academy of Child Psychiatry 24, 49-57.

Gehring, T. M. (1985). Socio-psychosomatic dysfunctions: A case study. Child Psychiatry and Human Development 15, 269-280.

Herzog, D. B., & Harper, G. (1981). Unexplained disability: Diagnostic dilemmas and principles of management. Clinical Pediatrics 20, 761-768.

Hodges, K., Kline, J. J., Barbero, G., & Woodruff, C. (1985). Anxiety in children with recurrent abdominal pain and their parents. Psychosomatics 26, 859, 862-866.

Hofer, M. A. (1984). Relationships as regulators: A psychobiologic perspective on bereavement. Psychosomatic Medicine 46, 183-197.

Ikemi, Y., & Ikemi, A. (1982). Some psychosomatic disorders in Japan in a cultural perspective. Psychothererapy and Psychosomatics 38, 231-238.

Jacobson, A. M., & Hauser, S. T. (1983). Behavioral and psychological aspects of diabetes. In M. Ellenberg & H. Rifkin (Eds.), Diabetes mellitus. New York: Medical Examination Publishing.

Johnson, S. B. (1980). Psychosocial factors in juvenile diabetes: A review. Journal of Behavioral Medicine 3, 95-116.

Juni, S. (1980). Reaction formation and over-control in enureses. American Journal of Psychoanalysis 40, 249-257.

Leaverton, D. R., White, C. A., McCormick, C. R., Smith, P., & Sheikholislam, B. (1980). Parental loss antecedent to childhood diabetes mellitus. Journal of the American Academy of Child Psychiatry 19, 678-689.

Lesse, S. (1981). Hypochondriacal and psychosomatic disorders masking depression in adolescents. American Journal of Psychotherapy 35, 356-367.

Levitan, H. L. (1980). Traumatic events in dreams of psychosomatic patients. Psychotherapy and Psychosomatics 33, 226-232.

Livingston, R., Taylor, J., & Crawford, S. (1988). A study of somatic complaints and psychiatric diagnosis in children. Journal of the American Academy of Child and Adolescent Psychiatry 27(2), 185-187.

McGrath, P. J., Goodman, J. T., Firestone, P., Shipman, R., & Peters, S. (1983). Recurrent abdominal pain: A psychogenic disorder? Archives of Disease in Childhood 58, 888-890.

Menahem, S., Lipton, G. L., & Caplan, G. (1981). The psychologically orientated pediatrician and the provision of psychoanalytic psychotherapy. Child Psychiatry and Human Development 12, 67-81.

Olness, K. N. (1986). Hypnotherapy in children. New approach to solving common pediatric problems. Postgraduate Medicine 79, 95-100, 105.

Panconesi, E. (1984). Psychosomatic dermatology. Clinics in Dermatolology 2, 94-179.

Parmelee, A. H., Howard, J., & Beckwith, L. (1984). Infant mental health and biological risk. Child Abuse and Neglect 8, 219-226.

Ratnoff, O. D. (1980). The psychogenic purpuras: A review of autoerythrocyte sensitization, auto sensitization to DNA, "hysterical" and factitial bleeding, and the religious stigmata. Seminars in Hematology 17, 192-213.

Rauste-von Wright, M., & von Wright, J. (1981). A longitudinal study of psychosomatic symptoms in healthy 11-18 year old girls and boys. Journal of Psychosomatic Research 25, 525-534.

Richtsmeier, A. J. (1984). Pitfalls in diagnosis of unexplained symptoms. Psychosomatics 25, 253-255.

Richtsmeier, A. J., & Waters, D. B. (1984). Somatic symptoms as family myth. American Journal of Diseases of Children 138, 855-857.

Sanders, K. (1984). Bion's 'protomental system' and psychosomatic illness in general practice. British Journal of Medical Psychology 57, 167-172.

Shafer, N., & Shafer, R. (1980). Factitious diseases including Munchausen's syndrome. New York State Journal of Medicine 80, 594-604.

Shanon, J. (1984). Holistic approach to diagnosis in psychosomatic dermatology. Clinics in Dermatology 2, 237-254.

Shuper, A., Mukamel, M., Mimouni, M., Lerman, M., & Varsano, I. (1983). Psychogenic cough. Archives of Disease in Childhood 58, 745-747.

Stams, U. K., Martin, C. H., & Tan, T. G. (1982). Psychogenic urinary retention in eight-year-old boy. Urology 20, 83-85.

Steiner, H., Walton, C. O., & Emslie, G. (1983). A psychosomatic unit for children and adolescents: Report on first year and ten months. Child Psychiatry and Human Development 14, 3-15.

Steinhausen, H. C. (1982). Locus of control among psychosomatically and chronically ill children and adolescents. Journal of Abnormal Child Psychology 10, 609-615.

Van Eerdewegh, M. M., Clayton, P. J., & Van Eerdewegh, P. (1985). The bereaved child: Variables influencing early psychopathology. British Journal of Psychiatry 147, 188-194.

Vandvik, I. H., & Seltzer, W. J. (1984). Evolution of child psychiatric teamwork in a somatic hospital. Psychotherapy and Psychosomatics 41, 77-84.

Wasserman, A. L., Whitington, P. F., & Rivara, F. P. (1988). Psychogenic basis for abdominal pain in children and adolescents. Journal of the American Academy of Child and Adolescent Psychiatry 27(2), 179-184.

Wilkinson, J. B. (1981). Hypnotherapy in the psychosomatic approach to illness: A review. Journal of the Royal Society of Medicine 74, 525-530.

Wolff, E. W., & Bayer, L. M. (1952). Psychosomatic disorders of childhood and adolescent. American Journal of Orthopsychiatry 22, 510-521.

Wolpe, J. (1980). Behavior therapy for psychosomatic disorders. Psychosomatics 21, 379-385.

4. Family Involvement in Psychophysiologic Disorders

Burbeck, T. (1979). An empirical investigation of the psychosomatogenic family model. Journal of Psychosomatic Research 23, 327-337.

Fielding, D., Moore, B., Dewey, M., Ashley, P., McKendrick T., & Pinkerton, P. (1985). Children with end-stage renal failure: Psychological effects on patients, siblings and parents. Journal of Psychosomatic Research 29, 457-465.

Haggerty, J. J. (1983). The psychosomatic family: An overview. Psychosomatics 24, 615-618, 623.

Minichin, S., Baker, L., Rosman, B., Liebman, R., Milman, L., & Todd, T. (1975). A conceptual model of psychosomatic illness in children. Archives of General Psychiatry 32, 1031-1038.

Plionis, E. M. (1977). Family functioning and childhood accident occurrence. American Journal of Orthopsychiatry 47, 250-263.

Smithells, R. W. (1979). Prenatal influences in psychosomatic disorders. Developmental Medicine and Child Neurology 21, 530-534.

Weakland, J. H. (1977). "Family somatics"--a neglected edge. Family Process 16, 263-272.

Wirsching, M., & Stierlin, H. (1979). Family dynamics and family psychotherapy of psychosomatic. Psychotherapy and Psychosomatics 32, 128-133.

5. Diagnostic Problems in Psychophysiologic Disorders

Freud, A. (1952). The role of bodily illness in the mental life of children. In R. S. Eissler, et al. (Eds.), Psychoanalytic study of the child (Vol. 7, pp. 69-81). New Haven: Yale University Press.

Herzog, D. B., & Harper, G. (1981). Unexplained disability: Diagnostic dilemmas and principles of management. Clinical Pediatrics 20, 761-768.

Hodges, K., Kline, J. J., Barbero, G., & Woodruff, C. (1985). Anxiety in children with recurrent abdominal pain and their parents. Psychosomatics 26, 859, 862-866.

McGrath, P. J., Goodman, J. T., Firestone, P., Shipman, R., & Peters, S. (1983). Recurrent abdominal pain: A psychogenic disorder? Archives of Disease in Childhood 58, 888-890.

Richtsmeier, A. J., & Waters, D. B. (1984). Somatic symptoms as family myth. American Journal of Diseases of Children 138, 855-857.

Shanon, J. (1984). Holistic approach to diagnosis in psychosomatic dermatology. Clinics in Dermatology 2, 237-254.

6. Failure to Thrive

Altemeier, W. A., O'Connor, S. M., Sherrod, K. B., & Vietze, P. M. (1985). Prospective study of antecedents for nonorganic failure to thrive. Journal of Pediatrics 106, 360-365.

Bell, L. S., & Woolston, J. L. (1985). The relationship of weight gain and caloric intake in infants with organic and nonorganic failure to thrive syndrome. Journal of the American Academy of Child Psychiatry 24, 447-452.

Chatoor, I., Schaefer, S., Dickson, L., & Egan, J. (1984). Non-organic failure to thrive: A developmental perspective. Pediatric Annals 13, 829-835, 838, 840-842.

Green, W. H., Campbell, M., & David, R. (1984). Psychosocial dwarfism: A critical review of the evidence. Journal of the American Academy of Child Psychiatry 23, 39-48.

Loewald, E. L. (1985). Psychotherapy with parent and child in failure-to-thrive. Analogies to the treatment of severely disturbed adults. In A. Solnit, et al. (Eds.), Psychoanalytic study of the child (Vol. 40, pp. 345-364). New Haven: Yale University Press.

Oates, R. K., Peacock, A., & Forrest, D. (1985). Long-term effects of nonorganic failure to thrive. Pediatrics 75, 36-40.

Reinhart, J. B., & Drash, S. L. (1969). Psychosocial dwarfism: Environmentally induced recovery. Psychosomatic Medicine 31, 165-172.

Singer, L. T., & Fagan, J. F. (1984). Cognitive development in the failure-to-thrive infant: A three-year longitudinal study. Journal of Pediatric Psychology 9, 363-383.

Skuse, D. H. (1985). Non-organic failure to thrive: A reappraisal. Archives of Disease in Childhood 60, 173-178.

Woolston, J. L. (1983). Eating disorders in infancy and early childhood. Journal of the American Academy of Child Psychiatry 22, 114-121.

7. Eating Disorders in Children and Adolescents

a. General Overview

Casper, R. C., Eckert, E. D., Halmi, K. A., Goldberg, S. C., & Davis, J. M. (1980). Bulimia. Its incidence and clinical importance in patients with anorexia nervosa. Archives of General Psychiatry 37, 1030-1035.

Casper, R. C., Offer, D., & Ostrov, E. (1981). The self-image of adolescents with acute anorexia nervosa. Journal of Pediatrics 98, 656-661.

de la Burde, B., & Reames, B. (1973). Prevention of pica, the major cause of lead poisoning in children. American Journal of Public Health 63, 737-743.

Jacobs, B. W., & Isaacs, S. (1986). Pre-pubertal anorexia nervosa: A retrospective controlled study. Journal of Child Psychology and Psychiatry 27, 237-250.

Lourie, R. S., & Millican, F. K. (1969). Pica. In J. G. Howells (Ed.), Modern perspective in international child psychiatry (pp. 455-470). Edinburgh: Oliver and Boyd.

Millican, F. K., Layman, E. M., Lourie, R. S., & Takahashi, L. Y. (1968). Study of an oral fixation: Pica. Journal of the American Academy of Child Psychiatry 7, 79-107.

Pyle, R. L., Mitchell, J. E., & Eckert, E. D. (1981). Bulimia: A report of 34 cases. Journal of Clinical Psychiatry 42, 60-64.

Ritvo, S. (1984). The image and uses of the body in psychic conflict. With special reference to eating disorders in adolescence. In A. Solnit, et al. (Eds.), Psychoanalytic study of the child (Vol. 39, pp. 449-469). New Haven: Yale University Press.

Rizzuto, A. M., Peterson, R. K., & Reed, M. (1981). The pathological sense of self in anorexia nervosa. Psychiatric Clinics of North America 4, 471-487.
Russell, G. F. (1985). Premenarchal anorexia nervosa and its sequelae. Journal of Psychiatric Research 19, 363-369.
Satter, E. M. (1986). Childhood eating disorders. Journal of the American Dietetic Association 86, 357-361.
Witt, E. D., Ryan, C., & Hsu, L. K. (1985). Learning deficits in adolescents with anorexia nervosa. Journal of Nervous and Mental Disease 173, 182-184.
Wortis, H., Rue, R., Heimer, C., Braine, M., Redlo, M., & Freedman, A. M. (1962). Children who eat noxious substances. Journal of the American Academy of Child Psychiatry 1, 536-547.

b. Anorexia Nervosa and Bulimia

Alessi, N. E., Krahn, D., Brehm, D., & Wittekindt, J. (1989). Prepubertal anorexia nervosa and major depressive disorder. Journal of the American Academy of Child and Adolescent Psychiatry 28, 380-384.
Andersen, A. E. (1984). Anorexia nervosa and bulimia in adolescent males. Pediatric Annals 13, 901-904, 907.
Andersen, A. E., & Mickalide, A. D. (1985). Anorexia nervosa and bulimia. Their differential diagnoses in 24 males referred to an eating and weight disorders clinic. Bulletin of the Menninger Clinic 49, 227-235.
Barcai, A. (1971). Family therapy in the treatment of anorexia nervosa. American Journal of Psychiatry 128, 286-290.
Berlin, I. N., Boatman, M. J., Sheimo, S. L., & Szurek, S. A. (1951). Adolescent alternation of anorexia and obesity. [Workshop, 1950]. American Journal of Orthopsychiatry 21, 387-419.
Biederman, J., Baldessarini, R. J., Harmatz, J. S., Rivinus, T. M., Arana, G. W., Herzog, D. B., & Schildkraut, J. J. (1986). Heterogeneity in anorexia nervosa. Biological Psychiatry 21, 213-216.
Biederman, J., Herzog, D. B., Rivinus, T. M., Harper, G. P., Ferber, R. A., Rosenbaum, J. F., Harmatz, J. S., & Tondorf, R. (1985). Amitriptyline in the treatment of anorexia nervosa: A double-blind, placebo-controlled study. Journal of Clinical Psychopharmacology 5, 10-16.
Bliss, E. L., & Branch, C. H. H. (1960). Anorexia nervosa. New York: Hoeber.
Bruch, H. (1970). Psychotherapy in primary anorexia nervosa. Journal of Nervous and Mental Disease 150, 51-67.
Bruch, H. (1981). Developmental considerations of anorexia nervosa and obesity. Canadian Journal of Psychiatry 26, 212-217.
Cantwell, D. P., Sturzenberger, S., Burroughs, J., Salkin, B., & Green, J. K. (1977). Anorexia nervosa. An affective disorder? Archives of General Psychiatry 34, 1087-1093.
Casper, R. C. (1984). Hypothalamic dysfunction and symptoms of anorexia nervosa. Psychiatric Clinics of North America 7, 201-213.

Chatoor, I., Egan, J., Getson, P., Menvielle, E., & O'Donnell, R. (1988). Mother-infant interactions in infantile anorexia nervosa. Journal of the American Academy of Child and Adolescent Psychiatry 27, 535-540.

Crisp, A. H. (1979). Early recognition and prevention of anorexia nervosa. Developmental Medicine and Child Neurology 21, 393-395.

Crisp, A. H. (1981). Therapeutic outcome in anorexia nervosa. Canadian Journal of Psychiatry 26, 232-235.

Drenowski, A., Yee, D. K., & Krahn, D. D. (1988). Bulimia in college women: Incidence and recovery rates. American Journal of Psychiatry 145, 753-755.

Eckert, E. C., Goldberg, S. C., Halmi, K. A., Casper, R. C., & Davis, J. M. (1979). Behavior therapy in anorexia nervosa. British Journal of Psychiatry 134, 55-59.

Fundudus, T. (1986). Anorexia nervosa in a pre-adolescent girl: A multimodal behaviour therapy approach. Journal of Child Psychology and Psychiatry 27, 261-273.

Garfinkel, P. E., & Garner, D. E. (1982). Anorexia nervosa: A multi-dimensional perspective. New York: Brunner/Mazel.

Garner, D. M., & Bemis, K. M. (1982). A cognitive-behavioral approach to anorexia nervosa. Cognitive Therapy and Research 6, 123-150.

Hall, A., Slim, E., Hawker, F., & Salmond, C. (1984). Anorexia nervosa: Long-term outcome in 50 female patients. British Journal of Psychiatry 145, 407-413.

Halmi, K. A., Eckert, E., LaDu, T. J., & Cohen, J. (1986). Anorexia nervosa: Treatment efficacy of cyproheptadine and amitriptyline. Archives of General Psychiatry 43, 177-181.

Halmi, K. A., Goldberg, S. C., Casper, R. C., Eckert, E. D., & Davis, J. M. (1979). Pretreatment predictors of outcome in anorexia nervosa. British Journal of Psychiatry 134, 71-78.

Hawley, R. M. (1985). The outcome of anorexia nervosa in younger subjects. British Journal of Psychiatry 146, 657-660.

Hendren, R. L. (1983). Depression in anorexia nervosa. Journal of the American Academy of Child Psychiatry 22, 59-62.

Hsu, L. K. G. (1980). Outcome of anorexia nervosa: A review of the literature (1954 to 1978). Archives of General Psychiatry 37, 1041-1046.

Hsu, L. K. G. (1982). Is there a disturbance in body image in anorexia nervosa? Journal of Nervous and Mental Disease 170, 305-307.

Huse, D. M., & Lucas, A. R. (1984). Dietary patterns in anorexia nervosa. American Journal of Clinical Nutrition 40, 251-254.

Isager, T., Brinch, M., Kreiner, S., & Tolstrup, K. (1985). Death and relapse in anorexia nervosa: Survival analysis of 151 cases. Journal of Psychiatric Research 19, 515-521.

Jaffe, A. C., & Singer, L. T. (1989). Atypical eating disorders in young children. International Journal of Eating Disorders 8, 575-582.

Jones, D. J., Fox, M. M., Babigian, H. M., & Hutton, H. E. (1980). Epidemiology of anorexia nervosa in Monroe County, New York: 1960-1976. Psychosomatic Medicine 42, 551-558.

Liebman, R., Sargent, J., & Silver, M. (1983). A family systems orientation to the treatment of anorexia nervosa. Journal of the American Academy of Child Psychiatry 22, 128-133.

Lippe, B. M. (1983). The physiologic aspects of eating disorders. Journal of the American Academy of Child Psychiatry 22, 108-113.

Lucas, A. R. (1981). Toward the understanding of anorexia nervosa as a disease entity. Mayo Clinic Proceedings 56, 254-264.

Lucas, A. R., Beard, C. M., O'Fallon, W. M., & Kurland, L. T. (1988). Anorexia nervosa in Rochester, Minnesota: A 45-year study. Mayo Clinic Proceedings 63, 433-442.

Lucas, A. R., & Callaway, C. W. (1985). Anorexia nervosa and bulimia. In J. E. Berk (Ed.), Bockus gastroenterology. Philadelphia: W. B. Saunders.

Maloney, M. J., & Klykylo, W. M. (1983). An overview of anorexia nervosa, bulimia, and obesity in children and adolescents. Journal of the American Academy of Child Psychiatry 22, 99-107.

Risen, S. E. (1982). The psychoanalytic treatment of an adolescent with anorexia nervosa. In A. Solnit, et al. (Eds.), Psychoanalytic study of the child (Vol. 37, pp. 433-459). New Haven: Yale University Press.

Rivinus, T. M., Biederman, J., Herzog, D. B., Kemper, K., Harper, G. P., Harmatz, J. S., & Houseworth, S. (1984). Anorexia nervosa and affective disorders: A controlled family history study. American Journal of Psychiatry 141, 1414-1418.

Selvini-Palazzoli, M. (1970). The families of patients with anorexia nervosa. In E. J. Anthony & C. Koupernik (Eds.), The child in his family (pp. 319-322). New York: Wiley.

Steinhausen, H. C., & Glanville, K. (1983). Follow-up studies of anorexia nervosa: A review of research findings. Psychological Medicine 13, 239-249.

Strober, M. (1980). Personality and symptomatological features in young, nonchronic anorexia nervosa patients. Journal of Psychosomatic Research 24, 353-359.

Swift, W. J. (1982). The long-term outcome of early onset anorexia nervosa. A critical review. Journal of the American Academy of Child Psychiatry 21, 38-46.

White, M. (1983). Anorexia nervosa: A transgenerational system perspective. Family Process 22, 255-273.

Yates, A. (1989). Current perspectives on the eating disorders: I. History, psychological and biological aspects. Journal of the American Academy of Child and Adolescent Psychiatry 28, 813-828.

c. Obesity in Children and Adolescents

Basseches, H. I., & Karp, S. A. (1984). Field dependence in young anorectic and obese women. Psychotherapy and Psychosomatics 41, 33-37.

Bonato, D. P., & Boland, F. J. (1983). Delay of gratification in obese children. Addictive Behavior 8, 71-74.

Boxer, G., Bauer, A., & Miller, B. (1988). Case study: Obesity-hypoventilation in childhood. Journal of the American Academy of Child and Adolescent Psychiatry 27 (5), 552-558.

Brownell, K. D., & Wadden, T. A. (1984). Confronting obesity in children: Behavioral and psychological factors. Pediatric Annals 13, 473-478, 480.

Bruch, H. (1970). Juvenile obesity: Its course and outcome. International Psychiatry Clinics 7, 231-254.

Bruch, H. (1981). Developmental consideration of anorexia nervosa and obesity. Canadian Journal of Psychiatry 26, 212-217.

Cecere, M. C. (1983). PIP (positive image program): A group approach for obese adolescents. Nursing Clinics of North America 18, 219-256.

Costanzo, P. R., & Woody, E. Z. (1979). Externality as a function of obesity in children: Pervasive style or eating-specific attribute? Journal of Personality and Social Psychology 37, 2286-2296.

Epstein, L. H., Wing, R. R., Steranchak, L., Dickson, B., & Michelson, J. (1980). Comparison of family-based behavior modification and nutrition education for childhood obesity. Journal of Pediatric Psychology 5, 25-36.

Garner, D. M., Garfinkel, P. E., & Moldofsky, H. (1978). Perceptual experiences in anorexia nervosa and obesity. Canadian Psychiatric Association Journal 23, 249-263.

Geller, S. E., Keane, T. M., & Scheirer, C. J. (1981). Delay of gratification, locus of control, and eating patterns in obese and nonobese children. Addictive Behavior 6, 9-14.

Harris, M. B., & Smith, S. D. (1983). The relationships of age, sex, ethnicity, and weight to stereotypes of obesity and self-perception. International Journal of Obesity 7, 361-371.

Hertzler, A. A. (1981). Obesity--impact of the family. Journal of the American Dietetic Association 79, 525-530.

Isbitsky, J. R., & White, D. R. (1981). Externality and locus of control in obese children. Journal of Psychology 107, 163-172.

Leon, G. R., Bemis, K. M., Meland, M., & Nussbaum, D. (1978). Aspects of body image perception in obese and normal-weight youngsters. Journal of Abnormal Child Psychology 6, 361-371.

Nathan, S., & Pisula, D. (1970). Psychological observations of obese adolescents during starvation treatment. Journal of the American Academy of Child Psychiatry 9, 722-740.

O'Brien, T. P., Walley, P. B., Anderson-Smith, S., & Drabman, R. S. (1982). Naturalistic observation of the snack-selecting behavior of obese and nonobese children. Addictive Behavior 7, 75-77.

Sobhany, M. S., & Rogers, C. S. (1985). External responsiveness to food and non-food cues among obese and non-obese children. International Journal of Obesity 9, 99-106.

Storz, N. S. (1982). Body image of obese adolescent girls in a high school and clinical setting. Adolescence 17, 667-672.

Strauss, C. C., Smith, K., Frame, C., & Forehand, R. (1985). Personal and interpersonal characteristics associated with childhood obesity. Journal of Pediatric Psychology 10, 337-343.
Tobias, A. L., & Gordon, J. B. (1980). Social consequences of obesity. Journal of the American Dietetic Association 76, 338-342.
Wadden, T. A., Foster, G. D., Brownell, K. D., & Finley, E. (1984). Self-concept in obese and normal-weight children. Journal of Consulting and Clinical Psychology 52, 1104-1105.
Worsley, A., Coonan, W., Leitch, D., & Crawford, D. (1984). Slim and obese children's perceptions of physical activities. International Journal of Obesity 8, 201-211.

d. Gastrointestinal Disease: Psychophysiological Aspects

Apley, J. (1967). The child with recurrent abdominal pain. Pediatric Clinics of North America 14, 63-72.
Davenport, C. W., Zrull, J. P., Kuhn, C. C., & Harrison, S. I. (1972). Cyclic vomiting. Journal of the American Academy of Child Psychiatry 11, 66-87.
Ein, S. H., Lynch, M. J., & Stephens, C. A. (1971). Ulcerative colitis in children under one year: A twenty-year review. Journal of Pediatric Surgery 6, 264-271.
Finch, S. M., & Hess, J. H. (1962). Ulcerative colitis in children. American Journal of Psychiatry 118, 819-826.
Gerbert, B. (1980). Psychological aspects of Crohn's disease. Journal of Behavioral Medicine 3, 41-58.
McDermott, J. F., & Finch, S. M. (1967). Ulcerative colitis in children: Reassessment of a dilemma. Journal of the American Academy of Child Psychiatry 6, 512-525.
Millar, T. P. (1969). Peptic ulcers in children. In J. G. Howells (Ed.), Modern perspective in international child psychiatry (pp. 471-493). Edinburgh: Oliver and Boyd.
Nowicki, S., & Strickland, B. R. (1973). A locus of control scale for children. Journal of Consulting and Clinical Psychology 40, 148-154.
Prugh, D. G., & Jordan, K. (1969). The management of ulcerative colitis in childhood. In J. G. Howells (Ed.), Modern perspective in international child psychiatry (pp. 494-530). Edinburgh: Oliver and Boyd.
Reinhart, J. B. (1982). Disorders of the gastrointestinal tract in children: Consultation-liaison experience. Psychiatric Clinics of North America 5, 387-397.
Steinhausen, H. C., & Kies, H. (1982). Comparative studies of ulcerative colitis and Crohn's disease in children and adolescents. Journal of Child Psychology and Psychiatry 23, 33-42.

8. Congenital Heart Disease

Bergman, A. (1967). The morbidity of cardiac nondisease in schoolchildren. New England Journal of Medicine 276, 1008-1013.

Galdston, R., & Gamble, W. J. (1969). On borrowed time: Observations on children with implanted cardiac pacemakers and their families. American Journal of Psychiatry 126, 104-108.

Glaser, H. H., Harrison, G. S., & Lynn, D. B. (1964). Emotional implications of congenital heart disease in children. Pediatrics 33, 367-379.

Green, M., & Levitt, E. E. (1962). Constriction of body image in children with congenital heart disease. Pediatrics 29, 438-441.

Josselyn, I. M., Simon, A. J., & Eells, E. (1955). Anxiety in children convalescing from rheumatic fever. American Journal of Orthopsychiatry 25, 109-119.

Lawler, K. A., Allen, M. T., Critcher, E. C., & Standard, B. A. (1981). The relationship of physiological responses to the coronary-prone behavior pattern in children. Journal of Behavioral Medicine 4, 203-216.

Linde, L. M. (1982). Psychiatric aspects of congenital heart disease. Psychiatric Clinics of North America 5, 399-406.

Matthews, K. A., & Avis, N. E. (1983). Stability of overt Type A behaviors in children: Results from a one-year longitudinal study. Child Development 54, 1507-1512.

Myers-Vando, R., Steward, M. S., Folkins, C. H., & Hines, P. (1979). The effects of congenital heart disease on cognitive development, illness causality concepts, and vulnerability. American Journal of Orthopsychiatry 49, 617-625.

Rausch de Traubenberg, N. (1973). Psychological aspects of congenital heart disease in the child. In E. J. Anthony & C. Koupernik (Eds.), The child in his family. Vol. 2. The impact of disease and death (pp. 75-83). New York: Wiley.

9. Rheumatoid Arthritis' Emotional Effect on Children and Adolescents

Beales, J. G., Keen, J. H., & Holt, P. J. (1983). The child's perception of the disease and the experience of pain in juvenile chronic arthritis. Journal of Rheumatology 10, 61-65.

Blom, G. E., & Nocholls, G. (1954). Emotional factors in children with rheumatoid arthritis. American Journal of Orthopsychiatry 24, 588-601.

Brazelton, T. B., Holder, R., & Talbot, B. (1953). Emotional aspects of rheumatic fever in children. Journal of Pediatrics 43, 339-358.

Litt, I. F., Cuskey, W. R., & Rosenberg, A. (1982). Role of self-esteem and autonomy in determining medication compliance among adolescents with juvenile rheumatoid arthritis. Pediatrics 69, 15-17.

Wilkinson, V. A. (1981). Juvenile chronic arthritis in adolescence: Facing the reality. International Rehabilitation Medicine 3, 11-17.

10. Asthma--Its Psychological Aspects

Aronsson, G., & Koivunen, E. (1985). Differences in personality between parents of asthmatic children and parents of non-asthmatic children. Journal of Psychosomatic Research 29, 177-182.

Conners, C. K. (1983). Psychological management of the asthmatic child. Clinical Reviews in Allergy 1, 163-177.

Cosper, M. R., & Erickson, M. T. (1985). The psychological, social, and medical needs of lower socioeconomic status mothers of asthmatic children. Journal of Asthma 22, 145-158.

Creer, T. L., Marion, R. J., & Creer, P. P. (1983). Asthma problem behavior checklist: Parental perceptions of the behavior of asthmatic children. Journal of Asthma 20, 97-104.

Dubo, S., McLean, J. A., Ching, A. Y. T., Wright, H. L., Kauffman, P. E., & Sheldon, J. M. (1961). A study of relationships between family situation, bronchial asthma, and personal adjustment in children. Journal of Pediatrics 59, 402-414.

Dunleavy, R. A., & Baade, L. E. (1980). Neuropsychological correlates of severe asthma in children 9-14 years old. Journal of Consulting and Clinical Psychology 48, 214-219.

Friedman, M. A. (1984). Psychological factors associated with pediatric asthma death: A review. Journal of Asthma 21, 97-117.

Fritz, G. K. (1983). Childhood asthma. Psychosomatics 24, 959-967.

Gauthier, Y., Fortin, C., Drapeau, P., Breton, J. J., Gosselin, J., Quintal, L., Weisnagel, J., & Lamarre, A. (1978). Follow-up study of 35 asthmatic preschool children. Journal of the American Academy of Child Psychiatry 17, 679-694.

Heilveil, I., & Schimmel, B. (1982). Self-esteem in asthmatic children. Journal of Asthma 19, 253-254.

Hilliard, J. P., Fritz, G. K., & Lewiston, N. J. (1982). Goal-setting behavior of asthmatic, diabetic and healthy children. Child Psychiatry and Human Development 13, 35-47.

Hilliard, J. P., Fritz, G. K., & Lewiston, N. J. (1985). Levels of aspiration of parents for their asthmatic, diabetic, and healthy children. Journal of Clinical Psychology 41, 587-597.

Hilton, S., Sibbald, B., Anderson, H. R., & Freeling, P. (1982). Evaluating health education in asthma--developing the methodology: Preliminary communication. Journal of the Royal Society of Medicine 75, 625-630.

Jackson, M. (1976). Psychopathology and psychotherapy in bronchial asthma. British Journal of Medical Psychology 49, 249-255.

Jurenec, G. S., & Ullman, D. G. (1984). Interrelationship of indices of emotional precipitants of asthma, psychological response to asthma, and symptom history in children. Journal of Asthma 21, 21-28.

Mrazek, D. A. (1986). Childhood asthma: Two central questions for child psychiatry. Journal of Child Psychology and Psychiatry 27, 1-5.

Piazzi, E. U. (1981). Comprehensive therapy of chronic asthma on a psychosomatic unit. Adolescence 16, 139-144.

Purcell, K., Brady, K., Chai, H., Muser, J., Molk, L., Gordon, N., & Means, J. (1969). The effect on asthma in children of experimental separation from the family. Psychosomatic Medicine 31, 144-164.

Sadler, J. E. (1982). Childhood asthma from the point of view of the liaison child psychiatrist. Psychiatric Clinics of North America 5, 333-343.
Staudenmayer, H. (1982). Medical manageability of psychosocial factors in childhood asthma. Journal of Chronic Diseases 35, 183-198.
Steiner, H., Fritz, G. K., Hilliard, J., & Lewiston, N. J. (1982). A psychosomatic approach to childhood asthma. Journal of Asthma 19, 111-121.
Steinhausen, H. C. (1983). Life events in relation to psychopathology among severely and chronically ill children and adolescents. Child Psychiatry and Human Development 13, 249-258.
Steinhausen, H. C., Schindler, H. P., & Stephan, H. (1983a). Comparative psychiatric studies on children and adolescents suffering from cystic fibrosis and bronchial asthma. Child Psychiatry and Human Development 14, 117-130.
Steinhausen, H. C., Schindler, H. P., & Stephan, H. (1983b). Correlates of psychopathology in sick children: An empirical model. Journal of the American Academy of Child Psychiatry 22, 559-564.
Stroudmire, A. (1985). Psychosomatic theory and pulmonary disease. Advances in Psychosomatic Medicine 14, 1-15.
Zlatich, D., Kenny, T. J., Sila, U., & Huang, S. W. (1982). Parent-child life events: Relation to treatment in asthma. Journal of Developmental and Behavioral Pediatrics 3, 69-72.

11. Epilepsy

Arlow, J. A. (1959). The structure of the deja vu experience. Journal of the American Psychoanalytic Association 7, 611-630.
Bandkler, B., Kaufman, I. C., et al. (1985). Role of sexuality in epilepsy. Psychosomatic Medicine 20, 227-234.
Berlin, I. N., & Yeager, C. L. (1951). Correlation of epileptic seizures, electroencephalograms and emotional state: Some preliminary observations in several children. American Journal of Disease of Children 81, 664-670.
Bernstein, N. R. (1969). Psychogenic seizure in adolescent girls. Behavioral Neuropsychiatry 1, 31-34.
Cohen, R. J., & Suter, C. (1982). Hysterical seizures: Suggestion as a provocative EEG test. Annals of Neurology 11, 391-395.
Dikmen, S., Temkin, N., Weiler, M., & Wyler, A. R. (1984). Behavioral effects of anticonvulsant prophylaxis: No effect of artifact? Epilepsia 25, 741-746.
Dodrill, C. B. (1979). Sex differences on the Halstead-Reitan Neuropsychological Battery and on other neuropsychological measures. Journal of Clinical Psychology 35, 236-241.
Ellenberg, J. H., Hirtz, D. G., & Nelson, K. B. (1986). Do seizures in children cause intellectual deterioration? New England Journal of Medicine 314, 1085-1088.
Gardner, D. L., & Goldberg, R. L. (1982-1983). Psychogenic seizures and loss. International Journal of Psychiatry and Medicine 12, 121-128.

Guberman, A. (1982). Psychogenic pseudoseizures in non-epileptic patients. Canadian Journal of Psychiatry 27, 401-404.

Heath, R. G., Dempsey, C. W., Fontana, C. J., & Fitzjarrell, A. T. (1980). Feedback loop between cerebellum and septal-hippocampal sites: Its role in emotion and epilepsy. Biological Psychiatry 15, 541-556.

Hermann, B. P., Dikmen, S., & Wilensky, A. J. (1982). Increased psychopathology associated with multiple seizure types: Fact or artifact? Epilepsia 23, 587-596.

LaBarbera, J. D., & Dozier, J. E. (1980). Hysterical seizures: The role of sexual exploitation. Psychosomatics 21, 897-903.

Master, D. R., & Lishman, W. A. (1984). Seizures, dyslexia, and dysgraphia of psychogenic origin. Archives of Neurology 41, 889-890.

McInytyre, D. C., & Wann, P. D. (1980). Cortical kindled convulsions: Disruption of inhibitory avoidance. Physiology and Behavior 25, 1-7.

Neutra, R., Levy, J. E., & Parker, D. (1977). Cultural expectations versus reality in Navajo seizure patterns and sick roles. Culture, Medicine and Psychiatry 1, 255-275.

O'Leary, D. S., Seidenberg, M., Berent, S., & Boll, T. J. (1981). Effects of age of onset of tonic-clonic seizures on neuropsychological performance in children. Epilepsia 22, 197-204.

Rosen, A. D., & Remmes, A. H. (1982). The visual evoked potential development of focal epilepsy. Journal of Neurological Science 53, 217-224.

Rothenberg, M. B., & Voeller, K. K. S. (1973). Psychosocial aspects of the management of seizures in children. Pediatrics 51, 1072-1082.

Sackellares, J. C., Giordani, B., Berent, S., Seidenberg, M., Dreifuss, F. E., Vanderzant, C. W., & Boll, T. J. (1985). Patients with pseudoseizures: Intellectual and cognitive performance. Neurology 35, 116-119.

Silver, L. B. (1982). Conversion disorder with pseudoseizures in adolescence: A stress reaction to unrecognized and untreated learning disabilities. Journal of the American Academy of Child Psychiatry 21, 508-512.

Wallace, S. J. (1984). Febrile convulsions: Their significance for later intellectual development and behaviour. Journal of Child Psychology and Psychiatry 25, 15-21.

12. Enuresis

Achenbach, T. M., & Lewis, M. (1971). A proposed model for clinical research and its application of encopresis and enureses. Journal of the American Academy of Child Psychiatry 10, 535-554.

Ambrosini, P. J. (1984). A pharmacological paradigm for urinary incontinence and enuresis. Journal of Clinical Psychopharmacology 4, 253-274.

Berg, I., Forsythe, I., & McGuire, R. (1982). Response of bedwetting to the enuresis alarm. Influence of psychiatric disturbance and maximum functional bladder capacity. Archives of Disease in Childhood 57, 394-396.

Bindelglas, P. M., & Dee, G. (1978). Enuresis treatment with imipramine hydrochloride: A 10-year follow-up study. American Journal of Psychiatry 135, 1549-1552.

Couchells, S. M., Johnson, S. B., Carter, R., & Walker, D. (1981). Behavioral and environmental characteristics of treated and untreated enuretic children and matched nonenuretic controls. Journal of Pediatrics 99, 812-816.

de Gatta, M. F., Garcia, M. J., Acosta, A., Rey, F., Gutierrez, J. R., & Dominguez-Gil, A. (1984). Monitoring of serum levels of imipramine and desipramine and individualization of does in enuretic children. Therapeutic Drug Monitor 6, 438-443.

Diamond, J. M., & Stein, J. M. (1983). Enuresis: A new look at stimulant therapy. Canadian Journal of Psychiatry 28, 395-397.

Dische, S., Yule, W., Corbett, J., & Hand, D. (1983). Childhood nocturnal enuresis: Factors associated with outcome of treatment with an enuresis alarm. Developmental Medicine and Child Neurology 25, 67-80.

Doleys, D. M., & Dolce, J. J. (1982). Toilet training and enuresis. Pediatric Clinics of North America 29, 297-313.

Esman, A. H. (1977). Nocturnal enuresis. Some current concepts. Journal of the American Academy of Child Psychiatry 16, 150-158.

Fielding, D., Berg, I., & Bell, S. (1978). An observational study of postures and limb movements of children who wet by day and at night. Developmental Medicine and Child Neurology 20, 453-461.

Foxman, B., Valdez, R. B., & Brook, R. H. (1986). Childhood enuresis: Prevalence, perceived impact, and prescribed treatments. Pediatrics 77, 482-487.

Fritz, G. K., & Anders, T. F. (1979). Enuresis: The clinical application of an etiologically based classification system. Child Psychiatry and Human Development 10, 103-113.

Fritz, G. K., & Armbrust, J. (1982). Enuresis and encopresis. Psychiatric Clinics of North America 5, 283-296.

Gillin, J. C., Rapoport, J. L., Mikkelsen, E. J., Langer, D., Vanskiver, C., & Mendelson, W. (1982). EEG sleep patterns in enuresis: A further analysis and comparison with normal controls. Biological Psychiatry 17, 947-953.

Glicklich, L. B. (1951). An historical account of enuresis. Pediatrics 8, 259-269.

Kaffman, M., & Elizur, E. (1977). Infants who become enuretics: A longitudinal study of 161 kibbutz children. Monographs of the Society for Research in Child Development (Vol. 42, pp. 1-61). Chicago: University of Chicago Press.

Kaplan, S. L., Briet, M., Gauthier, B., & Busner, J. (1989). A comparison of three nocturnal enuresis treatment methods. Journal of the American Academy of Child and Adolescent Psychiatry 28, 282-286.

May, H. J., Colligan, R. C., & Schwartz, M. S. (1983). Childhood enuresis. Important points in assessment, trends in treatment. Postgraduate Medicine 74, 111-119.

Mikkelsen, E. J., Brown, G. L., Minichiello, M. D., Millican, F. K., & Rapoport, J. L. (1982). Neurologic status in hyperactive, enuretic, encopretic, and normal boys. Journal of the American Academy of Child Psychiatry 21, 75-81.

O'Regan, S., Yazbeck, S., Hamberger, B., & Schick, E. (1986). Constipation a commonly unrecognized cause of enuresis. American Journal of Diseases of Children 140, 260-261.

Rapoport, J. L., Mikkelsen, E. J., & Zavadil, A. (1978). Plasma imipramine and desmethylimipramine concentration and clinical response in childhood enuresis. Psychopharmacology Bulletin 14, 60-61.

Rapoport, J. L., Mikkelsen, E. J., Zavadil, A., Nee, L., Gruenau, C., Mendelson, W., & Gillin, J. C. (1980). Childhood enuresis. II. Psychopathology, tricyclic concentration in plasma, and antienuretic effect. Archives of General Psychiatry 37, 1146-1152.

Romberger, J. A., & Offord, D. R. (1977). Psychosocial correlates of nocturnal enuresis among poor boys at a summer camp. Canadian Journal of Public Health 68, 499-502.

Schmitt, B. D. (1982). Daytime wetting (diurnal enuresis). Pediatric Clinics of North America 29, 9-20.

Shelov, S. P., Gundy, J., Weiss, J. C., McIntire, M. S., Olness, K., Staub, H. P., Jones, D. J., & Haque, M. (1981). Enuresis: A contrast of attitudes of parents and physicians. Pediatrics 66, 707-710.

Steinhausen, H. C., & Göbel, D. (1989). Enuresis in child psychiatric clinic patients. Journal of the American Academy of Child and Adolescent Psychiatry 28, 279-281.

13. Encopresis

Achenbach, T. M., & Lewis, M. (1971). A proposed model for clinical research and its application of encopresis and enuresis. Journal of the American Academy of Child Psychiatry 10, 535-554.

Amsterdam, B. (1979). Chronic encopresis: A system based psychodynamic approach. Child Psychiatry and Human Development 9, 137-144.

Bemporad, J. R., Pfeifer, C. M., Gibbs, L., Cortner, R. H., & Bloom, W. (1971). Characteristics of encopretic patients and their families. Journal of the American Academy of Child Psychiatry 10, 272-292.

Berg, I., Forsythe, I., Holt, P., & Watts, J. (1983). A controlled trial of 'Senokot' in faecal soiling treated by behavioural methods. Journal of Child Psychology and Psychiatry 24, 543-549.

Fritz, G. K., & Armbrust, J. (1982). Enuresis and encopresis. Psychiatric Clinics of North America 5, 283-296.

Halpern, W. I. (1977). The treatment of encopretic children. Journal of the American Academy of Child Psychiatry 16, 478-499.

Kisch, E. H., & Pfeffer, C. R. (1984). Functional encopresis: Psychiatric inpatient treatment. American Journal of Psychotherapy 38, 264-271.

Landman, G. B., & Rappaport, L. (1985). Pediatric management of severe treatment-resistant encopresis. Journal of Developmental and Behavioral Pediatrics 6, 349-351.

Levine, M. D., Mazonson, P., & Bakow, H. (1980). Behavioral symptom substitution in children cured of encopresis. American Journal of Diseases of Children 134, 663-667.

Loening-Baucke, V. A., & Cruikshank, B. M. (1986). Abnormal defecation dynamics in chronically constipated children with encopresis. Journal of Pediatrics 108, 562-566.

Margolies, R., & Gilstein, K. W. (1983-1984). A systems approach to the treatment of chronic encopresis. International Journal of Psychiatry and Medicine 13, 141-152.

Mikkelsen, E. J., Brown, G. L., Minichiello, M. D., Millican, F. K., & Rapoport, J. L. (1982). Neurologic status in hyperactive, enuretic, encopretic, and normal boys. Journal of the American Academy of Child Psychiatry 21, 75-81.

Protinsky, H., & Kersey, B. (1983). Psychogenic encopresis: A family therapy approach. Journal of Clinical Child Psychology 12, 192-197.

Wakefield, M. A., Woodbridge, C., Steward, J., & Croke, W. M. (1984). A treatment programme for faecal incontinence. Developmental Medicine and Child Psychology 26, 613-616.

Waksman, S. A. (1983). A multimodal treatment for secondary psychogenic encopresis: A case study. Psychological Reports 53, 271-273.

14. Disfigurement, Hair and Skin Disorders

Aleksandrowicz, M. K., & Mares, A. J. (1978). Trichotillomania and trichobezoar in an infant. Psychological factors underlying this symptom. Journal of the American Academy of Child Psychiatry 17, 533-539.

Arneson, S. W., & Triplett, J. L. (1978). How children cope with disfiguring changes in their appearance. MCN; American Journal of Maternal Child Nursing 3, 366-370.

Chalmers, A., Sayson, R., & Walters, K. (1982). Juvenile dermatomyositis: Medical, social and economic status in adulthood. Canadian Medical Association Journal 126, 31-33.

France, D. M. (1978). Atopic eczema and its management. Health Visitor 51, 294-295.

Fritz, G. K. (1979). Psychological aspects of atopic dermatitis. A viewpoint. Clinical Pediatrics 18, 360-364.

Galdston, R. (1974). The burning and the healing of children. In S. Chess & A. Thomas (Eds.), Annual progress in child psychiatry and child development: 1973 (pp. 464-478). New York: Brunner/Mazel.

Goodwin, J. M., Goodwin, J. S., & Kellner, R. (1979). Psychiatric symptoms in disliked medical patients. Journal of the American Medical Association 241, 1117-1120.

Hill-Beuf, A., & Porter, J. D. (1984). Children coping with impaired appearance: Social and psychologic influences. General Hospital Psychiatry 6, 294-301.

Knudson-Cooper, M. S. (1981). Adjustment to visible stigma: The case of the severely burned. Social Science and Medicine. Medical Anthropology 15B, 31-44.

Krishnan, K. R., Davidson, J. R., & Guajardo, C. (1985). Trichotillomania--a review. Comprehensive Psychiatry 26, 123-128.

Molinaro, J. R. (1978). The social fate of children disfigured by burns. American Journal of Psychiatry 135, 979-980.

Pines, D. (1980). Skin communication: Early skin disorders and their effect on transference and countertransference. International Journal of Psycho-Analysis 61, 315-323.

Saul, L. J., & Bernstein, C. (1941). The emotional settings of some attacks of urticaria. Psychosomatic Medicine 3, 349-369.

Schilder, R. (1936). Remarks on the psychophysiology of the skin. Psychoanalytic Review 23, 274-285.

Seligman, R. (1974). A psychiatric classification system for burned children. American Journal of Psychiatry 131, 41-46.

Silber, T. J., Chatoor, I., & White, P. H. (1984). Psychiatric manifestations of systemic lupus erythematosus in children and adolescents. A review. Clinical Pediatrics 23, 331-335.

15. Speech Disorders

Aram, D. M., Ekelman, B. L., Rose, D. F., & Whitaker, H. A. (1985). Verbal and cognitive sequelae following unilateral lesions acquired in early childhood. Journal of Clinical and Experimental Neuropsychology 7, 55-78.

Baker, L., & Cantwell, D. P. (1982). Developmental, social and behavioral characteristics of speech and language disordered children. Child Psychiatry and Human Development 12, 195-206.

Baumgartner, S. (1980). The social behavior of speech disordered children as viewed by parents. International Journal of Rehabilitation Research 3, 82-84.

Beitchman, J., Hood, J., Rochon, J., & Peterson, M. (1989). Empirical classification of speech/language impairment in children. II. Behavioral characteristics. Journal of the American Academy of Child and Adolescent Psychiatry 28 (1), 118-123.

Beitchman, J., Hood, J., Rochon, J., Peterson, M., Mantini, T., & Majumdar, S. (1989). Empirical classification of speech/language impairment in children. I. Identification of speech/language categories. Journal of the American Academy of Child and Adolescent Psychiatry 28 (1), 112-117.

Beitchman, J., Peterson, M., & Clegg, M. (1988). Speech and language impairment and psychiatric disorder. Child Psychiatry and Human Development 18, 191-207.

Blood, G. W., & Blood, I. M. (1984). Central auditory function in young stutterers. Perceptual and Motor Skills 59, 699-705.

Blood, I. M., & Blood, G. W. (1986). Relationship between specific disfluency variables and dichotic listening in stutterers. Perceptual and Motor Skills 62, 337-338.

Bloodstein, O., & Grossman, M. (1981). Early stutterings: Some aspects of their form and distribution. Journal of Speech and Hearing Research 24, 298-302.

Browne, E., Wilson, V., & Laybourne, P. C. (1963). Diagnosis and treatment of elective mutism in children. Journal of the American Academy of Child Psychiatry 2, 605-617.

Butterworth, B., Howard, D., & McLoughlin, P. (1984). The semantic deficit in aphasia: The relationship between semantic errors in auditory comprehension and picture naming. Neuropsychologia 22, 409-426.

Cantwell, D. P., Baker, L., & Mattison, R. (1981). Prevalence, type, and correlates of psychiatric diagnoses in 200 children with communication disorder. Journal of Developmental and Behavioral Pediatrics 2, 131-136.

Caparulo, B. K., & Cohen, D. J. (1977). Cognitive structure, language, and emerging social competence in autistic and aphasic children. Journal of the American Academy of Child Psychiatry 16, 620-645.

Conen, H., Davine, M., & Meloche-Kelly, M. (1989). Prevalence of unsuspected language disorders in a child psychiatric population. Journal of the American Academy of Child and Adolescent Psychiatry 28 (1), 107-111.

Conture, E. G. (1982). Youngsters who stutter: Diagnosis, parent counseling, and referral. Journal of Developmental and Behavioral Pediatrics 3, 163-169.

de Negri, M. (1980). Some critical motes about "the epilepsy-aphasia syndrome" in children. Brain and Development 2, 81-85.

Fuller, P., Newcombe, F., & Ounsted, C. (1983). Late language development in a child unable to recognize or produce speech sounds. Archives of Neurology 40, 165-168.

Gemelli, R. J. (1982). Classification of child stuttering: Part I. Transient developmental, neurogenic acquired, and persistent child stuttering. Child Psychiatry and Human Development 12, 220-253.

Hayden, T. L. (1980). Classification of elective mutism Journal of the American Academy of Child Psychiatry 19, 118-133.

Howlin, P. (1982). Echolalic and spontaneous phrase speech in autistic children. Journal of Child Psychology and Psychiatry 23, 281-293.

Kolvin, I., & Fundudis, T. (1981). Elective mute children: Psychological development and background factors. Journal of Child Psychology and Psychiatry 22, 219-232.

Mann, V. A., Sharlin, H. M., & Dorman, M. (1985). Children's perception of sibilants: The relation between articulation and perceptual development. Journal of Experimental Child Psychology 39, 252-264.

Mattison, R. E., Cantwell, D. P., & Baker, L. (1982). A practical method for screening psychiatric disorder in children with speech and language disorders. Journal of Abnormal Child Psychology 10, 25-32.

Metellus, J. (1980). The personality of patients with Brocas's aphasias. Annales Medico-Psychologiques (Paris) 138, 856-861.

Meyers, S. C., & Freeman, F. J. (1985). Interruptions as a variable in stuttering and disfluency. Journal of Speech and Hearing Research 28, 428-435.

Morton-Evans, A., & Hensley, R. (1978). Paired associate learning in early infantile autism and receptive developmental aphasia. Journal of Autism and Childhood Schizophrenia 8, 61-69.

Pohl, P. (1979). Dichotic listening in a child recovering from acquired aphasia. Brain and Language 8, 372-379.

Ruscello, D. M., Moreau, V. K., & Sholtis, D. (1980). Awareness of certain articulatory gestures in normal-speaking and articulatory-defective children. Journal of Communication Disorders 13, 59-64.

Schlesinger, H. S., & Meadow, K. P. (1972). Sound and sign: Childhood deafness and mental health. Berkeley: University of California Press.

Wall, M. J., & Myers, F. L. (1982). A review of linguistic factors associated with early childhood stuttering. Journal of Communication Disorders 15, 441-449.

16. Psychological Aspects of Malignant Diseases in Children and Adolescents

Copeland, D. R., Fletcher, J. M., Pfefferbaum-Levine, B., Jaffe, N., Ried, H., & Maor, M. (1985). Neuropsychological sequelae of childhood cancer in long-term survivors. Pediatrics 75, 745-753.

Crisp, A. H. (1970). Some psychosomatic aspects of neoplasia. British Journal of Medical Psychology 43, 313-331.

Hilgard, J. R., & LeBaron, S. (1982). Relief of anxiety and pain in children and adolescents with cancer: Quantitative measures and clinical observations. International Journal of Clinical and Experimental Hypnosis 30, 417-442.

Obetz, S. W., et al. (1980). Children who survive malignant disease: Emotional adaptation of the child and their families. In J. Schulman, M. J. Kupst, & C. C. Thomas (Eds.), The child with cancer: Clinical approaches to psychosocial care: Research in psychosocial aspects. Springfield, Ill.: Charles C. Thomas.

Pfefferbaum-Levine, B., Copeland, D. R., Fletcher, J. M., Ried, H. L., Jaffe, N., & McKinnon, W. R. (1984). Neuropsychologic assessment of long-term survivors of childhood leukemia. American Journal of Pediatric Hematology/Oncology 6, 123-128.

Van Dongen-Melman, J. E., & Sanders-Woudstra, J. A. (1986). Psychosocial aspects of childhood cancer: A review of the literature. Journal of Child Psychology and Psychiatry 27, 145-180.

Zeltzer, L., LeBaron, S., & Zeltzer, P. M. (1984). The effectiveness of behavioral intervention for reduction of nausea and vomiting in children and adolescents receiving chemotherapy. Journal of Clinical Oncology 2, 683-690.

17. Tics--Gilles de la Tourette Syndrome

Annibali, J. A., et al. (1986). Anorexia nervosa in a young male with Tourette's syndrome. Journal of Clinical Psychology 47, 324-326.

Baird, L., et al. (1986). A prevalence study of Gilles de la Tourette syndrome in North Dakota school-age children. Journal of the American Academy of Child Psychiatry 25, 552-553.

Belfer, M. L., & Kaban, L. B. (1982). Temporomandibular joint dysfunction with facial pain in children. Pediatrics 69, 564-567.

Grad, L. R., et al. (1987). Obsessive-compulsive symptomatology in children with Tourette's syndrome. Journal of the American Academy of Child and Adolescent Psychiatry 26, 69-73.

Lacey, D. J. (1986). Diagnosis of Tourette syndrome in childhood. Clinical Pediatrics 25, 433-435.

Lucas, A. R., Kaufman, P. E., & Morris, E. M. (1967). Gilles de la Tourette's disease: A clinical study of fifteen cases. Journal of the American Academy of Child Psychiatry 6, 700-722.

Madorsky, J. G., Radford, L. M., & Neumann, E. M. (1984). Psychosocial aspects of death and dying in Duchenne muscular dystrophy. Archives of Physical Medicine and Rehabilitation 65, 79-82.

Meares, R. (1971). Features which distinguish groups of spasmodic torticollis. Journal of Psychosomatic Research 15, 1-11.

Melnichuk, P. V., et al. (1985). Early diagnosis of Tourette's syndrome. Neuroscience and Behavioral Physiology 15, 45-47.

Silverstien, F., et al. (1985). Effect of clonidine on platelet alpha 2-adrenoreceptors and plasma norepinephrine of children with Tourette syndrome. Developmental Medicine and Child Neurology 27, 793-799.

Sollee, N. D., Lathma, E. E., Kindlon, D. J., & Bresnan, M. J. (1985). Neuropsychological impairment in Duchenne muscular dystrophy. Journal of Clinical and Experimental Neuropsychology 7, 486-496.

D. Attention Deficit Disorders with and without Hyperactivity

Larry Silver, M.D., Section Editor

Abikoff, H., & Gittelman, R. (1985). The normalizing effects of methylphenidate on the classroom behavior of ADDH children. Journal of Abnormal Child Psychology 13, 33-44.

Arnold, L. E., Christopher, J., Heustis, R., & Smeltzer, D. J. (1978). Methylphenidate vs. dextroamphetamine vs. caffeine in minimal brain dysfunction: Controlled comparison by placebo washout design with Bayes' analysis. Archives of General Psychiatry 35, 463-473.

Brown, R. T., Borden, K. A., & Clingerman, S. R. (1985). Pharmacotherapy in ADD adolescents with special attention to multimodality treatments. Psychopharmacology Bulletin 21, 192-211.

Cantwell, D. P. (1985). Hyperactive children have grown up. What have we learned about what happens to them? Archives of General Psychiatry 42, 1026-1028.

Comings, D. E., & Comings, B. G. (1984). Tourette's syndrome and attention deficit disorder with hyperactivity: Are they genetically related? Journal of the American Academy of Child Psychiatry 23, 138-146.

Conners, C. K. (1980). Food additives and hyperactive children. New York: Plenum Press.

Conners, C. K., & Taylor, E. (1980). Pemoline, methylphenidate, and placebo in children with minimal brain dysfunction. Archives of General Psychiatry 37, 922-930.

Firestone, P. (1982). Factors associated with children's adherence to stimulant medication. American Journal of Orthopsychiatry 52, 447-457.

Gardner, R. A. (1973). MBD: The family book about minimal brain dysfunction. New York: Jason Aronson.

Gardner, R. A. (1980). What every psychoanalyst should know about minimal brain dysfunction. Journal of the American Academy of Psychoanalysis 8, 403-426.

Gittelman, R., & Mannuzza, S. (1985). Diagnosing ADD-H in adolescents. Psychopharmacology Bulletin 21, 237-242.

Gualtieri, C. T., & Hicks, R. E. (1985). Neuropharmacology of methylphenidate and a neural substrate for childhood hyperactivity. Psychiatric Clinics of North America 8, 875-892.

Hechtman, L., Weiss, G., & Perlman, T. (1984a). Hyperactives as young adults: Past and current substance abuse and antisocial behavior. American Journal of Orthopsychiatry 54, 415-425.

Hechtman, L., Weiss, G., & Perlman, T. (1984b). Young adult outcome of hyperactive children who received long-term stimulant treatment. Journal of the American Academy of Child Psychiatry 23, 261-269.

Huestis, R. D., Arnold, L. E., & Smeltzer, D. J. (1975). Caffeine versus methylphenidate and d-amphetamine in minimal brain dysfunction: A double-blind comparison. American Journal of Psychiatry 132, 868-870.

Hunt, R. D., Brunstetter, R., & Silver, L. B. (1986). ADD: Recent advances. In J. Noshpitz (Ed.), Basic handbook of child psychiatry (Vol. 5, pp. 337-353). New York: Basic Books.

Lowe, T. L., Cohen, D. J., Detlor, J., Kremenitzer, M. W., & Shaywitz, B. A. (1982). Stimulant medications precipitate Tourette's syndrome. Journal of the American Medical Association 247, 1168-1169.

Mattes, J. A., & Gittelman, R. (1983). Growth of hyperactive children on maintenance regimen of methylphenidate. Archives of General Psychiatry 40, 317-321.

National Institutes of Health consensus development conference statement: Defined diets and childhood hyperactivity. (1983). American Journal of Clinical Nutrition 37, 161-165.

Rapoport, J. L., & Ferguson, H. B. (1981). Biological validation of the hyperkinetic syndrome. Developmental Medicine and Child Neurology 23, 667-682.

Reatig, N. (1984). Attention deficit disorder: A bibliography. Psychopharmacology Bulletin 20, 693-718.

Rutter, M. (1982). Syndromes attributed to "minimal brain dysfunction" in childhood. American Journal of Psychiatry 139, 21-33.

Satterfield, J. H., Hoppe, C. M., & Schell, A. M. (1982). A prospective study of delinquency in 110 adolescent boys with attention deficit disorder and 88 normal adolescent boys. American Journal of Psychiatry 139, 795-798.

Shaywitz, S. E., Hunt, R. D., Jatlow, P., Cohen, D. J., Young, J. G., Pierce, R. N., Anderson, G. M., & Shaywitz, B. A. (1982). Psychopharmacology of attention deficit disorder: Pharmacokinetic, neuroendocrine, and behavioral measures following acute and chronic treatment with methylphenidate. Pediatrics 69, 688-694.

Shaywitz, S. E., & Shaywitz, B. A. (1988). Attention deficit disorder: Current perspective. In J. F. Kavanagh & T. J. Truss, Jr. (Eds.), Learning disabilities: Proceedings of the National Conference (pp. 369-523). Parkton, Md.: York Press.

Silver, L. B. (1976). The playroom diagnostic evaluation of children with neurologically based learning disabilities. Journal of the American Academy of Child Psychiatry 15, 240-256.

Silver, L. B. (1981). The relationship between learning disabilities, hyperactivity, distractibility, and behavioral problems: A clinical analysis. Journal of the American Academy of Child Psychiatry 20, 385-397.

Weiss, G., Hechtman, L., Milroy, T., & Perlman, T. (1985). Psychiatric status of hyperactives as adults: A controlled prospective 15-year follow-up of 63 hyperactive children. Journal of the American Academy of Child Psychiatry 24, 211-220.

Wender, P. H., Reimherr, F. W., Wood, D., & Ward, M. (1985). A controlled study of methylphenidate in the treatment of attention deficit disorder, residual type, in adults. American Journal of Psychiatry 142, 547-552.

E. Learning and School Disorders

Lionel Hersov, M.D., F.R.C.P., D.P.M., Section Editor

Irving N. Berlin, M.D., Eli M. Bower, Ph.D., Ken Farley, M.D., Carl Feinstein, M.D., Larry Silver, M.D., and Peter Toscano, M.D., Associate Editors

1. Theories of Learning

Bandura, A. (1971). Social learning theory. New York: General Learning Press.

Berger, M. (1985). Development and childhood disorders. In M. Rutter & L. Hersov (Eds.), Child and adolescent psychiatry: Modern approaches (pp. 179-190). Oxford: Blackwell.

Bower, G. H., & Hilgard, E. R. (1981). Theories of learning. Englewood Cliffs, N.J.: Prentice-Hall.

Flavell, J. H. (1963). The developmental psychology of Jean Piaget. Princeton, N.J.: Van Nostrand.

Freud, A. (1954). Psychoanalysis and education. In R. S. Eissler, et al. (Eds.), Psychoanalytic study of the child (Vol. 9, pp. 9-15). New York: International Universities Press.

Hebb, D. O. (1976). Physiological learning theory. Journal of Abnormal Child Psychology 4, 309-314.

Hilgard, E. R., & Bower, G. H. (1975). Theories of learning. Englewood Cliffs, N.J.: Prentice-Hall.

Hobson, R. P. (1985). On ways of knowing in childhood. In M. Rutter & L. Hersov (Eds.), Child and adolescent psychiatry: Modern approaches (pp. 191-203). Oxford: Blackwell.

Holland, P. C. (1984). Origins of behavior in Pavlovian conditioning. In G. H. Bower (Ed.), The psychology of learning and motivation: Advances in research and theory (pp. 129-174). New York: Academic Press.

Mahoney, M. J., & Nezworksi, M. T. (1985). Cognitive-behavioral approaches to children's problems. Journal of Abnormal Child Psychology 13, 467-476.

Mowrer, O. H. (1950). Learning theory and personality dynamics: Selected papers. New York: Ronald Press.

Piaget, J. (1959). The language and thought of the child. New York: Humanities Press.

Piaget, J. (1967). Six psychological studies. New York: Vintage Books.

Skinner, B. F. (1950). Are theories of learning necessary? Psychological Review 57, 193-216.

Woody, C. D. (1986). Understanding the cellular basis of memory and learning. Annual Review of Psychology 37, 433-493.

2. Historical Review of Learning Problems

Berlin, I. N. (1960). Aspects of creativity and the learning process. American Imago 17, 83-99.

Berlin, I. N., & Szurek, S. A. (Eds.). (1965). Learning and its disorders. Clinical approaches to problems of childhood. The Langley Porter child psychiatry series (Vol. 1). Palo Alto: Science and Behavior Books.

Biber, B. (1961). Integration of mental health principles in the school setting. In G. Caplan (Ed.), Prevention of mental disorders in children (pp. 323-352). New York: Basic Books.

Hellman, I. (1954). Some observations on mothers of children with intellectual inhibitions. In R. S. Eissler, et al. (Eds.), Psychoanalytic study of the child (Vol. 9, pp. 259-273). New York: International Universities Press.

Holmes, D. (1965). A contribution to a psychoanalytic theory of work. In R. S. Eissler, et al. (Eds.), Psychoanalytic study of the child (Vol. 20, pp. 384-393). New York: International Universities Press.

Klein, E. (1949). Psychoanalytic aspects of school problems. In R. S. Eissler, et al. (Eds.), Psychoanalytic study of the child (Vol. 3/4, pp. 369-390). New York: International Universities Press.

Levy, D. M. (1955). Oppositional syndromes and oppositional behavior. Proceeding of the American Psychopathological Association 44, 204-226.

Liss, E. (1955). Motivations in learning. In R. S. Eissler, et al. (Eds.), Psychoanalytic study of the child (Vol. 10, pp. 100-116). New York: International Universities Press.

Mahler, M. S. (1950). Energy-economic considerations in the learning process. Quarterly Journal of Child Behavior 2, 233-236.

Nagera, H. (1967). The concepts of structure and structuralization: Psychoanalytic usage and implications for a theory of learning and creativity. In R. S. Eissler, et al. (Eds.), Psychoanalytic study of the child (Vol. 22, pp. 77-102). New York: International Universities Press.

Nirk, G. (1973). Observations on the relationship of emotional and cognitive development: A psychiatric contribution to compensatory education. Journal of the American Academy of Child Psychiatry 12, 93-107.

Pearson, G. H. (1952). A survey of learning difficulties in children. In R. S. Eissler, et al. (Eds.), Psychoanalytic study of the child (Vol. 7, pp. 322-386). New York: International Universities Press.

Peller, L. E. (1956). The school's role in promoting sublimation. In R. S. Eissler, et al. (Eds.), Psychoanalytic study of the child (Vol. 11, pp. 437-449). New York: International Universities Press.

Rubenstein, B. O., Falick, M. L., Levitt, M., & Ekstein, R. (1959). Learning problems. 2. Learning impotence: A suggested diagnostic category. American Journal of Orthopsychiatry 29, 315-323.

Sarnoff, I. (1956). Some psychological problems of the incipient artist. Mental Hygiene 40, 375-383.

Sperry, B., Staver, N., Reiner, B. S., & Ulrich, D. (1958). Renunciation and denial in learning difficulties. American Journal of Orthopsychiatry 28, 98-111.

Strang, R. (1957). Students' perception of factors affecting their studying. Mental Hygiene 41, 97-102.

3. General Learning Problems

Blom, G. E., Rudnick, M., & Searless, J. (1966). Some principles and practices in the psychoeducational treatment of emotionally disturbed children. Psychology in the Schools 3, 30-38.

Bryan, T. H. (1974). Learning disabilities: A new stereotype. Journal of Learning Disabilities 7, 304-309.

Cohen, S. (1966). Teaching emotionally disturbed children. Children 13, 232-236.

Ekanger, C. A., & Westervelt, G. (1967). Contributions of observation in naturalistic settings to clinical and educational practice. Journal of Special Education 1, 207-213.

Kounin, J. S., & Obradovic, S. (1968). Managing emotionally disturbed children in regular classrooms: A replication and extension. Journal of Special Education 2, 129-135.

Mahler, M. S. (1942). Psuedoimbecility: A magic cap of invisibility. Psychoanalytic Quarterly 11, 149-164.

Newman, C. J., & Krug, O. (1964). Problems in learning arithmetic in emotionally disabled children. Journal of the American Academy of Child Psychiatry 3, 412-429.

Redl, F. (1959). The life space interview. 1. Strategy and techniques of the life space

interview. American Journal of Orthopsychiatry 29, 1-18.
Sperry, B., Ulrich, D. N., & Staver, N. (1958). The relation of motility to boys' learning problems. American Journal of Orthopsychiatry 28, 640-646.
Switzer, J. (1963). A genetic approach to the understanding of learning problems. Journal of the American Academy of Child Psychiatry 2, 653-666.
Wimberger, H. C. (1966). Conceptual system for classification of psychogenic school underachievement. Journal of Pediatrics 69, 1092-1097.

4. Language and Reading Disorders

Bender, L. (1958). Problems in conceptualization and communication in children with developmental alexia. Proceedings of the American Psychopathological Association 46, 155-176.
Blom, G. E., Farley, G. K., & Guthals, C. (1970). The concept of body image and the remediation of body image disorders. Journal of Learning Disabilities 3, 440-447.
Eisenberg, L. (1966). Reading retardation: I. Psychiatric and sociologic aspects. Pediatrics 37, 352-365.
Frank, J., & Levinson, H. (1973). Dysmetric dyslexia and dyspraxia. Journal of the American Academy of Child Psychiatry 12, 690-701.
Fredman, G. (1989). Critical review of the classification of reading disorders. Newsletter of the Association for Child Psychology and Psychiatry 11, 5-10.
Galaburda, A. M., Sherman, G. F., Rosen, G. D., Aboitiz, F., & Geschwind, N. (1985). Developmental dyslexia: Four consecutive patients with cortical anomalies. Annals of Neurology 18, 222-233.
Johnson, D. J. (1988). Review of research on specific reading, writing, and mathematics disorders. In J. F. Kavanagh & T. J. Truss, Jr., Learning disabilities: Proceedings of the national conference. Parkton, Md.: York Press.
Millman, I. K., & Canter, S. M. (1972). Language disturbances in normal and pathological development: Comparisons and practical considerations. Journal of the American Academy of Child Psychiatry 11, 243-254.
Rabinovitch, R. D. (1959). Reading and learning disabilities. In S. Ariete (Ed.), American handbook of psychiatry (Vol. 1, pp. 857-869). New York: Basic Books.
Richardson, S. O. (1989). Developmental language disorder. In H. I. Kaplan & B. J. Sadock (Eds.), Comprehensive textbook of psychiatry (5th ed., pp. 1812-1817). Baltimore, Md.: Williams and Wilkins.
Shepherd, J. J., Charnow, D. A., & Silver, L. B. (1989). Developmental reading disorder. In H. I. Kaplan & B. J. Sadock (Eds.), Comprehensive textbook of psychiatry (5th ed., pp. 1790-1796). Baltimore, Md.: Williams and Wilkins.
Silver, A. A., & Hagin, R. A. (1960). Specific reading disability: Delineation of the syndrome and relationship to cerebral dominance. Comprehensive Psychiatry 1, 126-134.
Silver, A. A., & Hagin, R. A. (1964). Specific reading disability: Follow-up studies. American Journal of Orthopsychiatry 34, 95-102.

Stewart, R. S. (1950). Personality maladjustment and reading achievement. American Journal of Orthopsychiatry 20, 410-417.

Tallal, P. (1988). Developmental language disorders. In J. F. Kavanagh & T. J. Truss, Jr. (Eds.), Learning disabilities: Proceedings of the National Conference (pp. 181-272). Parkton, Md.: York Press.

5. Parents and School Problems

Blum, H. M., Boyle, M. H., & Offord, D. R. (1988). Single-parent families: Child psychiatric disorder and school performance. Journal of the American Academy of Child and Adolescent Psychiatry 27, 214-219.

Buxbaum, E. (1964). The parents' role in the etiology of learning disabilities. In R. S. Eissler, et al. (Eds.), Psychoanalytic study of the child (Vol. 19, pp. 421-447). New York: International Universities Press.

Hellman, I. (1954). Some observations on mothers of children with intellectual inhibitions. In R. S. Eissler, et al. (Eds.), Psychoanalytic study of the child (Vol. 9, pp. 259-273). New York: International Universities Press.

McCarthy, D. (1954). Language disorders and parent-child relationships. Journal of Speech and Hearing Disorders 19, 514-523.

Silver, L. B. (1989). Psychological and family problems associated with learning disabilities: Assessment and intervention. Journal of the American Academy of Child and Adolescent Psychiatry 28, 319-325.

Staver, N. (1953). The child's learning difficulty as related to the emotional problem of the mother. American Journal of Orthopsychiatry 23, 131-141.

Walker, D. R. (1959). Parents as "enablers" in helping the child with a school problem. Child Welfare 38(3), 11-16.

Ziegler, R., & Halden, L. (1988). Family therapy for learning disabled and attention-deficit disordered children. American Journal of Orthopsychiatry 58, 190-210.

6. An Overview of Learning Problems: Diagnosis and Treatment

Abelson, A. G., & Mutsch, M. A. (1985). A measure of adaptive behavior of learning disabled students. Perceptual and Motor Skills 61, 862.

Abrams, J. C. (1981). The psychologist-educator views the relationship of vision to reading and related learning disabilities. Journal of Learning Disabilities 14, 565-567.

Ackerman, P. T., Dykman, R. A., & Peters, J. E. (1977). Learning-disabled boys as adolescents: Cognitive factors and achievement. Journal of the American Academy of Child Psychiatry 16, 296-313.

Adelman, H. S., Taylor, L., & Nelson, P. (1982). Prevalence and treatment of learning problems in upper and lower income areas. American Journal of Orthopsychiatry 52, 719-742.

Aman, M. G. (1980). Psychotropic drugs and learning problems--a selective review. Journal of Learning Disabilities 13, 87-97.

Amerikaner, M., & Summerlin, M. L. (1982). Group counseling with learning disabled children: Effects of social skills and relaxation training on self-concept and classroom behavior. Journal of Learning Disabilities 15, 340-343.

Amerikaner, M. J., & Omizo, M. M. (1984). Family interaction and learning disabilities. Journal of Learning Disabilities 17, 540-543.

Anastas, J. W., & Reinherz, H. (1984). Gender differences in learning and adjustment problems in school: Results of a longitudinal study. American Journal of Orthopsychiatry 54, 110-122.

Anderson, M. A. (1985). Cooperative group tasks and their relationship to peer acceptance and cooperation. Journal of Learning Disabilities 18, 83-86.

Balk, D. (1983). Learned helplessness: A model to understand and overcome a child's extreme reaction to failure. Journal of School Health 53, 365-370.

Bennett, F. C., & Furukawa, C. T. (1984). Effects of conductive hearing loss on speech, language, and learning development. Clinical Reviews in Allergy 2, 377-385.

Berger, M., & Kennedy, H. (1975). Pseudobackwardness in children. Maternal attitudes as an etiological factor. In R. S. Eissler, et al. (Eds.), Psychoanalytic study of the child (Vol. 30, pp. 279-306). New York: International Universities Press.

Berk, R. A. (1983). The value of WISC-R profile analysis for the differential diagnosis of learning disabled children. Journal of Clinical Psychology 39, 133-136.

Berninger, V. W., & Colwell, S. O. (1985). Relationships between neurodevelopmental and educational findings in children aged 6 to 12 years. Pediatrics 75, 697-702.

Bognar, C. J., & Martin, W. B. (1982). A sociological perspective on diagnosing learning difficulties. Journal of Learning Disabilities 15, 347-351.

Breen, M. J., Carlson, M., & Lehman, J. (1985). The revised developmental test of visual-motor integration: Its relation to the VMI, WISC-R, and Bender Gestalt for a group of elementary aged learning disabled students. Journal of Learning Disabilities 18, 136-138.

Brent, D. A., & Howell, M. (1983). Data based on program evaluation in a project involving mental health consultation to schools. Journal of the American Academy of Child Psychiatry 22, 447-453.

Brodzinsky, D. M., Schechter, D. E., Braff, A. M., & Singer, L. M. (1984). Psychological and academic adjustment in adopted children. Journal of Consulting and Clinical Psychology 52, 582-590.

Brown, R. T., & Alford, N. (1984). Ameliorating attentional deficits and concomitant academic deficiencies in learning disabled children through cognitive training. Journal of Learning Disabilities 17, 20-26.

Bryan, T., Donahue, M., Pearl, R., & Herzog, A. (1984). Conversational interactions between mothers and learning-disabled or nondisabled children during a problem-solving task. Journal of Speech and Hearing Disorders 49, 64-71.

Carbo, M. (1983). Research in reading and learning style: Implications for exceptional children. Exceptional Children 49, 486-494.

Carter, J. L, & Russell, H. L. (1985). Use of EMG biofeedback procedures with learning disabled children in a clinical and an educational setting. Journal of Learning Disabilities 18, 213-216.

Ceci, S. J. (1984). A developmental study of learning disabilities and memory. Journal of Experimental Child Psychology 38, 352-371.

Cermak, L. S. (1983). Information processing deficits in children with learning disabilities. Journal of Learning Disabilities 16, 599-605.

Churton, M. W. (1985). Selected measures of physical fitness for a group of learning disabled children. Perceptual and Motor Skills 61, 678.

Cohen, N. J., Kolers, N., & Bradley, S. (1987). Predictors of the outcome of treatment in a therapeutic preschool. Journal of the American Academy of Child and Adolescent Psychiatry 26, 829-833.

Colbert, P., Newman, B., Ney, P., & Young, J. (1982). Learning disabilities as a symptom of depression in children. Journal of Learning Disabilities 15, 333-336.

Conners, C. K. (1979). Application of biofeedback to treatment of children. Journal of the American Academy of Child Psychiatry 18, 143-153.

Connolly, B. H. (1983). Lateral dominance in children with learning disabilities. Physical Therapy 63, 183-187.

Conrad, K. E., Cermak, S. A., & Drake, C. (1983). Differentiation of praxis among children. American Journal of Occupational Therapy 37, 466-473.

Copeland, A. P., & Reiner, E. M. (1984). The selective attention of learning-disabled children: Three studies. Journal of Abnormal Child Psychology 12, 455-470.

Cruickshank, W. M. (1983). Learning disabilities: Neurophysiological dysfunction. Journal of Learning Disabilities 16, 27-29.

Cruickshank, W. M. (1984). Definition: A major issue in the field of learning disabilities. Journal of Rehabilitation 50, 7-18.

Dainer, K. B., Klorman, R., Salzman, L. F., Hess, D. W., Davidson, P. W., & Michael, R. L. (1981). Learning-disordered children's evoked potentials during sustained attention. Journal of Abnormal Child Psychology 9, 79-94.

Demers, L. A. (1981). Effective mainstreaming for the learning disabled student with behavior problems. Journal of Learning Disabilities 14, 179-188, 203.

Denckla, M. B., Rudel, R. G., & Broman, M. (1981). Tests that discriminate between dyslexic and other learning-disabled boys. Brain and Language 13, 118-129.

Derr, A. M. (1985). Conservation and mathematics achievement in the learning disabled child. Journal of Learning Disabilities 18, 333-336.

Deshler, D. D., Schumaker, J. B., & Lenz, B. K. (1984). Academic and cognitive interventions for LD adolescents: Part I. Journal of Learning Disabilities 17, 108-117.

Dorr, D. (1989). Learning disabilities and personality disorders. Highland Highlights 28, 29-32.

Douglas, J. W., & Gear, R. (1976). Children of low birthweight in the 1946 national cohort: Bevahiour and educational achievement in adolescents. Archives of Disease in Childhood 51, 820-827.

Dudley-Marling, C. (1985). The pragmatic skills of learning disabled children: A review. Journal of Learning Disabilities 18, 193-199.

Duffey, J. B., Salvia, J., Tucker, J., & Ysseldyke, J. (1981). Nonbiased assessment: A need for operationalism. Exceptional Children 47, 427-434.

Dunn, R. (1983). Learning style and its relation to exceptionality at both ends of the spectrum. Exceptional Children 49, 496-506.

Durlak, J. A. (1985). Primary prevention of school maladjustment. Journal of Consulting and Clinical Psychology 53, 623-630.

Ely, D. L, Mostardi, R. A., Woebkenberg, N., & Worstell, D. (1981). Aerometric and hair trace metal content in learning-disabled children. Environmental Research 25, 325-339.

Epstein, J., Berg-Cross, G., & Berg-Cross, L. (1980). Maternal expectations and birth order in families with learning disabled and normal children. Journal of Learning Disabilities 13, 273-280.

Faerstein, L. M. (1986). Coping and defense mechanisms of mothers of learning disabled children. Journal of Learning Disabilities 19, 8-11.

Faigel, H. C. (1983). Learning disabilities in adolescents with high IQ scores. Journal of Developmental and Behavioral Pediatrics 4, 11-15.

Farnham-Diggory, S. (1980). Learning disabilities, a view from cognitive science. Journal of the American Academy of Child Psychiatry 19, 570-578.

Feagans, L. (1983). A current view of learning disabilities. Journal of Pediatrics 102, 487-493.

Feiring, C., & Taft, L. T. (1985). The gifted learning disabled child: Not a paradox. Pediatric Annals 14, 729-732.

Ferguson, H. B., & Mamen, M. (1985). Learning disabilities. Etiology, diagnosis, and management. Psychiatric Clinics of North America 8, 703-720.

Fincham, F., & Barling, J. (1978). Locus of control and generosity in learning disabled, normal achieving, and gifted children. Child Development 49, 530-533.

Fisk, J. L., & Rourke, B. P. (1983). Neuropsychological subtyping of learning-disabled children: History, methods, implications. Journal of Learning Disabilities 16, 529-531.

Fleisher, L. S., Soodak, L. C., & Jelin, M. A. (1984). Selective attention deficits in learning disabled children: Analysis of the data base. Exceptional Children 51, 136-141.

Fleischner, J. E., Garnett, K., & Silver, L. B. (1989). Developmental arithmetic disorder. In H. I. Kaplan & B. J. Sadock (Eds.), Comprehensive textbook of psychiatry (5th ed., pp. 1800-1804). Baltimore: Williams and Wilkins.

Frostig, M. (1980). Meeting individual needs of all children in the classroom setting. Journal of Learning Disabilities 13, 158-161.

Fuller, P. W., Guthrie, R. D., & Alvord, E. C. (1983). A proposed neuropathological basis for learning disabilities in children born prematurely. Developmental Medicine and Child Neurology 25, 214-231.

Gadow, K. D. (1983). Effects of stimulant drugs on academic performance in hyperactive and learning disabled children. Journal of Learning Disabilities 16, 290-299.

Galler, J. R., Ramsey, F., & Solimano, G. (1984). The influence of early malnutrition on subsequent behavioral development. III. Learning disabilities os a sequel to malnutrition. Pediatric Research 18, 309-313.

Geary, D. C., & Gilger, J. W. (1984). The Luria-Nebraska neuropsychological battery-children's revision: Comparison of learning disabled and normal children matched on full scale IQ. Perceptual and Motor Skills 58, 115-118.

Giordano, G. (1984). Analyzing and remediating writing disabilities. Journal of Learning Disabilities 17, 78-83.

Golden, G. S. (1984). Symposium on learning disorders. Controversial therapies. Pediatric Clinics of North America 31, 459-469.

Gottesman, R. L. (1980). Clinic, school, and parents: Working together. Journal of Learning Disabilities 13, 167-171.

Graham, S. (1985). Teaching basic academic skills to learning disabled students: A model of the teaching-learning process. Journal of Learning Disabilities 18, 528-534.

Hamill, J. S. (1984). Tactile defensiveness: A type of sensory integrative dysfunction. Journal of Rehabilitation 50, 95-96.

Harris, J. C., King, S. L., Reifler, J. P., & Rosenberg, L. A. (1984). Emotional and learning disorders in 6-12-year-old boys attending special schools. Journal of the American Academy of Child Psychiatry 23, 431-437.

Harris, K. R. (1986). The effects of cognitive-behavior modification on private speech and task performance during problem solving among learning-disabled and normally achieving children. Journal of Abnormal Child Psychology 14, 63-76.

Hazel, J. S., & Schumaker, J. B. (1988). Social skills and learning disabilities: Current issues and recommendations for future research. In J. F. Kavanagh & T. J. Truss, Jr. (Eds.), Learning disabilities: Proceedings of the national conference (pp. 293-354). Parkton, Md.: York Press.

Horn, W. F., O'Donnell, J. P., & Vitulano, L. A. (1983). Long-term follow-up studies of learning-disabled persons. Journal of Learning Disabilities 16, 542-555.

Hunt, R. D., & Cohen, D. J. (1984). Psychiatric aspects of learning difficulties. Pediatric Clinics of North America 31, 471-497.

Ivarie, J., Hogue, D., & Brulle, A. R. (1984). An investigation of mainstream teacher time spent with students labeled learning disabled. Exceptional Children 51, 142-149.

John, E. R., Prichep, L., Ahn, H., Easton, P., Fridman, J., & Kaye, H. (1983). Neurometric evaluation of cognitive dysfunctions and neurological disorders in children. Progress in Neurobiology 21, 239-290.

Johnson, L. S., Johnson, D. L., Olson, M. R., & Newman, J. P. (1981). The use of hypnotherapy with learning disabled children. Journal of Clinical Psychology 37, 291-299.

Kandt, R. S. (1984). Neurologic examination of children with learning disorders. Pediatric Clinics of North America 31, 297-315.

Kaufman, A. S. (1981). The WISC-R and learning disabilities assessment: State of the art. Journal of Learning Disabilities 14, 520-526.

Kistner, J., White, K., Haskett, M., & Robbins, F. (1985). Development of learning-disabled and normally achieving children's causal attributions. Journal of Abnormal Child Psychology 13, 639-647.

Kistner, J. A. (1985). Attentional deficits of learning-disabled children: Effects of rewards and practice. Journal of Abnormal Child Psychology 13, 19-31.

Krall, V., Sachs, H., Rayson, B., Lazar, B., Growe, G., & O'Connell, L. (1980). Effects of lead poisoning on cognitive test performance. Perceptual and Motor Skills 50, 483-486.

Lambert, N. M., & Sandoval, J. (1980). The prevalence of learning disabilities in a sample of children considered hyperactive. Journal of Abnormal Child Psychology 8, 33-50.

Lerner, J. W. (1989). Educational interventions in learning disabilities. Journal of the American Academy of Child and Adolescent Psychiatry 28, 326-331.

Levine, M. D., Clarke, S., & Ferb, T. (1981). The child as a diagnostic participant: Helping students describe their learning disorders. Journal of Learning Disabilities 14, 527-530.

Levine, M. D., & Zallen, B. G. (1984). The learning disorders of adolescence: Organic and nonorganic failure to strive. Pediatric Clinics of North America 31, 345-369.

Levy, F. (1982). Central auditory testing in learning disabled children. South African Journal of Communication Disorders 29, 23-34.

Lewandowski, L. J. (1985). Clinical syndromes among the learning disabled. Journal of Learning Disabilities 18, 177-178.

Lindquist, G. T. (1982). Preschool screening as a means of predicting later reading achievement. Journal of Learning Disabilities 15, 331-332.

Lindsay, G. A., & Wedell, K. (1982). The early identification of educationally 'at risk' children revisited. Journal of Learning Disabilities 15, 212-217.

Livingston, R. (1985). Depressive illness and learning difficulties: Research needs and practical implications. Journal of Learning Disabilities 18, 518-520.

Luchow, J. P., Crowl, T. K., & Kahn, J. P. (1985). Learned helplessness: Perceived effects of ability and effort on academic performance among EH and LD/EH children. Journal of Learning Disabilities 18, 470-474.

Ludlow, B. L., & Woodrum, D. T. (1985). Hypothesis testing and problem solving by learning disabled and nondisabled boys. Perceptual and Motor Skills 60, 160.

Margalit, M. (1982). Learning disabled children and their families: Strategies of extension of adaptation of family therapy. Journal of Learning Disabilities 15, 594-595.

Margalit, M. (1984). Leisure activities of learning disabled children as a reflection of their passive life style and prolonged dependency. Child Psychiatry and Human Development 15, 133-141.

Margalit, M., & Zak, I. (1984). Anxiety and self-concept of learning disabled children. Journal of Learning Disabilities 17, 537-539.

May, D. C., & Welch, E. (1984). Developmental placement: Does it prevent future learning problems? Journal of Learning Disabilities 17, 338-341.

McKay, H., Sinisterra, L., McKay, A., Gomez, H., & Lloreda, P. (1978). Improving cognitive ability in chronically deprived children. Science 200, 270-278.

McKibben, E., & King, J. (1983). Activity group counseling for learning-disabled children with behavior problems. American Journal of Occupational Therapy 37, 617-623.

Mishra, S. P. (1984). WISC-R performance patterns of learning-disabled children from Papago culture. Journal of Clinical Psychology 40, 1489-1492.

Modarressi, T. (1975). The effect of system intervention on the cognitive control of preschool children. Journal of Nervous and Mental Disease 160, 392-401.

Morrisson, D., Mantzicopoulos, P., & Carte, E. (1989). Pre-academic screening for learning and behavior problems. Journal of the American Academy of Child and Adolescent Psychiatry 28, 101-106.

Morrisson, D. C., Hinshaw, S. P., & Carte, E. T. (1985). Signs of neurobehavioral dysfunction in a sample of learning disabled children: Stability and concurrent validity. Perceptual and Motor Skills 61, 863-872.

Myklebust, H. R. (1983). Toward a science of learning disabilities. Journal of Learning Disabilities 16, 17-18.

Newberger, D. A. (1983a). Learning disabilities and competency-based instruction: Intertwined or poles apart? Journal of Learning Disabilities 16, 393-397.

Newberger, D. A. (1983b). Learning disabilities and competency-based instruction: Intertwined or poles apart? Part II. Journal of Learning Disabilities 16, 448-452.

O'Brien, J. (1982). School problems: School phobia and learning disabilities. Psychiatric Clinics of North America 5, 297-307.

Obrzut, J. E., Obrzut, A., Bryden, M. P., & Bartels, S. G. (1985). Information processing and speech lateralization in learning-disabled children. Brain and Language 25, 87-101.

Okabayashi, H., & Torrance, E. P. (1984). Role of style of learning and thinking and self directed learning readiness in the achievement of gifted students. Journal of Learning Disabilities 17, 104-107.

Omizo, M. M., & Williams, R. E. (1982). Biofeedback-induced relaxation training as an alternative for the elementary school learning-disabled child. Biofeedback and Self Regulation 7, 139-148.

Ottenbacher, K., Abbott, C., Haley, D., & Watson, P. J. (1984). Human figure drawing ability and vestibular processing dysfunction in learning-disabled children. Journal of Clinical Psychology 40, 1084-1089.

Pearl, R. (1985). Cognitive-behavioral interventions for increasing motivation. Journal of Abnormal Child Psychology 13, 443-453.

Pennington, B. F., Bender, B., Puck, M., Salbenblatt, J., & Robinson, A. (1982). Learning disabilities in children with sex chromosome anomalies. Child Development 53, 1182-1192.

Pickar, D. B. (1986). Psychosocial aspects of learning disabilities. A review of research. Bulletin of the Menninger Clinic 50, 22-32.

Pihl, R. O., & Niaura, R. (1982). Learning disability: An inability to sustain attention. Journal of Clinical Psychology 38, 632-634.

Polatajko, H. J. (1985). A critical look at vestibular dysfunction in learning-disabled children. Developmental Medicine and Child Neurology 27, 283-292.

Porges, S. W. (1984). Physiologic correlates of attention: A core process underlying learning disorders. Pediatric Clinics of North America 31, 371-385.

Rasmussen, F., Gustavson, K. H., & Bille, B. (1984). Familial minor neurodevelopmental disorders. Clinical Genetics 25, 148-154.

Ratcliffe, S. G. (1982). Speech and learning disorders in children with sex chromosome abnormalities. Developmental Medicine and Child Neurology 24, 80-84.

Reeves, W. H. (1980). Auditory learning disabilities and emotional disturbance: Diagnostic differences. Journal of Learning Disabilities 13, 199-202.

Rich, H. L. (1981). Educationally handicapped children's locus of control and reading achievement. Exceptional Children 48, 244-248.

Richardson, S. A., Koller, H., & Katz, M. (1986). Factors leading to differences in the school performance of boys and girls. Journal of Developmental and Behavioral Pediatrics 7, 49-55.

Richey, L. S., & Ysseldyke, J. E. (1983). Teachers' expectations for the younger siblings of learning disabled students. Journal of Learning Disabilities 16, 610-615.

Roit, M. L., & McKenzie, R. G. (1985). Disorders of written communication: An instructional priority for LD students. Journal of Learning Disabilities 18, 258-260.

Roth, F. P., & Spekman, N. J. (1986). Narrative discourse: Spontaneously generated stories of learning-disabled and normally achieving students. Journal of Speech and Hearing Disorders 51, 8-23.

Rothstein, A. (1982). An integrative perspective on the diagnosis of learning disorders. Journal of the American Academy of Child Psychiatry 21, 420-426.

Rourke, B. P. (1982). Central processing deficiencies in children: Toward a developmental neuropsychological model. Journal of Clincal Neuropsychology 4, 1-18.

Royce, J. M., Lazar, I., & Darlington, R. B. (1983). Minority families, early education, and later life chances. American Journal of Orthopsychiatry 53, 706-720.

Rubenstein, B., & Levitt, M. (1977). Learning disabilities as related to a special form of mothering. International Journal of Psycho-Analysis 58, 45-55.

Rudel, R. G. (1980). Learning disability. Diagnosis by exclusion and discrepancy. Journal of the American Academy of Child Psychiatry 19, 547-569.

Russell, R. A. (1984). The efficacy of hypnosis in the treatment of learning problems in children. International Journal of Psychosomatics 31, 23-32.

Sak, R. J., & Ruben, R. J. (1982). Effects of recurrent middle ear effusion in preschool years on language and learning. Journal of Developmental and Behavioral Pediatrics 3, 7-11.

Samuels, S. J., & Miller, N. L. (1985). Failure to find attention differences between learning disabled and normal children on classroom and laboratory tasks. Exceptional Children 51, 358-375.

Schneider, B. H. (1984). LD as they see it: Perceptions of adolescents in a special residential school. Journal of Learning Disabilities 17, 533-536.

Scholom, A., & Schiff, G. (1980). Relating infant temperament to learning disabilities. Journal of Abnormal Child Psychology 8, 127-132.

Sell, E. J., Gaines, J. A., Gluckman, C., & Williams, E. (1985). Early identification of learning problems in neonatal intensive care graduates. American Journal of Diseases of Children 139, 460-463.

Shapiro, B. K., Palmer, F. B., Wachtel, R. C., & Capute, A. J. (1984). Issues in the early identification of specific learning disability. Journal of Developmental and Behavioral Pediatrics 5, 15-20.

Shapiro, S., & Forbes, C. R. (1981). A review of involvement programs for parents of learning disabled children. Journal of Learning Disabilities 14, 499-504.

Shaywitz, S. E., Shaywitz, B. A., McGraw, K., & Groll, S. (1984). Current status of the neuromaturational examination as an index of learning disability. Journal of Pediatrics 104, 819-825.

Shepherd, M. J., Charnow, D. A., & Silver, L. B. (1989). Developmental expressive writing disorder. In H. I. Kaplan & B. J. Sadock (Eds.), Comprehensive textbook of psychiatry (5th ed., pp. 1796-1800). Baltimore: Williams and Wilkins.

Silver, A. A., & Hagin, R. A. (1985). Outcome of learning disabilities in adolescence. In S. C. Feinstein, et al. (Eds.), Adolescent psychiatry: Developmental and clinical studies (Vol. 12, pp. 197-213). Chicago: University of Chicago Press.

Silver, L. B. (1976). The playroom diagnostic evaluation of children with neurologically based learning disabilities. Journal of the American Academy of Child Psychiatry 15, 240-256.

Silver, L. B. (1981). The relationship between learning disabilities, hyperactivity, distractibility, and behavioral problems: A clinical analysis. Journal of the American Academy of Child Psychiatry 20, 385-397.

Silver, L. B. (1987). The "magic cure": A review of the current controversial approaches for treating learning disabilities. Journal of Learning Disabilities 20, 498-512.

Silver, L. B. (1989). Learning disabilities. Journal of the American Academy of Child and Adolescent Psychiatry 28, 309-313.

Siperstein, G. N., & Goding, M. J. (1985). Teachers' behavior toward LD and non-LD children: A strategy for change. Journal of Learning Disabilities 18, 139-144.

Sparrow, S. S., Blachman, B. A., & Chauncey, S. (1983). Diagnostic and prescriptive intervention in primary school education. American Journal of Orthopsychiatry 53, 721-729.

Stanton, H. E. (1981). A therapeutic approach to help children overcome learning difficulties. Journal of Learning Disabilities 14, 220-237.

Stevens, R., & Pihl, R. O. (1982). The identification of the student at-risk for failure. Journal of Clinical Psychology 38, 540-545.

Stevenson, D. T., & Romney, D. M. (1984). Depression in learning disabled children. Journal of Learning Disabilities 17, 579-582.

Stewart, J. M., & Spells, V. R. (1983). Learning disabilities with communicative disorders as related handicaps: A two year study. Journal of Communication Disorders 16, 345-355.

Swanson, H. L. (1984). Effect of cognitive effort on learning disabled and nondisabled readers' recall. Journal of Learning Disabilities 17, 67-74.

Switzer, L. S. (1985). Accepting the diagnosis: An educational intervention for parents of children with learning disabilities. Journal of Learning Disabilities 18, 151-153.

Tharp, R. G., & Gallimore, R. (1985). The logical status of metacognitive training. Journal of Abnormal Child Psychology 13, 455-466.

Thatcher, R. W., & Lester, M. L. (1985). Nutrition, environmental toxins and computerized EEG: A mini-max approach to learning disabilities. Journal of Learning Disabilities 18, 287-297.

Torgesen, J. K., & Young, K. A. (1983). Priorities for the use of microcomputers with learning disabled children. Journal of Learning Disabilities 16, 234-237.

Valett, R. E. (1983). Developing linguistic auditory memory patterns. Journal of Learning Disabilities 16, 462-466.

Vaughn, S. (1985). Why teach social skills to learning disabled students? Journal of Learning Disabilities 18, 588-591.

Vigilante, F. W. (1983). Working with families of learning disabled children. Child Welfare 62, 429-436.

Wang, M. C., & Birch, J. W. (1984). Comparison of a full-time mainstreaming program and a resource room approach. Exceptional Children 51, 33-40.

Weingartner, H., Langer, D., Grice, J., & Rapoport, J. L. (1982). Acquisition and retrieval of information in amphetamine-treated hyperactive children. Psychiatry Research 6, 21-29.

Weiss, E. (1984). Learning disabled children's understanding of social interactions of peers. Journal of Learning Disabilities 17, 612-615.

Weissbluth, M., Davis, A. T., Poncher, J., & Reiff, J. (1983). Signs of airway obstruction during sleep and behavioral, developmental, and academic problems. Journal of Developmental and Behavioral Pediatrics 4, 119-121.

Werner, E. E., & Smith, R. S. (1979). An epidemiologic perspective on some antecedents and consequences of childhood mental health problems and learning disabilities: A report from the Kauai longitudinal study. Journal of the American Academy of Child Psychiatry 18, 292-306.

Wiig, E. H. (1984). Psycholinguistic aspects of learning disorders: Identification and assessment. Pediatric Clinics of North America 31, 317-330.

Wiig, E. H., Becker-Redding, U., & Semel, E. M. (1983). A cross-cultural, cross-linguistic comparison of language abilities of 7- to 8- and 12- to 13-year-old children with learning disabilities. Journal of Learning Disabilities 16, 576-585.

Wong, B. Y. (1985). Issues in cognitive-behavioral interventions in academic skill areas. Journal of Abnormal Child Psychology 13, 425-441.

Wood, C., Powell, S., & Knight, R. C. (1984). Predicting school readiness: The validity of developmental age. Journal of Learning Disabilities 17, 8-15.

Ysseldyke, J. E. (1983). Current practices in making psychoeducational decisions about learning disabled students. Journal of Learning Disabilities 16, 226-233.

Zieffle, T. H., & Romney, D. M. (1985). Comparison of self-instruction and relaxation training in reducing impulsive and inattentive behavior of learning disabled children on cognitive tasks. Psychological Reports 57, 271-274.

Zinkus, P. W., & Gottlieb, M. I. (1980). Patterns of perceptual and academic deficits related to early chronic otitis media. Pediatrics 66, 246-253.

7. Special Education and Educational Issues

Howlin, P. (1985). Special educational treatment. In M. Rutter & L. Hersov (Eds.), Child and adolescent psychiatry: Modern approaches (pp. 851-870). Oxford: Blackwell.

Jensen, A. (1969). How much can we boost I.Q. and scholastic achievement. Harvard Educational Review 39, 1-123.

Kris, K. (1978). The school consultant as an object for externalization. In A. Solnit, et al. (Eds.), Psychoanalytic study of the child (Vol. 33, pp. 456-482). New Haven: Yale University Press.

Lazar, I., & Darlington, R. (1982). Lasting effects of early education. Monographs of the Society for Research in Child Development 47(1-2), 1-151.

Robins, L., Ratcliff, K., & West, P. (1979). School achievement in two generations: A study of 88 urban black families. In S. J. Shamsie (Ed.), New directions in children's mental health (pp. 105-130). New York: Spectrum Publications.

Sarason, S. B. (1984). Unexamined axioms in American schooling. Journal of Learning Disabilities 17, 180-181.

Swann, W. (Ed.). (1981). The practice of special education. New York: Guilford; Oxford: Blackwell.

Vitello, S. (1976). The institutionalization and deinstitutionalization of the mentally retarded in the United States. In L. Mann & D. A. Sobatino (Eds.), A third review of special education. New York: Grune & Stratton.

Werry, J. S. (1988). Drugs, learning and cognitive function in children: An update. Journal of Child Psychology and Psychiatry 29, 129-141.

Zigler, E., & Valentine, J. (1980). Project Head Start. A legacy of the War on Poverty. New York: The Free Press.

8. School Phobias

Berg, I., Casswell, G., Goodwin, A., Hullin, R., McGuire, R., & Tagg, G. (1985). Classification of severe school attendance problems. Psychological Medicine 15, 157-165.

Berg, I., & Fielding, D. (1978). An evaluation of hospital in-patient treatment in adolescent school phobia. British Journal of Psychiatry 132, 5-505.

Bernstein, G. A., & Garfinkel, B. D. (1986). School phobia: The overlap of affective and anxiety disorders. Journal of the American Academy of Child Psychiatry 25, 235-241.

Blagg, N. R., & Yule, W. (1984). The behavioural treatment of school refusal--a comparative study. Behavior Research and Therapy 22, 119-127.

Coolidge, J. C., Brodie, R. D., & Feeney, B. (1964). A 10 year follow-up of 66 school-phobic children. American Journal of Orthopsychiatry 34, 675-684.

Crumley, F. E. (1974). A school phobia in a three-generational family conflict. Journal of the American Academy of Child Psychiatry 13, 536-550.

Eisenberg, L. (1958). School phobia--a study in the communication of anxiety. American Journal of Orthopsychiatry 114, 712-718.

Gittelman-Klein, R., & Klein, D. F. (1980). Separation anxiety in school refusal and its treatment with drugs. In L. Hersov & I. Berg (Eds.), Out of school--modern perspectives in school refusal and truancy (pp. 321-341). Chichester: Wiley.

Hersov, L. (1985). School refusal. In M. Rutter & L. Hersov (Eds.), Child and adolescent psychiatry: Modern approaches (pp. 382-389). Oxford: Blackwell.

Hersov, L., & Berg, I. (1980). (Eds.). Out of school--modern perspectives in school refusal and truancy. Chichester: Wiley.

Hersov, L. A. (1980). Hospital in-patient and day-patient treatment of school refusal. In L. Hersov & I. Berg (Eds.), Out of school--modern perspectives in school refusal and truancy (pp. 303-320). Chichester: Wiley.

Hsia, H. (1984). Structural and strategic approach to school phobia/school refusal. Psychology in the Schools 21, 360-367.

Lansky, S. B., Lowman, J. T., Vats, T., & Gyulay, J. E. (1975). School phobia in children with malignant neoplasms. American Journal of Diseases of Children 129, 42-46.

Waldron, S., Shrier, D. K., Stone, B., & Tobin, F. (1975). School phobia and other childhood neuroses: A systematic study of the children and their families. American Journal of Psychiatry 132, 802-808.

F. Language Disorders

Larry Silver, M.D., Section Editor

Aram, D. M., & Nation, J. E. (1980). Preschool language disorders and subsequent language and academic difficulties. Journal of Communication Disorders 13, 159-170.

Bakker, D. J. (1983). Hemispheric specialization and specific reading retardation. In M. Rutter (Ed.), Developmental neuropsychiatry (pp. 498-506). New York: Guilford Press.

Beitchman, J. H., Hood, J., Rochon, J., & Peterson, M. (1989). Empirical classification of speech/language impairment in children: II. Behavioral characteristics. Journal of the American Academy of Child and Adolescent Psychiatry 28, 118-123.

Beitchman, J. H., Hood, J., Rochon, J., Peterson, M., Mantini, T., & Majumdar, S. (1989). Empirical classification of speech/language impairment in children: I. Identification of speech language categories. Journal of the American Academy of Child and Adolescent Psychiatry 28, 112-117.

Psychopathology: Disease and Disorder

Bartak, L., Rutter, M., & Cox, A. (1977). A comparative study of infantile autism and specific development receptive language disorders. Journal of Autism and Childhood Schizophrenia 7, 383-396.

Cantwell, D. P., & Baker, L. (1980a). Academic features in children with communication disorders. Journal of the American Academy of Child Psychiatry 19, 579-591.

Cantwell, D. P., & Baker, L. (1980b). Academic features in children with communication disorders. Journal of Pediatric Psychology 5, 161-178.

Cantwell, D. P., Baker, L., & Mattison, R. E. (1980). Psychiatric disorders in children with speech and language retardation. Factors associated with development. Archives of General Psychiatry 37, 423-426.

Childs, B., & Finnuci, J. M. (1983). Genetics, epidemiology, and specific reading disability. In M. Rutter (Ed.), Developmental neuropsychiatry (pp. 507-519). New York: Guilford Press.

Cohen, N. J., Davine, L., & Meloche-Kelly, M. (1989). Prevalence of unsuspected language disorders in a child psychiatric population. Journal of the American Academy of Child and Adolescent Psychiatry 28, 107-111.

Duane, D. D. (1979). The dyslexic child: Diagnostic implications. Pediatric Annals 8, 632-640.

Duane, D. D. (1989). Neurobiological correlates of learning disorders. Journal of the American Academy of Child and Adolescent Psychiatry 28, 314-318.

Duffy, F. H. (1988). Neurophysiological studies in dyslexia. In F. Plum (Ed.), Language, communication and the brain. New York: Raven Press.

Duffy, F. H., Denckla, M. B., Bartels, P. H., Sandini, G., & Kiessling, L. S. (1980). Dyslexia: Automated diagnosis by computerized classification of brain electrical activity. Annals of Neurology 7, 421-428.

Dyslexia: An appraisal of current knowledge. (1980). In A. L. Benton & D. Pearl (Eds.), Dyslexia: An appraisal of current knowledge (pp. 451-476). New York: Oxford University Press.

Frith, U. (1978). Spelling difficulties. Journal of Child Psychology and Psychiatry and Allied Disciplines 19, 279-285.

Gittelman, R. (1983). Treatment of reading disorders. In M. Rutter (Ed.), Developmental neuropsychiatry (pp. 520-541). New York: Guilford Press.

Gittelman, R., & Feingold, I. (1983). Children with reading disorders--I. Efficacy of reading remediation. Journal of Child Psychology and Psychiatry and Allied Disciplines 24, 167-191.

Gittelman, R., Klein, D. F., & Feingold, I. (1983). Children with reading disorders--II. Effects of methylphenidate in combination with reading remediation. Journal of Child Psychology and Psychiatry and Allied Disciplines 24, 193-212.

Johnson, D. J., & Myklebust, H. R. (1967). Learning disabilities: Educational principles and practices. New York: Grune & Stratton.

Lewis, D. O., Shanok, S, S., Balla, D. A., & Bard, B. (1980). Psychiatric correlates of severe reading disabilities in an incarcerated delinquent population. Journal of the American Academy of Child Psychiatry 19, 611-622.

Mattison, R. E., Cantwell, D. P., & Baker, L. (1982). A practical method for screening psychiatric disorders in children with speech and language disorders. Journal of Abnormal Child Psychology 10, 25-32.

Prior, M. R., Frolley, M., & Sanson, A. (1983). Language lateralization in specific reading retarded children and backward readers. Cortex 19, 149-163.

Russell, G. (1982). Writing and dyslexia--an historical analysis. Journal of Child Psychology and Psychiatry and Allied Disciplines 23, 383-400.

Rutter, M. (1974). Emotional disorder and educational underachievement. Archives of Disease in Childhood 49, 249-256.

Shaffer, D., Bijur, P., Chadwick, O. F., & Rutter, M. L. (1980). Head injury and later reading disability. Journal of the American Academy of Child Psychiatry 19, 592-610.

Shapiro, T. (1982). Language and the psychiatric diagnosis of preschool children. Psychiatric Clinics of North America 5, 309-319.

Silver, A. A., Hagin, R. A., DeVito, E., Kreeger, H., & Scully, E. (1976). A SEARCH battery for scanning kindergarten children for potential learning disability. Journal of the American Academy of Child Psychiatry 15, 224-239.

Stevenson, H. W., Stigler, J. W., Lucker, G. W., Lee, S., Hsu, C., & Kitamura, S. (1982). Reading disabilities: The case of Chinese, Japanese, and English children. Child Development 53, 1164-1181.

Stevenson, J., Richman, N., & Graham, P. (1985). Behaviour problems and language abilities at three years and behavioural deviance at eight years. Journal of Child Psychology and Psychiatry and Allied Disciplines 26, 215-230.

Stores, G., & Hart, J. (1976). Reading skills of children with generalized or focal epilepsy attending ordinary school. Developmental Medicine and Child Neurology 18, 705-716.

Sturge, C. (1982). Reading retardation and antisocial behaviour. Journal of Child Psychology and Psychiatry and Allied Disciplines 23, 21-31.

Tizard, B., Hughes, M., Carmichael, H., & Pinkerton, G. (1983). Language and social class. Is it a myth? Journal of Child Psychology and Psychiatry and Allied Disciplines 24, 533-542.

Yule, W. (1976). Dyslexia [Editorial]. Psychological Medicine 6, 165-167.

Yule, W., & Rutter, M. (1985). Reading and other learning difficulties. In M. Rutter & L. Hersov (Eds.), Child and adolescent psychiatry: Modern approaches (pp. 444-464). Oxford: Blackwell.

G. Reactions to Catastrophic Events

Spencer Eth, M.D., Section Editor
William Arroyo, M.D., Associate Editor

1. Effects of Severe Trauma on Children and Adolescents

Anthony, E. J. (1986). Terrorizing attacks on children by psychotic parents. Journal of the American Academy of Child Psychiatry 25, 326-335.

Bergen, M. E. (1958). The effect of severe trauma on a four-year-old child. In R. S. Eissler, et al. (Eds.), Psychoanalytic study of the child (Vol. 13, pp. 407-429). New York: International Universities Press.

Burgess, A. W. (1974). Family reaction to homicide. American Journal of Orthopsychiatry 45, 391-398.

Burgess, A. W., Hartman, C. R., McCausland, M. P., & Powers, P. (1984). Response patterns in children and adolescents exploited through sex rings and pornography. American Journal of Psychiatry 141, 656-662.

Burgess, A. W., & Holmstrom, L. L. (1975). Sexual trauma of children and adolescents: Pressure, sex and secrecy. Nursing Clinics of North America 10, 551-563.

Cain, A., & Fast, I. (1966). Children's disturbed reactions to parent suicide. American Journal of Orthopsychiatry 36, 873-880.

Chatoor, I., Conley, C., & Dickson, L. (1988). Food refusal after an incident of choking: A post-traumatic eating disorder. Journal of the American Academy of Child and Adolescent Psychiatry 27, 105-110.

Dallas, D. (1978). Savagery, show and tell. American Psychologist 33, 388-390.

Donaldson, M. A., & Gardner, R. (1985). Diagnosis and treatment of traumatic stress among women after childhood incest. In C. R. Figley (Ed.), Trauma and its wake (pp. 356-377). New York: Brunner/Mazel.

Eth, S., Arroyo, W., & Silverstein, S. (1985). Psychiatric crisis team response to violence in elementary school. In I. H. Berkovitz & J. S. Seliger (Eds.), Expanding mental health interventions in schools (pp. 55-62). Dubuque, Iowa: Kendall/Hunt.

Eth, S., & Pynoos, R. S. (1985). Psychiatric interventions with children traumatized by violence. In D. H. Schetky & E. P. Benedek (Eds.), Emerging issues in child psychiatry (pp. 285-309). New York: Brunner/Mazel.

Eth, S., Silverstein, S., & Pynoos, R. S. (1985). Mental health consultation to a preschool following the murder of a mother and child. Hospital and Community Psychiatry 36, 73-76.

Famularo, R., Kinscherff, R., & Fenton, T. (1988). Propranolol treatment for childhood post-traumatic stress disorder, acute type. American Journal of Diseases of Children 142, 1244-1247.

Gardner, G. E. (1971). Aggression and violence--enemies of precision learning in children. American Journal of Psychiatry 128, 445-450.

Goodwin, J. (1985). Post-traumatic symptoms in incest victims. In S. Eth & R. S. Pynoos (Eds.), Post-traumatic stress disorder in children (pp. 155-168). Washington: D.C.: American Psychiatric Press.

Green, A. H. (1983). Dimension of psychological trauma in abused children. Journal of the American Academy of Child Psychiatry 22, 231-237.

Green, A. H. (1985). Children traumatized by physical abuse. In S. Eth & R. S. Pynoos (Eds.), Post-traumatic stress disorder in children (pp. 133-154). Washington: D.C.: American Psychiatric Press.

Hershorn, M., & Rosenbaum, A. (1985). Children of marital violence: A closer look at the unintended victims. American Journal of Orthopsychiatry 55, 260-266.

Hughes, H., & Barad, S. (1983). Psychological functioning of children in a battered women's shelter. American Journal of Orthopsychiatry 53, 525-531.

Jackson, H. J., & King, H. J. (1981). The emotive imagery treatment of a child's trauma-induced phobia. Journal of Behavior Therapy and Experimental Psychiatry 12, 325-328.

Jaffe, P., Wolfe, D., Wilson, S., & Zak, L. (1986). Similarities in behavioral and social maladjustment among child victims and witnesses to family violence. American Journal of Orthopsychiatry 56, 142-146.

Jaffe, P., Wolfe, D., Wilson, S. K., & Zak, L. (1986). Family violence and child adjustment: A comparative analysis of girls' and boys' behavioral symptoms. American Journal of Psychiatry 143, 74-77.

Jones, D. P., & Krugman, R. D. (1986). Can a three-year-old child bear witness to her sexual assault and attempted murder. Child Abuse and Neglect 10, 253-258.

Katan, A. (1973). Children who were raped. In R. S. Eissler, et al. (Eds.), Psychoanalytic study of the child (Vol. 28, pp. 208-224). New York: International Universities Press.

Kluft, R. P. (1985). The natural history of multiple personality disorder. In R. P. Kluft (Ed.), Childhood antecedents of multiple personality (pp. 197-238). Washington, D.C.: American Psychiatric Press.

Lebovici, S. (1974). Observations on children who have witnessed the violent death of one of their parents. International Review of Psychoanalysis 1, 117-123.

Levine, M. (1975). Interpersonal violence and its effect on children. Medicine, Science and the Law 15, 172-176.

Lindberg, F. H., & Distad, L. J. (1985). Post-traumatic stress disorders in women who experienced childhood incest. Child Abuse and Neglect 9, 329-334.

Malmquist, C. P. (1985). Children who witness violence: Tortious aspects. Bulletin of the American Academy of Psychiatry and the Law 13, 221-231.

Malmquist, C. P. (1986). Children who witness parental murder: Post-traumatic aspects. Journal of the American Academy of Child Psychiatry 25, 320-325.

Marohn, R. C. (1974). Trauma and the delinquent. In S. C. Feinstein, et al. (Eds.), Adolescent psychiatry: Developmental and clinical studies (Vol. 3, pp. 354-361). Chicago: University of Chicago Press.

Ornitz, E. M., & Pynoos, R. S. (1989). Startle modulation in children with post-traumatic stress disorder. American Journal of Psychiatry 146, 866-870.

Pfouts, J., Schopler, J., & Henley, H. C. (1982). Forgotten victims of family violence. Social Work 27, 367-368.

Pruett, K. D. (1979). Home treatment for two infants who witnessed their mother's murder. Journal of the American Academy of Child Psychiatry 18, 647-657.

Pynoos, R. S., & Eth, S. (1984). The child as a witness to homicide. Journal of Social Issues 40, 87-108.

Pynoos, R. S., & Eth, S. (1985). Children traumatized by acts of personal violence. In S. Eth & R. S. Pynoos (Eds.), Post-traumatic stress disorder in children (pp. 17-44). Washington: D.C.: American Psychiatric Press.

Pynoos, R. S., & Eth, S. (1986a). Special intervention programs for child witnesses to violence. In M. Lystad (Ed.), Violence in the home: Interdisciplinary perspectives (pp. 193-216). New York: Brunner/Mazel.

Pynoos, R. S., & Eth, S. (1986b). Witness to violence: The child interview. Journal of the American Academy of Child Psychiatry 25, 306-319.

Rosenbaum, A., & O'Leary, K. (1981). Children: The unintended victims of marital violence. American Journal of Orthopsychiatry 51, 692-699.

Schetky, D. H. (1973). Preschoolers' responses to murder of their mothers by their fathers: Study of four cases. Bulletin of the American Academy of Psychiatry and the Law 6, 45-57.

Schetky, D. H., & Haller, L. (1983). Parental kidnapping. Journal of the American Academy of Child Psychiatry 22, 279-285.

Schoettle, U. C. (1980). Child exploitation: A study of child pornography. Journal of the American Academy of Child Psychiatry 19, 289-299.

Senior, N., Gladstone, T., & Nurcombe, B. (1982). Child snatching: A case report. Journal of the American Academy of Child Psychiatry 21, 579-583.

Shapiro, S. (1973). Preventative analysis following a trauma. A 4 1/2 year old girl witnesses a stillbirth. In R. S. Eissler, et al. (Eds.), Psychoanalytic study of the child (Vol. 28, pp. 249-285). New York: International Universities Press.

Shepherd, D., & Barraclough, B. (1976). The aftermath of parental suicide for children. British Journal of Psychiatry 129, 267-276.

Summit, R. C. (1983). The child sexual abuse accommodation syndrome. Child Abuse and Neglect 7, 177-193.

Terr, L. C. (1981a). Forbidden games: Post-traumatic child's play. Journal of the American Academy of Child Psychiatry 20, 741-760.

Terr, L. C. (1981b). Psychic trauma in children: Observations following the Chochilla school-bus kidnapping. American Journal of Psychiatry 138, 14-19.

Terr, L. C. (1983a). Child snatching: A new epidemic of an ancient malady. Journal of Pediatrics 103, 151-156.

Terr, L. C. (1983b). Chochilla revisited: The effects of psychic trauma four years after a schoolbus kidnapping. American Journal of Psychiatry 140, 1543-1550.

Terr, L. C. (1984). Time and trauma. In A. Solnit, et al. (Eds.), Psychoanalytic study of the child (Vol. 39, pp. 633-665). New Haven: Yale University Press.

Terr, L. C. (1988). What happens to early memories of trauma? A study of twenty children under age five at the time of documented traumatic events. Journal of the American Academy of Child and Adolescent Psychiatry 27, 96-104.

Terr, L. C. (1989). Treating psychic trauma in children. Journal of Traumatic Stress 2, 3-20.

Ulbirch, P., & Huber, J. (1981). Observing parental violence: Distribution and effects. Journal of Marriage and the Family 46, 623-631.

van der Kolk, B. A. (1985). Adolescent vulnerability to post-traumatic stress disorder. Psychiatry 48, 365-370.

Wolfe, D. A., Jaffe, P., Wilson, S. K., & Zak, L. (1985). Children of battered women: The relation of child behavior to family violence and maternal stress. Journal of Consulting and Clinical Psychology 53, 657-665.

Zeanah, C. H., & Burk, G. S. (1984). A young child who witnessed her mother's murder: Therapeutic and legal considerations. American Journal of Psychotherapy 38, 132-145.

2. Children of Holocaust Survivors

Aleksandrowicz, D. R. (1973). Children of concentration camp survivors. In E. J. Anthony & C. Koupernik (Eds.), The child in his family: The impact of disease and death (pp. 385-293). New York: Wiley.

Auerhahn, N. C., & Prelinger, E. (1983). Repetition in the concentration camp survivor and her child. International Review of Psychoanalysis 10, 31-46.

Axelrod, S., Schnipper, O. L., & Rau, J. H. (1980). Hospitalized offspring of Holocaust survivors: Problems and dynamics. Bulletin of the Menninger Clinic 44, 1-14.

Barocas, H. A. (1971). A note on the children of concentration camp survivors. Psychotherapy 8, 189-190.

Barocas, H. A., & Barocas, C. B. (1973). Manifestations of concentration camp effects on the second generation. American Journal of Psychiatry 130, 820-821.

Barocas, H. A., & Barocas, C. B. (1979). Wounds of the fathers: The next generation of Holocaust victims. International Review of Psychoanalysis 6, 331-341.

Barocas, H. A., & Barocas, C. B. (1980). Separation-individuation conflicts in children of Holocaust survivors. Journal of Contemporary Psychotherapy 11, 6-14.

Bergmann, M. S. (1983). Therapeutic issues in the treatment of Holocaust survivors and their children. American Journal of Social Psychiatry 1, 21-23.

Danieli, Y. (1985). The treatment and prevention of long-term effects and intergenerational transmission of victimization. In C. R. Figley (Ed.), Trauma and its wake (pp. 295-313). New York: Brunner/Mazel.

Epstein, A. W. (1982). Mental phenomenal across generations: the Holocaust. Journal of the American Academy of Psychoanalysis 10, 565-570.

Fogelman, E., & Savran, B. (1979). Therapeutic groups with children of Holocaust survivors. International Journal of Group Psychotherapy 29, 211-236.

Fogelman, E., & Savran, B. (1980). Brief group therapy with offspring of Holocaust survivors: Leaders' reactions. American Journal of Orthopsychiatry 50, 96-108.

Freyberg, J. T. (1980). Difficulties in separation-individuation as experienced by offspring of Nazi Holocaust survivors. American Journal of Orthopsychiatry 50, 87-95.

Furman, E. (1973). The impact of the Nazi concentration camps on the children of the survivors. In E. J. Anthony & C. Koupernik (Eds.), The child in his family: The impact of disease and death (pp. 379-384). New York: Wiley.

Grubrich-Simitis, I. (1981). Extreme traumatization as cumulative trauma: Psychoanalytic investigations of the effects of concentration camp experience in survivors and their children. In A. Solnit, et al. (Eds.), Psychoanalytic study of the child (Vol. 36, pp. 415-450). New Haven: Yale University Press.

Haley, S. A. (1984). The Vietnam veteran and his preschool child: Child rearing as a delayed stress in combat veterans. Journal of Contemporary Psychotherapy 14, 114-121.

Heller, D. (1982). Themes of culture and ancestry among children of concentration camp survivors. Psychiatry 45, 247-261.

Herzog, J. M. (1981). The aging survivor of the Holocaust. Father hurt and father hunger: The effect of a survivor father's waning years on his son. Journal of Geriatric Psychiatry 14, 211-223.

Kestenberg, J. S. (1980). Psychoanalyses of children of survivors from the Holocaust: Case presentations and assessment. Journal of the American Psychoanalytic Association 28, 775-804.

Klein, H. (1973). Children of the Holocaust: Mourning and bereavement. In E. J. Anthony & C. Koupernik (Eds.), The child in his family: The impact of disease and death (pp. 393-409). New York: Wiley.

Krell, R. (1982). Family therapy with children of concentration camp survivors. American Journal of Psychotherapy 36, 513-522.

Krell, R. (1984). Holocaust survivors and their children: Comments on psychiatric consequences and psychiatric terminology. Comprehensive Psychiatry 25, 521-528.

Laufer, M. (1973). The analysis of a child of survivors. In E. J. Anthony & C. Koupernik (Eds.), The child in his family: The impact of disease and death (pp. 263-273). New York: Wiley.

Levine, H. B. (1982). Toward a psychoanalytic understanding of children of survivors of the Holocaust. Psychoanalytic Quarterly 51, 70-92.

Link, N., Victor, B., & Binder, R. L. (1985). Psychosis in children of Holocaust survivors: Influence of the Holocaust in the choice of themes in their psychoses. Journal of Nervous and Mental Disease 173, 115-117.

Roden, R. G., & Roden, M. M. (1982). Children of Holocaust survivors. In S. C. Feinstein, et al. (Eds.), Adolescent psychiatry: Developmental and clinical studies (Vol. 10, pp. 66-72). Chicago: University of Chicago Press.

Rosenberger, L. (1973). Children of survivors. In E. J. Anthony & C. Koupernik (Eds.), The child in his family: The impact of disease and death (pp. 375-377). New York: Wiley.

Rosenheck, R. (1986). Impact of post-traumatic stress disorder of World War II on the next generation. Journal of Nervous and Mental Disease 174, 319-327.

Rosenheck, R., & Nathan, P. (1985). Secondary traumatization in children of Vietnam veterans. Hospital and Community Psychiatry 36, 538-539.

Russell, A., Plotkin, D., & Heapy, N. (1985). Adaptive abilities in nonclinical second-generation Holocaust survivors and controls: A comparison. American Journal of Psychotherapy 39, 564-679.

Rustin, S. L., & Lipsig, F. S. (1972). Psychotherapy with the adolescent children of concentration camp survivors. Journal of Contemporary Psychotherapy 4, 87-94.

Savran, B., & Fogelman, E. (1979). Therapeutic groups for children of Holocaust survivors. International Journal of Group Psychotherapy 29, 211-215.

Sigal, J. J., Silver, D., Rakoff, V., & Ellin, B. (1973). Some second generation effects of survival of the Nazi persecution. American Journal of Orthopsychiatry 43, 320-327.

Solkoff, N. (1981). Children of survivors of the Nazi Holocaust: A critical review of the literature. American Journal of Orthopsychiatry 51, 29-42.

Wilson, A., & Fromm, E. (1982). Aftermath of the concentration camp: The second generation. American Academy of Psychoanalysis 10, 289-313.

Zlotogorski, Z. (1983). Offspring of concentration camp survivors: The relationship of perceptions of family cohesion and adaptability to levels of ego functioning. Comprehensive Psychiatry 24, 345-354.

3. Stress and Holocaust Victims and Their Children

Gyomroi-Ludowyk, E. (1963). The analysis of a young concentration camp victim. In R. S. Eissler, et al. (Eds.), Psychoanalytic study of the child (Vol. 18, pp. 484-510). New York: International Universities Press.

Klein, H. (1974). Child victims of the Holocaust. Journal of Clinical Child Psychology 3, 44-47.

Moskovitz, S. (1982). Love despite hate. Child survivors of the Holocaust and their adult lives. New York: Schocken.

Moskovitz, S. (1985). Longitudinal follow up of child survivors of the Holocaust. Journal of the American Academy of Child Psychiatry 24, 401-407.

Rotenberg, L. (1985). A child survivor/psychiatrist's personal adaptation. Journal of the American Academy of Child Psychiatry 24, 385-389.

Solomon, Z., Kutler, M., & Mikulincer, M. (1988). Combat-related post-traumatic stress disorder among second-generation Holocaust survivors: Preliminary findings. American Journal of Psychiatry 145, 865-868.

Spero, M. H. (1980). Psychophysiological sequelae of Holocaust trauma in a Jewish child. American Journal of Psychoanalysis 40, 53-66.

4. Psychiatric Disorders in Holocaust Victims and Their Children

Gyomroi-Ludowyk, E. (1963). The analysis of a young concentration camp victim. In R. S. Eissler, et al. (Eds.), Psychoanalytic study of the child (Vol. 18, pp. 484-510). New York: International Universities Press.

Kinzie, J. D., Sack, W., Angell, R., Clarke, G., & Ben, R. (1989). A three-year follow-up of Cambodian young people traumatized as children. Journal of the American Academy of Child and Adolescent Psychiatry 28, 501-504.

Klein, H. (1974). Child victims of the Holocaust. Journal of Clinical Child Psychology 3, 44-47.

Krell, R. (1988). Survivors of childhood experiences in Japanese concentration camps. American Journal of Psychiatry 145, 383-384.

Moskovitz, S. (1982). Love despite hate. Child survivors of the Holocaust and their adult lives. New York: Schocken.

Moskovitz, S. (1985). Longitudinal follow up of child survivors of the Holocaust. Journal of the American Academy of Child Psychiatry 24, 401-407.

Robinson, S., & Hemmendinger, J. (1982). Psychosocial adjustment 30 years later of people who were in Nazi concentration camps as children. In N. Milgram (Ed.), Stress and anxiety (pp. 397-399). Washington, D.C.: Hemisphere.

Rotenberg, L. (1985). A child survivor/psychiatrist's personal adaptation. Journal of the American Academy of Child Psychiatry 24, 385-389.

Spero, M. H. (1980). Psychophysiological sequelae of Holocaust trauma in a Jewish child. American Journal of Psychoanalysis 40, 53-66.

Sterba, E. (1968). The effects of persecution on adolescents. In H. Krystal (Ed.), Massive psychic trauma (pp. 51-59). New York: International Universities Press.

5. Physical Shock as Trauma

Anthony, E. J. (1986). Terrorizing attacks on children by psychotic parents. Journal of the American Academy of Child Psychiatry 25, 326-335.

Bergen, M. E. (1958). The effect of severe trauma on a four-year-old child. In R. S. Eissler, et al. (Eds.), Psychoanalytic study of the child (Vol. 13, pp. 407-429). New York: International Universities Press.

Black, D., & Kaplan, T. (1988). Father kills mother: Issues and problems encountered by a child psychiatric team. British Journal of Psychiatry 153, 624-630.

Burgess, A. W. (1974). Family reaction to homicide. American Journal of Orthopsychiatry 45, 391-398.

Burgess, A. W., Hartman, C. R., McCausland, M. P., & Powers, P. (1984). Response patterns in children and adolescents exploited through sex rings and pornography. American Journal of Psychiatry 141, 656-662.

Burgess, A. W., & Holmstrom, L. L. (1975). Sexual trauma of children and adolescents: Pressure, sex and secrecy. Nursing Clinics of North America 10, 551-563.

Cain, A., & Fast, I. (1966). Children's disturbed reactions to parent suicide. American Journal of Orthopsychiatry 36, 873-880.

Dallas, D. (1978). Savagery, show and tell. American Psychologist 33, 388-390.

Donaldson, M. A., & Gardner, R. (1985). Diagnosis and treatment of traumatic stress among women after childhood incest. In C. R. Figley (Ed.), Trauma and its wake (pp. 356-377). New York: Brunner/Mazel.

Eth, S. (1989). The adolescent witness to homicide. In E. P. Benedek & D. G. Cornell (Eds.), Juvenile homicide. Washington, D. C.: American Psychiatric Press.

Eth, S., Arroyo, W., & Silverstein, S. (1985). Psychiatric crisis team response to violence in elementary school. In I. H. Berkovitz & J. S. Seliger (Eds.), Expanding mental health interventions in schools (pp. 55-62). Dubuque, Iowa: Kendall/Hunt.

Eth, S., & Pynoos, R. S. (1985). Psychiatric interventions with children traumatized by violence. In D. H. Schetky & E. P. Benedek (Eds.), Emerging issues in child psychiatry (pp. 285-309). New York: Brunner/Mazel.

Eth, S., Silverstein, S., & Pynoos, R. S. (1985). Mental health consultation to a preschool following the murder of a mother and child. Hospital and Community Psychiatry 36, 73-76.

Goodwin, J. (1985). Post-traumatic symptoms in incest victims. In S. Eth & R. S. Pynoos (Eds.), Post-traumatic stress disorder in children (pp. 155-168). Washington, D.C.: American Psychiatric Press.

Goodwin, J. (1988). Post-traumatic symptoms in abused children. Journal of Traumatic Stress 1, 475-488.

Green, A. H. (1985). Children traumatized by physical abuse. In S. Eth & R. S. Pynoos (Eds.), Post-traumatic stress disorder in children (pp. 133-154). Washington, D.C.: American Psychiatric Press.

Hershorn, M., & Rosenbaum, A. (1985). Children of marital violence: A closer look at the unintended victims. American Journal of Orthopsychiatry 55, 260-266.

Hughes, H., & Barad, S. (1983). Psychological functioning of children in a battered women's shelter. American Journal of Orthopsychiatry 53, 525-531.

Hughes, H. M. (1988). Psychological and behavioral correlates of family violence in child winessses and victims. American Journal of Orthopsychiatry 58, 77-90.

Jackson, H. J., & King, H. J. (1981). The emotive imagery treatment of a child's trauma-induced phobia. Journal of Behavior Therapy and Experimental Psychiatry 12, 325-328.

Jaffe, P., Wolfe, D., Wilson, S., & Zak, L. (1986). Similarities in behavioral and social maladjustment among child victims and witnesses to family violence. American Journal of Orthopsychiatry 56, 142-146.

Jones, D. P., & Krugman, R. D. (1986). Can a three-year-old child bear witness to her sexual assault and attempted murder. Child Abuse and Neglect 10, 253-258.

Katan, A. (1973). Children who were raped. In R. S. Eissler, et al. (Eds.), Psychoanalytic study of the child (Vol. 28, pp. 208-224). New York: International Universities Press.

Kiser, L. J., Ackerman, B. J., Brown, E., Edwards, N. B., McColgan, E., Pugh, R., & Pruitt, D. B. (1988). Post-traumatic stress disorder in young children: A reaction to purported sexual abuse. Journal of the American Academy of Child and Adolescent Psychiatry 27, 645-649.

Lindberg, F. H., & Distad, L. J. (1985). Post-traumatic stress disorders in women who experienced childhood incest. Child Abuse and Neglect 9, 329-334.

Malmquist, C. P. (1986). Children who witness parental murder: Post-traumatic aspects. Journal of the American Academy of Child Psychiatry 25, 320-325.

Marohn, R. C. (1974). Trauma and the delinquent. In S. C. Feinstein, et al. (Eds.), Adolescent psychiatry: Developmental and clinical studies (Vol. 3, pp. 354-361). Chicago: University of Chicago Press.

McLeer, S. V., Deblinger, E., Atkins, M. S., Foa, E. B., & Ralphe, D. L. (1988). Post-traumatic stress disorder in sexually abused children. Journal of the American Academy of Child and Adolescent Psychiatry 27, 650-654.

Pfouts, J., Schopler, J., & Henley, H. C. (1982). Forgotten victims of family violence. Social Work 27, 367-368.

Pruett, K. D. (1979). Home treatment for two infants who witnessed their mother's murder. Journal of the American Academy of Child Psychiatry 18, 647-657.

Pynoos, R. S., & Eth, S. (1985). Children traumatized by acts of personal violence. In S. Eth & R. S. Pynoos (Eds.), Post-traumatic stress disorder in children (pp. 17-44). Washington, D.C.: American Psychiatric Press.

Pynoos, R. S., & Eth, S. (1986a). Special intervention programs for child witnesses to violence. In M. Lystad (Ed.), Violence in the home: Interdisciplinary perspectives (pp. 193-216). New York: Brunner/Mazel.

Pynoos, R. S., & Eth, S. (1986b). Witness to violence: The child interview. Journal of the American Academy of Child Psychiatry 25, 306-319.

Pynoos, R. S., Frederick, C., Naderk, K., Arroyo, W., Steinberg, A., Eth, S., Nunez, F., & Fairbanks, L. (1987). Life threat and post traumatic stress in school-age children. Archives of General Psychiatry 44, 1057-1063.

Pynoos, R. S., & Nader, K. (1988a). Children who witness the sexual assaults of their mothers. Journal of the American Academy of Child and Adolescent Psychiatry 27, 567-572.

Pynoos, R. S., & Nader, K. (1988b). Psychological first aid and treatment approach to children exposed to community violence. Journal of Traumatic Stress 1, 445-474.

Pynoos, R. S., & Nader, K. (1989). Children's memory and proximity to violence. Journal of the American Academy of Child and Adolescent Psychiatry 28, 236-241.

Schetky, D. H., & Haller, L. (1983). Parental kidnapping. Journal of the American Academy of Child Psychiatry 22, 279-285.

Schoettle, U. C. (1980). Child exploitation: A study of child pornography. Journal of the American Academy of Child Psychiatry 19, 289-299.

Senior, N., Gladstone, T., & Nurcombe, B. (1982). Child snatching: A case report. Journal of the American Academy of Child Psychiatry 21, 579-583.

Shapiro, S. (1973). Preventative analysis following a trauma. A 4 1/2 year old girl witnesses a stillbirth. In R. S. Eissler, et al. (Eds.), Psychoanalytic study of the child (Vol. 28, pp. 249-285). New York: International Universities Press.

Terr, L. C. (1981a). Forbidden games: Post-traumatic child's play. Journal of the American Academy of Child Psychiatry 20, 741-760.

Terr, L. C. (1981b). Psychic trauma in children: Observations following the Chochilla school-bus kidnapping. American Journal of Psychiatry 138, 14-19.

Terr, L. C. (1983). Chochilla revisited: The effects of psychic trauma four years after a schoolbus kidnapping. American Journal of Psychiatry 140, 1543-1550.

Terr, L. C. (1984). Time and trauma. In A. Solnit, et al. (Eds.), Psychoanalytic study of the child (Vol. 39, pp. 633-665). New Haven: Yale University Press.

Utterback, J., & Caldwell, J. (1989). Proactive and reactive approaches to PTSD in the aftermath of campus violence. Journal of Traumatic Stress 2, 171-184.

van der Kolk, B. A. (1985). Adolescent vulnerability to post-traumatic stress disorder. Psychiatry 48, 365-370.

Wolfe, D. A., Jaffe, P., Wilson, S. K., & Zak, L. (1985). Children of battered women: The relation of child behavior to family violence and maternal stress. Journal of Consulting and Clinical Psychology 53, 657-665.

Zeanah, C. H., & Burk, G. S. (1984). A young child who witnessed her mother's murder: Therapeutic and legal considerations. American Journal of Psychotherapy 38, 132-145.

6. Psychiatric Disorders in Children and Adolescents after a Natural Disaster

Adams, P. R., & Adams, G. R. (1984). Mount Saint Helen's ashfall. Evidence for a disaster stress reaction [volcano]. American Psychologist 39, 252-260.

Benedek, E. P. (1985). Children and disaster: Emerging issues. Psychiatric Annals 15, 168-172.

Blaufarb, H., & Levine, J. (1972). Crisis intervention in an earthquake. Social Work 17, 16-19.

Bloch, D. A., Silber, E., & Perry, S. E. (1956). Some factors in the emotional reaction of children to disaster. American Journal of Psychiatry 113, 416-422.

Blom, G. E. (1986). A school disaster--intervention and research aspects [building collapse]. Journal of the American Academy of Child Psychiatry 25, 336-345.

Burke, J. D., Borus, J. F., Burns, B. J., Millstein, K. H., & Beasley, M. C. (1982). Changes in children's behavior after a natural disaster [blizzard]. American Journal of Psychiatry 139, 1010-1014.

Burke, J. D., Moccia, P., Borus, J. F., & Burns, B. J. (1986). Emotional distress in fifth-grade children ten months after a natural disaster [blizzard]. Journal of the American Academy of Child Psychiatry 25, 536-541.

Cohen, R., & Ahearn, F. L. (1980). Handbook for mental health care of disaster victims. Baltimore: Johns Hopkins University Press.

Cornely, P., & Bromet, E. (1986). Prevalence of behavior problems in three-year-old children living near Three Mile Island: A comparative analysis. Journal of Child Psychology and Psychiatry and Allied Disciplines 27, 489-498.

Crabbs, M. A. (1981). School mental health services following an environmental disaster. Journal of School Health 51, 165-167.

Dollinger, S. J., O'Donnell, J. P., & Stanley, A. A. (1984). Lightning strike disaster: Effects on children's fears and worries [lightning]. Journal of Consulting and Clinical Psychology 52, 1028-1038.

Earls, F., Smith, E., Reich, W., & Jung, K. G. (1988). Investigating psychopathological consequences of a disaster in children: A pilot study incorporating a structured diagnostic interview. Journal of the American Academy of Child and Adolescent Psychiatry 27, 90-95.

Galante, R., & Foa, D. (1986). An epidemiological study of psychic trauma and treatment effectiveness for children after a natural disaster. Journal of the American Academy of Child Psychiatry 25, 357-363.

Gislason, I. L., & Call, J. (1982). Dog bite in infancy: Trauma and personality development. Journal of the American Academy of Child Psychiatry 21, 203-207.

Handford, H. A., Mayes, S. D., Mattison, R. E., Humphrey, F. J., Bagnato, S., Bixler, E. O., & Kales, J. D. (1986). Child and parent reaction the Three Mile Island nuclear accident. Journal of the American Academy of Child Psychiatry 25, 346-356.

Lindy, J. D., Grace, M. C., & Green, B. L. (1981). Survivors: Outreach to a reluctant population. American Journal of Orthopsychiatry 51, 468-478.

Maclean, G. (1977). Psychic trauma and traumatic neurosis. Play therapy with a four-year-old boy. Canadian Psychiatric Association Journal 22, 71-76.

Maclean, G. (1980). Addendum to a case of traumatic neurosis: Consideration of family dynamics. Canadian Journal of Psychiatry 25, 506-508.

McIntire, M. S., & Sadeghi, E. (1977). The pediatrician and mental health in a community-wide disaster. Clinical Pediatrics 16, 702-705.

Milgram, N. A., Toubiana, Y. H., Klingman, A., Raviv, A., & Goldstein, I. (1988). Situational exposure and personal loss in children's acute and chronic stress reactions to a school bus disaster. Journal of Traumatic Stress 1, 339-352.

Miller, J. A., Turner, J. G., & Kimball, E. (1981). Big Thompson flood victims: One year later. Family Relations 30, 111-116.

Newman, C. J. (1976). Children of disaster: Clinical observations at Buffalo Creek. American Journal of Psychiatry 133, 306-312.

Piotrowski, C. (1985). Use of the semantic differential technique in research on disaster: A methodological note. Psychological Reports 56, 527-530.

Piotrowski, C., & Dunham, F. Y. (1983). Locus of control orientation and perception of "hurricane" in fifth graders. Journal of General Psychology 109, 119-127.

Schwebel, M., & Schwebel, B. (1981). Children's reactions to the treat of nuclear plant accidents. American Journal of Orthopsychiatry 51, 260-270.

Silber, E., Perry, S. E., & Bloch, D. A. (1958). Patterns of parent-child interaction in a disaster. Psychiatry 21, 159-168.

Titchener, J. L., & Kapp, F. T. (1976). Family and character change at Buffalo Creek. American Journal of Psychiatry 133, 295-299.

Wilkenson, C. B. (1983). Aftermath of a disaster: The collapse of the Hyatt Regency Hotel skywalks. American Journal of Psychiatry 140, 1134-1139.

7. Post-Traumatic Effects

Anthony, E. J. (1986). The response to overwhelming stress: Some introductory comments. Journal of the American Academy of Child Psychiatry 25, 299-305.

Brett, E. A., & Ostroff, R. (1985). Imagery and post-traumatic stress disorder. American Journal of Psychiatry 142, 417-424.

Coddington, R. D. (1972). The significance of life events as etiologic factors in the diseases of children. II: A study of a normal population. Journal of Psychosomatic Research 16, 205-213.

Dowling, S. (1982). Dreams and dreaming in relation to trauma in childhood. International Journal of Psycho-Analysis 63, 157-166.

Esman, A. (1983). The "stimulus barrier." In A. Solnit, et al. (Eds.), Psychoanalytic study of the child (Vol. 38, pp. 193-207). New Haven: Yale University Press.

Eth, S., & Pynoos, R. S. (1985a). Developmental perspective in psychic trauma in childhood. In C. R. Figley (Ed.), Trauma and its wake (pp. 36-52). New York: Brunner/Mazel.

Eth, S., & Pynoos, R. S. (1985b). Post-traumatic stress disorder in children. Washington, D.C.: American Psychiatric Press.

Ettedgui, E., & Bridges, M. (1985). Post-traumatic stress disorder. Psychiatric Clinics of North America 8, 89-103.

Figley, C. R. (Ed.). (1985). Trauma and its wake: The study and treatment of post-traumatic stress. New York: Brunner/Mazel.

Frederick, C. J. (1985). Children traumatized by catastrophic situations. In S. Eth & R. S. Pynoos (Eds.), Post-traumatic stress disorder in children (pp. 71-100). Washington, D.C.: American Psychiatric Press.

Freud, A. (1967). Comments on psychic trauma. In A. Freud (Ed.), The writings of Anna Freud (pp. 221-241). New York: International Universities Press.

Garmezy, N. (1986). Children under severe stress: Critique and commentary. Journal of the American Academy of Child Psychiatry 25, 384-392.

Garmezy, N., Masten, A. S., & Tellegen, A. (1984). The study of stress and competence in children: A building block for developmental psychopathology. Child Development 55, 97-111.

Garmezy, N., & Rutter, M. (1985). Acute reactions to stress. In M. Rutter & L. Hersov (Eds.), Child and adolescent psychiatry (pp. 152-176). Oxford: Blackwell.

Khan, M. M. R. (1963). The concept of cumulative trauma. In R. S. Eissler, et al. (Eds.), Psychoanalytic study of the child (Vol. 18, pp. 286-306). New York: International Universities Press.

Krystal, H. (1978). Trauma and affects. In A. Solnit, et al. (Eds.), Psychoanalytic study of the child (Vol. 33, pp. 81-116). New Haven: Yale University Press.

Levy, D. (1939). Release therapy. American Journal of Orthopsychiatry 9, 713-736.

Pruett, K. D. (1984). A chronology of defensive adaptations to severe psychological trauma. In A. Solnit, et al. (Eds.), Psychoanalytic study of the child (Vol. 39, pp. 591-612). New Haven: Yale University Press.

Ruben, M. (1974). Trauma in the light of clinical experience. In R. S. Eissler, et al. (Eds.), Psychoanalytic study of the child (Vol. 29, pp. 369-387). New York: International Universities Press.

Rutter, M. (1981). Stress, coping and development: Some issues and some questions. Journal of Child Psychology and Psychiatry and Allied Disciplines 22, 323-356.

Sandler, I. N., & Block, M. (1979). Life stress and maladaptation of children. American Journal of Community Psychology 7, 425-440.

Saussure, J. D. (1982). Dreams and dreaming in relation to trauma in childhood. International Journal of Psycho-Analysis 63, 167-175.

Terr, L. C. (1983a). Life attitudes, dreams and psychic trauma in a group of normal children. Journal of the American Academy of Child Psychiatry 22, 221-230.

Terr, L. C. (1983b). Play therapy and psychic trauma: A preliminary report. In C. Schaefer & K. O'Connor (Eds.), Handbook of play therapy (pp. 308-319). New York: Wiley-Interscience.

Terr, L. C. (1983c). Time sense following psychic trauma: A clinical study of ten adults and twenty children. American Journal of Orthopsychiatry 53, 244-261.
Terr, L. C. (1984). Child at acute risk: Psychic trauma. In L. Grinspoon (Ed.), Psychiatry update (pp. 104-120). Washington, D.C.: American Psychiatric Press.
Terr, L. C. (1985a). Psychic trauma in children and adolescents. Psychiatric Clinics of North America 8, 815-835.
Terr, L. C. (1985b). Remembered images in psychic trauma: One explanation for the supernatural. In A. Solnit, et al. (Eds.), Psychoanalytic study of the child (Vol. 40, pp. 493-533). New York: International Universities Press.
Titchener, J. L., & Kapp, F. T. (1976). Family and character change at Buffalo Creek. American Journal of Psychiatry 133, 295-299.
Yates, A. (1983). Stress management in childhood. Clinical Pediatrics 22, 131-135.

H. Children in the Hospital

Jay Tarnow, M.D., Section Editor

Andres Pumariega, M.D., Associate Editor

1. General Issues

Adams, M. A. (1976). A hospital play program: Helping children with serious illness. American Journal of Orthopsychiatry 46, 416-424.
Adams, P. L. (1968). Techniques for pediatric consultation. In J. J. Schwab (Ed.), Handbook of psychiatric consultation (pp. 107-123). New York: Appleton-Century-Crofts.
Albertini, R. (1979). Use of paradoxical injunction with a hospitalized adolescent. Hospital and Community Psychiatry 30, 163-164.
Alger, I., Linn, S., & Beardslee, W. (1985). Puppetry as a therapeutic tool for hospitalized children. Hospital and Community Psychiatry 36, 129-130.
Azarnoff, P., & Woody, P. D. (1981). Preparation of children for hospitalization in acute care hospitals in the United States. Pediatrics 68, 361-368.
Bailey, W. E., & Moure, D. A. (1980). Group meetings for families of burn victims. Topics in Clinical Nursing 2, 67-75.
Barbero, G. J. (1984). Children with recurrent hospitalizations: A problem of disabled children, parents, and physicians. Journal of Developmental and Behavioral Pediatrics 5, 319-324.
Bauman, S. (1981). Physical aspects of the self. A review of some aspects of body image development in childhood. Psychiatric Clinics of North America 4, 455-470.
Baxter, J. E. (1978). Recognition and management of emotional problems associated with end-stage kidney disease. Journal of Dialysis 2, 175-212.
Bear, D. M., & Defio, P. (1977). Quantitative analysis of interictal behavior in temporal lobe epilepsy. Archives of Neurology 34, 454-467.

Bell, T. S., Ellenberg, L., & McComb, J. G. (1985). Neuropsychological outcome after severe pediatric near-drowning. Neurosurgery 17, 604-608.

Bergman, A. S., & Fritz, G. K. (1981). Psychiatric and social work collaboration in pediatric chronic illness hospital. Social Work in Health Care 7, 45-55.

Berlin, I. N. (1978). Developmental issues in the psychiatric hospitalization of children. American Journal of Psychiatry 135, 1044-1048.

Bolian, G. (1971). Psychiatric consultation within a community of sick children: Lessons from a children's hospital. Journal of the American Academy of Child Psychiatry 10, 293-307.

Brett, A. (1983). Preparing children for hospitalization: A Classroom teaching approach. Journal of School Health 53, 561-563.

Brewster, A. B. (1982). Chronically ill hospitalized children's concepts of their illness. Pediatrics 69, 355-362.

Brown, J. K. (1977). Migraine and migraine equivalents in children. Developmental Medicine and Child Neurology 19, 683-692.

Burstein, S., & Meichenbaum, D. (1979). The work of worrying in children undergoing surgery. Journal of Abnormal Child Psychology 7, 121-132.

Carty, R. M. (1980). Observed behaviors of preschoolers to intensive care. Pediatric Nursing 6, 21-25.

Coddington, R. D. (1972). The significance of life events as etiological factors in the diseases of children. II. A study of normal populations. Journal of Psychosomatic Research 16, 205.

Cofer, D. H., & Nir, Y. (1975). Theme-focused group therapy on a pediatric ward. International Journal of Psychiatry and Medicine 6, 541-550.

Coffey, H., & Koch, C. R. (1975). Psycho-social care of the paralyzed child: A technique in intensive care nursing. Pediatric Nursing 1, 21-23.

Cooper, J. E. (1976). Pets in hospitals. British Medical Journal 1, 698-700.

Craft, M. J., Wyatt, N., & Sandell, B. (1985). Behavior and feeling changes in siblings of hospitalized children. Clinical Pediatrics 24, 374-378.

Crittenden, M. R., Holliday, M. A., Piel, C. F., & Potter, D. E. (1985). Intellectual development of children with renal insufficiency and end state disease. International Journal of Pediatric Nephrology 6, 275-280.

Cyntryn, L., Moore, P. V. P., & Robinson, M. E. (1973). Psychological adjustment of children with cystic fibrosis. In E. J. Anthony & C. J. Koupernik (Eds.), The child in his family. New York: Wiley.

Dittemore, I. L. (1983). Behavioral responses in the early recovery of a severely burned 4 year old child. Maternal-Child Nursing Journal 12, 21-34.

Drotar, D. (1981). Adaptational problems of children and adolescents with cystic fibrosis. Journal of Pediatric Psychology 8, 45-50.

Drotar, D., Doershuk, C. F., Stern, R. C., Boat, T. F., Boyer, W., & Matthews, L. (1981). Psychosocial functioning of children with cystic fibrosis. Pediatrics 67, 338-343.

Duff, R. S., Cook, C. D., Margolis, C. Z., Lattanzi, W. E., & Landwirth, J. (1975). A review of pediatric inpatient care. American Journal of Diseases of Children 129, 1422-1432.

Eisendrath, S. E. (1981). Psychiatric liaison support groups for general hospital staff. Psychosomatics 22, 685-694.

Elkins, P. D., & Roberts, M. C. (1985). Reducing medical fears in a general population of children: A comparison of three audio-visual modeling procedures. Journal of Pediatric Psychology 10, 65-75.

Erickson, M. P. (1978). Hospital care of the ill child with mental retardation. Developmental Medicine and Child Neurology 20, 674-677.

Fassler, D. (1985). The fear of needles in children. American Journal of Orthopsychiatry 55, 371-377.

Faust, J., & Melamed, B. G. (1984). Influence of arousal, previous experience, and age on surgery preparation of same day of surgery and in-hospital pediatric patients. Journal of Consulting and Clinical Psychology 52, 359-365.

Fennell, R. S., Rasbury, W. C., Fennell, E. B., & Morris, M. K. (1984). Effects of kidney transplantation on cognitive performance in a pediatric population. Pediatrics 74, 273-278.

Ferguson, B. F. (1979). Preparing young children for hospitalization: A comparison of two methods. Pediatrics 64, 656-664.

Ferrari, M. (1984). Chronic illness: Psychosocial effects on siblings. I. Chronically ill boys. Journal of Child Psychology and Psychiatry and Allied Disciplines 25, 459-476.

Fielding, D., Moore, B., Dewey, M., Ashley, P., McKendrick, T., & Pinkerton, P. (1985). Children with end-stage renal failure. Psychological effects on patients, siblings and parents. Journal of Psychosomatic Research 29, 457-465.

Fine, S. H., & Tonkin, R. S. (1982). Limited psychiatric consultation to an adolescent medicine unit. Child Psychiatry and Human Development 13, 48-54.

Fiser, D. H., Stanford, G., & Dorman, D. J. (1984). Services for parental stress reduction in a pediatric ICU. Critical Care Medicine 12, 504-507.

Foust, L. A. (1980). The concerns of a ten year old boy threatened with body image disruption due to reconstructive craniofacial surgery. Maternal-Child Nursing Journal 9, 37-48.

Freud, A. (1952). The role of bodily illness in the mental life of the child. In R. S. Eissler, et al., The psychoanalytic study of the child (pp. 69-81). New York: International Universities Press.

Freud, W. E. (1980). Notes on some psychological aspects of neonatal intensive care. In S. Greenspan & G. Pollock (Eds.), The course of life: Psychoanalytic contributions towards understanding personality development (pp. 257-270). Bethesda, Md.: National Institute of Mental Health.

Gabriel, H. P., & Danilowicz, D. (1978). Postoperative responses in 'prepared' child after cardiac surgery. British Heart Journal 40, 1046-1051.

Gaiter, J. L., & Johnson, A. (1984). Contact with intensive care infants: Father's sex type, infant preference, and frequency of visits. In J. D. Call, E. Galenson, & R. L. Tyson (Eds.), Frontiers of infant psychiatry (pp. 385-394). New York: Basic Books.

Galligan, A. C. (1975). Books for the hospitalized child. American Journal of Nursing 75, 2164-2166.

Gardner, G. (1977). Hypnosis with infants and preschool children. American Journal of Clinical Hypnosis 19, 158-162.

Gauthier, Y., et al. (1978). The mother-child relationship and the development of autonomy and self-assertion in young asthmatic children. Journal of the American Academy of Child Psychiatry 17, 679-694.

Gersten, J. C., Langner, T. S., Eisenberg, J. G., et al. (1977). An evaluation of the etiologic role of stressful life-change events in psychological disorders. Journal of Health and Social Behavior 18, 228.

Graham, P. J., et al. (1967). Childhood asthma: A psychosomatic disorder? Some epidemiological considerations. British Journal of Preventive and Social Medicine 21, 78-85.

Grupe, W. E., Greifer, I., Greenspan, S. I., Leavitt, L. A., & Wolff, G. (1986). Psychosocial development in children with renal insufficiency. American Journal of Kidney Diseases 7, 324-328.

Hardgrove, C. B., & Kermoian, R. (1978). Parent-inclusive pediatric units: A survey of policies and practices. American Journal of Public Health 68, 847-850.

Hofmann, A. D., Becker, R. D., & Bagriel, H. P. (1976). The hospitalized adolescent (pp. 139-146). New York: The Free Press.

Hollenbeck, A. R., Susman, E. J., Nannis, E. D., Strope, B. E., Hersh, S. P., Levine, A. S., & Pizzo, P. A. (1980). Children with serious illness: Behavioral correlates of separation and isolation. Child Psychiatry and Human Development 11, 3-11.

Houts, C. B., Turbett, J. A., Arnold, L. E., & Kruse, E. (1985). Cost of medical/surgical pediatric hospital days preventable by psychiatric treatment. Journal of the American Academy of Child Psychiatry 24, 227-230.

Hughes, M. C. (1982). Chronically ill children in groups: Recurrent issues and adaptations. American Journal of Orthopsychiatry 52, 704-711.

Hunt, A. D. (1974). On the hospitalization of children: An historical approach. Pediatrics 54, 542-546.

Jackson, E. B. (1942). Treatment of the young child in the hospital. American Journal of Orthopsychiatry 12, 56-67.

Jessner, L., Blom, G. E., & Waldfogel, S. (1952). Emotional implications of tonsillectomy and adenoidectomy on children. In R. S. Eissler, et al. (Eds.), Psychoanalytic study of the child (Vol. 7, pp. 126-169). New York: International Universities Press.

Jessop, D. J., & Stein, R. E. (1985). Uncertainty and its relation to the psychological and social correlates of chronic illness. Social Science and Medicine 20, 993-999.

Johnson, J. E., Kirchoff, K. T., & Endress, M. P. (1975). Altering children's distress behavior during orthopedic cast removal. Nursing Research 24, 404-419.

Johnson, M. R., Gershowitz, M., & Stabler, B. (1981). Maternal compliance and children's self-concept in cystic fibrosis. Journal of Developmental and Behavioral Pediatrics 2, 5-8.

Jonsen, A. R., Phibbs, R. H., Tooley, W. H., & Garland, M. J. (1977). Critical issues in newborn intensive care: A conference report and policy proposal. In J.

L. Schwartz & L. H. Schwartz (Eds.), Vulnerable infants: A psychosocial dilemma (pp. 312-334). New York: McGraw-Hill.

Kashani, J. H., Barbero, G. J., & Bolander, F. D. (1981). Depression in hospitalized pediatric patients. Journal of the American Academy of Child Psychiatry 20, 123-134.

Kavanagh, C. (1983). Psychological intervention with the severely burned child: Report of an experimental comparison of two approaches and their effects on psychological sequelae. Journal of the American Academy of Child Psychiatry 22, 145-156.

Kellerman, J., Ellenberg, L., Zeltzer, L., Dash, J., & Rigler, D. (1980). Psychological effects of illness in adolescence. I. Anxiety, self esteem, and perception of control. Journal of Pediatrics 97, 126-131.

Kemph, J., Bermann, E. A., & Copolillo, H. P. (1969). Kidney transplant and shifts in family dynamics. American Journal of Psychiatry 125, 1485-1490.

Klaus, M. H., & Kennell, J. H. (1976). The impact of early separation or loss on family development. St. Louis, Miss.: C.V. Mosby.

Knight, R. B., Atkins, A., Eagle, C. J., Evans, N., Finkelstein, J. W., Fukushima, D., Katz, J., & Weiner, H. (1979). Psychological stress, ego defenses, and cortisol production in children hospitalized for elective surgery. Psychosomatic Medicine 41, 40-49.

Kutsanei, J., Lou-Meyer, M., & Christ, G. H. (1978). Factors affecting coping of adolescents and infants on a reverse isolation unit. Social Work in Health Care 4, 125-137.

LeBow, H., Schiller, M., Caplan, G., & Selinger, D. (1983). The integration of the emotional and surgical treatment of children hospitalized on a pediatric-surgical ward. Child Psychiatry and Human Development 13, 180-188.

Lesser, S., & Easser, B. (1972). Personality differences in the perpetually handicapped. Journal of the American Academy of Child Psychiatry 11, 458-466.

Levy, D. M. (1945). Psychic trauma of operations in children and a note on combat neurosis. American Journal of Diseases of Children 69, 7-25.

Lewis, B. L., & Khaw, K. T. (1982). Family functioning as a mediating variable affecting psychosocial adjustment of children with cystic fibrosis. Journal of Pediatrics 101, 636-340.

Liakopoulou, M., Patterson, A., Samaraweera, S., & Finnegan, L. (1983). Developmental interventions in infancy during lengthy hospitalizations. Journal of Developmental and Behavioral Pediatrics 4, 213-217.

Liebman, R., Minuchin, S., & Baker, L. (1974). The use of structural family therapy in the treatment of intractable asthma. American Journal of Psychiatry 131, 535-540.

Linn, S., Beardslee, W., & Patenaude, A. F. (1986). Puppet therapy with pediatric bone marrow transplant patients. Journal of Pediatric Psychology 11, 294-301.

Magreb, P. R. (Ed.). (1978). Psychological management of pediatric problems. Early life conditions and chronic diseases. Baltimore: University Park Press.

McBride, M. M., & Sack, W. H. (1980). Emotional management of children with acute respiratory failure in the intensive care unit: A case study. Heart and Lung 9, 98-102.

McDonnell, L. (1979). Paraverbal therapy in pediatric cases with emotional complications. American Journal of Orthopsychiatry 49, 44-52.

McGraw, M. E., & Haka-Ikse, K. (1985). Neurologic-developmental sequelae of chronic renal failure in infancy. Journal of Pediatrics 106, 579-583.

Minde, K., et al. (1972). How they grow up: 41 physically handicapped children and their families. American Journal of Psychiatry 128, 1554-1560.

Moore, C. L. (1981). Hypnosis: An adjunct to pediatric consultation. American Journal of Clinical Hypnosis 23, 211-216.

Moore, N. (1965). Behavioral therapy in bronchial asthma: A controlled study. Journal of Psychosomatic Research 9, 257.

Mrazek, D. A. (1984). Effects of hospitalization on early child development. In R. N. Ende & R. J. Harmon (Eds.), Continuities and discontinuities in development. New York: Plenum Press.

Nagera, H. (1978). Children's reactions to hospitalization and illness. Child Psychiatry and Human Development 9, 3-19.

Orr, D. P., Weller, S. C., Satterwhite, B., & Pless, I. B. (1984). Psychosocial implications of chronic illness in adolescence. Journal of Pediatrics 104, 152-157.

Perrin, E. C., & Gerrity, P. S. (1981). There's a demon in your belly. Children: Understanding of illness. Pediatrics 67, 841.

Peterson, L., & Ridley-Johnson, R. (1984). Preparation of well children in the classroom: An unexpected contrast between the academic lecture and filmed modeling methods. Journal of Pediatric Psychology 9, 349-361.

Peterson, L., Ridley-Johnson, R., Tracey, K., & Mullins, L. L. (1984). Developing cost-effective presurgical preparation: A comparative analysis. Journal of Pediatric Psychology 9, 439-455.

Peterson, L., & Shigetomi, C. (1982). One-year follow-up of elective surgery child patients receiving preoperative preparation. Journal of Pediatric Psychology 7, 43-48.

Petrillo, M., & Sanger, S. (1980). Play in the hospital. In M. Petrillo & S. Sanger (Eds.), Emotional care of hospitalized children: An environmental approach (pp. 208-231. Philadelphia: Lippincott.

Pfeffer, C. R. (1979). A model for acute psychiatric inpatient treatment of latency-age children. Hospital and Community Psychiatry 30, 547-551.

Pilowsky, I., Bassett, D. L., Begg, M. W., & Thomas, P. G. (1982). Childhood hospitalization and chronic intractable pain in adults: A controlled retrospective study. International Journal of Psychiatry and Medicine 12, 75-84.

Potter, P. C., & Roberts, M. C. (1984). Children's perceptions of chronic illness: The roles of disease symptoms, cognitive development, and information. Journal of Pediatric Psychology 9, 13-27.

Powazek, M., Goff, J. R., Schyving, J., & Paulson, M. A. (1978). Emotional reactions of children to isolation in a cancer hospital. Journal of Pediatrics 92, 834-837.

Pozanski, E. O., Miller, E., Salguero, C., & Kelsh, R. C. (1978). Quality of life for long-term survivors of end-stage renal disease. Journal of the American Medical Association 239, 2343-2347.

Prugh, D. G. (1967). Children's reactions to illness, hospitalization, and surgery. In A. M. Freedman & H. I. Kaplan (Eds.), Comprehensive textbook of psychiatry. (pp. 1369-1376). Baltimore: Williams and Wilkins.

Prugh, D. G., Staub, E. M., Sands, H. H., Kirschbaum, R. M., & Lenihan, E. A. (1953). A study of the emotional reactions of children and families to hospitalization and illness. American Journal of Orthopsychiatry 23, 70-106.

Pumariega, A. J., & Snow, S. S. (1985). Multi-level intervention on behalf of a catastrophically ill child. Family Systems Medicine 13, 325-332.

Quinby, S., & Bernstein, N. R. (1971). Identity problems and the adaptation of nurses to severely burned children. American Journal of Psychiatry 128, 91-95.

Quinton, D., & Rutter, M. (1976). Early hospital admissions and later disturbances of behavior: An attempted replication of Douglas' findings. Developmental Medicine and Child Neurology 18, 447-459.

Robertson, J., & Robertson, J. (1971). Young children in brief separation. In R. S. Eissler, et al. (Eds.), Psychoanalytic study of the child (Vol. 26, pp. 264-315). New York: International Universities Press.

Sabbeth, B. F. (1984). Understanding the impact of chronic childhood illness on families. Pediatric Clinics of North America 31, 47-57.

Sabbeth, B. F., & Leventhal, J. M. (1984). Marital adjustment to chronic childhood illness: A critique of the literature. Pediatrics 73, 762-768.

Sadler, E. (1975). The long-term hospitalization of asthmatic children. Pediatric Clinics of North America 22, 173-183.

Salzinger, S., Antrobus, J., & Glick, J. (1980). The ecosystem of the "sick" child. New York: Academic Press.

Sampson, T. F. (1975). The child in renal failure: Emotional impact of treatment on the child and his family. Journal of the American Academy of Child Psychiatry 14, 462-476.

Sanders, S. (1975). Corrective social interaction therapy: Role modeling. American Journal of Orthopsychiatry 45, 875-883.

Sarles, R. M. (1975). The use of hypnosis with hospitalized children. Journal of Clinical Child Psychology 4, 36-38.

Schowalter, J. E. (1971). The utilization of child psychiatry on the pediatric adolescent ward. Journal of the American Academy of Child Psychiatry 10, 684-699.

Schowalter, J. E. (1977). Psychological reactions to physical illness and hospitalization in adolescence: A survey. Journal of the American Academy of Child Psychiatry 16, 500-516.

Senn, M. J. E. (1945). Emotional aspects of convalescence. The Child 10, 24-28.

Sherman, M. (1982). The neonatal intensive care unit. Psychiatric Clinics of North America 5, 433-443.

Silber, T. (1983). Chronic illness in adolescents: A sociological perspective. Adolescence 18, 675-677.

Solnit, A. J. (1960). Hospitalization: An aid to physical and psychological health in childhood. American Journal of Diseases of Children 99, 155-163.

Spinetta, J., & Deasy-Spinetta, P. (1981). Talking with children with a life-threatening illness: A handbook for health care professionals. Rockville, Md.: Cystic Fibrosis Foundation.

Spinetta, J. J., & Deasy-Spinetta, P. (1981). Emotional aspects of life-threatening illness in children: A handbook for parents. Rockville, Md.: Cystic Fibrosis Foundation.

Steinhausen, H. C. (1981). Chronically ill and handicapped children and adolescents: Personality studies in relation to disease. Journal of Abnormal Child Psychology 9, 291-297.

Steinhausen, H. C., Schindler, H. P., & Stephan, H. (1983). Correlates of psychopathology in sick children: An empirical model. Journal of the American Academy of Child Psychiatry 22, 559-564.

Stoddard, F. J. (1982). Body image development in the burned child. Journal of the American Academy of Child Psychiatry 21, 502-507.

Tarnow, J. (1984). Pediatric and adolescent parents in rehabilitation. In D. W. Krueger (Ed.), Emotional rehabilitation of physical trauma and disability. New York: Spectrum Publications.

Tarnow, J. D., & Gutstein, S. E. (1983). Children's preparatory behavior for elective surgery. Journal of the American Academy of Child Psychiatry 22, 365-369.

Thompson, R. H., & Stanford, G. (1981). Child life in hospitals: Theory and practice. Springfield, Ill.: Charles C. Thomas.

Tisza, V. B., et al. (1971). The use of a play program for hospitalized children. Journal of the American Academy of Child Psychiatry 10, 156-186.

Toker, E. (1971). Psychiatric aspects of cardiac surgery in a child. Journal of the American Academy of Child Psychiatry 10, 156-186.

Visintainer, M. A., & Wolfer, J. A. (1975). Psychological preparation for surgery pediatric patients: The effects on children's and parents' stress responses and adjustment. Pediatrics 56, 187-202.

Woolston, J. L., & Schowalter, J. E. (1980). Behavior modification protocols on a pediatric adolescent unit. Pediatrics 66, 355-358.

2. Children with Diabetes

Allen, D. A., Tennen, H., McGrade, B. J., Affleck, G., & Ratzan, S. (1983). Parent and child perceptions of the management of juvenile diabetes. Journal of Pediatric Psychology 8, 129-141.

Chase, H. P., & Jackson, G. G. (1981). Stress and sugar control in children with insulin-dependent diabetes mellitus. Journal of Pediatrics 98, 1011-1013.

Greydanus, D. E., & Hofmann, A. D. (1979). Psychological factors in diabetes mellitus. A review of the literature with emphasis on adolescence. American Journal of Diseases of Children 133, 1061-1066.

Gross, A. M., & Johnson, W. G. (1981). The diabetes assertiveness test: A measure of social coping skills in pre-adolescent diabetics. Diabetes Educator 7, 26-27.

Hilliard, J. P., Fritz, G. K., & Lewiston, N. J. (1985). Levels of aspiration of parents for their asthmatic, diabetic, and healthy children. Journal of Clinical Psychology 41, 587-597.

Holmes, C. S., & Richman, L. C. (1985). Cognitive profiles of children with insulin-dependent diabetes. Journal of Developmental and Behavioral Pediatrics 6, 323-326.

Ingersoll, G. M., Orr, D. P., Herrold, A. J., & Golden, M. P. (1986). Cognitive maturity and self-management among adolescents with insulin-dependent diabetes mellitus. Journal of Pediatrics 108, 620-623.

Kovacs, M., Feinberg, T. L., Paulauskas, S., Finkelstein, R., Pollock, M., & Crouse-Novak, M. (1985). Initial coping responses and psychosocial characteristics of children with insulin-dependent diabetes mellitus. Journal of Pediatrics 106, 827-834.

Leaverton, D. R., White, C. A., McCormick, C. R., Smith, P., & Sheikholislam, B. (1980). Parental loss antecedent to child diabetes mellitus. Journal of the American Academy of Child Psychiatry 19, 678-689.

Lustman, P. J., Amado, H., & Wetzel, R. D. (1983). Depression in diabetics: A critical appraisal. Comprehensive Psychiatry 24, 65-74.

Moffatt, M. E., & Pless, I. B. (1983). Locus of control in juvenile diabetic campers: Changes during camp, and relationship to camp staff assessments. Journal of Pediatrics 103, 146-150.

Orr, D. P., Golden, M. P., Myers, G., & Marrero, D. G. (1983). Characteristics of adolescents with poorly controlled diabetes referred to a tertiary care center. Diabetes Care 6, 170-175.

Potter, P. C., & Roberts, M. C. (1984). Children's perceptions of chronic illness: The roles of disease symptoms, cognitive development, and information. Journal of Pediatric Psychology 9, 13-27.

Ryan, C., Vega, A., & Drash, A. (1985). Cognitive deficits in adolescents who developed diabetes early in life. Pediatrics 75, 921-927.

Sullivan, B. J. (1979a). Adjustment in diabetic adolescent girls. II. Adjustment, self-esteem, and depression in diabetic adolescent girls. Psychosomatic Medicine 41, 127-138.

Sullivan, B. J. (1979b). Adjustment in diabetic adolescent girls. I. Development of the Diabetic Adjustment Scale. Psychosomatic Medicine 41, 119-126.

Tarnow, J., & Silberman S. (1981-1982). The psychophysiologic aspects of stress in juvenile diabetes mellitus. International Journal of Psychiatry and Medicine 11, 25-44.

Tarnow, J., & Tomlinson, N. (1978). Juvenile diabetes: Impact on the child and family. Psychosomatics 19, 487-491.

White, K., Kolman, M. L., Wexler, P., Polin, G., & Winter, R. J. (1984). Unstable diabetes and unstable families: A psychosocial evaluation of diabetic children with recurrent ketoacidosis. Pediatrics 73, 749-755.

3. Children with Injuries and Burns

Atkinson, J. H., Stewart, N., & Gardner, D. (1980). The family meeting in critical care settings. Journal of Trauma 20, 43-46.

Beales, J. G. (1983). Factors influencing the expectation of pain among patients in a children's burn unit. Burns, Including Thermal Injury 9, 187-192.

Bernstein, N. R. (1983). Child psychiatry and burn care. Journal of the American Academy of Child Psychiatry 22, 202-204.

Braverman, M. (1980). Onset of psychotraumatic reactions. Journal of Forensic Sciences 25, 821-825.

Caldwell, E. (1978). The psychologic impact of trauma. Nursing Clinics of North America 13, 247-254.

Dittemore, I. L. (1983). Behavioral responses in the early recovery of a severely burned 4 year old child. Maternal-Child Nursing Journal 12, 21-34.

Eyles, P., Browne, G., Byrne, C., Brown, B., Pennock, M., Truscott, D., & Dabbs, R. (1984). Methodological problems in studies of burn survivors and their psychosocial prognosis. Burns, Including Thermal Injury 10, 427-433.

Goodstein, R. K. (1985). Burns: An overview of clinical consequences affecting patient, staff, and family. Comprehensive Psychiatry 26, 43-57.

Halliday, G. (1982). Direct alteration of a traumatic nightmare. Perceptual and Motor Skills 54, 413-414.

Henker, F. O. (1979). Body-image conflict following trauma and surgery. Psychosomatics 20, 812-815, 819-820.

Kavanagh, C. (1983). A new approach to dressing change in the severely burned child and its effect on burn-related psychopathology. Heart and Lung 12, 612-619.

Knudson-Cooper, M. S., & Leuchtag, A. K. (1982). The stress of a family move as a precipitating factor in children's burn accidents. Journal of Human Stress 8, 32-38.

Langley, J. (1984). Injury control--psychosocial considerations. Journal of Child Psychology and Psychiatry and Allied Disciplines 25, 349-356.

Molinaro, J. R. (1978). The social fate of children disfigures by burns. American Journal of Psychiatry 135, 979-980.

Ravenscroft, K. (1979). Psychological considerations for the child with multiple trauma. In K. Ravenscroft (Ed.), The injured child: Surgical management (pp. 31-42). Chicago: Year Book Medical Publishers.

Ravenscroft, K. (1982a). The burn unit. Psychiatric Clinics of North America 5, 419-432.

Ravenscroft, K. (1982b). Psychiatric consultation to the child with acute physical trauma. American Journal of Orthopsychiatry 52, 298-307.

Rheiner, N. W., Aslakson, M. A., Morin, P., & Patach, D. (1981). Investigation of compliance in the severely injured: A literature review. Rehabilitation Nursing 6, 12-15.

Sawyer, M. G., Minde, K., & Zuker, R. (1983). The burned child--scarred for life? A study of the psychosocial impact of a burn injury at different developmental stages. Burns, Including Thermal Injury 9, 205-213.

Stoddard, F. J. (1982). Body image development in the burned child. Journal of the American Academy of Child Psychiatry 21, 502-507.

Tarnow, J. (1984). Pediatric and adolescent patients in rehabilitation. In D. W. Krueger (Ed.), Emotional rehabilitation of physical trauma and disability. New York: Spectrum Publications.

Wright, L., & Fulwiler, R. (1974). Long range emotional sequelae of burns: Effects on children and their mothers. Pediatric Research 8, 931-934.

4. Children with Cancer

Adams, D. W. (Ed.). (1980). Childhood malignancy: The psychosocial care of the child and his family. Springfield, Ill.: Charles C. Thomas.

Barbarin, O. A., & Chesler, M. A. (1984). Relationships with the medical staff and aspects of satisfaction with care expressed by parents of children with cancer. Journal of Community Health 9, 302-313.

Beardslee, C., & Neff, E. J. (1982). Body related concerns of children with cancer as compared with the concerns of other children. Maternal-Child Nursing Journal 11, 121-134.

Bernstein, I. L., Webster, M. M., & Bernstein, I. D. (1982). Food aversions in children receiving chemotherapy for cancer. Cancer 50, 2961-2963.

Binger, C. M. (1984). Psychosocial intervention with the child cancer patient and family. Psychosomatics 25, 899-902.

Blanchard, C. G., Ruckdeschel, J. C., Blanchard, E. B., Arena, J. G., Saunders, N. L., & Malloy, E. D. (1983). Interactions between oncologists and patients during rounds. Annals of Internal Medicine 99, 694-699.

Brouwers, P., Riccardi, R., Poplack, D., & Fedio, P. (1984). Attentional deficits in long-term survivors of childhood acute lymphoblastic leukemia (ALL). Journal of Clinical Neuropsychology 6, 325-336.

Brunnquell, D., & Hall, M. D. (1982). Issues in the psychological care of pediatric oncology patients. American Journal of Orthopsychiatry 52, 32-44.

Cairns, N. U., Clark, G. M., Smith, S. D., & Lansky, S. B. (1979). Adaptation of siblings to childhood malignancy. Journal of Pediatrics 95, 484-487.

Clopper, R. R., Meyer, W. J., Udvarhelyi, G. B., Money, J., Aarabi, B., Mulvihill, J. J., & Piasio, M. (1977). Postsurgical IQ and behavioral data on twenty patients with a history of childhood craniopharyngioma. Psychoneuroendocrinology 2, 365-372.

Eiser, C. (1979). Psychological development of the child with leukemia: A review. Journal of Behavioral Medicine 2, 141-157.

Eiser, C. (1980). How leukaemia affects a child's schooling. British Journal of Social and Clinical Psychology 19, 365-368.

Eiser, C. (1981). Psychological sequelae of brain tumours in childhood: A retrospective study. British Journal of Clinical Psychology 20, 35-38.

Ellenberg, L., Kellerman, J., Dash, J., Higgins, G., & Zeltzer, L. (1980). Use of hypnosis for multiple symptoms in an adolescent girl with leukemia. Journal of Adolescent Health Care 1, 132-136.

Frydman, M. I. (1980). Perception of illness severity and psychiatric symptoms in parents of chronically ill children. Journal of Psychosomatic Research 24, 361-369.

Gilder, R., Buschman, P. R., Sitarz, A. L., & Wolff, J. A. (1978). Group therapy with parents of children with leukemia. American Journal of Psychotherapy 32, 276-287.

Goff, J. R., Anderson, H. R., & Cooper, P. F. (1980). Distractibility and memory deficits in long-term survivors of acute lymphoblastic leukemia. Journal of Developmental and Behavioral Pediatrics 1, 158-163.

Gogan, J. L., Koocher, G. P., Fine, W. E., Foster, D. J., & O'Malley, J. E. (1979). Pediatric cancer survival and marriage: Issues affecting adult adjustments. American Journal of Orthopsychiatry 49, 423-430.

Henning, J., & Fritz, G. K. (1983). School reentry in childhood cancer. Psychosomatics 24, 261-269.

Hilgard, J. R., & LeBaron, S. (1982). Relief of anxiety and pain in children and adolescents with cancer: Quantitative measures and clinical observations. International Journal of Clinical and Experimental Hypnosis 30, 417-442.

Jacobs, T. J., & Charles, E. (1980). Life events and the occurrence of cancer in children. Psychosomatic Medicine 42, 11-24.

Johnson, F. L., Rudolph, L. A., & Hartmann, J. R. (1979). Helping the family cope with childhood cancer. Psychosomatics 20, 241, 245-247, 251.

Kalnins, I. V., Churchill, M. P., & Terry, G. E. (1980). Concurrent stresses in families with a leukemic child. Journal of Pediatric Psychology 5, 81-92.

Kashani, J., & Hakami, N. (1982). Depression in children and adolescents with malignancy. Canadian Journal of Psychiatry 27, 474-477.

Katz, E. R., Kellerman, J., & Siegel, S. E. (1980). Behavioral distress in children with cancer undergoing medical procedures: Developmental considerations. Journal of Consulting and Clinical Psychology 48, 356-365.

Kellerman, J. (Ed.). (1980). Psychological aspects of cancer in children. Springfield, Ill.: Charles C. Thomas.

Koocher, G. P., & O'Malley, J. E. (1980). (Eds.). The Damocles syndrome: Psychosocial consequences of surviving childhood cancer. New York: McGraw-Hill.

Koocher, G. P., O'Malley, J. E., Gogan, J. L., & Foster, D. J. (1980). Psychological adjustment among pediatric survivors. Journal of Child Psychology and Psychiatry and Allied Disciplines 21, 163-173.

Kupst, M. J., Schulman, J. L., Maurer, H., Honig, G., Morgan, E., & Fochtman, D. (1984). Coping with pediatric leukemia: A two-year follow-up. Journal of Pediatric Psychology 9, 149-163.

Lansky, S. B., Stephenson, L., Weller, E., Cairns, G. F., & Cairns, N. U. (1982). Failure to thrive during infancy in siblings of pediatric cancer patients. American Journal of Pediatric Hematology/Oncology 4, 361-366.

Levenson, P. M., Copeland, D. R., Morrow, J. R., Pfefferbaum, B., & Silberberg, Y. (1983). Disparities in disease-related perceptions of adolescent cancer patients and their parents. Journal of Pediatric Psychology 8, 33-45.

Maguire, P. (1985). The psychological impact of cancer. *British Journal of Hospital Medicine* *34*, 100-103.

Michielutte, R., & Diseker, R. A. (1982). Children's perceptions of cancer in comparison to other chronic illnesses. *Journal of Chronic Diseases* *35*, 843-852.

Morrow, G. R., Hoagland, A., & Carnrike, C. L. (1981). Social support and parental adjustment to pediatric cancer. *Journal of Consulting and Clinical Psychology* *49*, 763-765.

National Cancer Institute. (1979). *Coping with childhood cancer: A resource for health professionals*. Bethesda, Md: Department of Health and Human Services.

O'Malley, J. E., Foster, D., Koocher, G., & Slavin, L. (1980). Visible physical impairment and psychological adjustment among pediatric cancer survivors. *American Journal of Psychiatry* *137*, 94-96.

O'Malley, J. E., Koocher, G., Foster, D., & Slavin, L. (1979). Psychiatric sequelae of surviving childhood cancer. *American Journal of Orthopsychiatry* *49*, 608-616.

Pfefferbaum, B., Lindamood, M. M., & Wiley, F. M. (1977). Pediatric bone marrow transplantation: Psychosocial aspects. *American Journal of Psychiatry* *134*, 1299-1301.

Pfefferbaum, B., & Lucas, R. H. (1979). Management of acute psychologic problems in pediatric oncology. *General Hospital Psychiatry* *1*, 214-219.

Pfefferbaum-Levine, B., Copeland, D. R., Fletcher, J. M., Ried, H. L., Jaffe, N., & McKinnon, W. R. (1984). Neuropsychologic assessment of long-term survivors of childhood leukemia. *American Journal of Pediatric Hematology/Oncology* *6*, 123-128.

Schulman, J. L., & Kupst, M. J. (Eds.). (1980). *The child with cancer: Clinical approaches to psychosocial care--research in psychological aspects*. Springfield, Ill.: Charles C. Thomas.

Spiegel, D. (1985). The use of hypnosis in controlling cancer pain. *CA: A Cancer Journal for Clinicians* *35*, 221-231.

Spinetta, J. J. (1982). Behavioral and psychological research in childhood cancer. An overview. *Cancer* *50*, 1939-1943.

Spinetta, J. J., & Deasy-Spinetta, P. (Eds.). (1981). *Living with childhood cancer*. St. Louis: C.V. Mosby.

Van Dongen-Melman, J. E. W. M., & Sanders-Woudstra, J. A. (1986). Psychosocial aspects of childhood cancer: A review of the literature. *Journal of Child Psychology and Psychiatry and Allied Disciplines* *27*, 145-180.

Zeltzer, L., LeBaron, S., & Zeltzer, P. M. (1984). The effectiveness of behavioral intervention for reduction of nausea and vomiting in children and adolescents receiving chemotherapy. *Journal of Clinical Oncology* *2*, 683-690.

Zwartjes, W. J., & Zwartjes, G. (1980). The child with cancer: Clinical approaches to psychosocial care. In W. J. Zwartjes & G. Zwartjes (Eds.), *Research in psychological aspects*. Springfield, Ill.: Charles C. Thomas.

I. Death and Dying

John E. Schowalter, M.D., Section Editor

1. Overview

Betz, C. L., & Poster, E. C. (1984). Children's concepts of death: Implications for pediatric practice. Nursing Clinics of North America 19, 341-349.

Brown, L. K., & Fritz, G. K. (1988). Children's knowledge and attitudes about AIDS. Journal of the American Academy of Child and Adolescent Psychiatry 27, 504-508.

Clyman, R. I., Green, C., Rowe, J., Mikkelsen, C., & Ataide, L. (1980). Issues concerning parents after the death of their newborn. Critical Care Medicine 8, 215-218.

Eth, S., Silverstein, S., & Pynoos, R. S. (1985). Mental health consultation to a preschool following the murder of a mother and child. Hospital and Community Psychiatry 36, 73-76.

Evans, N. S. (1976). Mourning as a family secret. Journal of the American Academy of Child Psychiatry 15, 502-509.

Fischoff, J., & O'Brien, N. (1976). After the child dies. Journal of Pediatrics 88, 140-146.

Fritz, G. K., & Williams, J. R. (1988). Issues of adolescent development for survivors of childhood cancer. Journal of the American Academy of Child and Adolescent Psychiatry 27, 712-715.

Fritz, G. K., Williams, J. R., & Amylon, M. (1988). After treatment ends: Psychosocial sequelae in pediatric cancer survivors. American Journal of Orthopsychiatry 58, 552-561.

Greenham, D. E., & Lohmann, R. A. (1982). Children facing death: Recurring patterns of adaptation. Health and Social Work 7, 89-94.

Johnson, P. A. (1982). After a child's parent has died. Child Psychiatry and Human Development 12, 160-170.

Krell, R., & Rabkin, L. (1979). The effects of sibling death on the surviving child: A family perspective. Family Process 18, 471-477.

Lang, D. (1981). Death education: An integral part of school health education. Health Education 12, 38-39.

Lansdown, R., & Benjamin, G. (1985). The development of the concept of death in children aged 5-9 years. Child: Health, Care and Development 11, 13-20.

Lewis, E. (1979). Mourning by the family after a stillbirth or neonatal death. Archives of Disease in Childhood 54, 303-306.

McIntosh, N., & Eldridge, C. (1984). Neonatal death--the neglected side of neonatal care? Archives of Disease in Childhood 59, 585-587.

Naylor, A. (1982). Premature mourning and failure to mourn: Their relationship to conflict between mothers and intellectually normal children. American Journal of Orthopsychiatry 52, 679-687.

Orbach, I., Carlson, G., Feshbach, S., & Ellenberg, L. (1984). Attitudes toward life and death in suicidal, normal, and chronically ill children: An extended replication. Journal of Consulting and Clinical Psychology 52, 1020-1027.
Orbach, I., Gross, Y., Glaubman, H., & Berman, D. (1985). Children's perception of death in humans and animals as a function of age, anxiety and cognitive ability. Journal of Child Pschology and Psychiatry and Allied Disciplines 26, 453-463.
Pettle, M., & Lansdown, R. G. (1986). Adjustment to the death of a sibling. Archives of Disease in Childhood 61, 278-283.
Rait, D. S., Jacobsen, P. B., Lederberg, M. S., & Holland, J. C. (1988). Characteristics of psychiatric consultations in a pediatric cancer center. American Journal of Psychiatry 145, 363-364.
Rando, T. A. (1983). An investigation of grief and adaptation in parents whose children have died from cancer. Journal of Pediatric Psychology 8, 3-20.
Reilly, T. P., Hasazi, J. E., & Bond, L. A. (1983). Children's conceptions of death and personal mortality. Journal of Pediatric Psychology 8, 21-31.
Speece, M. W., & Brent, S. B. (1984). Children's understanding of death: A review of three components of a death concept. Child Development 55, 1671-1686.
Spinetta, J., & Maloney, J. (1975). Death anxiety in the outpatient leukemic child. Pediatrics 56, 1035-1037.
Sternlicht, M. (1980). The concept of death in preoperational retarded children. Journal of Genetic Psychology 137, 157-164.
Trent, B. (1985). Helping children cope with death. Canadian Medical Association Journal 133, 1157-1161.

2. Historical Aspects

Agee, J. (1963). A death in the family. New York: Avon.
Anthony, E. J., & Koupernik, C. J. (Eds.). (1974). The child in his family. Vol. 2. The impact of disease and death. New York: Wiley.
Anthony, S. (1972). The discovery of death in childhood and after. New York: Basic Books.
Bergman, A. B., & Schulte, C. J. A. (1967). Care of the child with cancer. Pediatrics 40, 487-546.
Binger, C. M., Ablin, A. R., Feuerstein, R. C., Kushner, J. H., Zoger, S., & Mikkelsen, C. (1969). Childhood leukemia: Emotional impact on patient and family. New England Journal of Medicine 280, 414-418.
Bowlby, J. (1960). Grief and mourning in infancy and early childhood. In R. S. Eissler, et al. (Eds.), Psychoanalytic study of the child (Vol. 15, pp. 9-52). New York: International Universities Press.
Cain, A. C., Fast, I., & Erickson, M. E. (1964). Children's disturbed reactions to the death of a sibling. American Journal of Orthopsychiatry 34, 741-752.
Evans, A. E. (1968). If a child must die. New England Journal of Medicine 278, 138-142.

Freud, A. (1960). Discussion of Dr. John Bowlby's paper. In R. S. Eissler, et al. (Eds.), Psychoanalytic study of the child (Vol. 15, pp. 53-62). New York: International Universities Press.

Freud, S. (1957). Mourning and melancholia. In E. Jones (Ed.), Collected papers. Standard edition (pp. 243-260). New York and London: Hogarth Press.

Friedman, S. B., Chodoff, P., Mason, J. W., & Hamburg, D. A. (1963). Behavioral observations on parents anticipating the death of a child. Pediatrics 32, 610-625.

Futterman, E. H., & Hoffman, I. (1970). Transient school phobia in a leukemic child. Journal of the American Academy of Child Psychiatry 9, 477-494.

Green, M. (1967). Care of the child with a long-term, life-threatening illness: Some principles of management. Pediatrics 39, 441-445.

Green, M., & Solnit, A. J. (1964). Reactions to the threatened loss of a child: A vulnerable child syndrome. Pediatric management of the dying child. Part III. Pediatrics 34, 58-66.

Griffith, J. A., Fagri, P. J., Kies, M. S., & Sinibaldi, M. R. (1974). Three medical students confront death on a pediatric ward: A case report. Journal of the American Academy of Child Psychiatry 13, 72-77.

Heuscher, J. E. (1967). Death in a fairy-tale. Diseases of the Nervous System 28, 462-468.

Karon, M., & Varnick, J. (1968). An approach to the emotional support of fatally ill children. Clinical Pediatrics 7, 274-280.

Kennell, J. H., Slyter, H., & Klaus, M. H. (1970). The mourning response of parents to the death of a newborn infant. New England Journal of Medicine 283, 344-349.

Knudson, A. G., & Natterson, J. M. (1960). Participation of parents in the hospital care of fatally ill children. Pediatrics 26, 482-490.

Koocher, G. P. (1974). Talking with children about death. American Journal of Orthopsychiatry 44, 404-411.

Lindemann, E. (1944). Symptomatology and management of acute grief. American Journal of Psychiatry 101, 141-148.

McDonald, M. (1964). A study of the reactions of nursery school children to the death of a child's mother. In R. S. Eissler, et al. (Eds.), Psychoanalytic study of the child (Vol. 19, pp. 358-376). New York: International Universities Press.

Nagera, H. (1970). Children's reactions to the death of important objects: A developmental approach. In R. S. Eissler, et al. (Eds.), Psychoanalytic study of the child (Vol. 25, pp. 360-400). New York: International Universities Press.

Ross, E. K. (1969). On death and dying. New York: Macmillan.

Schowalter, J. E. (1971). The utilization of child psychiatry on a pediatric adolescent ward. Journal of the American Academy of Child Psychiatry 10, 684-699.

Solnit, A. J., & Green, M. (1959). Psychologic considerations in the management of deaths on pediatric hospital services. I. The doctor and the child's family. Pediatrics 24, 106-112.

Vernick, J., & Karon, M. (1965). Who's afraid of death on leukemia ward? American Journal of Diseases of Children 109, 393-397.

3. Death and its Effects on Family Members

Balk, D. (1983). Effects of sibling death on teenagers. Journal of School Health 53, 14-18.

Breier, A., Kelsoe, J. R., Jr., Kirwin, P. D., Beller, S. A., Wolkowitz, O. M., & Pickar, D. (1988). Early parental loss and development of adult psychopathology. Archives of General Psychiatry 45, 987-993.

Brent, D. A. (1983). A death in the family: The pediatrician's role. Pediatrics 72, 645-651.

Burgess, A. W., & Hazelwood, R. R. (1983). Autoerotic asphyxial deaths and social network response. American Journal of Orthopsychiatry 53, 166-170.

Cohen, G. J. (1984). Children dead on arrival: Predictors of short-term family follow-up. American Journal of Emergency Medicine 2, 315-320.

Corder, B. F., Ball, B. C., Haizlip, T. M., Rollins, R., & Beaumont, R. (1976). Adolescent parricide: A comparison with other adolescent murder. American Journal of Psychiatry 133, 957-961.

Davidson, G. W. (1985). Stillbirth, neonatal death, and sudden infant death syndrome. Issues in Comprehensive Pediatric Nursing 8, 243-257.

Elizur, E., & Kaffman, M. (1982). Children's bereavement reactions following death of the father: II. Journal of the American Academy of Child Psychiatry 21, 474-480.

Lauer, M. E., Mulhern, R. K., Bohne, J. B., & Camitta, B. M. (1985). Children's perceptions of their sibling's death at home or hospital: The precursors of differential adjustment. Cancer Nursing 8, 21-27.

Lyman, R. D., Wurtele, S. K., & Wilson, D. R. (1985). Psychological effects on parents of home and hospital apnea monitoring. Journal of Pediatric Psychology 10, 439-448.

Mulhern, R. K., Lauer, M. E., & Hoffmann, R. G. (1983). Death of a child at home or in the hospital: Subsequent psychological adjustment of the family. Pediatrics 71, 743-747.

Payton, J. B., & Krocker-Tuskan, M. (1988). Children's reactions to loss of parent through violence. Journal of the American Academy of Child and Adolescent Psychiatry 27, 563-566.

Post, S. (1982). Adolescent parricide in abusive families. Child Welfare 61, 445-455.

Segal, S., Fletcher, M., & Meekison, W. G. (1986). Survey of bereaved parents. Canadian Medical Association Journal 134, 38-42.

Tennant, C. (1988). Parental loss in childhood. Archives of General Psychiatry 45, 1045-1050.

Walwork, E., & Ellison, P. H. (1985). Follow-up of families of neonates in whom life support was withdrawn. Clinical Pediatrics 24, 14-20.

Yates, T. T., & Bannard, J. R. (1988). The "haunted" child: Grief, hallucinations and family dynamics. Journal of the American Academy of Child and Adolescent Psychiatry 27, 573-581.

4. The Process of Grieving

Birtchnell, J. (1981). In search of correspondences between age at psychiatric breakdown and parental age at death--'anniversary reactions.' British Journal of Medical Psychology 54, 111-120.

Bowlby, J. (1982). Attachment and loss: Retrospect and prospect. American Journal of Orthopsychiatry 52, 664-678.

Davidson, G. W. (1985). Stillbirth, neonatal death, and sudden infant death syndrome. Issues in Comprehensive Pediatric Nursing 8, 243-257.

Dorner, S., & Atwell, J. D. (1985). Family adjustment to the early loss of a baby born with spina bifida. Developmental Medicine and Child Neurology 27, 461-466.

Elizur, E., & Kaffman, M. (1983). Factors influencing the severity of childhood bereavement reactions. American Journal of Orthopsychiatry 53, 668-676.

Evans, N. S. (1976). Mourning as a family secret. Journal of the American Academy of Child Psychiatry 15, 502-509.

Furman, E. (1983). Studies in childhood bereavement. Canadian Journal of Psychiatry 28, 241-247.

Gath, A. (1985). Parental reactions to loss and disappointment: The diagnosis of Down's syndrome. Developmental Medicine and Child Neurology 27, 392-400.

Kessler, S., Kessler, H., & Ward, P. (1984). Psychological aspects of genetic counseling. III. Management of guilt and shame. American Journal of Medical Genetics 17, 673-697.

Lewis, S. N. (1983). Maternal anxiety following bereavement by cot death and emotional security of subsequent infants. Child Psychiatry and Human Development 14, 55-61.

Mahon, E. (1985). Some aspects of separation and loss in therapy with disturbed children. American Journal of Psychoanalysis 45, 35-51.

Mandell, F., McAnulty, E., & Reece, R. M. (1980). Observations of paternal response to sudden unanticipated infant death. Pediatrics 65, 221-225.

Miles, M. S. (1985). Helping adults mourn the death of a child. Issues in Comprehensive Pediatric Nursing 8, 219-241.

Mulhern, R. K., Lauer, M. E., & Hoffmann, R. G. (1983). Death of a child at home or in the hospital: Subsequent psychological adjustment of the family. Pediatrics 71, 743-747.

Rando, T. A. (1983). An investigation of grief and adaptation in parents whose children have died from cancer. Journal of Pediatric Psychology 8, 3-20.

Roback, H. B., Roback, E., & LaBarbera, J. D. (1984). Epidemic grieving at a birthday party: A case of mass hysteria. Journal of Developmental and Behavioral Pediatrics 5, 86-89.

Schulman, J. L., & Rehm, J. L. (1983). Assisting the bereaved. Journal of Pediatrics 102, 992-998.

Weller, E. B., Weller, R. A., Fristad, M. A., Cain, S. E., & Bowers, J. M. (1988). Should children attend their parent's funeral? Journal of the American Academy of Child and Adolescent Psychiatry 27, 559-562.

5. Long-Term Bereavement in Holocaust Survivors

Fogelman, E., & Savran, B. (1980). Brief group therapy with offspring of Holocaust survivors: Leaders' reactions. American Journal of Orthopsychiatry 50, 96-108.

Freyberg, J. T. (1980). Difficulties in separation-individuation as experienced by offspring of Nazi Holocaust survivors. American Journal of Orthopsychiatry 50, 87-95.

Gay, M., & Shulman, S. (1978). Comparison of children of Holocaust survivors with children of the general population in Israel. Are children of Holocaust-survivor parents more disturbed than others? Mental Health and Society 5, 252-256.

Kappy, M. S. (1984). The longest illness. Effects of nuclear war in children. American Journal of Diseases of Children 138, 293-298.

Kestenberg, J. (1985). Child survivors of the Holocaust--40 years later: Reflections and commentary. Journal of the American Academy of Child Psychiatry 24, 408-412.

Krell, R. (1985). Child survivors of the Holocaust: 40 years later. Introduction. Journal of the American Academy of Child Psychiatry 24, 378-380.

Moskovitz, S. (1985). Longitudinal follow-up of child survivors of the Holocaust. Journal of the American Academy of Child Psychiatry 24, 401-407.

Solkoff, N. (1981). Children of the survivors of the Nazi Holocaust: A critical review of the literature. American Journal of Orthopsychiatry 51, 29-42.

6. Caring for the Dying Child

Corr, C. A., & Corr, D. M. (1985). Pediatric hospice care. Pediatrics 76, 774-780.

Duff, R. S. (1979). Guidelines for deciding care of critically ill or dying patients. Pediatrics 64, 17-23.

Jeffrey, P., & Lansdown, R. (1982). The role of the special school in the care of the dying child. Developmental Medicine and Child Neurology 24, 693-697.

LeBaron, S., & Zeltzer, L. K. (1985). The role of imagery in the treatment of dying children and adolescents. Journal of Behavioral and Developmental Pediatrics 6, 252-258.

Maisami, M., Sohmer, B. H., & Coyle, J. T. (1985). Combined use of tricyclic antidepressants and neuroleptics in the management of terminally ill children: A report on three cases. Journal of the American Academy of Child Psychiatry 24, 487-489.

Martinson, I. M. (1979). Caring for the dying child. Nursing Clinics of North America 14, 467-474.

Mulhern, R. K., Lauer, M. E., & Hoffmann, R. G. (1983). Death of a child at home or in the hospital: Subsequent psychological adjustment of the family. Pediatrics 71, 743-747.

Sack, W. H., Fritz, G., Krener, P. G., & Sprunger, L. (1984). Death and the pediatric house officer revisited. Pediatrics 73, 676-681.

Watchko, J. F. (1983). Decision making on critically ill infants by parents. American Journal of Diseases of Children 137, 795-798.

7. Psychosocial Support in Grieving

Behnke, M., Setzer, E., & Mehta, P. (1984). Death counseling and psychosocial support by physicians concerning dying children. Journal of Medical Education 59, 906-908.

Benfield, D. G., Leib, S. A., & Vollman, J. H. (1978). Grief response of parents to neonatal death and parent participation in deciding care. Pediatrics 62, 171-177.

Cohen-Sandler, R., Berman, A. L., & King, R. A. (1982). Life stress and symptomatology: Determinants of suicidal behavior in children. Journal of the American Academy of Child Psychiatry 21, 178-186.

LaRoche, C., Lalinec-Michaud, M., Engelsmann, F., Fuller, N., Copp, M., McQuade-Soldatos, L., & Azima, R. (1984). Grief reactions to perinatal death--a follow-up study. Canadian Journal of Psychiatry 29, 14-19.

Plank, E. N., & Plank, R. (1978). Children and death: As seen through the art and autobiographies. In A. Solnit, et al. (Eds.), Psychoanalytic study of the child (Vol. 33, pp. 593-620). New Haven: Yale University Press.

J. Abuse and Neglect

Arthur Green, M.D., Section Editor

1. General Issues

Adams-Tucker, C. (1982). Proximate effects of sexual abuse in childhood: A report on 28 children. American Journal of Psychiatry 139, 1252-1256.

Adams-Tucker, C. (1984a). Early treatment of child incest victims. American Journal of Psychotherapy 38, 505-516.

Adams-Tucker, C. (1984b). The unmet psychiatric needs of sexually abused youths: Referrals from a child protection agency and clinical evaluations. Journal of the American Academy of Child Psychiatry 23, 659-667.

Adams-Tucker, C. (1985). Defense mechanisms used by sexually abused children. Children Today 14, 8-12, 34.

Altemeier, W. A., O'Connor, S., Vietze, P., Sandler, H., & Sherrod, K. (1984). Prediction of child abuse: A prospective study of feasibility. Child Abuse and Neglect 8, 393-400.

Altemeier, W. A., Vietze, P. M., Sherrod, K. B., Sandler, H. M., Falsey, S., & O'Connor, S. (1979). Prediction of child maltreatment during pregnancy. Journal of the American Academy of Child Psychiatry 18, 205-218.

Anderson, S. C., & Lauderdale, M. L. (1982). Characteristics of abusive parents: A look at self-esteem. Child Abuse and Neglect 6, 285-293.

Appelbaum, A. S. (1977). Developmental retardation in infants as a concomitant of physical child abuse. Journal of Abnormal Child Psychology 5, 417-423.

Ayoub, C., & Pfeifer, D. (1979). Burns as a manifestation of child abuse and neglect. American Journal of Diseases of Children 133, 910-914.

Psychopathology: Disease and Disorder

Azar, S. T., Robinson, D. R., Hekimian, E., & Twentyman, C. T. (1984). Unrealistic expectations and problem-solving ability in maltreating and comparison mothers. Journal of Consulting and Clinical Psychology 52, 687-691.

Baker, A. W., & Duncan, S. P. (1985). Child sexual abuse: A study of prevalence in Great Britain. Child Abuse and Neglect 9, 457-467.

(1985). The battered-child syndrome by C. Henry Kempe, Frederick N. Silverman, Brandt F. Steele, William Droegemueller and Henry K. Silver. Landmark article 1962, Journal of the American Medical Association. Child Abuse and Neglect 9, 143-154.

Bauer, W. D., & Twentyman, C. T. (1985). Abusing, neglectful, and comparison mothers' responses to child-related and non-child-related stressors. Journal of Consulting and Clinical Psychology 53, 335-343.

Beal, D., Melowski, F., & Hamilton, A. (1984). A cross-validation of Paulson's discriminant function-derived scales for identifying "at risk: child-abusive parents." Suicide and Life-Threatening Behavior 14, 270-274.

Blumberg, M. L. (1981). Depression in abused and neglected children. American Journal of Psychotherapy 35, 372-355.

Bousha, D. M., & Twentyman, C. T. (1984). Mother-child interactional style in abuse, neglect, and control groups: Naturalistic observations in the home. Journal of Abnormal Psychology 93, 106-114.

Bowlby, J. (1984). Violence in the family as a disorder of the attachment and caregiving systems. American Journal of Psychoanalysis 44, 9-27, 29-31.

Bowman, E. S., Blix, S., & Coons, P. M. (1985). Multiple personality in adolescence: RElationship to incestual experiences. Journal of the American Academy of Child Psychiatry 24, 109-114.

Brooks, B. (1985). Sexually abused children and adolescent identity development. American Journal of Psychotherapy 39, 401-410.

Brown, G. W. (1983). Multiple personality disorder as perpetrator of child abuse. Child Abuse and Neglect 7, 123-126.

Burgess, A. W., Groth, A. N., & McCausland, M. P. (1981). Child sex initiation rings. American Journal of Orthopsychiatry 51, 110-119.

Burgess, A. W., McCausland, M. P., & Wolbert, W. A. (1981). Children's drawings as indicators of sexual trauma. Perspectives in Psychiatric Care 19, 50-58.

Call, J. D. (1984). Child abuse and neglect in infancy: Sources of hostility within the parent-infant dyad and disorders of attachment in infancy. Child Abuse and Neglect 8, 185-202.

Cantwell, H. B. (1983). Vaginal inspection as it relates to child sexual abuse in girls under thirteen. Child Abuse and Neglect 7, 171-176.

Carter, J. E., & McCormick, A. Q. (1983). Whiplash shaking syndrome: Retinal hemorrhages and computerized axial tomography of the brain. Child Abuse and Neglect 7, 279-286.

Chan, D. A., Salcedo, J. R., Atkins, D. M., & Ruley, E. J. (1986). Munchausen syndrome by proxy: A review and case study. Journal of Pediatric Psychology 11, 71-80.

Christoffel, K. K., Zieserl, E. J., & Chiaramonte, J. (1985). Should child abuse and neglect be considered when a child dies unexpectedly? American Journal of Diseases of Children 139, 876-880.

Cohen, F. S., & Densen-Gerber, J. (1982). A study of the relationship between child abuse and drug addiction in 178 patients: Preliminary results. Child Abuse and Neglect 6, 383-387.

Crittenden, P. M. (1985). Maltreated infants: Vulnerability and resilience. Journal of Child Pschology and Psychiatry and Allied Disciplines 26, 85-96.

De Jong, A. R. (1985). The medical evaluation of sexual abuse in children. Hospital and Community Psychiatry 36, 509-512.

De Jong, A. R., Emmett, G. A., & Hervada, A. R. (1982). Sexual abuse of children. Sex-, race-, and age-dependent variations. American Journal of Diseases of Children 136, 129-134.

Derdeyn, A. P. (1977). A case for permanent foster placement of dependent, neglected, and abused children. American Journal of Orthopsychiatry 47, 604-614.

Dietrich, K. N., Starr, R. H., & Weisfeld, G. E. (1983). Infant maltreatment: Caretaker-infant interactions and developmental consequences at different levels of parenting failure. Pediatrics 72, 532-540.

Egeland, B., & Brunnquell, D. (1979). An at-risk approach to the study of child abuse: Some preliminary findings. Journal of the American Academy of Child Psychiatry 18, 219-235.

Egeland, B., & Sroufe, L. A. (1981). Attachment and early maltreatment. Child Development 52, 44-52.

Egeland, B., Sroufe, L. A., & Erickson, M. (1983). The developmental consequence of different patterns of maltreatment. Child Abuse and Neglect 7, 459-469.

Egeland, B., & Vaughn, B. (1981). Failure of "bond formation" as a cause of abuse, neglect, and maltreatment. American Journal of Orthopsychiatry 51, 78-84.

Estroff, T. W., Herrera, C., Gaines, R., Shaffer, D., Gould, M., & Green, A. H. (1984). Maternal psychopathology and perception of child behavior in psychiatrically referred and child maltreatment families. Journal of the American Academy of Child Psychiatry 23, 649-652.

Fagan, J., & McMahon, P. P. (1984). Incipient multiple personality in children. Four cases. Journal of Nervous and Mental Disease 172, 26-36.

Fanshel, D. (1981). Decision-making under uncertainty: Foster care for abused or neglected children. American Journal of Public Health 71, 685-686.

Finkelhor, D., & Browne, A. (1985). The traumatic impact of child sexual abuse: A conceptualization. American Journal of Orthopsychiatry 55, 530-541.

Frank, Y., Zimmerman, R., & Leeds, N. M. (1985). Neurological manifestations in abused children who have been shaken. Developmental Medicine and Child Neurology 27, 312-316.

Friedrich, W. N., Tyler, J. D., & Clark, J. A. (1985). Personality and psychophysiological variables in abusive, neglectful, and low-income control mothers. Journal of Nervous and Mental Disease 173, 449-460.

Frodi, A., & Smetana, J. (1984). Abused, neglected, and nonmaltreated preschoolers' ability to discriminate emotions in others: The effects of IQ. Child Abuse and Neglect 8, 459-465.

Frodi, A. M., & Lamb, M. E. (1980). Child abusers' responses to infant smiles and cries. Child Development 51, 238-241.

Fromuth, M. E. (1986). The relationship of childhood sexual abuse with later psychological and sexual adjustment in a sample of college women. Child Abuse and Neglect 10, 5-15.

Gaensbauer, T. J., & Sands, K. (1979). Distorted affective communications in abused/neglected infants and their potential impact on caretakers. Journal of the American Academy of Child Psychiatry 18, 236-250.

George, C., & Main, M. (1979). Social interactions of young abused children: Approach, avoidance, and aggression. Child Development 50, 306-318.

Giarretto, H. (1982). A comprehensive child sexual abuse treatment program. Child Abuse and Neglect 6, 263-278.

Giblin, P. T., Starr, R. H., & Agronow, S. J. (1984). Affective behavior of abused and control children: Comparisons of parent-child interactions and the influence of home environment variables. Journal of Genetic Psychology 144, 69-82.

Gomes-Schwartz, B., Horowitz, J. M., & Sauzier, M. (1985). Severity of emotional distress among sexually abused preschool, school-age, and adolescent children. Hospital and Community Psychiatry 36, 503-508.

Goodwin, J., Cormier, L., & Owen, J. (1983). Grandfather-granddaughter incest: A trigenerational view. Child Abuse and Neglect 7, 163-170.

Green, A. H. (1976). A psychodynamic approach to the study and treatment of child-abusing parents. Journal of the American Academy of Child Psychiatry 15, 414-429.

Green, A. H. (1978a). Psychiatric treatment of abused children. Journal of the American Academy of Child Psychiatry 17, 356-371.

Green, A. H. (1978b). Psychopathology of abused children. Journal of the American Academy of Child Psychiatry 17, 92-103.

Green, A. H. (1978c). Self-destructive behavior in battered children. American Journal of Psychiatry 135, 579-582.

Green, A. H. (1979a). Child abuse and neglect. Introduction. Journal of the American Academy of Child Psychiatry 18, 201.

Green, A. H. (1979b). Child-abusing fathers. Journal of the American Academy of Child Psychiatry 18, 270-282.

Green, A. H. (1979c). Expanding psychiatry's role in child abuse treatment. Hospital and Community Psychiatry 30, 702-705.

Green, A. H. (1981). Core affective disturbance in abused children. Journal of the American Academy of Psychoanalysis 9, 435-446.

Green, A. H. (1984). Child abuse by siblings. Child Abuse and Neglect 8, 311-317.

Gruber, K. J., & Jones, R. J. (1983). Identifying determinants of risk of sexual victimization of youth: A multivariate approach. Child Abuse and Neglect 7, 17-24.

Hawkins, W. E., & Duncan, D. F. (1985). Perpetrator and family characteristics related to child abuse and neglect: Comparison of substantiated and unsubstantiated reports. Psychological Reports 56, 407-410.

Helfer, R. E. (1984). The epidemiology of child abuse and neglect. Pediatric Annals 13, 745-751.

Heller, J. R., & Derdeyn, A. P. (1979). Child custody consultation in abuse and neglect: A practical guide. Child Psychiatry and Human Development 9, 171-179.

Herrenkohl, E. C., & Herrenkohl, R. C. (1979). A comparison of abused children and their nonabused siblings. Journal of the American Academy of Child Psychiatry 18, 260-269.

Herrenkohl, E. C., Herrenkohl, R. C., Toedter, L., & Yanushefski, A. M. (1984). Recent studies in child abuse. Parent-child interactions in abusive and nonabusive families. Journal of the American Academy of Child Psychiatry 23, 641-648.

Hyman, C. A. (1977). A report on the psychological test results of battering parents. British Journal of Social and Clinical Psychology 16, 221-224.

In, P. A., & McDermott, J. F. (1976). The treatment of child abuse. Play therapy with a 4-year-old child. Journal of the American Academy of Child Psychiatry 15, 430-440.

Johnson, R. L., & Shrier, D. K. (1985). Sexual victimization of boys. Experience at adolescent medicine clinic. Journal of Adolescent Health Care 6, 372-376.

Jones, J. G., Butler, H. L., Hamilton, B., Perdue, J. D., Stern, H. P., & Woody, R. C. (1986). Munchausen syndrome by proxy. Child Abuse and Neglect 10, 33-40.

Justice, B., Calvert, A., & Justice, R. (1985). Factors mediating child abuse as a response to stress. Child Abuse and Neglect 9, 359-363.

Kempe, C. H. (1976). Approaches to preventing child abuse. The health visitors concept. American Journal of Diseases of Children 130, 941-947.

King, J. M., & Taitz, L. S. (1985). Catch up growth following abuse. Archives of Disease in Childhood 60, 1152-1154.

Koski, M. A., & Ingram, E. M. (1977). Child abuse and neglect: Effect on Bayley scale scores. Journal of Abnormal Child Psychology 5, 79-91.

Kunkel, B. E. (1983). The alienation response of children abused in out-of-home placement. Child Abuse and Neglect 7, 479-484.

LaBarbera, J. D., & Dozier, J. E. (1980). Hysterical seizures: The role of sexual exploitation. Psychosomatics 21, 897-903.

Lamphear, V. S. (1985). The impact of maltreatment on children's psychosocial adjustment: A review of the research. Child Abuse and Neglect 9, 251-263.

Lewis, D. O., Shanok, S. S., & Balla, D. A. (1979). Perinatal difficulties, head and face trauma, and child abuse in the medical histories of seriously delinquent children. American Journal of Psychiatry 136, 419-423.

Lewis, D. O., Shanok, S. S., Pincus, J. H., & Glaser, G. H. (1979). Violent juvenile delinquents: Psychiatric, neurological, psychological, and abuse factors. Journal of the American Academy of Child Psychiatry 18, 307-319.

Lynch, M. A. (1985). Child abuse before Kempe: An historical literature review. Child Abuse and Neglect 9, 7-15.

Main, M., & Goldwyn, R. (1984). Predicting rejection of her infant from mother's representation of her own experience: Implications for the abused-abusing intergenerational cycle. Child Abuse and Neglect 8, 203-217.

McCord, J. (1983). A forty year perspective on effects of child abuse and neglect. Child Abuse and Neglect 7, 265-270.

McGuire, L. S., & Wagner, N. N. (1978). Sexual dysfunction in women who were molested as children: One response pattern and suggestions for treatment. Journal of Sex and Marital Therapy 4, 11-15.

Milner, J. S., & Robertson, K. R. (1985). Development of a random response scale for the child abuse potential inventory. Journal of Clinical Psychology 41, 639-643.

Monane, M., Leichter, D., & Lewis, D. O. (1984). Physical abuse in psychiatrically hospitalized children and adolescents. Journal of the American Academy of Child Psychiatry 23, 653-658.

Money, J., Annecillo, C., & Kelley, J. F. (1983). Growth of intelligence: Failure and catch-up associated respectively with abuse and rescue in the syndrome of abuse dwarfism. Psychoneuroendocrinology 8, 309-319.

Mrazek, D. A. (1983). Long-term follow-up of an adolescent perpetrator of sexual abuse. Child Abuse and Neglect 7, 239-240.

Nelson, H. B., & Martin, C. A. (1985). Increased child abuse in twins. Child Abuse and Neglect 9, 501-515.

Oates, R. K. (1984). Personality development after physical abuse. Archives of Disease in Childhood 59, 147-150.

Oppenheimer, R., Howells, K., Palmer, R. L., & Chaloner, D. A. (1985). Adverse sexual experience in childhood and clinical eating disorders: A preliminary description. Journal of Psychiatric Research 19, 357-361.

Panton, J. H. (1979). MMPI profile configurations associated with incestuous and non-incestuous child molesting. Psychological Reports 45, 335-338.

Paperny, D. M., & Deisher, R. W. (1983). Maltreatment of adolescents: The relationship to a predisposition toward violent behavior and delinquency. Adolescence 18, 499-506.

Parish, R. A., Myers, P. A., Brandner, A., & Templin, K. H. (1985). Developmental milestones in abused children, and their improvement with a family-oriented approach to the treatment of child abuse. Child Abuse and Neglect 9, 245-250.

Pelton, L. H. (1978). Child abuse and neglect: The myth of classlessness. American Journal of Orthopsychiatry 48, 608-617.

Perlmutter, L. H., Engel, T., & Sager, C. J. (1982). The incest taboo: Loosened sexual boundaries in remarried families. Journal of Sex and Marital Therapy 8, 83-96.

Petrovich, M., & Templer, D. I. (1984). Heterosexual molestation of children who later became rapists. Psychological Reports 54, 810.

Pierce, R., & Pierce, L. H. (1985). The sexually abused child: A comparison of male and female victims. Child Abuse and Neglect 9, 191-199.

Polansky, N. A., Gaudin, J. M., Ammons, P. W., & Davis, K. B. (1985). The psychological ecology of the neglectful mother. Child Abuse and Neglect 9, 265-275.

Prodgers, A. (1984). Psychopathology of the physically abusing parent: A comparison with the borderline syndrome. Child Abuse and Neglect 8, 411-424.

Pruitt, D. L., & Erickson, M. T. (1985). The child abuse potential inventory: A study of concurrent validity. Journal of Clinical Psychology 41, 104-111.

Robertson, K. R., & Milner, J. S. (1983). Construct validity of the child abuse potential inventory. Journal of Clinical Psychology 39, 426-429.

Rogers, S., & LeUnes, A. (1979). A psychometric and behavioral comparison of delinquents who were abused as children with their non-abused peers. Journal Clinical Psychology 35, 470-472.

Rosenthal, P. A., & Doherty, M. B. (1984). Serious sibling abuse by preschool children. Journal of the American Academy of Child Psychiatry 23, 186-190.

Rossman, P. G. (1985). The aftermath of abuse and abandonment: A treatment approach for ego disturbance in female adolescence. Journal of the American Academy of Child Psychiatry 24, 345-352.

Runyan, D. K., Gould, C. L., Trost, D. C., & Loda, F. A. (1982). Determinants of foster care placement for the maltreated child. Child Abuse and Neglect 6, 343-350.

Russell, D. E. (1983). The incidence and prevalence of intrafamilial and extrafamilial sexual abuse of female children. Child Abuse and Neglect 7, 133-146.

Russell, D. E. (1984). The prevalence and seriousness of incestuous abuse: Stepfathers vs. biological fathers. Child Abuse and Neglect 8, 15-22.

Ryan, G. (1986). Annotated bibliography: Adolescent perpetrators of sexual molestation of children. Child Abuse and Neglect 10, 125-131.

Sahler, O. J. (1980). Adolescent parenting: Potential for child abuse and neglect? Pediatric Annals 9, 120-125.

Sankey, C. G., Elmer, E., Halechko, A. D., & Schulberg, P. (1985). The development of abused and high-risk infants in different treatment modalities: Residential versus in-home care. Child Abuse and Neglect 9, 237-243.

Schneider-Rosen, K., Braunwald, K. G., Carlson, V., & Cicchetti, D. (1985). Current perspectives in attachment theory: Illustration from the study of maltreated infants. Monographs of the Society for Research in Child Development (Vol. 50, pp. 194-210). Chicago: University of Chicago Press.

Schneider-Rosen, K., & Cicchetti, D. (1984). the relationship between affect and cognition in maltreated infants: Quality of attachment and the development of visual self-recognition. Child Development 55, 648-658.

Scholettle, U. C. (1980). Child exploitation: A study of child pornography. Journal of the American Academy of Child Psychiatry 19, 289-299.

Sedney, M. A., & Brooks, B. (1984). Factors associated with a history of childhood sexual experience in a nonclinical female population. Journal of the American Academy of Child Psychiatry 23, 215-218.

Shanok, S. S., & Lewis, D. O. (1981). Medical histories of abused delinquents. Child Psychiatry and Human Development 11, 222-231.

Shengold, L. (1985). The effects of child abuse as seen in adults: George Orwell. Psychoanalytic Quarterly 54, 20-45.

Shorkey, C. T., & Armendariz, J. (1985). Personal worth, self-esteem, anomia, hostility and irrational thinking of abusing mothers: A multivariate approach. Journal of Clinical Psychology 41, 414-421.

Slade, B., Steward, M. S., Morrison, T. L., & Abramowitz, S. I. (1984). Locus of control, persistence, and use of contingency information in physically abused children. Child Abuse and Neglect 8, 447-457.

Smetana, J. G., Kelly, M., & Twentyman, C. T. (1984). Abused, neglected, and nonmaltreated children's conceptions of moral and social-conventional transgressions. Child Development 55, 277-287.

Solnit, A. J. (1984). Theoretical and practical aspects of risks and vulnerabilities in infancy. Child Abuse and Neglect 8, 133-144.

Summit, R. C. (1983). The child sexual abuse accommodation syndrome. Child Abuse and Neglect 7, 177-193.

Susman, E. J., Trickett, P. K., Iannotti, R. J., Hollenbeck, B. E., & Zahn-Waxler, C. (1985). Child-rearing patterns in depressed, abusive, and normal mothers. American Journal of Orthopsychiatry 55, 237-251.

Szykula, S. A., & Fleischman, M. J. (1985). Reducing out-of-home placements of abused children: Two controlled field studies. Child Abuse and Neglect 9, 277-283.

Tarter, R. E., Hegedus, A. M., Winsten, N. E., & Alterman, A. I. (1984). Neuropsychological, personality, and familial characteristics of physically abused delinquents. Journal of the American Academy of Child Psychiatry 23, 668-674.

Waller, D. A. (1983). Obstacles to the treatment of Munchausen by proxy syndrome. Journal of the American Academy of Child Psychiatry 22, 80-85.

Webster-Stratton, C. (1985). Comparison of abusive and nonabusive families with conduct-disordered children. American Journal of Orthopsychiatry 55, 59-69.

Wharton, R., & Mandell, F. (1985). Violence on television and imitative behavior: Impact on parenting practices. Pediatrics 75, 1120-1123.

Wilbur, C. B. (1984). Multiple personality and child abuse. An overview. Psychiatric Clinics of North America 7, 3-7.

Wolfe, D. A., & Mosk, M. D. (1983). Behavioral comparisons of children from abusive and distressed families. Journal of Consulting and Clinical Psychology 51, 702-708.

Wolock, I., & Horowitz, B. (1984). Child maltreatment as a social problem: The neglect of neglect. American Journal of Orthopsychiatry 54, 530-543.

Yates, A. (1981). Narcissistic traits in certain abused children. American Journal of Orthopsychiatry 51, 55-62.

2. Families Involved in Abuse--Causes and Treatment

Ayoub, C., & Jacewitz, M. M. (1982a). Families at risk of poor parenting: A descriptive study of sixty at risk families in a model prevention program. Child Abuse and Neglect 6, 413-422.

Ayoub, C., & Jacewitz, M. M. (1982b). Families at risk of poor parenting: A model for service delivery, assessment, and intervention. Child Abuse and Neglect 6, 351-358.

Barber-Madden, R. (1983). Training day care program personnel in handling child abuse cases: Intervention and prevention outcomes. Child Abuse and Neglect 7, 25-32.

Barth, R. P., Ash, J. R., & Hacking, S. (1986). Identifying, screening and engaging high-risk clients in private non-profit child abuse prevention programs. Child Abuse and Neglect 10, 99-109.

Blythe, B. J. (1983). A critique of outcome evaluation in child abuse treatment. Child Welfare 62, 325-335.

Cohn, A. H. (1979). An evaluation of three demonstration child abuse and neglect treatment programs. Journal of the American Academy of Child Psychiatry 18, 283-291.

Conte, J. R., Rosen, C., Saperstein, L., & Shermack, R. (1985). An evaluation of a program to prevent the sexual victimization of young children. Child Abuse and Neglect 9, 319-328.

Crimmins, D. B., Bradlyn, A. S., Lawrence, S., & Kelly, J. A. (1984). A training technique for improving the parent-child interaction skills of an abusive-neglectful mother. Child Abuse and Neglect 8, 533-539.

Dale, P., & Davies, M. (1985). A model of intervention in child-abusing families: A wider systems view. Child Abuse and Neglect 9, 449-455.

Daniel, J. H., Hampton, R. L., & Newberger, E. H. (1983). Child abuse and accidents in black families: A controlled comparative study. American Journal of Orthopsychiatry 53, 645-653.

Gabinet, L. (1983). Child abuse treatment failures reveal need for redefinition of the problem. Child Abuse and Neglect 7, 395-402.

3. Prevention of Child Abuse

Garbarino, J. (1980). Changing hospital childbirth practices: A developmental perspective on prevention of child maltreatment. American Journal of Orthopsychiatry 50, 588-597.

Helfer, R. E. (1982). A review of the literature on the prevention of child abuse and neglect. Child Abuse and Neglect 6, 251-261.

Howze, D. C., & Kotch, J. B. (1984). Disentangling life events, stress and social support: Implications for the primary prevention of child abuse and neglect. Child Abuse and Neglect 8, 401-409.

Isaacs, C. D. (1982). Treatment of child abuse: A review of the behavioral interventions. Journal of Applied Behavior Analysis 15, 273-294.

Kempe, C. H. (1978). Child abuse--the pediatrician's role in child advocacy and preventive pediatrics. American Journal of Diseases of Children 132, 255-260.

Kempe, C. H. (1982). Changing approaches to treatment of child abuse and neglect. Child Abuse and Neglect 6, 491-493.

Koverola, C., Manion, I., & Wolfe, D. (1985). A microanalysis of factors associated with child-abusive families: Identifying individual treatment priorities. Behavior Research and Therapy 23, 499-506.

Lally, J. R. (1984). Three views of child neglect: Expanding visions of preventive intervention. Child Abuse and Neglect 8, 243-254.

Lealman, G. T., Haigh, D., Phillips, J. M., Stone, J., & Ord-Smith, C. (1983). Prediction and prevention of child abuse--an empty hope? Lancet 1, 1423-1424.

Long, K. A. (1986). Cultural considerations in the assessment and treatment of intrafamilial abuse. American Journal of Orthopsychiatry 56, 131-136.

Magnus, P. D. (1979). Prevention of child abuse: Pediatrician's role. Pediatrics 64, 550-551.

Martin, H. P. (1984). Intervention with infants at risk for abuse or neglect. Child Abuse and Neglect 8, 255-260.

Murphy, J. F., Jenkins, J., Newcombe, R. G., & Sibert, J. R. (1981). Objective birth data and the prediction of child abuse. Archives of Disease in Childhood 56, 295-297.

O'Connor, S., Vietze, P. M., Sherrod, K. B., Sandler, H. M., & Altemeier, W. A. (1980). Reduced incidence of parenting inadequacy following rooming-in. Pediatrics 66, 176-182.

Pawl, J. H. (1984). Strategies of intervention. Child Abuse and Neglect 8, 261-270.

Piussan, C., Pautard, J. C., Gineston, B., Lenaerts, C., Boudailliez, B., & Goldfarb, A. (1985). Long-term follow-up of abused children (apropos of 65 cases). Child Abuse and Neglect 9, 71-80.

Resnick, G. (1985). Enhancing parental competencies for high risk mothers: An evaluation of prevention effects. Child Abuse and Neglect 9, 479-489.

Rosenberg, M. S., & Reppucci, N. D. (1985). Primary prevention of child abuse. Journal of Consulting and Clinical Psychology 53, 576-585.

Rosenstein, P. J. (1978). Family outreach: A program for the prevention of child neglect and abuse. Child Welfare 57, 519-525.

Savells, J. (1983). Child abuse in residential institutions and community programs for intervention and prevention. Child Abuse and Neglect 7, 473-475.

Siegel, E., Bauman, K. E., Schaefer, E. S., Saunders, M. M., & Ingram, D. D. (1980). Hospital and home support during infancy: Impact on maternal attachment, child abuse and neglect, and health care utilization. Pediatrics 66, 183-190. .

Solnit, A. J. (1980). Child abuse: Least harmful, most protective intervention. Pediatrics 65, 170-171.

Swan, H. L., Press, A. N., & Briggs, S. L. (1985). Child sexual abuse prevention: Does it work? Child Welfare 64, 395-405.

Volpe, R. (1984). A psychoeducational program dealing with child abuse for elementary school children. Child Abuse and Neglect 8, 511-517.

Wolfe, D. A., MacPherson, T., Blount, R., & Wolfe, V. V. (1986). Evaluation of a brief intervention for education school children in awareness of physical and sexual abuse. Child Abuse and Neglect 10, 85-92.

Wolfe, D. A., Sandler, J., & Kaufman, K. (1981). A competency-based parent training program for child abusers. Journal of Consulting and Clinical Psychology 49, 633-640.

4. Child Abuse and the Law

Benedek, E. P. (1982). The role of the child psychiatrist in court cases involving child victims of sexual assault. Journal of the American Academy of Child Psychiatry 21, 519-520.

Borgman, R. (1981). Antecedents and consequences of parental rights termination for abused and neglected children. Child Welfare 60, 391-404.

Bross, D. C. (1982). Medical care neglect. Child Abuse and Neglect 6, 375-381.

Burnstein, M. H. (1981). Child abandonment: Historical, sociological and psychological perspectives. Child Psychiatry and Human Development 11, 213-221.

Craft, J. L., & Clarkson, C. D. (1985). Case disposition recommendations of attorneys and social workers in child abuse investigations. Child Abuse and Neglect 9, 165-174.

Finkelhor, D. (1983). Removing the child--prosecuting the offender in cases of sexual abuse: Evidence from the national reporting system for child abuse and neglect. Child Abuse and Neglect 7, 195-205.

Frankel, S. A. (1978). Intervention with overtly rejecting parents. A suggestion for a collaborative legal and psychiatric approach. Journal of the American Academy of Child Psychiatry 17, 498-504.

Guyer, M. J. (1982). Child abuse and neglect statutes: Legal and clinical implications. American Journal of Orthopsychiatry 52, 73-81.

Kaplan, S. J. (1981). Psychiatric consultation to attorneys for abused and neglected children. Bulletin of the American Academy of Psychiatry and the Law 9, 140-148.

Mehta, M. N. (1982). Physical abuse of abandoned children in India. Child Abuse and Neglect 6, 171-175.

Smith, S. R., & Meyer, R. G. (1984). Child abuse reporting laws and psychotherapy: A time for reconsideration. International Journal of Law and Psychiatry 7, 351-366.

Tyler, A. H. (1984). Abuse in the investigation and treatment of intrafamilial child sexual abuse. Child Abuse and Neglect 8, 47-53.

Wasserman, S., & Rosenfeld, A. (1985). Decision-making in child abuse and neglect. Bulletin of the American Academy of Psychiatry and the Law 13, 259-271.

Weiss, E. H., & Berg, R. F. (1982). Child victims of sexual assault: Impact of court procedures. Journal of the American Academy of Child Psychiatry 21, 513-518.

K. Sexual Abuse

Irving N. Berlin, M.D., Section Editor

1. Effects on the Small Child

Cahill, M. E. (1977). Sexually abused children: Fact, not fiction. Proceedings of the House of Representatives, Subcommittee on Crime. Serial #12, 95th Congress, First Session.

Finkelhor, D. (1979). Sexually victimized children. New York: The Free Press.

Finkelhor, D., et al. (1986). A source book on child sexual abuse. Beverly Hills: Sage.

Fish-Murray, C., Koby, E., & Van der Kolk, B. (1987). Evolving ideas: The effect of abuse on children's thoughts in psychological trauma. In B. Van der Kolk (Ed.), Child abuse and psychological trauma. Washington, D.C.: American Psychiatric Press.

Groth, A. N. (1982). Patterns of sexual assault against children and adolescents. In A. W. Burgess, et al. (Eds.), Sexual assault of children and adolescents (p. 15). Lexington, Mass.: Lexington Books.

Jaffe, A. C., Dynneson, L., & Ten Bensel, R. W. (1975). Sexual abuse of children: An epidemiological study. American Journal of Diseases of Children 129, 689-692.

Justice, B., & Justice, R. (1979). The broken taboo: Sex in the family. New York: Human Sciences Press.

Lourie, I. S. (1984). The locus of emotional harm in incest: The study on non-victims of incestuous families. Clinical Proceedings, Children's Hospital National Medical Center 4, 46-51.

Reinhart, M. A. (1987). Sexually abused boys. Child Abuse and Neglect 11, 229-236.

Russell, D. (1983). The incidence and prevalence of intra-familial and extra-familial sexual abuse of female children. Child Abuse and Neglect 7, 133-146.

Sgroi, S. M., Blick, L. C., & Porter, F. S. (1982). A conceptual framework for child sexual abuse. In S. M. Sgroi (Ed.), Handbook of clinical intervention in child sexual abuse. Lexington, Mass.: Lexington Books.

Weeks, R. B. (1976). The sexually exploited child. Southern Medical Journal 69, 848-850.

2. Effects on the Older Child and Adolescent

Emslie, G. H., & Rosenfeld, A. A. (1983). Incest reported by children and adolescents hospitalized for severe psychiatric problems. American Journal of Psychiatry 140, 708-711.

Lourie, I. S. (1979). Family dynamics and the abuse of adolescents. Child Abuse and Neglect 3, 967-974.

Sansonelt-Hayden, H., Hayley, G., Marniage, K., & Fini, S. (1987). Sexual abuse and psychopathology in hospitalized adolescents. Journal of the American Academy of Child and Adolescent Psychiatry 26, 753-757.

3. Long-Term Effects of Sexual Abuse

Fromuth, M. E. (1986). The relationship of childhood sexual abuse with later psychological and sexual adjustment in a sample of college women. Child Abuse and Neglect 10, 5-16.

Gelinas, D. J. (1983). The persisting negative effects of incest. Psychiatry 46, 13.

Goodwin, J. M. (1985). Post traumatic symptoms in incest victims. In S. Eth & R. S. Pynoos (Eds.), Post-traumatic stress disorder in children (pp. 157-168). Washington, D.C.: American Psychiatric Press.

Green, A. H. (1985). Children traumatized by physical abuse. In S. Eth & R. S. Pynoos (Eds.), Post-traumatic stress disorder in children (pp. 135-154). Washington, D.C.: American Psychiatric Press.

Greenspan, S. I., Lourie, R. S., & Nover, R. A. (1979). A developmental approach to the classification of psychopathology in infancy and early childhood. In N. D. Noshpitz, Basic handbook of child psychiatry. Vol. 3. New York: Basic Books.

Summit, R. C. (1983). The child abuse accommodation syndrome. Journal of Child Abuse and Neglect 7, 177-193.

4. Diagnosis and Legal Aspects of Establishing Sexual Abuse

Benedek, E. P., & Schetky, D. H. (1985). Allegations of sexual abuse in custody and visitation disputes. In D. H. Schetky & E. P. Benedek (Eds.), Emerging issues in child psychiatry and the law. New York: Brunner/Mazel.

Benedek, E. P., & Schetky, D. H. (1987a). Problems in validating allegations of sexual abuse. Part 1: Factors affecting perception and recall of events. Journal of the American Academy of Child and Adolescent Psychiatry 26, 912-915.

Benedek, E. P., & Schetky, D. H. (1987b). Problems in validating allegations of sexual abuse. Part 2: Clinical evaluation. Journal of the American Academy of Child and Adolescent Psychiatry 26, 916-921.

Borke, H. (1973). The development of empathy in Chinese and American children between three and six year of age: A cross-cultural study. Developmental Psychology 9, 102-108.

Borke, H. (1978). Piaget's view of social interaction and the theoretical construct of empathy. In L. S. Siegel & C. J. Brainerd (Eds.), Alternatives to Piaget: Critical essays on the theory. New York: Academic Press.

Brant, R. S. J. (1984). Dilemmas in court-ordered evaluation of sexual abuse charges during custody and visitation proceedings. Paper presented at the 31st Annual Meeting of the American Academy of Child Psychiatry, Toronto, Ontario, Canada.

Bresse, P., Stearns, G., Bess, B., & Packer, L. (1986). Allegations of child sexual abuse in child custody disputes: A therapeutic assessment model. American Journal of Orthopsychiatry 56, 560-576.

Brown, A. L. (1975). The development of memory: Knowing about and knowing how to know. In H. W. Teese (Ed.), Advances in child development and behavior (Vol. 10, pp. 103-152). New York: Academic Press.

Bulkley, J. (1981). Child sexual abuse and the law. Washington, D.C.: American Bar Association.

Burgess, A. W., Holmstrom, L. L., & McCausland, M. P. (1978). Counseling young victims and their families. In A. W. Burgess, A. N. Groth, L. L. Holmstrom, & S. M. Sgroi (Eds.), Sexual assault of children and adolescents. Lexington, Mass.: Lexington Books.

Cantwell, H. (1981). Vaginal inspection as it related to child sexual abuse in girls under thirteen. Child Abuse and Neglect 7, 171-176.

Chance, J. E., & Goldstein, A. C. (1984). Face-recognition memory: Implications for children's eyewitness testimony. Journal of Social Issues 40, 69-85.

Cohen, R., & Harnick, M. S. (1980). The susceptibility of the child witness to suggestion. Law and Human Behavior 4, 201-210.

Dale, P. S., Loftus, E. F., & Rathburn, E. (1978). The influence of the form of the question on the eyewitness testimony of preschool children. Journal of Psycholinguist Research 7, 269-277.

Dejong, A. R. (1985). The medical evaluation of sexual abuse in children. Hospital and Community Psychiatry 36, 509-512.

Finkel, M. (1988). The medical evaluation of sexual abuse. In D. Schetky & A. Green (Eds.), Child sexual abuse: A guide for health care and legal professionals. New York: Brunner/Mazel.

Goodman, G. S. (1984). The child witness: Conclusions and future directions for research and legal practice. Journal of Social Issues 40, 157.

Graham, M. H. (1985). Indicia of reliability and face-to-face confrontation: Emerging issues in child sexual abuse prosecuting. University of Miami Law Review 40, 19-95.

Green, A. H. (1986a). Did he or didn't he? True and false allegations of sexual abuse in child custody disputes. Journal of the American Academy of Child Psychiatry 25, 449-457.

Green, A. H. (1986b). True and false allegations of sexual abuse in child custody disputes. Journal of the American Academy of Child and Adolescent Psychiatry 25, 449-456.

Groth, A. N. (1979). Men who rape: The psychology of the offender. New York: Plenum Press.

Hibbard, R. A., Roghmann, K., & Hoekelman, R. A. (1987). Genitalia in children's drawings: An association with sexual abuse. Pediatrics 79, 129-137.

Jampole, L., & Weber, M. K. (1987). An assessment of the behavior of sexually abused and nonsexually abused children with anatomically correct dolls. Child Abuse and Neglect 11, 187-192.

Johnson, M. K., & Foley, M. A. (1984). Differentiating fact from fantasy: The reliability of children's memories. Journal of Social Issues 40, 33-50.

Neisser, U. (1984). The control of information pickup in selective looking. In A. D. Pick (Ed.), Perception and its development: A tribute to Eleanor Gibson (pp. 201-219). Hillsdale, N.J.: Erlbaum.

Packard, W. S., & Rosner, R. (1985). Psychiatric evaluation of sex offenders. Journal of Forensic Sciences 30, 715-720.

Riskind, J. H., Beck, A. T., Berchick, R. J., Brown, G., & Steer, R. A. (1987). Reliability of DSM-III diagnoses for major depression and generalized anxiety disorder using the SCID. Archives of General Psychiatry 44, 817-820.

Rosenfeld, A., Bailey, R., Siegel, B., & Bailey, G. (1986). Determining incestuous contact between parent and child: Frequency of children touching parents' genitals in a nonclinical population. Journal of the American Academy of Child Psychiatry 25, 481-485.

Schetky, D. H., et al. (1987). Proposed standards for the evaluation of sexually abused children. Washington, D.C.: American Academy of Child and Adolescent Psychiatry.

Schuman, D. (1984). False accusation of physical and sexual abuse. Bulletin of the American Academy of Psychiatry and the Law 14, 5-21.

Sgroi, S. M. (1978). Comprehensive examination for child sexual assault: Diagnostic, therapeutic, and child protection issues. In A. W. Burgess, A. N. Groth, L. L. Holmstrom, & S. M. Sgroi (Eds.), Sexual assault of children and adolescents. Lexington, Mass.: Lexington Books.

Terr, L. (1980). The child as a witness. In E. P. Benedek & D. H. Schetky (Eds.), Child psychiatry and the law. New York: Brunner/Mazel.

White, S., Strom, G., Santill, G., & Halpin, B. (1986). Interviewing young sexual abuse victims with anatomically correct dolls. Child Abuse and Neglect 10, 519-529.

Yates, A. A., Beutler, L., & Crago, M. (1985). Drawings by child victims of abuse. Child Abuse and Neglect 9, 183-189.

Yates, A. A., & Terr, L. (1988). Debate: Anatomically correct dolls: Should they be used as the basis for expert testimony. Journal of the American Academy of Child and Adolescent Psychiatry 27, 2-3, 254-257, 387-388.

5. Characteristics of the Sexual Abuser

Becker, J. V., Rathner, J., & Kaplan, M. (1987). Adolescent sexual offenders: Demographics, criminal and sexual histories, and recommendations for reducing future offenses. Journal of Interpersonal Violence 1, 431-445.

Fehrenbach, P. A., Smith, W., Monastersky, C., & Beisher, R. W. (1986). Adolescent sex offenders: Offender and offense characteristics. American Journal of Orthopsychiatry 56, 225-233.

Giarretto, H., Giarretto, A., & Sgroi, S. M. (1978). Coordinated community treatment of incest. In A. W. Burgess, A. N. Groth, L. L. Holmstrom, & S. M.

Sgroi (Eds.), Sexual assault of children and adolescents (pp. 231-240). Lexington, Mass.: Lexington Books.

Groth, A. N. (1977). The adolescent sexual offender and his prey. International Journal of Offender Therapy and Comparative Criminology 21, 249-345.

Groth, A. N. (1982). The incest offender. In S. M. Sgroi (Ed.), Handbook of clinical intervention in child sexual abuse (pp. 214-240). Lexington, Mass.: Lexington Books.

Kavoussi, R. J., Kaplan, M., & Becker, J. J. (1988). Psychiatric diagnosis in adolescent sex offenders. Journal of the American Academy of Child and Adolescent Psychiatry 27, 241-243.

Lewis, D. O., Shanok, S. S., & Pincus, J. H. (1979). Juvenile male sexual assaulters. American Journal of Psychiatry 139, 1194-1196.

McManus, M., Alessi, N. E., Grapentime, W. L., & Brickman, A. (1984). Psychiatric disturbance in serious delinquents. Journal of the American Academy of Child and Adolescent Psychiatry 23, 602-615.

Ryan, G. (1986). Annotated bibliography: Adolescent perpetrators and sexual molestation of children. Child Abuse and Neglect 10, 125-132.

Tinklenberg, J. R., Murphy, P., Murphy, P. L., & Pefferbaum, A. (1981). Drugs and criminal assaults by adolescents: A replication study. Journal of Psychoactive Drugs 13, 277-287.

Vinogradov, S., Dishotsky, N. I., Doty, A. K., & Tinklenberg, J. R. (1988). Patterns of behavior in adolescent rape. American Journal of Orthopsychiatry 58(2), 179-187.

6. Multiple Personality

Erickson, M. H. (1980). The clinical discovery of a dual personality. In E. L. Rossi (Ed.), The collected papers of Milton H. Erickson (Vol. 3, pp. 261-270). New York: Irvington.

Fagan, J., & McMahon, P. (1984). Incipient multiple personality in children. Four cases. Journal of Nervous and Mental Disease 172, 26-36.

Goodwin, J. M. (1985). Credibility problems in multiple personality disorder patients and abused children. In R. P. Kluft (Ed.), Childhood antecedents of multiple personality (pp. 2-19). Washington, D. C.: American Psychiatric Press.

Greaves, G. B. (1980). Multiple personality: 165 years after Mary Reynolds. Journal of Nervous and Mental Disease 168, 577-596.

Horwitz, R. P., & Braun, B. G. (1984). Are multiple personality disorders borderline? Psychiatric Clinics of North America 7, 69-87.

Khan, M. (1967). The concept of cumulative trauma. In R. S. Eissler, et al. (Eds.), Psychoanalytic study of the child (Vol. 18, pp. 54-88). New York: International Universities Press.

Kluft, R. P. (1984a). Aspects of the treatment of multiple personality disorder. Psychiatric Annals 14, 51-55.

Kluft, R. P. (1984b). Multiple personality in childhood. Psychiatric Clinics of North America 7, 121-134.

Kluft, R. P. (1984c). Treatment of multiple personality disorder. Psychiatric Clinics of North America 7, 9-28.

Kluft, R. P. (1985). Childhood multiple personality disorder: Predictors, clinical findings and treatment results. In R. P. Kluft (Ed.), Childhood antecedents of multiple personality. Washington, D.C.: American Psychiatric Press.

Kluft, R. P. (1986). Treating children who have multiple personality disorder. In B. G. Braun (Ed.), Treatment of multiple personality disorder (pp. 81-105). Washington, D.C.: American Psychiatric Press.

Putnam, F. (1987). The diagnosis and treatment of multiple personality disorder. New York: Guilford Press.

Putnam, F. W., Guroff, J. J., Silberman, E. K., et al. (1986). The clinical phenomenology of multiple personality disorder: 100 recent cases. Journal of Clinical Psychiatry 47, 285-293.

Spiegel, D. (1984). Multiple personality as a post traumatic stress disorder. Psychiatric Clinics of North America 7, 101-110.

Stern, C. R. (1984). The etiology of multiple personalities. Psychiatric Clinics of North America 7, 149-160.

Wilbur, C. B. (1984). Multiple personality and child abuse. Psychiatric Clinics of North America 7, 3-8.

7. Treatment of the Sexually Abused and Family

Adams-Tucker, C. (1984). Early treatment of child incest victims. American Journal of Psychotherapy 38, 505-516.

Anderson, L., & Shafer, G. (1979). The character disordered family: A community treatment model for family sexual abuse. American Journal of Orthopsychiatry 10, 436-445.

Becker, J. V., Kaplan, M., & Kavoussi, R. K. (1989). Measuring the effectiveness of treatment for the aggressive adolescent sex offender. Annals of the New York Academy of Sciences 227, 67-80.

Berliner, L., & Stevens, D. (1982). Clinical issues in child sexual abuse. In J. Contee & D. Shore (Eds.), Social work and child sexual abuse (pp. 93-108). New York: Haworth Press.

Brownell, K., & Barlow, D. (1976). Measurement and treatment of two sexual deviations in one person. Journal of Behavior Therapy and Experimental Psychiatry 7, 349-354.

Burgess, A. W., Holmstrom, L. L., & McCausland, M. P. (1978). Counseling young victims and their families. In A. W. Burgess, A. N. Groth, L. L. Holmstrom, & S. M. Sgroi (Eds.), Sexual assault of children and adolescents (pp. 181-204). Lexington, Mass.: Lexington Books.

Jones, D. H. (1986). Individual psychotherapy for the sexually abused child. Child Abuse and Neglect 10, 377-386.

Giarretto, H., Giarretto, A., & Sgroi, S. M. (1978). Coordinated community treatment of incest. In A. W. Burgess, A. N. Groth, L. L. Holmstrom, & S. M.

Sgroi (Eds.), Sexual assault of children and adolescents (pp. 231-240). Lexington, Mass.: Lexington Books.

Karpel, M. A. (1980). Family secrets: I. Conceptual and ethical issues in the relational concept: II. Ethical and practical considerations in therapeutic management. Family Process 19, 295.

Naitove, C. E. (1982). Arts therapy with sexually abused children. In S. M. Sgroi (Ed.), Handbook of clinical intervention in child sexual abuse. Lexington, Mass.: Lexington Books.

Porter, F. S., Blick, L. C., & Sgroi, S. M. (1982). Treatment of the sexually abused child. In S. M. Sgroi (Ed.), Handbook of clinical intervention in child sexual abuse. Lexington, Mass.: Lexington Books.

Sgroi, S. M. (Ed.). (1982). Handbook of clinical intervention in child sexual abuse. Lexington, Mass.: Lexington Books.

8. Treatment of the Abuser and Family

Abel, G. G., Mittelman, M., & Becker, J. V. (1985). Sex offenders: Results of assessment and recommendations for treatment. In S. Ben-Aron, S. Hucker, & C. Webster (Eds.), Clinical criminology: Current concepts (pp. 191-205). Toronto: M and M Graphics.

Berlin, F. S., & Meinecke, C. F. (1981). Treatment of sex offenders with antiandrogenic medication: Conceptualization, review of treatment modalities and preliminary findings. American Journal of Psychiatry 138, 601-607.

Bradford, J. M. (1985). Organic treatments for the male sexual offender. Behavioral Sciences and the Law 3, 355-375.

Knopp, F. H. (1986). Report on nationwide survey of juvenile and adult sex offender treatment programs and providers. New York: Safer Society Press.

Marshall, W. L. (1973). The modification of sexual fantasies: A combined treatment approach to the reduction of deviant sexual behavior. Behavior and Research Therapy 11, 557-564.

Marshall, W. L., & Barbaree, H. E. (1978). The reduction of deviant arousal: Satiation treatment for sexual aggressors. Criminal Justice Behavior 5, 294-303.

Smets, A. C., & Cebula, D. E. (1987). A group treatment program for adolescent sex offenders: Five steps toward resolution. Child Abuse and Neglect 11, 247-254.

Sgroi, S. M. (1982a). An approach to case management. In S. M. Sgroi (Ed.), Handbook of clinical intervention in child sexual abuse. Lexington, Mass.: Lexington Books.

Sgroi, S. M. (1982b). Family treatment. In S. M. Sgroi (Ed.), Handbook of clinical intervention in child sexual abuse. Lexington, Mass.: Lexington Books.

Silver, S. (1976). Outpatient treatment for sexual offenders. Social Work 21, 134-140.

Stember, C. J. (1980). Art therapy: A new use in the diagnosis and treatment of sexually abused children. In K. MacFarlane (Ed.), Sexual abuse of children:

Selected readings. Washington, D.C.: National Center on Child Abuse and Neglect.

Summit R. (1978). Sexual abuse, the psychotherapist and the team concept. In A. H. Green (Ed.), Dealing with sexual child abuse. Vol. 2. Chicago: National Committee for the Prevention of Child Abuse.

9. Books for Children and Parents on Sexual Abuse

Adams, C., & Fay, J. (1981). No more secrets: Protecting your child from sexual assault. San Luis Obispo, Calif.: Impact Publishers.

Bassett, K. (1980). My very own special body book. Redding, Calif.: Hawthorne.

Krause, E. (1983a). For Pete's sake, tell! Second in a series of books for parents to help children avoid sexual abuse. Oregon City, Oreg.: Krause House.

Krause, E. (1983b). Speak up, say no. A book for adults to help children avoid sexual abuse. Oregon City, Oreg.: Krause House.

Loontjens, L. (1984). Talking to children/talking to parents about sexual assault. Santa Cruz, Calif.: Network.

L. Child Psychosis and Autism

Peter E. Tanguay, M.D., Section Editor

1. Historical Review of Childhood Schizophrenia and Autism

Bateson, G., Jackson, D. D., Haley, J., & Weakland, J. (1956). Toward a theory of schizophrenia. Behavioral Science 1, 251-264.

Bender, L. (1942). Childhood schizophrenia. Nervous Child 1, 138-140.

Bender, L. (1947). Childhood schizophrenia: Clinical study of one hundred schizophrenic children. American Journal of Orthopsychiatry 17, 40-56.

Bender, L. (1973). The life course of children with schizophrenia. American Journal of Psychiatry 130, 783-786.

Bergman, P., & Escalona, S. K. (1949). Unusual sensitivities in very young children. In R. S. Eissler, et al. (Eds.), Psychoanalytic study of the child (Vol. 3/4, pp. 333-352). New York: International Universities Press.

Berlin, I. N., & Szurek, S. A. (1973). Parental blame: An obstacle in psychotherapeutic work with schizophrenic children and their families. In S. A. Szurek & I. N. Berlin (Eds.), Clinical studies in childhood psychoses (pp. 115-126). New York: Brunner/Mazel.

Bettelheim, B. (1967). The empty fortress: Infantile autism and the birth of the self. New York: The Free Press.

Bowlby, J. (1969). Attachment and loss. Vol. 1. Attachment. New York: Basic Books.

Bradley, C. (1941). Schizophrenia in childhood. New York: Macmillan.

Bradley, C. (1942). Biography of a schizophrenic child. Nervous Child 1, 141-171.

Creak, M. (1964). Schizophrenic syndrome in childhood: Further progress report of a working party. Developmental Medicine and Child Neurology 6, 530-535.

Creak, M., & Ini, S. (1960). Families of psychotic children. Journal of Child Psychology and Psychiatry and Allied Disciplines 1, 156-175.

Despert, J. L. (1938). Schizophrenia in children. Psychiatric Quarterly 12, 366-371.

Despert, J. L. (1965). The emotionally disturbed child--then and now. New York: Vantage Press.

Ekstein, R. (1966). Children of time and space, of action and impulse. New York: Appleton-Century-Crofts.

Ekstein, R., & Wallerstein, J. (1954). Observations on the psychology of borderline and psychotic children. In R. S. Eissler, et al. (Eds.), Psychoanalytic study of the child (Vol. 9, pp. 344-369). New York: International Universities Press.

Fish, B. (1959). Longitudinal observations of biological deviations in a schizophrenic infant. American Journal of Psychiatry 116, 25-31.

Fish, B. (1966). The prediction of schizophrenia in infancy: II. A ten-year follow-up report of predictions made at one month of age. Proceedings of the American Psychopathological Association 54, 335-353.

Fish, B., & Hagin, R. (1973). Visual-motor disorders in infants at risk for schizophrenia. Archives of General Psychiatry 28, 900-904.

Fish, B., Shapiro, T., Campbell, M., & Wile, R. (1968). A classification of schizophrenic children under five years. American Journal of Psychiatry 124, 1415-1423.

Fish, B., Shapiro, T., Halpern, F., & Wile, R. (1965). The prediction of schizophrenia in infancy: III. A ten-year follow-up report of neurological and psychological development. American Journal of Psychiatry 121, 768-775.

Goldfarb, W. (1961). Childhood schizophrenia. Cambridge: Harvard University Press.

Hermelin, B. (1966). Recent psychological research. In J. K. Wing (Ed.), Early childhood autism: Clinical, educational and social aspects (pp. 159-173). Oxford: Pergamon Press.

Kanner, L. (1943). Autistic disturbances of affective contact. Nervous Child 2, 217-250.

Kolvin, I. (1971). Studies in the childhood psychoses. I. Diagnostic criteria and classification. British Journal of Psychiatry 118, 381-384.

Kolvin, I., Garside, R. F., & Kidd, J. S. H. (1971). Studies in the childhood psychoses. IV. Parental personality and attitude and childhood psychoses. British Journal of Psychiatry 118, 403-406.

Kolvin, I., Humphrey, M., & McNay, A. (1971). Studies in the childhood psychoses. British Journal of Psychiatry 118, 415-419.

Kolvin, I., Ounsted, C., Humphrey, M., & McNay, A. (1971). Studies in the childhood psychoses. II. The phenomenology of childhood psychoses. British Journal of Psychiatry 118, 385-395.

Kolvin, I., Ounsted, C., Richardson, L. M., & Garside, R. F. (1971). Studies in the childhood psychoses. III. The family and social background in childhood psychoses. British Journal of Psychiatry 118, 396-402.

Kolvin, I., Ounsted, C., & Roth, M. (1971). Studies in the childhood psychoses. V. Cerebral dysfunction and childhood psychoses. British Journal of Psychiatry 118, 407-414.

Kysar, J. E. (1968). The two camps in child psychiatry: A report from a psychiatrist-father of an autistic and retarded child. American Journal of Psychiatry 125, 103-109.

Lotter, V. (1966). Epidemiology of autistic conditions in young children. I. Prevalence. Social Psychiatry 1, 124-137.

Mahler, M. S. (1952). On childhood psychosis and schizophrenia: Autistic and symbiotic infantile psychoses. In R. S. Eissler, et al. (Eds.), Psychoanalytic study of the child (Vol. 7, pp. 286-305). New York: International Universities Press.

Mahler, M. S. (1963). Thoughts about development and individuation. In R. S. Eissler, et al. (Eds.), Psychoanalytic study of the child (Vol. 18, pp. 307-324). New York: International Universities Press.

Mahler, M. S. (1965). On early infantile psychosis: The symbiotic and autistic syndromes. Journal of the American Academy of Child Psychiatry 4, 554-568.

Ornitz, E. M., & Ritvo, E. R. (1968). Perceptual inconstancy in early infantile autism: The syndrome of early infant autism and its variants including certain cases of childhood schizophrenia. Archives of General Psychiatry 18, 76-98.

Potter, H. W. (1933). Schizophrenia in children. American Journal of Psychiatry 89, 1253-1270.

Rimland, B. (1964). Infantile autism: The syndrome and its implications for a neural theory of behavior. New York: Appleton-Century-Crofts.

Rutter, M. (1968). Concepts of autism: A review of research. Journal of Child Psychology and Psychiatry and Allied Disciplines 9, 1-25.

Rutter, M. (1969). A tri-axial classification of mental disorders in childhood: An international study. Journal of Child Psychology and Psychiatry and Allied Disciplines 10, 41-61.

Rutter, M. (1972). Childhood schizophrenia reconsidered. Journal of Autism and Childhood Schizophrenia 2, 315-337.

Rutter, M., Greenfield, D., & Lockyer, L. (1967). A five to fifteen year follow-up study of infantile psychosis. II. Social and behavioural outcome. British Journal of Psychiatry 113, 1183-1189.

Rutter, M., & Lockyer, L. (1967). A five to fifteen year follow-up study of infantile psychosis. I. Description of sample. British Journal of Psychiatry 113, 1169-1182.

Schopler, E., & Reichler, R. J. (1972). How well do parents understand their own psychotic child. Journal of Autism and Childhood Schizophrenia 2, 387-400.

Schou, M. (1959). Lithium in psychiatric therapy: Stock-taking after ten years. Psychopharmacologia 1, 65-78.

Shapiro, T., Fish, B., & Ginsberg, G. L. (1972). The speech of a schizophrenic child from two to six. American Journal of Psychiatry 128, 1408-1413.

Spitz, R. A. (1945). Hospitalism. An inquiry into the genesis of psychiatric conditions in early childhood. In R. S. Eissler, et al. (Eds.), Psychoanalytic study of the child (Vol. 1, pp. 53-74). New York: International Universities Press.

Vaillant, G. E. (1962). John Haslam on early infantile autism. American Journal of Psychiatry 119, 376.

Wing, J. K. (1966). Diagnosis, epidemiology, etiology. In J. K. Wing (Ed.), Early childhood autism: Clinical, educational and social aspects (pp. 3-49). Oxford: Pergamon Press.

Wing, L. (1971). Autistic children. London: Constable.

Wing, L. (1972). Autistic children: A guide for parents and professionals. New York: Brunner/Mazel.

2. Etiologic Factors in Autism and Childhood Psychosis

Aarkrog, T., & Mortensen, K. V. (1985). Schizophrenia in early adolescence. A study illustrated by long-term cases. Acta Psychiatrica Scandinavica 72, 422-429.

Bartak, L., & Rutter, M. (1976). Differences between mentally retarded and normally intelligent autistic children. Journal of Autism and Childhood Schizophrenia 6, 109-120.

Bartak, L., Rutter, M., & Cox, A. (1977). A comparative study of infantile autism and specific developmental receptive language disorders. III. Discriminant function analysis. Journal of Autism and Childhood Schizophrenia 7, 383-396.

Beitchman, J. H. (1983). Childhood schizophrenia: A review and comparison with adult onset schizophrenia. Psychiatric Journal of the University of Ottawa 8, 25-37.

Beitchman, J. H. (1985). Childhood schizophrenia. A review and comparison with adult-onset schizophrenia. Psychiatric Clinics of North America 8, 793-814.

Campbell, M., Hardesty, A. S., Breuer, H., & Polevoy, N. (1978). Childhood psychosis in perspective. A follow-up of 10 children. Journal of the American Academy of Child Psychiatry 17, 14-28.

Campbell, M., Rosenbloom, S., Perry, R., George, A. E., Kricheff, I. I., Anderson, L., Small, A. M., & Jennings, S. J. (1982). Computerized axial tomography in young autistic children. American Journal of Psychiatry 139, 510-512.

Cantor, S., Evans, J., Pearce, J., & Pezzot-Pearce, T. (1982). Computerized axial tomography in young autistic children. American Journal of Psychiatry 139, 758-762.

Caparulo, B. K., Cohen, D. J., Rothman, S. L., Young, J. G., Katz, J. D., Shaywitz, S. E., & Shaywitz, B. A. (1981). Computed tomographic brain scanning in children with developmental neuropsychiatric disorders. Journal of the American Academy of Child Psychiatry 20, 338-357.

Cohen, D. J., Caparulo, B. K., Gold, J. R., Waldo, M. C., Shaywitz, B. A., Ruttenberg, B. A., & Rimland, B. (1978). Agreement in diagnosis: Clinical assessment and behavior rating scales for pervasively disturbed children. Journal of the American Academy of Child Psychiatry 17, 589-603.

Dawson, G. (1983). Lateralized brain dysfunction in autism: Evidence from the Halstead-Reitan neuropsychological battery. Journal of Autism and Developmental Disorders 13, 269-286.

DeMyer, M. K. (1975). The nature of the neuropsychological disability in autistic children. Journal of Autism and Childhood Schizophrenia 5, 109-128.

Eggers, C. (1982). Psychoses in childhood and adolescence. Acta Paedopsychiatrica 48, 81-98.

Freeman, B. J., & Ritvo, E. R. (1984). The syndrome of autism: Establishing the diagnosis and principles of management. Pediatric Annals 13, 284-290, 294-296.

Freeman, B. J., Ritvo, E. R., Tonick, I., Guthrie, D., & Schroth, P. (1981). Behavior observation system for autism: Analysis of behaviors among autistic, mentally retarded, and normal children. Psychological Reports 49, 199-208.

Gillberg, C. (1984). Autistic children growing up: Problems during puberty and adolescence. Developmental Medicine and Child Neurology 26, 125-129.

Green, W. H., Campbell, M., Hardesty, A. S., Grega, D. M., Padron-Gayol, M., Shell, J., & Erlenmeyer-Kimling, L. (1984). A comparison of schizophrenic and autistic children. Journal of the American Academy of Child Psychiatry 23, 399-409.

Harcherik, D. F., Cohen, D. J., Ort, S., Paul, R., Shaywitz, B. A., Volkmar, F. R., Rothman, S. L., & Leckman, J. F. (1985). Computed tomographic brain scanning in four neuropsychiatric disorders of childhood. American Journal of Psychiatry 142, 731-734.

Hertzig, M. E., & Walker, H. A. (1975). Symptom formation as an expression of disordered information processing in schizophrenic children. Journal of Autism and Childhood Schizophrenia 5, 13-24.

Howells, J. G., & Guirguis, W. R. (1984). Childhood schizophrenia 20 years later. Archives of General Psychiatry 41, 123-128.

Lotter, V. (1974). Factors related to outcome in autistic children. Journal of Autism and Childhood Schizophrenia 4, 263-277.

Massie, H. N. (1978). The early natural history of childhood psychosis. Ten cases studied by analysis of family home movies of the infancies of the children. Journal of the American Academy of Child Psychiatry 17, 29-45.

Ornitz, E. M., & Ritvo, E. R. (1976). The syndrome of autism: A critical review. American Journal of Psychiatry 133, 609-621.

Parks, S. L. (1983). The assessment of autistic children: A selective review of available instruments. Journal of Autism and Developmental Disorders 13, 255-267.

Petty, L. K., Ornitz, E. M., Michelman, J. D., & Zimmerman, E. G. (1984). Autistic children who become schizophrenic. Archives of General Psychiatry 41, 129-135.

Prizant, B. M., & Rydell, P. J. (1984). Analysis of functions of delayed echolalia in autistic children. Journal of Speech and Hearing Research 27, 183-192.

Rutter, M. (1978). Diagnosis and definition of childhood autism. Journal of Autism and Childhood Schizophrenia 8, 139-161.

Schopler, E. (1982). Evolution in understanding and treatment of autism. Triangle 21, 51-57.

Sherman, M., Shapiro, T., & Glassman, M. (1983). Play and language in developmentally disordered preschoolers: A new approach to classification. Journal of the American Academy of Child Psychiatry 22, 511-524.

Wing, L. (1981). Asperger's syndrome: A clinical account. Psychological Medicine 11, 115-129.

Zappella, M. (1985). Rett syndrome: A significant proportion of girls affected by autistic behavior. Brain and Development 7, 307-312.

3. Diagnostic Factors in Autism and Childhood Psychosis

Cantwell, D. P., Baker, L., & Rutter, M. (1977). Families of autistic and dysphasic children. II. Mothers' speech to the children. Journal of Autism and Childhood Schizophrenia 7, 313-327.

Chess, S. (1977). Follow-up report on autism in congenital rubella. Journal of Autism and Childhood Schizophrenia 7, 69-81.

Maurer, R. G., & Damasio, A. R. (1982). Childhood autism from the point of view of behavioral neurology. Journal of Autism and Developmental Disorders 12, 195-205.

Stubbs, E. G., Ash, E., & Williams, C. P. (1984). Autism and congenital cytomegalovirus. Journal of Autism and Developmental Disorders 14, 183-189.

Wing, L., & Ricks, D. M. (1976). The aetiology of childhood autism: A criticism of the Tinbergen's ethological theory. Psychological Medicine 6, 533-543.

4. Genetic and Environmental Factors

August, G. J., & Lockhart, L. H. (1984). Familial autism and the fragile-X chromosome. Journal of Autism and Developmental Disorders 14, 197-204.

Erlenmeyer-Kimling, L., & Cornblatt, B. (1984). Biobehavioral risk factors in children of schizophrenic parents. Journal of Autism and Developmental Disorders 14, 357-374.

Folstein, S., & Rutter, M. (1977). Infantile autism: A genetic study of 21 twin pairs. Journal of Child Psychology and Psychiatry and Allied Disciplines 18, 297-321.

Garmezy, N. (1974). Children at risk: The search for the antecedents of schizophrenia. Part II: Ongoing research programs, issues, and intervention. Schizophrenia Bulletin 1, 55-125.

Garmezy, N., & Streitman, S. (1974). Children at risk: The search for the antecedents of schizophrenia. Part I: Conceptual models and research methods. Schizophrenia Bulletin 1, 14-90.

Gillberg, C., & Wahlstrom, J. (1985). Chromosome abnormalities in infantile autism and other childhood psychoses: A population study of 66 cases. Developmental Medicine and Child Neurology 27, 293-304.

Goldfarb, W., Spitzer, R. L., & Endicott, J. (1976). A study of psychopathology of parents of psychotic children by structured interview. Journal of Autism and Childhood Schizophrenia 6, 327-338.

Goldstein, M. J., & Doane, J. A. (1982). Family factors in the onset, course, and treatment of schizophrenic spectrum disorders: An update on current research. Journal of Nervous and Mental Disease 170, 692-700.

Hagerman, R. J., Jackson, A. W., Levitas, A., Rimland, B., & Braden, M. (1986). An analysis of autism in fifty males with the fragile X syndrome. American Journal of Medical Genetics 23, 359-374.

Harvey, P. D., Weintraub, S., & Neale, J. M. (1982). Speech competence of children vulnerable to psychopathology. Journal of Abnormal Child Psychology 10, 373-387.

Koegel, R. L., Schreibman, L., O'Neill, R. E., & Burke, J. C. (1983). The personality and family-interaction characteristics of parents of autistic children. Journal of Consulting and Clinical Psychology 51, 683-692.

Marcus, J., Hans, S. L., Byhouwer, B., & Norem, J. (1985). Relationships among neurological functioning, intelligence quotients, and physical anomalies. Schizophrenia Bulletin 11, 101-108.

Marcus, J., Hans, S. L., Mednick, S. A., Schulsinger, F., & Michelsen, N. (1985). Neurological dysfunctioning in offspring of schizophrenics in Israel and Denmark. A replication analysis. Archives of General Psychiatry 42, 753-761.

Minton, J., Campbell, M., Green, W. H., Jennings, S., & Samit, C. (1982). Cognitive assessment of siblings of autistic children. Journal of the American Academy of Child Psychiatry 21, 256-261.

Neuchterlein, K. H. (1986). Childhood precursors of adult schizophrenia. Journal of Child Psychology and Psychiatry and Allied Disciplines 27, 133-144.

Ritvo, E. R., Spence, M. A., Freeman, B. J., Mason-Brothers, A., Mo, A., & Marazita, M. L. (1985). Evidence for autosomal recessive inheritance in 46 families with multiple incidences of autism. American Journal of Psychiatry 142, 187-192.

Sigman, M., Mundy, P., Sherman, T., & Ungerer, D. S. (1986). Social interactions of autistic, mentally retarded and normal children and their caregivers. Journal of Child Psychology and Psychiatry 27(5), 647-656.

Sohlberg, S. C. (1985). Personality and neuropsychological performance of high-risk children. Schizophrenia Bulletin 11, 48-60.

5. Some Epidemiological Considerations

Ragins, N., Schachter, J., Elmer, E., Preisman, R., Bowes, A. E., & Harway, V. (1975). Infants and children at risk for schizophrenia. Environmental and developmental observations. Journal of the American Academy of Child Psychiatry 14, 150-177.

Wing, L. (1980). Childhood autism and social class: A question of selection? British Journal of Psychiatry 137, 410-417.

Wing, L., Yeates, S. R., Brierley, L. M., & Gould, J. (1976). The prevalence of early childhood autism: Comparison of administrative and epidemiological studies. Psychological Medicine 6, 89-100.

6. Cultural and Social Aspects of Autism

Lotter, V. (1980). Cross cultural perspectives on childhood autism. Journal of Tropical Pediatrics 26, 131-133.

Mundy, P., Sigman, M., Ungerer, D. S., & Sherman, T. (1986). Defining the social deficits of autism: The contribution of non-verbal communication measures. Journal of Child Psychology and Psychiatry 27(5), 657-669.

Prior, M. R., Gajzago, C. C., & Knox, D. T. (1976). An epidemiological study of autistic and psychotic children in the four eastern states of Australia. Australian and New Zealand Journal of Psychiatry 10, 173-184.

Ragins, N., Schachter, J., Elmer, E., Preisman, R., Bowes, A. E., & Harway, V. (1975). Infants and children at risk for schizophrenia. Environmental and developmental observations. Journal of the American Academy of Child Psychiatry 14, 150-177.

Wing, L. (1980). Childhood autism and social class: A question of selection? British Journal of Psychiatry 137, 410-417.

Wing, L., Yeates, S. R., Brierley, L. M., & Gould, J. (1976). The prevalence of early childhood autism: Comparison of administrative and epidemiological studies. Psychological Medicine 6, 89-100.

7. Communication in Autism

Attwood, A., Frith, U., & Hermelin, B. (1988). The understanding and use of interpersonal gestures by autistic and Downs syndrome children. Journal of Autism and Developmental Disorders 18, 241-257.

Baltaxe, C. A. M., & Guthrie, D. (1987). The use of primary sentence stress by normal, aphasic, and autistic children. Journal of Autism and Developmental Disorders 17(2).

Baltaxe, C. A. M., & Simmons, J. Q. (1987). Communication deficits in the adolescent with autism, schizophrenia, and language-learning disabilities. In T. L. Layton (Ed.), Language and treatment of autistic and developmentally disordered children. Springfield, Ill.: Charles C. Thomas.

Bartolucci, G., & Pierce, S. J. (1977). A preliminary comparison of phonological development in autistic, normal, and mentally retarded subjects. British Journal of Disorders of Communication 12, 137-147.

Bemporad, J. R. (1979). Adult recollections of a formerly autistic child. Journal of Autism and Developmental Disorders 9, 179-197.

Cantwell, D. P., & Baker, L. (1978a). Imitations and echoes in autistic and dysphasic children. Journal of the American Academy of Child Psychiatry 17, 614-624.

Cantwell, D. P., & Baker, L. (1978b). The language environment of autistic and dysphasic children. Journal of the American Academy of Child Psychiatry 17, 604-613.

Caparulo, B. K., & Cohen, D. J. (1977). Cognitive structures, language, and emerging social competence in autistic and aphasic children. Journal of the American Academy of Child Psychiatry 16, 620-645.

Christ, A. E. (1977). Cognitive assessment of the psychotic child. A Piagetian framework. Journal of the American Academy of Child Psychiatry 16, 227-237.

Fish, B. (1976). An approach to prevention in infants at risk for schizophrenia. Developmental deviations from birth to 10 years. Journal of the American Academy of Child Psychiatry 15, 62-82.

Prizant, B. M., & Rydell, P. J. (1984). Analysis of functions of delayed echolalia in autistic children. Journal of Speech and Hearing Research 27, 183-292.

Wetherby, A. M. (1986). Ontogeny of communicative functions in autism. Journal of Autism and Developmental Disorders 16(3).

8. Family Issues in Autism

August, G. J., & Lockhart, L. H. (1984). Familial autism and the fragile-X chromosome. Journal of Autism and Developmental Disorders 14, 197-204.

Cantwell, D. P., Baker, L., & Rutter, M. (1979). Families of autistic and dysphasic children. I. Family life and interaction patterns. Archives of General Psychiatry 36, 682-687.

Curcio, F., & Paccia, J. (1987). Conversations with autistic children: Contingent relationships between features of adult input and children's response adequacy. Journal of Autism and Developmental Disorders 16(3).

Erlenmeyer-Kimling, L., & Cornblatt, B. (1984). Biobehavioral risk factors in children of schizophrenic parents. Journal of Autism and Developmental Disorders 14, 357-374.

Folstein, S., & Rutter, M. (1977). Infantile autism: A genetic study of 21 twin pairs. Journal of Child Psychology and Psychiatry and Allied Disciplines 18, 297-321.

Garmezy, N. (1974). Children at risk: The search for the antecedents of schizophrenia. Part II: Ongoing research programs, issues, and intervention. Schizophrenia Bulletin 1, 55-125.

Garmezy, N., & Streitman, S. (1974). Children at risk: The search for the antecedents of schizophrenia. Part I: Conceptual models and research methods. Schizophrenia Bulletin 1, 14-90.

Gillberg, C., & Wahlstrom, J. (1985). Chromosome abnormalities in infantile autism and other childhood psychoses: A population study of 66 cases. Developmental Medicine and Child Neurology 27, 293-304.

Goldfarb, W., Spitzer, R. L., & Endicott, J. (1976). A study of psychopathology of parents of psychotic children by structured interview. Journal of Autism and Childhood Schizophrenia 6, 327-338.

Goldstein, M. J., & Doane, J. A. (1982). Family factors in the onset, course, and treatment of schizophrenic spectrum disorders: An update on current research. Journal of Nervous and Mental Disease 170, 692-700.

Hagerman, R. J., Jackson, A. W., Levitas, A., Rimland, B., & Braden, M. (1986). An analysis of autism in fifty males with the fragile X syndrome. American Journal of Medical Genetics 23, 359-374.

Harvey, P. D., Weintraub, S., & Neale, J. M. (1982). Speech competence of children vulnerable to psychopathology. Journal of Abnormal Child Psychology 10, 373-387.
Koegel, R. L., Schreibman, L., O'Neill, R. E., & Burke, J. C. (1983). The personality and family-interaction characteristics of parents of autistic children. Journal of Consulting and Clinical Psychology 51, 683-692.
MacCrimmon, D. J., Cleghorn, J. M., Asarnow, R. F., & Steffy, R. A. (1980). Children at risk for schizophrenia. Clinical and attentional characteristics. Archives of General Psychiatry 37, 671-674.
Marcus, J., Hans, S. L., Byhouwer, B., & Norem, J. (1985). Relationships among neurological functioning, intelligence quotients, and physical anomalies. Schizophrenia Bulletin 11, 101-108.
Marcus, J., Hans, S. L., Mednick, S. A., Schulsinger, F., & Michelsen, N. (1985). Neurological dysfunctioning in offspring of schizophrenics in Israel and Denmark. A replication analysis. Archives of General Psychiatry 42, 753-761.
Minton, J., Campbell, M., Green, W. H., Jennings, S., & Samit, C. (1982). Cognitive assessment of siblings of autistic children. Journal of the American Academy of Child Psychiatry 21, 256-261.
Neuchterlein, K. H. (1986). Childhood precursors of adult schizophrenia. Journal of Child Psychology and Psychiatry and Allied Disciplines 27, 133-144.
Ritvo, E. R., Spence, M. A., Freeman, B. J., Mason-Brothers, A., Mo, A., & Marazita, M. L. (1985). Evidence for autosomal recessive inheritance in 46 families with multiple incidences of autism. American Journal of Psychiatry 142, 187-192.
Sohlberg, S. C. (1985). Personality and neuropsychological performance of high-risk children. Schizophrenia Bulletin 11, 48-60.
Sohlberg, S. C., & Yaniv, S. (1985). Social adjustment and cognitive performance of high-risk children. Schizophrenia Bulletin 11, 61-65.
Winters, K. C., Stone, A. A., Weintraub, S., & Neale, J. M. (1981). Cognitive and attentional deficits in children vulnerable to psychopathology. Journal of Abnormal Child Psychology 9, 435-453.

9. Cognitive Assessment in Autism

Baron-Cohen, S., Leslie, A. M., & Frith, U. (1985). Does the autistic child have a "theory of mind"? Cognition 21, 37-46.
Caparulo, B. K., & Cohen, D. J. (1977). Cognitive structures, language, and emerging social competence in autistic and aphasic children. Journal of the American Academy of Child Psychiatry 16, 620-645.
Christ, A. E. (1977). Cognitive assessment of the psychotic child. A Piagetian framework. Journal of the American Academy of Child Psychiatry 16, 227-237.
Curcio, F. (1978). Sensorimotor functioning and communication in mute autistic children. Journal of Autism and Childhood Schizophrenia 8, 281-292.
Dalgleish, B. (1975). Cognitive processing and linguistic reference in autistic children. Journal of Autism and Childhood Schizophrenia 5, 353-361.

Fein, D., Waterhouse, L., Lucci, D., Pennington, B., & Humes, M. (1985). Handedness and cognitive functions in pervasive developmental disorders. Journal of Autism and Developmental Disorders 15, 323-333.

Freeman, B. J., Ritvo, E. R., Needleman, R., & Yokota, A. (1985). The stability of cognitive and linguistic parameters in autism: A five-year prospective study. Journal of the American Academy of Child Psychiatry 24, 459-464.

Fulkerson, S. C., & Freeman, W. M. (1980). Perceptual-motor deficiency in autistic children. Perceptual and Motor Skills 50, 331-336.

Hobson, R. P. (1987). The autistic child's recognition of age- and sex-related characteristics of people. Journal of Autism and Developmental Disorders 17(1).

Hoffmann, W. L., & Prior, M. R. (1982). Neuropsychological dimensions of autism in children: A test of the hemispheric dysfunction hypotheses. Journal of Clinical Neuropsychology 4, 27-41.

Sloate, P. L., & Voyat, G. (1983). Cognitive and affective features in childhood psychosis. American Journal of Psychotherapy 37, 376-386.

Sohlberg, S. C., & Yaniv, S. (1985). Social adjustment and cognitive performance of high-risk children. Schizophrenia Bulletin 11, 61-65.

10. Some Characteristics of Autism, Schizophrenia, and Psychoses in Childhood

Bergman, A., Schwartzman, M., Sloate, P., & Wilson, A. (1983). The oral deadlock: Treatment of a psychotic child. Journal of the American Psychoanalytic Association 31, 443-465.

Berlin, I. N., & Critchley, D. L. (1982). The work of play for parents of schizophrenic children. Child Psychiatry and Human Development 13, 111-119.

Cantwell, D. P., & Baker, L. (1978). The language environment of autistic and dysphasic children. Journal of the American Academy of Child Psychiatry 17, 604-613.

Cantwell, D. P., Baker, L., & Rutter, M. (1977). Families of autistic and dysphasic children. II. Mothers' speech to the children. Journal of Autism and Childhood Schizophrenia 7, 313-327.

Cantwell, D. P., Baker, L., & Rutter, M. (1979). Families of autistic and dysphasic children. I. Family life and interaction patterns. Archives of General Psychiatry 36, 682-687.

Galenson, E. (1984). Psychoanalytic approach to psychotic disturbances in very young children: A clinical report. Hillside Journal of Clinical Psychiatry 6, 221-240.

Harris, S. L., Handleman, J. S., & Palmer, C. (1985). Parents and grandparents view the autistic child. Journal of Autism and Developmental Disorders 15, 127-137.

Harris, S. L., Wolchik, S. A., & Weitz, S. (1981). The acquisition of language skills by autistic children: Can parents do the job? Journal of Autism and Developmental Disorders 11, 373-384.

Luckoff, D., Snyder, K., Ventura, J., & Nuechterlein, K. H. (1984). Life events, familial stress, and coping in the developmental course of schizophrenia. Schizophrenia Bulletin 10, 258-292.

Marcus, L. M. (1977). Patterns of coping in families of psychotic children. American Journal of Orthopsychiatry 47, 388-399.

Marcus, L. M., Lansing, M., Andrews, C. E., & Schopler, E. (1978). Improvement of teaching effectiveness in parents of autistic children. Journal of the American Academy of Child Psychiatry 17, 625-639.

Pollner, M., & McDonald-Wikler, L. (1985). The social construction of unreality: A case study of a family's attribution of competence to a severely retarded child. Family Process 24, 241-257.

Runco, M. A., & Schreibman, L. (1983). Parental judgments of behavior therapy efficacy with autistic children: A social validation. Journal of Autism and Developmental Disorders 13, 237-248.

Sameroff, A. J., & Seifer, R. (1983). Familial risk and child competence. Child Development 54, 1254-1268.

Schopler, E., Mesibov, G., & Baker, A. (1982). Evaluation of treatment for autistic children and their parents. Journal of the American Academy of Child Psychiatry 21, 262-267.

Sullivan, R. C. (1978). The hostage parent. Journal of Autism and Childhood Schizophrenia 8, 233-234.

Sullivan, R. C. (1979). Siblings of autistic children. Journal of Autism and Developmental Disorders 9, 287-298.

Walker, E., & Emory, E. (1983). Infants at risk for psychopathology: Offspring of schizophrenic parents. Child Development 54, 1269-1285.

11. Sensory-Motor Processing in Autism and Schizophrenia

Asarnow, R. F., & Sherman, T. (1984). Studies of visual information processing in schizophrenic children. Child Development 55, 249-261.

Baron-Cohen, S., Leslie, A. M., & Frith, U. (1985). Does the autistic child have a "theory of mind"? Cognition 21, 37-46.

Benaroya, S., Wesley, S., Ogilvie, H., Klein, L. S., & Meaney, M. (1977). Sign language and multisensory input training of children with communication and related developmental disorders. Journal of Autism and Childhood Schizophrenia 7, 23-31.

Carr, E. G., Pridal, C., & Dores, P. A. (1984). Speech versus sign comprehension in autistic children: Analysis and prediction. Journal of Experimental Child Psychology 37, 587-597.

Cobrinik, L. (1980). Visuo-motor dissociation in severely disturbed children: A study of Bender-Gestalt test performance. Acta Paedopsychiatrica 45, 353-363.

Curcio, F. (1978). Sensorimotor functioning and communication in mute autistic children. Journal of Autism and Childhood Schizophrenia 8, 281-292.

Dawson, G., & McKissick, F. C. (1984). Self-recognition in autistic children. Journal of Autism and Developmental Disorders 14, 383-394.

Fulkerson, S. C., & Freeman, W. M. (1980). Perceptual-motor deficiency in autistic children. Perceptual and Motor Skills 50, 331-336.

Herman, J., Mirsky, A. F., Ricks, N. L., & Gallant, D. (1977). Behavioral and electrographic measures of attention in children at risk for schizophrenia. Journal of Abnormal Psychology 86, 27-33.

Kiernan, C. (1983). The use of nonvocal communication techniques with autistic individuals. Journal of Child Psychology and Psychiatry and Allied Disciplines 24, 339-375.

Langdell, T. (1978). Recognition of faces: An approach to the study of autism. Journal of Child Psychology and Psychiatry and Allied Disciplines 19, 255-268.

Masterton, B. A., & Biederman, G. B. (1983). Proprioceptive versus visual control in autistic children. Journal of Autism and Developmental Disorders 13, 141-152.

O'Connor, N., & Hermelin, B. (1983). Peripheral and central handicap and encoding. Journal of Child Psychology and Psychiatry and Allied Disciplines 24, 39-48.

Reynolds, B. S., Newsom, C. D., & Lovaas, O. I. (1974). Auditory overselectivity in autistic children. Journal of Abnormal Child Psychology 2, 253-263.

Ricks, D. M., & Wing, L. (1975). Language, communication, and the use of symbols in normal and autistic children. Journal of Autism and Childhood Schizophrenia 5, 191-221.

Schachter, J., Kerr, J., Lachin, J. M., & Faer, M. (1975). Newborn offspring of a schizophrenic parent: Cardiac reactivity to auditory stimuli. Psychophysiology 12, 483-492.

Shah, A., & Frith, U. (1983). An islet of ability in autistic children: A research note. Journal of Child Psychology and Psychiatry and Allied Disciplines 24, 613-620.

Spiker, D., & Ricks, M. (1984). Visual self-recognition in autistic children: Developmental relationships. Child Development 55, 214-225.

Volkmar, F., Sparrow, S. S., Rende, R. D., & Cohen, D. J. (1989). Facial perception in autism. Journal of Child Psychology and Psychiatry 30, 591-598.

Weeks, S. J., & Hobson, R. P. (1987). The salience of facial expression for autistic children. Journal of Child Psychology and Psychiatry 28(1), 137-152.

12. Neuroanatomical, Neurophysiologic, and Neurochemical Findings in Autism

Arnold, G., & Schwartz, S. (1983). Hemispheric lateralization of language in autistic and aphasic children. Journal of Autism and Developmental Disorders 13, 129-139.

Bannon, M., Quanbury, A., & Cantor, S. (1981). The gait of hypotonic schizophrenic children. Developmental Medicine and Child Neurology 23, 770-777.

Cohen, D. J., Caparulo, B., & Shaywitz, B. (1976). Primary childhood aphasia and childhood autism: Clinical, biological, and conceptual observations. Journal of the American Academy of Child Psychiatry 15, 604-645.

Cohen, D. J., & Johnson, W. T. (1977). Cardiovascular correlates of attention in normal and psychiatrically disturbed children. Blood pressure, peripheral blood flow, and peripheral vascular resistance. Archives of General Psychiatry 34, 561-567.

Cohen, D. J., Shaywitz, B. A., Johnson, W. T., & Bowers, M. (1974). Biogenic amines in autistic and atypical children. Cerebrospinal fluid measures of homovanillic acid and 5-hydroxyindoleacetic acid. Archives of General Psychiatry 31, 845-853.

Cohen, D. J., & Young, J. G. (1977). Neurochemistry and child psychiatry. Journal of the American Academy of Child Psychiatry 16, 353-411.

Courchesne, E. R., Yeung-Courchesne, B. A., Press, G. A., Hesselink, J. R., & Jernigan, T. L. (1987). Hypoplasia of cerebellar vermal lobules VI and VII in autism. Vermal Hypoplasia in Autism 318(21), 1349-1354.

Creasey, H., Rumsey, J. M., Schwartz, M., Duara, R., Rapoport, J., & Rapoport, S. (1987). Brain morphometry in autistic men as measured by volumetric computed tomography. Archives of Neurology 43, 669-672.

DeMyer, M. K. (1975). The nature of the neuropsychological disability in autistic children. Journal of Autism and Childhood Schizophrenia 5, 109-128.

Gaffney, G. R., & Tsai, L. Y. (1987). Brief report: Magnetic resonance imaging of high level autism. Journal of Autism and Developmental Disorders 17(3).

Gaffney, G. R., Tsai, L. Y., Kuperman, S., Minchin, S. (1987). Cerebellar structure in autism. American Journal of Diseases of Children 141, 1330-1332.

Gillberg, C., Terenius, L., & Lonnerholm, G. (1985). Endorphin activity in childhood psychosis. Spinal fluid levels in 24 cases. Archives of General Psychiatry 42, 780-783.

Hoffmann, W. L., & Prior, M. R. (1982). Neuropsychological dimensions of autism in children: A test of the hemispheric dysfunction hypothesis. Journal of Clinical Neuropsychology 4, 27-41.

Jacobson, R., LeConteur, A., Howlin, P., & Rutter, M. (1988). Selective subcortical abnormalities in autism. Psychological Medicine 18, 39-48.

James, A. L., & Barry, R. J. (1980). A review of psychophysiology in early onset psychosis. Schizophrenia Bulletin 6, 506-525.

Lowe, T. L., Cohen, D. J., Miller, S., & Young, J. G. (1981). Folic acid and B12 in autism and neuropsychiatric disturbances of childhood. Journal of the American Academy of Child Psychiatry 20, 104-111.

Mauer, R. G., & Damasio, A. R. (1979). Vestibular dysfunction in autistic children. Developmental Medicine and Child Neurology 21, 656-659.

Mundy, P., & Sigman, M. (1989). The theoretical implication of joint attention deficits in autism. Development and Psychopathology 1, 173-183.

Neufeld, A., & Fantuzzo, J. W. (1984). Contingent application of a protective device to treat the severe self-biting behavior of a disturbed autistic child. Journal of Behavior Therapy and Experimental Psychiatry 15, 79-83

Ornitz, E. M. (1983). The functional neuroanatomy of infantile autism. International Journal of Neuroscience 19, 85-124.

Ornitz, E. M., Brown, M. B., Mason, A., & Putnam, N. H. (1974). Effect of visual input on vestibular nystagmus in autistic children. Archives of General Psychiatry 31, 369-375.

Rumsey, J. M., & Hamburger, S. D. (1989). Neuropsychological findings in high-functioning men and infantile autism, residual state. Journal of Clinical and Experimental Neuropsychology 10(2), 201-221.

Yuwiler, A., Ritvo, E., Geller, E., Glousman, R., Schneiderman, G., & Matsuno, D. (1975). Uptake and efflux of serotonin from platelets of autistic and nonautistic children. Journal of Autism and Childhood Schizophrenia 5, 83-98.

13. Treatment of Autistic and Psychotic Children

Campbell, M., & Cohen, I. L. (1978). Treatment of infantile autism. Comprensive Therapy 4, 33-37.

Critchley, D. L., & Berlin, I. N. (1979). Day treatment of young psychotic children and their parents: Interdisciplinary issues and problems. Child Psychiatry and Human Development 9, 227-237.

Critchley, D. L., & Berlin, I. N. (1981). Parent participation in milieu treatment of young psychotic children. American Journal of Orthopsychiatry 51, 149-155.

Ekstein, R., & Nelson, T. (1981). The birth of the psychotherapeutic dialogue and the self. From the autistic prelogue and monologue to the interpersonal dialogue and plurilogue. Psychiatric Clinics of North America 4, 533-548.

Galenson, E. (1984). Psychoanalytic approach to psychotic disturbances in very young children: A clinical report. Hillside Journal of Clinical Psychiatry 6, 221-240.

Gilpin, D. C. (1976). Psychotherapy of borderline psychotic children. American Journal of Psychotherapy 30, 483-496.

Koegel, R. L., & Rincover, A. (1974). Treatment of psychotic children in a classroom environment: I. Learning in a large group. Journal of Applied Behavior Analysis 7, 45-59.

Koegel, R. L., Russo, D. C., & Rincover, A. (1977). Assessing and training teachers in the generalized use of behavior modification with autistic children. Journal of Applied Behavior Analysis 10, 197-205.

Lester, E. P., & LaRoche, C. (1978). Schizophreniform psychosis of childhood: Therapeutic considerations. Comprehensive Psychiatry 19, 153-159.

Lovaas, O. I., Schreibman, L., & Koegel, R. L. (1974). A behavior modification approach to the treatment of autistic children. Journal of Autism and Childhood Schizophrenia 4, 111-129.

Margolies, P. J. (1977). Behavioral approaches to the treatment of early infantile autism: A review. Psychological Bulletin 84, 249-264.

Paul, R., & Cohen, D. J. (1984). Outcomes of severe disorders of language acquisition. Journal of Autism and Developmental Disorders 14, 405-421.

Risks and benefits in the treatment of autistic children. (1978). Journal of Autism and Childhood Schizophrenia 8, 99-113.

Rutter, M. (1985). The treatment of autistic children. Journal of Child Psychology and Psychiatry and Allied Disciplines 26, 193-214.

Rutter, M., & Sussenwein, F. (1971). A developmental and behavioral approach to the treatment of preschool autistic children. Journal of Autism and Childhood Schizophrenia 1, 376-397.

Sugar, M., Stuckey, B., Salley, P., Oppliger, S., & Stretch, J. J. (1975). Use of college-student companions for psychotic children to avoid hospitalization. Journal of the American Academy of Child Psychiatry 14, 249-267.

Volkmar, F. R., Hoder, E. L., & Cohen, D. J. (1985). Compliance, 'negativism,' and the effects of treatment structure in autism: A naturalistic, behavioral study. Journal of Child Psychology and Psychiatry and Allied Disciplines 26, 865-877.

14. Pharmacological Treatment

American Academy of Pediatrics Committee on Nutrition (1976). Megavitamin therapy for childhood psychoses and learning disabilities. Pediatrics 58, 910-912.

Anderson, L. T., Campbell, M., Grega, D. M., Perry, R., Small, A. M., & Green, W. H. (1984). Haloperidol in the treatment of infantile autism: Effects on learning and behavioral symptoms. American Journal of Psychiatry 141, 1195-1202.

August, G. J., Raz, N., & Baird, T. D. (1985). Effects of fenfluramine on behavioral, cognitive, and affective disturbances in autistic children. Journal of Autism and Developmental Disorders 15, 97-107.

Campbell, M. (1975). Pharmacotherapy in early infantile autism. Biological Psychiatry 10, 399-423.

Campbell, M., Adams, P., Small, A. M., et al. (1988). Efficacy and safety of fenfluramine in autistic children. Journal of the American Academy of Child and Adolescent Psychiatry 27, 434-439.

Campbell, M., Cohen, I. L., & Anderson, L. T. (1981). Pharmacotherapy for autistic children: A summary of research. Canadian Journal of Psychiatry 26, 265-273.

Campbell, M., & Palij, M. (1985). Behavioral and cognitive measures used in psychopharmacological studies of infantile autism. Psychopharmacology Bulletin 21, 1047-1053.

Geller, E., Ritvo, E. R., Freeman, B. J., & Yuwiler, A. (1982). Preliminary observations on the effect of fenfluramine on blood serotonin and symptoms in three autistic boys. New England Journal of Medicine 307, 165-169.

Gualtieri, C. T. (1986). Fenfluramine and autism: Careful reappraisal is in order [Editorial]. Journal of Pediatrics 108, 417-419.

Martineau, J., Barthelemy, C., Garreau, B., & Lelord, G. (1985). Vitamin B6, magnesium, and combined B6-Mg: Therapeutic effects in childhood autism. Biological Psychiatry 20, 467-478.

McDaniel, K. D. (1986a). Pharmacologic treatment of psychiatric and neurodevelopmental disorders in children and adolescents (Part 2). Clinical Pediatrics 25, 143-146.

McDaniel, K. D. (1986b). Pharmacologic treatment of psychiatric and neurodevelopmental disorders in children and adolescents (Part 3). Clinical Pediatrics 25, 198-204.

Ornitz, E. M. (1985). Should autistic children be treated with haloperidol? [Letter]. American Journal of Psychiatry 142, 883-884.

Petty, L. K., & Spar, C. J. (1980). Haloperidol-induced tardive dyskinesia in a 10-year-old girl. American Journal of Psychiatry 137, 745-746.
Ritvo, E. R., Freeman, B. J., Geller, E., & Yuwiler, A. (1983). Effects of fenfluramine on 14 outpatients with the syndrome of autism. Journal of the American Academy of Child Psychiatry 22, 549-558.
Volkmar, F. R., Paul, R., Cohen, D. J., & Shaywitz, B. A. (1983). Irritability in autistic children treated with fenfluramine [Letter]. New England Journal of Medicine 309, 187.

15. Miscellaneous References

Arboleda, C., & Holzman, P. S. (1985). Thought disorder in children at risk for psychosis. Archives of General Psychiatry 41(10), 1004-1013.
Barr, M. W. (1898). Some notes on echolalia, with the report of an extraordinary case. Journal of Nervous and Mental Disease 25, 21-30.
Campbell, M., & Palij, M. (1985). Behavioral and cognitive measures used in psychopharmacological studies of infantile autism. Psychopharmacology Bulletin 21(4), 1047-1053.
Courchesne, E., Courchesne, R. Y., Hicks, G., & Lincoln, A. J. (1985). Functioning of the brain-stem auditory pathway in non-retarded autistic individuals. Electroencephalography and Clinical Neurophysiology 61(6), 491-501.
Dawson, G., & Adams, A. (1984). Imitation and social responsiveness in autistic children. Journal of Abnormal Child Psychology 12, 209-225.
Hartman, E., Mitchell, W., Brune, P., & Greenwald, D. (1985). Vulnerability to schizophrenia: Childhood indicators predict adult outcome. Psychopharmacology Bulletin 21(3), 503-508.
Hobson, R. P. (1986). The autistic child's appraisal of expressions of emotion: A further study. Journal of Child Psychology and Psychiatry 27(5), 671-680.
Koegel, R. K. (1982). Education and understanding autistic children. ??, Md.: College Hill.
Lancy, D. F., & Goldstein, G. I. (1982). The use of nonverbal Piagetian tasks to assess the cognitive development of autistic children. Child Development 53, 1233-1241.
McGillivray, B. C., Herbst, D. S., Dill, F. J., Sandercock, H. J., & Tixchler, B. (1986). Infantile autism: An occasional manifestation of fragile (X) mental retardation. American Journal of Medical Genetics 23(1-2), 353-358.
Nuechterlein, K. H. (1986). Childhood precursors of adult schizophrenia. Journal of Child Psychology and Psychiatry and Allied Disciplines 27(2), 133-144.
Rubinstein, B., & Shaffer, D. (1985). Organicity in child psychiatry. Signs, symptoms, and syndromes. Psychiatric Clinics of North America 8(4), 755-777.
Rumsey, J. M., Rapoport, J. L., & Sceery, W. R. (1985). Autistic children as adults: Psychiatric, social, and behavioral outcomes. Journal of the American Academy of Child Psychiatry 24(4), 465-473.

Rutter, M., & Sandberg, S. (1985). Epidemiology of child psychiatric disorder: Methodological issues and some substantive findings [Review]. Child Psychiatry and Human Development 15(4), 209-233.

Rutter, M. L. (1986). Child psychiatry: The interface between clinical and developmental research. Psychological Medicine 16(1), 151-169.

Sigman, M., & Ungerer, J. (1981). Sensorimotor skills and language comprehension in autistic children. Journal of Abnormal Child Psychology 9, 149-165.

Sigman, M., & Ungerer, J. A. (1984). Attachment behaviors in autistic children. Journal of Autism and Developmental Disorders 14, 231-244.

Tager-Flusberg, H. (1985). Basic level and superordinate level categorization by autistic, mentally retarded, and normal children. Journal of Experimental Child Psychology 40, 450-469.

Tanguay, P., & Asarnow, R. (1985). Schizophrenia in children. In J. O. Cavenar (Ed.), Psychiatry. New York: Lippincott.

Tanguay, P. E., & Cantor, S. (1986). Schizophrenia in children. Journal of the American Academy of Child Psychiatry 25, 591-594.

Tsiantis, J., Macri, I., & Maratos, O. (1986). Schizophrenia in children: A review of European research. Schizophrenia Bulletin 12(1), 101-119.

Volkmar, F. R., Paul, R., & Cohen, D. J. (1985). The use of "Asperger's syndrome" [Letter]. Journal of Autism and Developmental Disorders 15(4), 437-439.

Wing, L. (1985). Autistic children. New York: Brunner/Mazel.

Zappella, M. (1985). Rett syndrome: A significant proportion of girls affected by autistic behavior. Brain and Development 7(3), 307-312.

16. Recent Books

Rutter, M., & Schopler, E. (Eds.). (1978). Autism. A reappraisal of concepts and treatment. New York: Plenum Press.

Schopler, E., & Mesibov, G. (Eds.). (1984). The effects of autism on the family. New York: Plenum Press.

Schopler, E., & Mesibov, G. (Eds.). (1985). Communication problems in autism. New York: Plenum Press.

Schopler, E., & Mesibov, G. (Eds.). (1986). Social behavior in autism. New York: Plenum Press.

M. Borderline Conditions and Narcissism

Paulina K. Kernberg, M.D. and Joseph D. Noshpitz, M.D., Section Coeditors
Efrain Bleiberg, M.D., Associate Editor

1. Narcissism

Akhtar, S., & Thomson, J. A. (1982). Narcissistic personality disorder. American Journal of Psychiatry 139(1), 12-20.

Amsterdam, B. K., & Levitt, M. (1980). Consciousness of self and painful self consciousness. In A. Solnit, et al. (Eds.), Psychoanalytic study of the child (Vol. 35, pp. 67-83). New Haven: Yale University Press.

Auerbach, J. S. (1984). Validation for two scales of narcissistic personality disorder. Journal of Personality Assessment 48(6), 649-653.

Bach, S. (1977). On the narcissistic state of consciousness. International Journal of Psycho-Analysis 58, 209-233.

Bach, S., & Schwartz, L. (1972). A dream of the Marquis de Sade: Psychoanalytic reflections of narcissistic trauma, decompensation and the reconstitution of delusional self. Journal of the American Psychoanalytic Association 20(3), 451-475.

Balint, M. (1960). Primary narcissism and primary love. Psychoanalytic Quarterly 29, 6-43.

Bane, A. (1979). The question of narcissistic personality disorders: Self pathology in children. Bulletin of the Hampstead Clinic 2(4), 209-218.

Benson, R. M. (1980). Narcissistic guardians: Developmental aspects of transitional objects, imaginary companions, and career fantasies. In S. C. Feinstein, et al. (Eds.), Adolescent psychiatry: Developmental and clinical studies (Vol. 8, pp. 253-264). Chicago: University of Chicago Press.

Berkowitz, D. A., Shapiro, R., Zinner, J., et al. (1974). Family contributions to narcissistic disturbances in adolescents. International Review of Psychoanalysis 1, 353-362.

Blatt, S. J. (1983). Narcissism and egocentrism and concepts in individual and cultural development. Psychoanalysis and Contemporary Thought 6(2), 291-303.

Bleiberg, E. (1984). Narcissistic disorders in children. Bulletin of the Menninger Clinic 48(6), 501-517.

Blos, P. (1972). The function of the ego ideal in adolescence. In R. S. Eissler, et al. (Eds.), Psychoanalytic study of the child (Vol. 27, pp. 93-97). New York: International Universities Press.

Brody, W. M. (1965). On the dynamics of narcissism: Externalization and early ego development. In R. S. Eissler, et al. (Eds.), Psychoanalytic study of the child (Vol. 20, pp. 165-193). New York: International Universities Press.

Burch, C. A. (1985). Identity foreclosure in early adolescence: A problem in narcissistic equilibrium. In S. C. Feinstein, et al. (Eds.), Adolescent psychiatry: Developmental and clinical studies (Vol. 12, pp. 145-161). Chicago: University of Chicago Press.

Burstein, B. (1982). Narcissistic personalities in D.S.M. III. Comprehensive Psychiatry 23(5), 409-420.

Carvalho, R. R. (1982). Paternal deprivation in relation to narcissistic damage. Journal of Analytic Psychology 27(4), 341-356.

Collins, J. K., & La Ganza, S. (1982). Self-recognition of the face: A study of adolescent narcissism. Journal of Youth and Adolescence 11(4), 317-328.

Diagnostic and statistical manual of mental disorders (3rd ed.). (1980). Washington, D.C.: American Psychiatric Association.

Dysart, D. (1977). Transference, cure, and narcissism. Journal of the American Academy of Psychoanalysis 5(1), 17-29.

Egan, J., & Kernberg, P. F. (1984). Pathological narcissism in childhood. Journal of the American Psychoanalytic Association 32(1), 39-62.

Emde, R. E. (1982). The experience of self: Aspects of its formation, expansion, and vulnerability. In A. Solnit, et al. (Eds.), Psychoanalytic study of the child (Vol. 37, pp. 143-168). New Haven: Yale University Press.

Erlich, H. S., & Blatt, S. J. (1985). Narcissism and object love: The metapsychology of experience. In A. Solnit, et al. (Eds.), Psychoanalytic study of the child (Vol. 40, pp. 57-80). New Haven: Yale University Press.

Fast, I. (1985). Infantile narcissism and the active infant. Psychoanalytic Psychology 2(2), 153-170.

Forman, M. (1980). Narcissistic personality disorder as a regression to a preoedipal phase of phallic narcissism. Hillside Journal of Clinical Psychiatry 3(1), 45-59.

Freud, S. (1914). On narcissism. In E. Jones (Ed.), Collected papers. Standard edition (Vol. 14, pp. 67-102). New York and London: Hogarth Press.

Freud, S. (1981). Libidinal types. In E. Jones (Ed.), Collected papers. Standard edition (Vol. 21). New York and London: Hogarth Press.

Friedrich, W. N., & Wheeler, K. K. (1982). The abusing parent revisited: A decade of psychological research. Journal of Nervous and Mental Disease 170(10), 577-587.

Goldberg, A. (Ed.). (1978). The psychology of the self. New York: International Universities Press.

Greene, M. A. (1984). The self-psychology of Heinz Kohut: A synopsis and critique. Bulletin of the Menninger Clinic 48, 37-53.

Hamilton, V. (1982). Narcissus and Oedipus. London, Boston & Henley: Routledge & Kegan Paul.

Havelock, E. (1898). Autoerotism: A psychological study. Alienist and Neurologist 19, 260-299.

Imber, R. R. (1984). Reflections on Kohut and Sullivan. Contemporary Psychoanalysis 20(2), 363-380.

Jacobson, E. (1976). The self and the object world. New York: International Universities Press.

Joffe, W., & Sandler, J. (1967). Some conceptual problems involved in the consideration of disorders of narcissism. Journal of Child Psychotherapy 2, 55-56.

Kernberg, O. F. (1975). Borderline conditions and pathological narcissism, New York: Jason Aronson.

Kernberg, O. F. (1982). An ego psychology and object relations approach to the narcissistic personality. In L. Grinspoon (Ed.), Psychiatry 1982: The American Psychiatric Association's annual review of psychiatry. Washington, D.C.: American Psychiatric Association.

Kernberg, P. (1981). The hysterical personality in child and adolescent analysis. In E. J. Anthony (Ed.), Three clinical faces of childhood (pp. 27-58). New York: Wiley.

Kernberg, P. (1989). Narcissistic personality disorder in childhood. Psychiatric Clinics of North Amercia 12(3), 671-694.

Khantzian, E., & Mack, J. E. (1983). Self-preservation and the care of the self: Ego instincts reconsidered. In A. Solnit, et al. (Eds.), Psychoanalytic study of the child (Vol. 38, pp. 209-232). New Haven: Yale University Press.

Kohut, H. (1968). The psychoanalytic treatment of narcissistic personality disorders: Outline of a systematic approach. In R. S. Eissler, et al. (Eds.), Psychoanalytic study of the child (Vol. 23, pp. 86-123). New York: International Universities Press.

Kohut, H. (1971). The analysis of the self. New York: International Universities Press.

Kohut, H. (1972). Thoughts on narcissism and narcissistic rage. In R. S. Eissler, et al. (Eds.), Psychoanalytic study of the child (Vol. 27, pp. 360-400). New York: International Universities Press.

Kohut, H., & Wolf, E. S. (1978). The disorders of the self and their treatment. International Journal of Psycho-Analysis 59, 413-425.

Kris, A. O. (1983). Determinants of free association in narcissistic phenomena. In A. Solnit, et al. (Eds.), Psychoanalytic study of the child (Vol. 38, pp. 439-458). New Haven: Yale University Press.

Lasch, C. (1978). The culture of narcissism: American life in an age of diminishing expectation. New York: Norton.

Laufer, M. E. (1981). The adolescent's use of the body in object relationships and in the transference: A comparison of borderline and narcissistic modes of functioning. In A. Solnit, et al. (Eds.), Psychoanalytic study of the child (Vol. 36, pp. 163-180). New Haven: Yale University Press.

Lederman, R. (1986). Pathological sexuality and paucity of symbolization in narcissistic disorder. Journal of Analytic Psychology 31, 23-43.

Lewis, M., & Brooks, J. (1978). Self-knowledge and emotional development. In M. Lewis & A. Rosenblum (Eds.), The development of affect (pp. 205-226). New York: Plenum Press.

Lewis, M., & Brooks-Gun, J. (1979). Social cognition and the acquisition of self. New York: Plenum Press.

Lichtenberg, J. D. (1975). The development of the sense of self. Journal of the American Psychoanalytic Association 5, 453-484.

Lichtenberg, J. D. (1978). Is there a line of development of narcissism? International Review of Psychoanalysis 5, 435-447.

Loewenstein, S. (1977). An overview of the concept of narcissism. Social Casework 58, 136-142.

Lynch, V. J. (1976). Narcissistic loss and depression in late adolescence. Perspectives in Psychiatric Care 14, 133-135.

Mahler, M. (1968). On human symbiosis and the vicissitudes of individuation. New York: International Universities Press.

Mahler, M. S., & Kaplan, L. (1977). Development aspects in the assessment of narcissistic or so-called borderline personalities. In P. Hartocollis (Ed.),

Borderline personality disorders: The concept, the syndrome, the patient (pp. 71-85). New York: International Universities Press.
McCarthy, J. B. (1978). Narcissism and the self in homicidal adolescents. American Journal of Psychoanalysis 38, 19-29.
Mendelbaum, A. (1980). Family characteristics of patients with borderline and narcissistic disorders. Bulletin of the Menninger Clinic 44, 201-211.
Mishne, J. (1979). Parental abandonment: A unique form of loss and narcissistic injury. Clinical Social Work Journal 7, 15-33.
Mitchell, S. A. (1986). The wings of Icarus: Illusion and the problem of narcissism. Contemporary Psychoanalysis 22, 107-132.
Mollon, P. (1984a). The fragile self: Narcissistic disturbance and the protective function of depression. British Journal of Medical Psychology 57, 137-145.
Mollon, P. (1984b). Shame in relation to narcissistic disturbance. British Journal of Medical Psychology 57, 207-214.
Moore, B. E., & Fine, N. D. (Eds.). (1967). A glossary of psychoanalytic terms and concepts. New York: American Psychoanalytic Association.
Niederland, W. G. (1956). Clinical observations of the "little man" phenomenon. In R. S. Eissler, et al. (Eds.), Psychoanalytic study of the child (Vol. 11, pp. 381-395). New York: International Universities Press.
Noshpitz, J. (1984). Narcissism and aggression. American Journal of Psychotherapy 38, 17-34.
Noshpitz, J., & Loughman, S. (1983). A narcissistic reaction in a six-year-old girl with a seizure disorder. American Journal of Psychotherapy 37, 533-543.
Ornstein, A. (1981). Self pathology in childhood: Developmental and clinical considerations. Psychiatric Clinics of North America 4, 435-453.
Ornstein, A. (1984). Oedipal self-object transferences: A clinical example. In J. D. Lichtenberg & S. Kaplan (Eds.), Reflections on self-psychology. New York: International Universities Press.
Ornstein, P. (1974). On narcissism. Annual of Psychoanalysis 2, 127-149.
Pine, F. (1982). The experience of self: Aspects of its formation, expansion and vulnerability. In A. Solnit, et al. (Eds.), Psychoanalytic study of the child (Vol. 37, pp. 143-168). New Haven: Yale University Press.
Reich, A. (1960). Pathologic forms of self-esteem regulation. In R. S. Eissler, et al. (Eds.), Psychoanalytic study of the child (Vol. 15, pp. 215-232). New York: International Universities Press.
Richards, A. D. (1981). Self-theory, conflict theory, and the problem of hypochondriasis. In A. Solnit, et al. (Eds.), Psychoanalytic study of the child (Vol. 36, pp. 319-337). New Haven: Yale University Press.
Rinsley, D. B. (1980a). The developmental etiology of borderline and narcissistic disorders. Bulletin of the Menninger Clinic 44, 127-134.
Rinsley, D. B. (1980b). Diagnosis and treatment of borderline and narcissistic children and adolescents. Bulletin of the Menninger Clinic 44, 147-170.
Rinsley, D. B. (1982). Borderline and other self disorders. New York: Aronson.

Rinsley, D. B. (1988). Overview of borderline and narcissistic disorders. Paper presented at the meeting of the Association of Adolescent Psychiatry, Seattle, Wash.

Robbins, M. (1982). Narcissistic personality as a symbiotic character disorder. International Journal of Psycho-Analysis 63, 457-473.

Roth, B. E. (1982). Six types of borderline and narcissistic patients: An initial typology. International Journal of Group Psychotherapy 32, 9-27.

Rothstein, A. (1980). Toward a critique of the psychology of the self. Psychoanalytic Quarterly 49, 423-455.

Rothstein, A. (1984). Fear of humiliation. Journal of the American Psychoanalytic Association 32, 99-116.

Rubenstein, B., & Levitt, M. (1980-1981). The creative process and the narcissistic personality disorder. International Journal of Psychoanalytic Psychotherapy 8, 461-482.

Rubins, J. L. (1983). Narcissism and the narcissistic personality: A holistic reappraisal. American Journal of Psychoanalysis 43, 3-20.

Sabo, S. (1977). Narcissism as a function of culture. In A. Solnit, et al. (Eds.), Psychoanalytic study of the child (Vol. 32, pp. 155-172). New Haven: Yale University Press.

Schwaber, E. (1980). Self-psychology and the concept of psychopathology. In A. Goldberg (Ed.), Advances in self-psychology. New York: International Universities Press.

Segal, H. (1983). Some clinical implications of Melanie Klein's work: Emergence from narcissism. International Journal of Psycho-Analysis 64, 269-276.

Settlage, C. (1980). The psychoanalytic understanding of narcissistic and borderline personality disorders: Advances in developmental theory. In R. F. Lax, S. Bach, & J. Burland (Eds.), Rapprochement: The critical subphase of separation-individuation (pp. 77-100). New York: Jason Aronson.

Sherick, I. (1983). Adoption and disturbed narcissism: A case illustration of a latency boy. Journal of the American Psychoanalytic Association 31, 487-513.

Sours, J. A. (1980). Starving to death in a sea of objects: Anorexia nervosa syndrome. New York: Jason Aronson.

Speigel, L. A. (1959). The self, the sense of self, and perception. In R. S. Eissler, et al. (Eds.), Psychoanalytic study of the child (Vol. 14, pp. 81-109). New York: International Universities Press.

Spruiell, V. (1975a). Adolescent narcissism and group psychotherapy. In M. Sugar (Ed.), The adolescent in group and family therapy. New York: Brunner/Mazel.

Spruiell, V. (1975b). Narcissistic transformations in adolescence. International Journal of Psychoanalytic Psychotherapy 4, 518-536.

Stamm, J. L. (1972). Infantile trauma, narcissistic injury and agoraphobia. Psychiatric Quarterly 46, 254-272.

Stechler, G., & Kaplan, S. (1980). The development of the self: A psychoanalytic perspective. In A. Solnit, et al. (Eds.), Psychoanalytic study of the child (Vol. 35, pp. 85-105). New Haven: Yale University Press.

Stern, D. N. (1982). The early development of schemas of self, or other, and of various experience of "self with other." In J. D. Lichtenberg & S. Kaplan (Eds.), Reflections on self-psychology. New York: International Universities Press.
Tolpin, M. (1978). Self-objects and oedipal objects: A crucial developmental distinction. In A. Solnit, et al. (Eds.), Psychoanalytic study of the child (Vol. 33, pp. 667-687). New Haven: Yale University Press.
Tylim, I. (1978). Narcissistic transference and countertransference in adolescent treatment. In A. Solnit, et al. (Eds.), Psychoanalytic study of the child (Vol. 33, pp. 279-292). New Haven: Yale University Press.
Tyson, R. L. (1983). Some narcissistic consequences of object loss: A developmental view. Psychoanalytic Quarterly 52, 205-224.
van der Waals, H. G. (1965). Problems of narcissism. Bulletin of the Menninger Clinic 29, 293-311.
Volkan, V. D. (1973). Transitional fantasies in the analysis of a narcissistic personality. Journal of the American Psychoanalytic Association 21, 351-376.
Waelder, R. (1925). The psychosis, their mechanisms and accessibility to influence. International Journal of Psychoanalysis 6, 259-281.
Willock, B. (1986). Narcissistic vulnerability in the hyperaggressive child: The disregarded (unloved, uncared-for) self. Psychoanalytic Psychology 3, 59-80.
Winnicott, D. W. (1965). Ego distortions in terms of true and false self. In D. W. Winnicott (Ed.), The maturation process and the facilitating environment (pp. 140-152). New York: International Universities Press.
Wylie, H. W. (1974). Threads in the fabric of a narcissistic disorder. Journal of the American Psychoanalytic Association 22, 310-328.
Yates, A. (1981). Narcissistic traits in certain abused children. American Journal of Orthopsychiatry 51, 55-62.
Zander, K. (1986). "The fragile princess": Midway in the narcissistic borderline personality continuum. Perspectives in Psychiatric Care 22, 77-84.

2. Borderline Syndromes

Bemporad, J., et al. (1982). Borderline syndromes in childhood: Criteria for diagnosis. American Journal of Psychiatry 139(5), 506-602.
Blum, H. F. (1974). The borderline childhood of the Wolf Man. Journal of the American Psychoanalytic Association 22, 721-742.
Chethik, M., & Fast, I. (1970). A function of fantasy in the borderline child. American Journal of Orthopsychiatry 40, 742-756.
Crumley, F. E. (1981). Adolescent suicide attempts and borderline personality disorder. Southern Medical Journal 174(5), 546-549.
Ekstein, R., & Wallerstein, J. (1954). Observations on the psychology of borderline and psychotic children. In R. S. Eissler, et al. (Eds.), Psychoanalytic study of the child (Vol. 9, pp. 344-369). New York: International Universities Press.
Engel, M. (1963). Psychological testing of borderline psychotic children. Archives of General Psychiatry 20(8), 426-434.

Fast, I., & Chethik, M. (1972). Some aspects of object relationships in borderline children. International Journal of Psycho-Analysis 53, 479-485.

Frijlin-Schreuder, E. C. M. (1969). Borderline states in children. In R. S. Eissler, et al. (Eds.), Psychoanalytic study of the child (Vol. 24, pp. 307-327). New York: International Universities Press.

Geleerd, E. R. (1958). Borderline states in childhood and adolescence. In R. S. Eissler, et al. (Eds.), Psychoanalytic study of the child (Vol. 13, pp. 279-295). New York: International Universities Press.

Kernberg, O. (1978). The diagnosis of borderline conditions in adolescence. In S. Feinstein & P. Giovacchini (Eds.), Adolescent psychiatry (Vol. 6, pp. 298-319). Chicago: University of Chicago Press.

Kernberg, P. F. (1979). Psychoanalytic profile of the borderline adolescent. In S. C. Feinstein, et al. (Eds.), Adolescent psychiatry: Developmental and clinical studies (Vol. 8, pp. 234-256). Chicago: University of Chicago Press.

Kernberg, P. F. (1983). Borderline conditions: Childhood and adolescent aspects. In K. S. Robson (Ed.), The borderline child--approaches to etiology, diagnosis and treatment (pp. 101-119). New York: McGraw-Hill.

Leichtman, M., & Nathan, S. (1983). A clinical approach to the psychological testing of borderline children. In K. S. Robson (Ed.), The borderline child--approaches to etiology, diagnosis and treatment (pp. 121-170). New York: McGraw-Hill.

Masterson, J. F., Lulow, W. V., & Costello, J. L. (1982). The test of time: Borderline adolescent to functioning adult. In S. C. Feinstein, et al. (Eds.), Adolescent psychiatry: Developmental and clinical studies (Vol. 10, pp. 494-522). Chicago: University of Chicago Press.

Ornstein, A. (1981). Self-pathology in children: Developmental and clinical considerations. Psychiatric Clinics of North America 4, 435-453.

Petti, T. A., & Unis, A. (1981). Imipramine treatment of borderline children: Case reports with a controlled study. American Journal of Psychiatry 138(4), 515-518.

Pfeffer, C. R. (1982). Clinical observations of suicidal behavior in a neurotic, a borderline, and a psychotic child: Common processes of symptom formation. Child Psychiatry and Human Development 13(2), 120-134.

Pine, F. (1974). On the concept of "borderline" in children. In R. S. Eissler, et al. (Eds.), Psychoanalytic study of the child (Vol. 26, pp. 341-368). New York: International Universities Press.

Pine, F. (1980). On phase-characteristic pathology of the school-age child: Disturbances of personality development and organization (borderline conditions) of learning and behavior. In S. I. Greenspan & G. H. Pollock (Eds.), The course of life: Psychoanalytic contributions toward understanding personality development (pp. 165-203). Washington, D.C.: National Institute of Mental Health.

Rinsley, D. B. (1980a). The developmental etiology of borderline and narcissistic disorders. Bulletin of the Menninger Clinic 44, 127-134.

Rinsley, D. B. (1980b). Diagnosis and treatment of borderline and narcissistic children and adolescents. Bulletin of the Menninger Clinic 44, 147-170.

Rinsley, D. B. (1981). Borderline psychopathology: The concepts of Masterson and Rinsley and beyond. In S. C. Feinstein, et al. (Eds.), Adolescent psychiatry: Developmental and clinical studies (Vol. 9, pp. 259-274). Chicago: University of Chicago Press.

Rosenfeld, S. K., & Sprince, M. D. (1963). An attempt to formulate the meaning of the concept "borderline." In R. S. Eissler, et al. (Eds.), Psychoanalytic study of the child (Vol. 18, pp. 603-635). New York: International Universities Press.

Schwartzberg, A. Z. (1978). Overview of borderline syndrome in adolescence. In S. C. Feinstein, et al. (Eds.), Adolescent psychiatry: Developmental and clinical studies (Vol. 6, pp. 286-297). Chicago: University of Chicago Press.

Settlage, C. (1980). The psychoanalytic understanding of narcissistic and borderline personality disorders: Advances in developmental theory. In R. F. Lax, S. Bach, & J. Burland (Eds.), Rapprochement: The critical subphase of separation-individuation (pp. 77-100). New York: Jason Aronson.

Simon, J. I. (1984). The borderline syndrome in adolescents. Adolescence 19, 505-520.

Shapiro, E. R., Zinner, J., Shapiro, R. I., & Berkowitz, D. (1975). The influence of family experience on borderline personality development. International Review of Psychoanalysis 2, 399-412.

Smith, F. H., Bemporad, J. R., & Harrison, G. (1982). Aspects of the treatment of borderline children. American Journal of Psychotherapy 36(2), 181-197.

Soloff, H. P., & Millward, J. W. (1983). Developmental histories of borderline patients. Comprehensive Psychiatry 24(6), 574-588.

Volkan, V. D. (1979). The glass bubble of the narcissistic patient in advances. In L. J. Capponi (Ed.), Psychotherapy of the borderline patient. New York: Jason Aronson.

Weil, A. P. (1953). Certain severe disturbances of ego development in childhood. In R. S. Eissler, et al. (Eds.), Psychoanalytic study of the child (Vol. 8, pp. 271-286). New York: International Universities Press.

N. Mental Retardation

Andrew Russell, M.D., Section Editor

Steven Forness, Ed.D., Fred Frankel, Ph.D., Connie Kasasi, Marian Sigman, Ph.D., Alexander Tymchuck, Ph.D., and Mario Valente, M.D., Associate Editors

1. Historical Aspects of Mental Retardation

Hightower-Vandamm, M. D. (1979). Developmental disabilities act: An historic perspective. Part 2. American Journal of Occupational Therapy 33, 421-423.

Kraft, I. (1961). Edouard Sequin and the 19th century moral treatment of idiots. Bulletin of the History of Medicine 35, 393-418.

Lakin, K., Krantz, G., Bruininks, R., Clumpner, J., & Hill, B. (1982). One hundred years of data on populations of public residential facilities for mentally retarded

people. American Journal of Mental Deficiency 87, 1-8.
Scheerenberger, R. C. (1983). A history of mental retardation. Baltimore: Brooks.
Shattuck, R. (1980). The forbidden experiment: The story of the wild boy of Aveyron. New York: McGraw-Hill.
Woolfson, R. C. (1984). Historical perspective on mental retardation. American Journal of Mental Deficiency 89, 231-235.

2. Etiology of Mental Retardation

Akuffo, E. O., & Sylvester, P. E. (1983). Head injury and mental handicap. Journal of the Royal Society of Medicine 76, 545-549.
Baird, P. A., & Sadovnick, A. D. (1988). Maternal age-specific rates for Down's syndrome: Changes over time. American Journal of Medical Genetics 29, 917-928.
Bovicelli, L., Orsini, L. F., Rizzo, N., Montacuti, V., & Bacchetta, M. (1982). Reproduction in Down syndrome. Obstetrics and Gynecology 59, 13S-17S.
Burack, J. A., Hodapp, R. M., & Ziger, E. (1988). Issues in the classification of mental retardation: Differentiating among organic etiologies. Journal of Child Psychology and Psychiatry and Allied Disciplines 28(6), 766-779.
Coleman, M., Brubaker, J., Hunter, K., & Smith, G. (1988). Rett syndrome--a survey of North American patients. Journal of Mental Deficiency Research 32, 117-124.
Crandall, B. F. (1977). Genetic disorders and mental retardation. American Journal of Child Psychiatry 16, 88-108.
Crandall, B. F. (1989). Update on genetics and mental retardation. Psychiatric Annals 19(4), 197-204.
Crandall, B. F., & Matsumoto, M. (1986). Routine amniotic fluid AFP assay: Experience with 40,000 pregnancies. American Journal of Medical Genetics 24, 143-149.
Crnic, L. S. (1984). Nutrition and mental development. American Journal of Mental Deficiency 88, 526-533.
Crocker, A., & Cohen, H. J. (1988). Guidelines on developmental services for children and adults with HIV infection. Unpublished manuscript, American Association of University Affiliated Programs for Persons with Developmental Disabilities. Silver Springs, Maryland.
de la Cruz, F. F. (1985). Fragile X syndrome. American Journal of Mental Deficiency 90, 19-123.
Deykin, E. Y., & MacMahon, B. (1979). The incidence of seizures among children with autistic symptoms. American Journal of Psychiatry 136, 471-479.
Falloon, J., Eddy, J., Wiener, L., & Pizzo, P. (1989). Human immunodeficiency virus infection in children. Journal of Pediatrics 114, 1-30.
Fulroth, R., Phillips, B., & Durand, D. (1989). Perinatal outcome of infants exposed to cocaine and/or heroin in utero. American Journal of Diseases of Children 143, 905-910.

Gal, P., & Sharpless, M. K. (1984). Fetal drug exposure--behavioral teratogenesis. Drug Intelligence and Clinical Pharmacy 18, 186-201.

Gillberg, C., Ohlson, V. A., Wahlstrom, J., Steffenburg, S., & Bux, K. (1988). Monozygotic female twins with autism and fragile-X syndrome (AFRAX). Journal of Child Psychology and Psychiatry and Allied Disciplines 29, 447-452.

Gomez, M. (Ed.). (1979). Tuberous sclerosis. New York: Raven Press.

Greenswag, L. (1987). Adults with Prader-Willi Syndrome: A survey of 232 cases. Developmental Medicine and Child Neurology 29, 145-152.

Hagberg, B., Aicardi, J., Dias, K., & Ramos, O. (1983). A progressive syndrome of autism, dementia, ataxia, and loss of purposeful hand use in girls. Rett's syndrome: Report of 35 cases. Annals of Neurology 14, 471-479.

Hagerman, R. J., & McBogg, P. M. (1983). (Eds.). The fragile X syndrome: Diagnosis, biochemistry, and intervention. Dillon, Colo.: Spectra Publishing.

Hershey, D. W., Crandall, B. F., & Perdue, S. (1986). Combining maternal age and serum AFP to predict the risk of Down's syndrome. Obstetrics and Gynecology 68, 177.

Kemper, M. B., Hagerman, R. J., & Altshul-Stark, D. (1988). American Journal of Medical Genetics 30, 191-200.

Kirman, B. H. (1985). Mental retardation: Medical aspects. In M. Rutter & L. Hersov (eds.), Child and adolescent psychiatry: Modern approaches. Oxford: Blackwell.

Nichols, P. L. (1984). Familial mental retardation. Behavior Genetics 14, 161-170.

Opitz, J. (Ed.). (1986). X-linked mental retardation [Special issue]. American Journal of Medical Genetics 23, 1-738.

Payton, J. B., Steele, M. W., Wenger, S. L., & Minshew, N. J. (1989). The fragile X marker and autism in perspective. Journal of the American Academy of Child and Adolescent Psychiatry 28, 417-421.

(1988). The Rett syndrome diagnostic criteria work group. Diagnostic criteria for Rett syndrome. Annals of Neurology 23, 425-428.

Riccardi, V. (1986). Neurofibromatosis: Phenotype, natural history and pathogenesis. Baltimore: Johns Hopkins University Press.

Shoumaker, R. D., Bennett, D. R., Bray, P. F., & Curless, R. G. (1974). Clinical and EEG manifestations of an unusual aphasic syndrome in children. Neurology 24, 10-16.

Smalley, S. L., Asarnow, R. F., & Spence, M. A. (1988). Autism and genetics. A decade of research. Archives of General Psychiatry 45(10), 953-961.

Streissguth, A. P. (1986). The behavioral teratology of alcohol: Performance, behavioral, and intellectual deficits in prenatally exposed children. In J. R. West (Ed.), Alcohol and brain development. New York: Oxford University Press.

Streissguth, A. P., Landesman-Dwyer, S., Martin, J. C., & Smith, D. W. (1980). Teratogenic effects of alcohol in humans and laboratory animals. Science 209, 353-361.

Taylor, D. J., Howie, P. W., Davidson, J., Davidson, D., & Drillien, C. M. (1985). Do pregnancy complications contribute to neurodevelopmental disability? Lancet 1, 713-716.

Vining, E., Accardo, P., Rubenstein, J. E., Farrell, S., & Roizen, N. J. (1976). Cerebral palsy. American Journal of Diseases of Children 130, 643-649.

Wisniewski, K. E., Wisniewski, H. M., & Wen, G. Y. (1985). Occurrence of neuropathological changes and dementia of Alzheimer's disease in Down's syndrome. Annals of Neurology 17, 278-282.

3. Ethics of Treatment

Allen, D. (1989). The effects of deinstitutionalization on people with mental handicaps: A review. Mental Handicap Research 2, 18-37.

Baumeister, A. A. (1981). Mental retardation policy and research: The unfulfilled promise. American Journal of Mental Deficiency 85, 449-456.

Braddock, D. (1986). From Roosevelt to Reagan: Federal spending for mental retardation and developmental disabilities. American Journal of Mental Deficiency 90, 479-489.

Braddock, D., & Heller, T. (1985). The closure of mental retardation institutions. I: Trends in the United States. Mental Retardation 23, 168-177.

Castellani, P. J. (1986). Symposium overview: Policy perspectives on the economics of mental retardation: The new environment of developmental services. Mental Retardation 24, 5-9.

Craig, E., & McCarver, R. B. (1984). Community placement and adjustment of deinstitutionalized clients: Issues and findings. International Review of Research in Mental Retardation 12, 95-122.

Cushna, B., Szymanski, L. S., & Tanguay, P. E. (1980). Professional roles and unmet manpower needs. In L. S. Szymanski & P. E. Tanguay (Eds.), Emotional disorders of mentally retarded persons. Baltimore: University Park Press.

Dokecki, P. R., & Zaner, R. M. (1986). Ethics of dealing with persons with severe handicaps: Toward a research agenda. Baltimore: Paul H. Brookes.

Edgerton, R. B. (1988). Aging in the community--a matter of choice. American Journal of Mental Retardation 92, 331-335.

Emerson, E., Cummings, R., Barrett, S., Hughes, H., McCook C., & Toogood, A. (1988). Challenging behavior and community services: 2. Who are the people who challenge services? Mental Handicaps 16, 16-19.

Shepperdson, B. (1983). Abortion and euthanasia of Down's syndrome children--the parents' view. Journal of Medical Ethics 9, 152-157.

Shepperdson, B. (1985). Changes in the characteristics of families with Down's syndrome children. Journal of Epidemiology and Community Health 39, 320-324.

Vitello, S. J., & Soskin, R. M. (1985). Mental retardation: Its social and legal context. Englewood Cliffs, N.J.: Prentice-Hall.

Wynne, M. E., & Rogers, J. J. (1985). Variables discriminating residential placement of severely handicapped children. American Journal of Mental Deficiency 89, 515-523.

4. Cognitive Capacities and Social Behavior

Ando, H., & Yoshimura, I. (1978). Prevalence of maladaptive behavior in retardedchildren as a function of IQ and age. Journal of Abnormal Child Psychology 6, 345-349.

Becker, S., & Glidden, L. M. (1979). Imitation in EMR boys: Model competency and age. American Journal of Mental Deficiency 83, 360-366.

Berry, H. K., O'Grady, D. J., Perlmuttter, L. J., & Bofinger, M. K. (1979). Intellectual development and academic achievement of children treated early for phenylketonuria. Developmental Medicine and Child Neurology 21, 311-320.

Blacher, J. (1982). Assessing social cognition in young mentally retarded and nonretarded children. American Journal of Mental Deficiency 86, 473-484.

Cicchetti, D., & Serafica, F. (1981). The interplay among behavioral systems: Illustration from the study of attachment, affiliation, and wariness in young Down's syndrome children. Developmental Psychology 17, 326-339.

Connolly, J. A. (1978). Intelligence levels of Down's syndrome children. American Journal of Mental Deficiency 83, 193-196.

Cunningham, C. C., Glenn, S. M., Wilkinson, P., & Sloper, P. (1985). Mental ability, symbolic play and receptive and expressive language of young children with Down's syndrome. Journal of Child Psychology and Psychiatry and Allied Disciplines 26, 255-265.

Dewart, M. H. (1979). Language comprehension processes of mentally retarded children. American Journal of Mental Deficiency 84, 177-183.

Edgerton, R. B. (1984). The participant-observer approach to research in mental retardation. American Journal of Mental Deficiency 88, 498-505.

Forness, S. R., Guthrie, D., & MacMillan, D. L. (1982). Classroom environments as they relate to mentally retarded children's observable behavior. American Journal of Mental Deficiency 87, 259-265.

Freeman, B. J., Guthrie, D., Ritvo, E., Schroth, P., Glass, R., & Frankel, F. (1979). Behavior observation scale: Preliminary analysis of the similarities and differences between autistic and mentally retarded children. Psychological Reports 44, 519-524.

Gath, A., & Gumley, D. (1984). Down's syndrome and the family: Follow-up of children first seen in infancy. Developmental Medicine and Child Neurology 26, 500-508.

Guralnick, M. J., & Groom, J. M. (1985). Correlates of peer-related social competence of developmentally delayed preschool children. American Journal of Mental Deficiency 90, 140-150.

Kahn, J. V. (1976). Moral and cognitive development of moderately retarded, mildly retarded, and nonretarded individuals. American Journal of Mental Deficiency 81, 209-214.

Koller, H., Richardson, S. A., & Katz, M. (1988a). Marriage in a young adult mentally retarded population. Journal of Mental Deficiency Research 32, 93-102.

Koller, H., Richardson, S. A., & Katz, M. (1988b). Peer relationships of mildly retarded young adults living in the community. Journal of Mental Deficiency Research 32, 321-332.

Kosari, C., Sigman, M., Mundy, P., & Yirmiya, N. (1988). Caregiver interactions with autistic children. Journal of Abnormal Child Psychology 16, 45-56.

Krupski, A. (1979). Are retarded children more distractible? Observational analysis of retarded and nonretarded children's classroom behavior. American Journal of Mental Deficiency 84, 1-10.

LaVeck, B., & Brehm, S. S. (1978). Individual variability among children with Down's syndrome. Mental Retardation 16, 135-137.

Libb, J. W., Myers, G. J., Graham, E., & Bell, B. (1983). Correlates of intelligence and adaptive behaviour in Down's syndrome. Journal of Mental Deficiency Research 27, 205-210.

Mink, I. T., Meyers, C. E., & Nihira, K. (1984). Taxonomy of family life styles: II. Homes with slow-learning children. American Journal of Mental Deficiency 89, 111-123.

Ramey, C. T., Yeates, K. O., & Short, E. J. (1984). The plasticity of intellectual development: Insights from preventive intervention. Child Development 55, 1913-1925.

Sigelman, C. K., Budd, E. C., Winer, J. L., Schoenrock, C. J., & Martin, P. W. (1982). Evaluating alternative techniques of questioning mentally retarded persons. American Journal of Mental Deficiency 86, 511-518.

Siperstein, G. N., & Bak, J. J. (1985). Effects of social behavior on children's attitudes toward their mildly and moderately mentally retarded peers. American Journal of Mental Deficiency 90, 319-327.

Weisz, J. (1982). Learned helplessness and the retarded child. In E. Zigler & D. Balla (Eds.), Mental retardation: The developmental difference controversy. Hillsdale, N.J.: Erlbaum.

Whorton, J. E., & Algozzine, R. F. (1978). A comparison of intellectual achievement, and adaptive behavior levels for students who are mildly retarded. Mental Retardation 16, 320-321.

Wilson, R. S., & Matheny, A. P. (1976). Retardation and twin concordance in infant mental retardation. Behavior Genetics 6, 353-358.

Wing, L. (1981). Language, social, and cognitive impairments in autism and severe mental retardation. Journal of Autism and Developmental Disorders 11, 31-44.

Zigler, E., & Balla, D. A. (1982). Motivational and personality factors in the performance of the retarded. In E. Zigler & D. Balla (Eds.), Mental retardation: The developmental-difference controversy. Hillsdale, N.J.: Erlbaum.

5. Psychopharmacological Treatment of Retardation

Aman, M. G. (1982). Stimulant drug effects in developmental disorders and hyperactivity--toward a resolution of disparate findings. Journal of Autism and Developmental Disorders 12, 385-398.

Psychopathology: Disease and Disorder

Aman, M. G., Field, C. J., & Bridgman, G. D. (1985). City-wide survey of drug patterns among non-institutionalized mentally retarded persons. Applied Research in Mental Retardation 6, 159-171.

Aman, M. G., & Singh, N. N. (1980). The usefulness of thioridazine for treating childhood disorders--fact or folklore? American Journal of Mental Deficiency 84, 331-338.

Aman, M. G., & Singh, N. N. (1988). Psychopharmacology of the developmental disabilities. New York: Springer-Verlag.

Aman, M. G., Singh, N. N., Stewart, A. W., & Field, C. J. (1985). The aberrant behavior checklist: A behavior rating scale for the assessment of treatment effects. American Journal of Mental Deficiency 89, 485-491.

Aman, M. G., & White, A. J. (1988). Thioridazine dose effects with reference to stereotypic behavior in mentally retarded residents. Journal of Autism and Developmental Disorders 18, 355-366.

Campbell, M., Adams, P., Small, A. M., Curren, E. L., Overall, J. E., Anderson, L. T., Lynch, N., & Perry, R. (1988). Efficacy and safety of fenfluramine in autistic children. Journal of the American Academy of Child and Adolescent Psychiatry 27, 434-439.

Gadow, K. D. (1985). Prevalence and efficacy of stimulant drug use with mentally retarded children and youth. Psychopharmacology Bulletin 21, 291-303.

Gualtieri, C. T., Lefler, W. H., Guimond, M., & Staye, J. I. (1982). Corneal and lenticular opacities in mentally retarded young adults treated with thioridazine and chlorpromazine. American Journal of Psychiatry 139, 1178-1180.

Hagerman, R. J., Murphy, M. A., & Whittenberger, M. D. (1988). A controlled trial of stimulant medication in children with the fragile X syndrome. American Journal of Medical Genetics 30, 377-392.

Hill, B. K., Balow, E. A., & Bruininks, R. H. (1985). A national study of prescribed drugs in institutions and community residential facilities for mentally retarded people. Psychopharmacology Bulletin 21, 279-284.

Jacobson, J. W. (1988). Problem behavior and psychiatric impairment within a developmentally disabled population. III: Psychotropic medication. Research in Developmental Disabilities 9, 23-38.

Lipman, R. S., DiMascio, A., Reatig, N., & Kirson, T. (1978). Psychotropic drugs and mentally retarded children. In M. A. Lipton, A. DiMascio, & K. F. Killam (Eds.), Psychopharmacology: A generation of progress. New York: Raven Press.

Lipman, R. S., & Nibble, E. D. (1986). Methodological issues in treatment research in the mentally retarded. Psychopharmacology Bulletin 22, 1045-1085.

Singh, N. N., & Aman, M. G. (1981). Effects of thioridazine dosage on behavior of mentally retarded persons. American Journal of Mental Deficiency 85, 580-587.

Singh, N. N., & Millichamp, C. J. (1984). Effects of medication on the self-injurious behavior of mentally retarded persons Psychiatric Aspects of Mental Retardation Review 3, 13-16.

Sprague, R. L. (1978). Principles of clinical trials and social, ethical, and legal issues of drug use in children. In J. S. Werry (Ed.), Pediatric psychopharmacology: The use of behavior modifying drugs in children. New York: Brunner/Mazel.

Sprague, R. L., Kalachnik, J. E., Breuning, S. E., et al. (1984). The dyskinesia identification system--coldwater (DIS-CO): A tardive dyskinesia rating scale for the developmentally disabled. Psychopharmacology Bulletin 20, 328-338.

Stone, R. K., Alvarez, W. F., & May, J. E. (1988). Dyskinesia, antipsychotic-drug exposure and risk factors in a developmentally disabled population. Pharmacology, Biochemistry and Behavior 29, 45-51.

Szymanski, L. S. (1978). Psychiatric diagnostic evaluation of mentally retarded individuals. Journal of the American Academy of Child Psychiatry 17, 67-87.

Varley, C. K., & Trupin, E. W. (1982). Double-blind administration of methylphenidate to mentally retarded children with attention deficit disorder: A preliminary study. American Journal of Mental Deficiency 86, 560-566.

Zimmermann, R. L., & Heistad, G. T. (1982). Studies of the long term efficacy of antipsychotic drugs in controlling the behavior of institutionalized retardates. Journal of the American Academy of Child Psychiatry 21, 136-143.

6. Education and Its Effects on Mentally Retarded Children

Burton, T. A., & Hirshoren, A. (1979). The education of severely and profoundly retarded children: Are we sacrificing the child to the concept? Exceptional Children 45, 598-602.

Carlberg, C., & Kavale, K. (1980). The efficacy of special versus regular class placement for exceptional children: A meta-analysis. Journal of Special Education 14, 294-309.

Forness, S. R., Guthrie, D., & MacMillan, D. L. (1982). Classroom environments as they relate to mentally retarded children's observable behavior. American Journal of Mental Deficiency 87, 259-265.

Forness, S. R., & Kavale, K. A. (1984). Education of the mentally retarded: A note on policy. Education and Training of the Mentally Retarded 19, 239-245.

Forness, S. R., & MacMillan, D. L. (1989). Mental retardation and the special education system. Psychiatric Annals 19(4), 190-196.

Haywood, H. C. (1979). What happened to mild and moderate mental retardation? American Journal of Mental Deficiency 83, 429-431.

Knoff, H. M. (1984). Placement decisions revisited: IQ doesn't always tip the scale. Exceptional Children 51, 122-128.

Linden, B., & Forness, S. R. (1986). Post-school adjustment of mentally retarded persons with psychiatric disorders: A ten-year follow-up. Education and Training of the Mentally Retarded 21, 196-203.

MacMillan, D. L. (1982). Mental retardation in school and society. Boston: Little, Brown.

MacMillan, D. L., & Borthwick, S. (1980). The new educable mentally retarded population: Can they be mainstreamed? Mental Retardation 18, 155-158.

Polloway, E. A., Epstein, M. H., Patton, J. R., Cullinan, D., & Luebke, J. (1986). Demographic, social, and behavioral characteristics of students with educable mental retardation. Education and Training of the Mentally Retarded 21, 27-34.

Russell, A. T., & Forness, S. R. (1985). Behavioral disturbances in mentally retarded children in TMR and EMR classrooms. American Journal of Mental Deficiency 89, 338-344.

Stainback, W., Stainback, S., Courtnage, L., & Jaben, T. (1985). Facilitating mainstreaming by modifying the mainstream. Exceptional Children 52, 144-152.

7. Training Parents and Staff to Work with Retarded Children and Adolescents

Baker, B., Heifetz, L., & Murphy, D. (1980). Behavioral training for parents of mentally retarded children. American Journal of Mental Deficiency 85, 31-38.

Baker, B. L., & Brightman, R. P. (1984). Training parents of retarded children: Program-specific outcomes. Journal of Behavior Therapy and Experimental Psychiatry 15, 255-260.

Breiner, J., & Beck, S. (1984). Parents as change agents in the management of their developmentally delayed children's non-compliant behaviors: A critical review. Applied Research in Mental Retardation 5, 259-278.

Burgio, L. D., Page, T. J., & Capriotti, R. M. (1985). Clinical behavioral pharmacology: Methods for evaluating medications and contingency management. Journal of Applied Behavior Analysis 18, 45-59.

Cowart, J., Iwata, B., & Poynter, H. (1984). Generalization and maintenance in training parents of the mentally retarded. Applied Research in Mental Retardation 5, 233-244.

Davidson, N. A., Hemingway, M. J., & Wysocki, T. (1984). Reducing the use of restrictive procedures in a residential facility. Hospital and Community Psychiatry 35, 164-167.

Delamater, A. M., Conners, C. K., & Wells, K. C. (1984). A comparison of staff training procedures: Behavioral applications in the child psychiatric inpatient setting. Behavior Modification 8, 39-58.

Edgerton, R. B. (1984). The participant-observer approach to research in mental retardation. American Journal of Mental Deficiency 88, 498-505.

Frankel, F., & Simmons, J. Q. (1985). Behavioral treatment approaches to pathological unsocialized physical aggression in young children. Journal of Child Psychology and Psychiatry and Allied Disciplines 26, 525-551.

Gair, D. S., Hersch, C., & Wiesenfeld, S. (1980). Successful psychotherapy of severe emotional disturbance in a young retarded boy. Journal of the American Academy of Child Psychiatry 19, 257-269.

Gorman-Smith, D., & Matson, J. L. (1985). A review of treatment research for self-injurious and stereotyped responding. Journal of Mental Deficiency Research 29, 295-308.

Helm, D., & Kozloff, M. (1986). Research on parent training: Shortcomings and remedies. Journal of Autism and Developmental Disorders 16, 1-22.

Hornby, G., & Singh, N. N. (1984). Behavioural group training with parents of mentally retarded children. Journal of Mental Deficiency Research 28, 43-52.

Konarski, E., & Diorio, M. (1985). A quantitative review of self-help research with the severely and profoundly mentally retarded. Applied Research in Mental Retardation 6, 229-245.

Matson, J. L. (1981). Assessment and treatment of clinical fears in mentally retarded children. Journal of Applied Behavior Analysis 14, 287-294.

Matson, J. L., & Gorman-Smith, D. (1986). A review of treatment research for aggressive and disruptive behavior in the mentally retarded. Applied Research in Mental Retardation 7, 95-103.

Morrison, T. L., & Newcomer, B. L. (1975). Effects of directive vs. nondirective play therapy with institutionalized mentally retarded children. American Journal of Mental Deficiency 79, 666-669.

Piper, M. C., & Pless, I. B. (1980). Early intervention for infants with Down syndrome: A controlled trial. Pediatrics 65, 463-468.

Richman, G. S., Reiss, M. L., Bauman, K. E., & Bailey, J. S. (1984). Teaching menstrual care to mentally retarded women: Acquisition, generalization, and maintenance. Journal of Applied Behavior Analysis 17, 441-551.

Robertson, I., Richardson, A. M., & Youngson, S. C. (1984). Social skills training with mentally handicapped people: A review. British Journal of Clinical Psychology 23, 241-264.

Seitz, V., Rosenbaum, L., & Apfel, N. (1985). Effects of family support intervention: A ten year follow-up. Child Development 56, 376-391.

Simeonsson, R. J., Cooper, D. H., & Scheiner, A. P. (1982). A review and analysis of the effectiveness of early intervention programs. Pediatrics 69, 635-641.

Wilson, P. G., Reid, D. H., Phillips, J. F., & Burgio, L. D. (1984). Normalization of institutional mealtimes for profoundly retarded persons: Effects and noneffects of teaching family-style dining. Journal of Applied Behavior Analysis 17, 189-201.

Wing, L. (1985). Services for severely retarded children and adolescents. In M. Rutter & L. Hersov (Eds.), Child and adolescent psychiatry: Modern approaches. Oxford: Blackwell.

Zigler, E. (1981). A plea to end the use of patterning treatment for retarded children. American Journal of Orthopsychiatry 51, 388-390.

8. Role of the Family in Promoting Optimal Function

Bernheimer, L. P., Young, M. S., & Winton, P. J. (1983). Stress over time: Parents with young handicapped children. Journal of Developmental and Behavioral Pediatrics 4, 177-181.

Blacher, J. (1984). Sequential stages of parental adjustment to the birth of a child with handicaps: Fact or artifact? Mental Retardation 22, 55-68.

Blacher, J., & Meyers, C. E. (1983). A review of attachment formation and disorder of handicapped children. American Journal of Mental Deficiency 87, 359-371.

Byrne, E. A., & Cunningham, C. C. (1985). The effects of mentally handicapped children on families--a conceptual review. Journal of Child Psychology and Psychiatry and Allied Disciplines 26, 847-864.

Carr, J. (1988). Six weeks to twenty-one years old--a longitudinal study of children with Down's syndrome and their families. Journal of Child Psychology and Psychiatry and Allied Disciplines 29, 407-432.

Cassidy, S. B., Pagon, R. A., Pepin, M., & Blumhagen, J. D. (1983). Family studies in tuberous sclerosis. Evaluation of apparently unaffected parents. Journal of the American Medical Association 249, 1302-1304.

Crawley, S. B., & Spiker, D. (1983). Mother-child interactions involving two-year-olds with Down's syndrome: A look at individual differences. Child Development 54, 1312-1323.

Crnic, K. A., Friedrich, W. N., & Greenberg, M. T. (1983). Adaptation of families with mentally retarded children. A model of stress, coping, and family ecology. American Journal of Mental Deficiency 88, 125-138.

Cunningham, C. E., Reuler, E., Blackwell, J., & Deck, J. (1981). Behavioral and linguistic developments in the interactions of normal and retarded children with their mothers. Child Development 52, 62-70.

Doernberg, N. L. (1982). Issues in communication between pediatricians and parents of young mentally retarded children. Pediatric Annals 11, 438-439, 442-444.

Emde, R. N., & Brown, C. (1978). Adaptation to the birth of a Down's syndrome infant: Grieving and maternal attachment. Journal of the American Academy of Child Psychiatry 17, 299-323.

Ferguson, P. M., Ferguson, D. I., & Jones, D. (1988). Generations of hope: Parental perspectives on the transitions of their children with severe retardation from school to adult life. Journal of the Association of Persons with Severe Handicaps 12, 177-187.

Friedrich, W. N. (1979). Predictors of the coping behavior of mothers of handicapped children. Journal of Consulting and Clinical Psychology 47, 1140-1141.

Gath, A., & Gumley, D. (1984). Down's syndrome and the family: Follow-up of children first seen in infancy. Developmental Medicine and Child Neurology 26, 500-508.

Holroyd, J., & McArthur, D. (1976). Mental retardation and stress on the parents: A contrast between Down's syndrome and childhood autism. American Journal of Mental Deficiency 80, 431-436.

Morrison, G. M., & Zetlin, A. (1988). Perceptions of communication, cohesion, and adaptability in families of adolescents with and without learning handicaps. Journal of Abnormal Child Psychology 16, 675-686.

Piper, M. C., & Ramsay, M. K. (1980). Effects of early home environments on the mental development of Down syndrome infants. American Journal of Mental Deficiency 85, 39-44.

Rubin, A. L., & Rubin, R. L. (1980). The effects of physician counseling technique on parent reactions to mental retardation diagnosis. Child Psychiatry and Human Development 10, 213-221.

Shepperdson, B. (1985). Changes in the characteristics of families with Down's syndrome in children. Journal of Epidemiology and Community Health 39, 320-324.

Sorce, J. F., & Emde, R. N. (1982). The meaning of infant emotional expressions: Regularities in caregiving responses in normal and Down's syndrome infants. Journal of Child Psychology and Psychiatry and Allied Disciplines 23, 145-158.

Wikler, L., Wasow, M., & Hatfield, E. (1981). Chronic sorrow revisited: Parent vs. professional depiction of the adjustment of parents of mentally retarded children. American Journal of Orthopsychiatry 51, 63-70.

9. Psychiatric Aspects of Mental Retardation in Children

Beck, D., Carlson, G., Russell, A., & Brownfield, F. (1987). Use of depression rating instruments in developmentally and educationally delayed adolescents. Journal of the American Academy of Child Psychiatry 26, 97-100.

Chess, S. (1977). Evolution of behavior disorder in a group of mentally retarded children. Journal of the American Academy of Child Psychiatry 16, 5-18.

Corbett, J. A. (1985). Mental retardation: Psychiatric aspects. In M. Rutter & L. Hersov (Eds.), Child and adolescent psychiatry: Modern approaches. Oxford: Blackwell.

Eaton, L. F., & Menolascino, F. J. (1982). Psychiatric disorders in the mentally retarded: Types, problems, and challenges. American Journal of Psychiatry 139, 1297-1303.

Freeman, B. J., Guthrie, D., Ritvo, E., Schroth, P., Glass, R., & Frankel, F. (1979). Behavior observation scale: Preliminary analysis of the similarities and differences between autistic and mentally retarded children. Psychological Reports 44, 519-524.

Ghaziuddin, M. (1988). Behavioral disorder in the mentally handicapped: The role of life events. British Journal of Psychiatry 152, 683-686.

Jacobson, J. W. (1982). Problem behavior and psychiatric impairment within a developmentally disabled population: Behavior frequency. Applied Research in Mental Retardation 3, 121-139.

Kazdin, A., Matson, J., & Senatore, V. (1983). Assessment of depression in mentally retarded adults. American Journal of Psychiatry 140, 1040-1043.

Koller, H., Richardson, S. W., Katz, M., & McKaren, J. (1983). Behavior disturbance since childhood among a 5 year birth cohort of all mentally retarded young adults in a city. American Journal of Mental Deficiency 87, 386-395.

Lund, J. (1988). Psychiatric aspects of Down's syndrome. Acta Paediatrica Scandinavica 78, 369-374.

Matson, J. L., Barrett, R., & Helsel, W. J. (1988). Depression in mentally retarded children. Research in Developmental Disabilities 9, 39-46.

McCracken, J. T., & Diamond, R. P. (1988). Bipolar disorder in mentally retarded adolescents. Journal of the American Academy of Child and Adolescent Psychiatry 27, 494-499.

Newton, J. T., & Sturmey, P. (1988). The aberrant behavior checklist--a British replication and extension of its psychometric properties. Journal of Mental Deficiency Research 32, 87-92.

Reiss, A. L., Hagerman, R. J., Vinogradov, S., Abrams, M., & King, R. J. (1988). Psychiatric disability in female carriers of the fragile X chromosome. Archives of General Psychiatry 45, 25-30.

Reynolds, W. M., & Baker, J. A. (1988). Assessment of depression in persons with mental retardation. American Journal of Mental Retardation 93, 93-103.

Richardson, S. A., Koller, H., & Katz, M. (1985). Continuities an change in behavior disturbance: A follow-up study of mildly retarded young people. American Journal of Orthopsychiatry 55, 220-229.

Watson, J. E., Aman, M. G., & Singh, N. N. (1988). The psychopathology instrument for mentally retarded adults: Psychometric characteristics, factor structure, and relationship to subject characteristics. Research in Developmental Disabilities 9, 277-290.

10. Epidemiology of Mental Retardation in Children

Corbett, J. A. (1977). Population studies of mental retardation. In P. J. Graham (Ed.), Epidemiological approaches in child psychiatry. London: Academic Press.

Rantakallio, P., & Von Wendt, L. (1986). Mental retardation and subnormality in a birth cohort of 12,000 children in northern Finland. American Journal of Mental Deficiency 90, 361-380.

Rutter, M., & Shaffer, D. (1980). DSM III: A step forward or back in terms of the classification of child psychiatric disorders. Journal of the American Academy of Child Psychiatry 19, 371-394.

Tarjan, G., Tizard, J., Rutter, M., Begab, M., Brooke, E. M., de la Cruz, F., Lin, H., et al. (1972). Classification and mental retardation: Issues arising in the firth W.H.O. seminar on psychiatric diagnosis, classification, and statistics. American Journal of Psychiatry 128, 34-45.

Tarjan, G., Wright, S. W., Eyman, R. K., & Keeran, C. V. (1973). Natural history of mental retardation: Some aspects of epidemiology. American Journal of Mental Deficiency 77, 359-379.

Zigler, E., & Hodapp, R. M. (1986a). Definition and classification of mental retardation. In E. Zigler & R. M. Hodapp (Eds.), Understanding mental retardation. Cambridge: Cambridge University Press.

Zigler, E., & Hodapp, R. M. (1986b). How many retarded people are there? In E. Zigler & R. M. Hodapp (Eds.), Understanding mental retardation. Cambridge: Cambridge University Press.

11. Miscellaneous References

de la Cruz, F. F., & La Veck, G. D. (Eds.). (1973). Human sexuality and the mentally retarded. New York: Brunner/Mazel.

Edgerton, R. M. (1984). The participant-observer approach to research in mental retardation. American Journal of Mental Deficiency 88, 498-505.

Lennox, D. B., Miltenberger, R. G., Spengler, P., & Erfanian, N. (1988). Decelerative treatment practices with persons who have mental retardation: A

review of five years of literature. American Journal of Mental Retardation 92, 492-501.
Mercer, J. R. (1973). Labeling the mentally retarded: Clinical and social system perspectives on mental retardation. Berkeley: University of California Press.
Zigler, E., & Hodapp, R. M. (Eds.). (1986). Understanding mental retardation. Cambridge: Cambridge University Press.

O. Adolescent Psychopathology and Special Problems

Lois T. Flaherty, M.D., Section Editor

Michael G. Kalogerakis, M.D., Spyros J. Monopolis, M.D., and Richard M. Sarles, M.D., Associate Editors

1. Overview of Adolescent Development

Abramowitz, R. H., Petersen, A. C., & Schulenberg, J. E. (1984). Changes in self-image during early adolescence. New Directions for Mental Health Services 21, 19-28.
Adams, G. R. (1985). Family correlates of female adolescents' ego-identity development. Journal of Adolescence 8, 69-82.
Adams, G. R., & Fitch, S. A. (1981). Ego stage and identity status development: A cross-lag analysis. Journal of Adolescence 4, 163-171.
Adler, I., & Kandel, D. B. (1981). Cross-cultural perspectives on developmental stages in adolescent drug use. Journal of Studies on Alcohol 42, 701-715.
Baumrind, D., & Moselle, K. A. (1985). A developmental perspective on adolescent drug abuse. Advances in Alcohol and Substance Abuse 4, 41-67.
Benson, R. M. (1980). Narcissistic guardians: Developmental aspects of transitional objects, imaginary companions, and career fantasies. In S. C. Feinstein, et al. (Eds.), Adolescent psychiatry: Developmental and clinical studies (Vol. 8, pp. 253-264. Chicago: University of Chicago Press.
Berkowitz, D. A. (1979). The disturbed adolescent and his family: Problems of individuation. Journal of Adolescence 2, 27-39.
Berlin, I. N. (1978). Some implications of the developmental process for treatment of depression in adolescence. Journal of Adolescence 1, 135-145.
Berndt, D. J., Kaiser, C. F., & Van Aalst, F. (1982). Depression and self-actualization of gifted adolescents. Journal of Clinical Psychology 38, 142-150.
Beveridge, M., Spencer, J, & Mittler, P. (1979). Self-blame and communication failure in retarded adolescents. Journal of Child Psychology and Psychiatry and Allied Disciplines 20, 129-138.
Brandt, L. M. (1983). The fairy tale as paradigm of the separation-individuation crisis: Implications for treatment of the borderline adolescent. In S. C. Feinstein, et al. (Eds.), Adolescent psychiatry: Developmental and clinical studies (Vol. 11, pp. 75-91). Chicago: University of Chicago Press.

Brooks, B. (1985). Sexually abused children and adolescent identity development. American Journal of Psychotherapy 39, 401-410.
Broughton, J. M. (1981). The divided self in adolescence. Human Development 24, 13-32.
Burch, C. A. (1985). Identity foreclosure in early adolescence: A problem of narcissistic equilibrium. In S. C. Feinstein, et al. (Eds.), Adolescent psychiatry: Developmental and clinical studies (Vol. 12, pp. 145-161). Chicago: University of Chicago Press.
Calderone, M. S. (1985). Adolescent sexuality: Elements and genesis. Pediatrics 76, 699-703.
Carneiro Leao, I. (1986). Identification and its vicissitudes as observed in adolescence. International Journal of Psycho-Analysis 67, 65-75.
Chassin, L., Presson, C. C., Young, R. D., & Light, R. (1981). Self-concepts of institutionalized adolescents: A framework for conceptualizing labeling effects. Journal of Abnormal Psychology 90, 143-151.
Chassin, L., Tetzloff, C., & Hershey, M. (1985). Self-image and social-image factors in adolescent alcohol use. Journal of Studies on Alcohol 46, 39-47.
Clarke, A. D., & Clarke, A. M. (1984). Constancy and change in the growth of human characteristics. Journal of Child Psychology and Psychiatry and Allied Disciplines 25, 191-210.
Clarke, B. A. (1983). Improving adolescent parenting through participant modeling and self-evaluation. Nursing Clinics of North America 18, 303-311.
Coleman, E. (1981-1982). Developmental stages of the coming out process. Journal of Homosexuality 7, 31-43.
Copeland, A. D. (1981). The impact of pregnancy on adolescent psychosocial development. In S. C. Feinstein, et al. (Eds.), Adolescent psychiatry: Developmental and clinical studies (Vol. 9, pp. 244-253). Chicago: University of Chicago Press.
Daniels, D., Dunn, J., Furstenberg, F. F., & Plomin, R. (1985). Environmental differences within the family and adjustment differences within pairs of adolescent siblings. Child Development 56, 764-774.
Dien, D. S. (1983). Big me and little me: A chinese perspective on self. Psychiatry 46, 281-286.
Dion, K. L., & Earn, B. M. (1975). The phenomenology of being a target of prejudice. Journal of Personality and Social Psychology 32, 944-950.
Elkind, D. (1985). Cognitive development and adolescent disabilities. Journal of Adolescent Health Care 6, 84-89.
Elson, M., & Kramer, J. F. (1980). Introduction--vulnerable youth: Hope, despair, and renewal. In S. C. Feinstein, et al. (Eds.), Adolescent psychiatry: Developmental and clinical studies (Vol. 8, pp. 267-269). Chicago: University of Chicago Press.
Esman, A. (1986). Giftedness and creativity in children and adolescents. In S. C. Feinstein, et al. (Eds.), Adolescent psychiatry: Developmental and clinical studies (Vol. 13, pp. 62-84). Chicago: University of Chicago Press.

Esman, A. H. (1980). Adolescent psychopathology and the rapprochement phenomenon. In S. C. Feinstein, et al. (Eds.), Adolescent psychiatry: Developmental and clinical studies (Vol. 8, pp. 320-331) . Chicago: University of Chicago Press.

Esman, A. H. (1985). A developmental approach to the psychotherapy of adolescents. In S. C. Feinstein, et al. (Eds.), Adolescent psychiatry: Developmental and clinical studies (Vol. 12, pp. 119-133). Chicago: University of Chicago Press.

Faust, M. S. (1977). Somatic development of adolescent girls. Monographs of the Society for Research in Child Development (Vol. 41, pp. 1-90). Chicago: University of Chicago Press.

Galler, J. R., Ramsey, F., & Solimano, G. (1985a). A follow-up study of the effects of early malnutrition on subsequent development. I. Physical growth and sexual maturation during adolescence. Pediatric Research 19, 518-523.

Galler, J. R., Ramsey, F., & Solimano, G. (1985b). A follow-up study of the effects of early malnutrition on subsequent development. II. Fine motor skills in adolescence. Pediatric Research 19, 524-527.

Garbarino, J., Sebes, J., & Schellenbach, C. (1984). Families at risk for destructive parent-child relations in adolescence. Child Development 55, 174-183.

Gilberg, A. L. (1977). Gender-specific therapy problems in male youths. American Journal of Psychoanalysis 37, 253-255.

Grant, T. N., & Domino, G. (1976). Masculinity-femininity in fathers of creative male adolescents. Journal of Genetic Psychology 129, 19-27.

Grotevant, H. D., & Cooper, C. R. (1985). Patterns of interaction in family relationships and the development of identity exploration in adolescence. Child Development 56, 415-428.

Guyer, M. J., Harrison, S. I., & Rieveschl, J. L. (1982). Developmental rights to privacy and independent decision-making. Journal of the American Academy of Child Psychiatry 21, 298-302.

Hauser, S. T., Jacobson, A. M., Noam, G., & Powers, S. (1983). Ego development and self-image complexity in early adolescence. Longitudinal studies of psychiatric and diabetic patients. Archives of General Psychiatry 40, 325-332.

Henderson, A. F. (1984). Homosexuality in the college years: Developmental differences between men and women. Journal of American College Health 32, 216-219.

Hill, J. P. (1981). The development of the self-concept during the adolescent years. Commentary. Monographs of the Society for Research in Child Development 46, 62-67.

Holzman, P. S. (1980). Discussion--vulnerable youth: Hope, despair, and renewal. In S. C. Feinstein, et al. (Eds.), Adolescent psychiatry: Developmental and clinical studies (Vol. 8, pp. 309-314). Chicago: University of Chicago Press.

Javaid, G. A. (1983). The sexual development of the adolescent daughter of a homosexual mother. Journal of the American Academy of Child Psychiatry 22, 196-201.

Keating, D. P., Keniston, A. H., Manis, F. R., & Bobbitt, B. L. (1980). Development of the search-processing parameter. Child Development 51, 39-44.

Laufer, M. (1976). The central masturbation fantasy, the final sexual organization, and adolescence. In R. S. Eissler, et al. (Eds.), Psychoanalytic study of the child (Vol. 31, pp. 297-316). New York: International Universities Press.
Laufer, M. E. (1982). Female masturbation in adolescence and the development of the relationship to the body. International Journal of Psycho-Analysis 63, 295-302.
Litt, I. F. (1985). Know thyself--adolescents self-assessment of compliance behavior. Pediatrics 75, 693-696.
Mac Vicar, K., & Dillon, M. (1980). Childhood and adolescent development of ten female prostitutes. Journal of the American Academy of Child Psychiatry 19, 145-159.
Manning, M. L. (1983). Three myths concerning adolescence. Adolescence 18, 823-829.
McCausland, M. P. (1979). Sexual development and sexual abuse: Emergencies in adolescents. Pediatric Clinics of North America 26, 895-901.
Miller, T. W. (1984). Paternal absence and its effect on adolescent self-esteem. International Journal of Social Psychiatry 30, 293-296.
Mitchell, J. J. (1975). Moral growth during adolescence. Adolescence 10, 221-226.
Nichtern, S. (1980). The missing adolescent. In S. C. Feinstein, et al. (Eds.), Adolescent psychiatry: Developmental and clinical studies (Vol. 8, pp. 54-64). Chicago: University of Chicago Press.
Noam, G. G., Hauser, S. T., Santostefano, S., Garrison, W., Jacobson, A. J., Powers, S. I., & Mead, M. (1984). Ego development and psychopathology: A study of hospitalized adolescents. Child Development 55, 184-194.
Norvell, M., & Guy, R. F. (1977). A comparison of self-concept in adopted and non-adopted adolescents. Adolescence 12, 443-448.
Offer, D., Ostrov, E., & Howard, K. I. (1986). Self-image, delinquency and help-seeking behavior among normal adolescents. In S. C. Feinstein, et al. (Eds.), Adolescent psychiatry: Developmental and clinical studies (Vol. 13, pp. 121-137). Chicago: University of Chicago Press.
Ostrov, E., Offer, D., & Hartlage, S. (1984). The quietly disturbed adolescent. New Directions for Mental Health Services 21, 73-81.
Rosenheim, E., & Gaoni, B. (1977). Defensive passivity in adolescence. Adolescence 12, 449-459.
Schowalter, J. E. (1983). Psyche and some of physical illness during adolescence. Psychosomatics 24, 453-461.
Shestowsky, B. J. (1983). Ego identity development and obesity in adolescent girls. Adolescence 18, 551-559.
Silverman, R., & Zigmond, N. (1983). Self-concept in learning disabled adolescents. Journal of Learning Disabilities 16, 478-482.
Slater, E. J., Stewart, K. J., & Linn, M. W. (1983). The effects of family disruption on adolescent males and females. Adolescence 18, 931-942.
Spruiell, V. (1975). Narcissistic transformations in adolescence. International Journal of Psychoanalytic Psychotherapy 4, 518-536.

Steiner-Adair, C. (1986). The body politic: Normal female adolescent development and the development of eating disorders. Journal of the American Academy of Psychoanalysis 14, 95-114.

Tyson, P. (1982). A developmental line of gender identity, gender role, and choice of love object. Journal of the American Psychoanalytic Association 30, 61-86.

2. Developmental Disabilities in Adolescence

Abram, D. M., Ekelman, B. L., & Nation, J. E. (1984). Preschoolers with language disorders: 10 year later. Journal of Speech and Hearing Research 27, 232-244.

Brier, N. M., & Demb, H. B. (1980). Psychotherapy with the developmentally disabled adolescent. Journal of Developmental and Behavioral Pediatrics 1, 19-23.

Grinnell, S. W., Scott-Hartnett, D., & Glasier, J. L. (1983). Language disorders. Journal of the American Academy of Child Psychiatry 22, 580-581.

Intagliata, J., & Doyle, N. (1984). Enhancing social support for parents of developmentally disabled children: Training in interpersonal problem solving skills. Mental Retardation 22, 4-11.

McDaniel, K. D. (1986). Pharmacologic treatment of psychiatric and neurodevelopmental disorders in children and adolescents. Part 1. Clinical Pediatrics 25, 65-71.

Paul R., Cohen, D. J., & Caparulo, B. K. (1983). A longitudinal study of patients with severe developmental disorders of language learning. Journal of the American Academy of Child Psychiatry 22, 525-534.

3. Communication Problems in Adolescence

Culton, G. L. (1986). Speech disorders among college freshmen: A 13-year survey. Journal of Speech and Hearing Disorders 51, 3-7.

Holmes, D. R., & McKeever, W. F. (1979). Material specific serial memory deficit in adolescent dyslexics. Cortex 15, 51-62.

LaVigna, G. W. (1977). Communication training in mute autistic adolescents using the written word. Journal of Autism and Childhood Schizophrenia 7, 13-49.

Munford, P. R., Reardon, D., Liberman, R. P., & Allen, L. (1976). Behavioral treatment of hysterical coughing and mutism: A case study. Journal of Consulting and Clinical Psychology 44, 1008-1014.

Nardi, T. J., & Di Scipio, W. J. (1977). The Ganser syndrome in an adolescent Hispanic-black female. American Journal of Psychiatry 134, 453-454.

Richman, L. C. (1983). Self-reported social, speech, and facial concerns and personality adjustment of adolescents with cleft lip and palate. Cleft Palate Journal 20, 108-112.

Ross, B. M., & Hoemann, H. (1975). The attainment of formal operations: A comparison of probability concepts in deaf and hearing adolescents. Genetic Psychology Monographs 91, 61-119.

Rustin, L. (1978). An intensive group programme for adolescent stammerers. British

Journal of Disorders of Communication 13, 85-92.
Saniga, R. D., & Carlin, M. F. (1985). Selective attention in a vocal abuse population. Journal of Communication Disorders 18, 118-131.
Sarno, M. T., Buonaguro, A., & Levita, E. (1986). Characteristics of verbal impairment in closed head injured patients. Archives of Physical Medicine and Rehabilitation 67, 400-405.
Zinkus, P. W., & Gottlieb, M. I. (1983). Patterns of auditory processing and articulation deficits in academically deficient juvenile delinquents. Journal of Speech and Hearing Disorders 48, 36-40.

4. Psychopathology and Treatment by Psychopharmacology and Psychotherapy

Apprey, M. (1982). The effort to separate in a pubertal Mormon convert: A terminal profile. Child Psychiatry and Human Development 12, 142-152.
Barlow, D. H., & Seidner, A. L. (1983). Treatment of adolescent agoraphobics: Effects on parent-adolescent relations. Behavior Research and Therapy 21, 519-526.
Barrow, J. C. (1982). Coping-skills training: A brief therapy approach for students with evaluative anxiety. Journal of American College Health 30, 269-274.
Berg, I., Butler, A., & Hall, G. (1976). The outcome of adolescent school phobia. British Journal of Psychiatry 128, 80-85.
Braddock, L. E. (1982). Dysmorphobia in adolescence: A case report. British Journal of Psychiatry 140, 199-201.
Brende, J. O, & Rinsley, D. B. (1979). Borderline disorder, altered states of consciousness, and glossolalia. Journal of the American Academy of Psychoanalysis 7, 165-188.
Croghan, L. M. (1981). Conceptualizing the critical elements in a rapid desensitization to school anxiety: A case study. Journal of Pediatric Psychology 6, 165-170.
Edwards, J. G., & Goldie, A. (1983). Placebo-controlled trial of mianserin and maprotiline in primary depressive illness: A preliminary report. British Journal of Clinical Pharmacology 15(Suppl.), 239S-248S.
Egeland, J. A., & Hostetter, A. M. (1983). Amish study, I: Affective disorders among the Amish, 1976-1980. American Journal of Psychiatry 140, 56-61.
Framrose, R. (1978). Out-patient treatment of severe school phobia. Journal of Adolescence 1, 353-361.
Goldberg, C. (1977). School phobia in adolescence. Adolescence 12, 499-509.
Green, D. (1980). A behavioural approach to the treatment of obsessional rituals: An adolescent case study. Journal of Adolescence 3, 297-306.
Gross, M., & Huerta, E. (1980). Functional convulsions masked as epileptic disorders. Journal of Pediatric Psychology 5, 71-79.
Kestenbaum, C. J. (1978). Some practical considerations in the assessment and treatment of adolescent girls with separation problems. Journal of the American Academy of Psychoanalysis 6, 353-368.
Munich, R. L. (1977). Depersonalization in a female adolescent. International Journal

of Psychoanalytic Psychotherapy 6, 187-197.

Oberfield, R. A., Reuben, R. N., & Burkes, L. J. (1983). Interdisciplinary approach to conversion disorders in adolescent girls. Psychosomatics 24, 983-989.

Pincus, S. H., Poliandro, E. J., & Jaffe, L. R. (1983). A somaticizing adolescent: An approach to evaluation and therapy. Journal of Adolescent Health Care 4, 174-177.

Ramm, E., Marks, I. M., Yuksel, S., & Stern, R. S. (1982). Anxiety management training for anxiety states: Positive compared with negative self-statements. British Journal of Psychiatry 140, 367-373.

Rapoport, J., Elkins, R., & Mikkelsen, E. (1980). Clinical controlled trial of chlorimipramine in adolescents with obsessive-compulsive disorder. Psychopharmacology Bulletin 16, 61-63.

Ritvo, S. (1981). Anxiety, symptom formation, and ego autonomy. In A. Solnit, et al. (Eds.), Psychoanalytic study of the child (Vol. 36, pp. 339-364). New Haven: Yale University Press.

Rosenthal, S., & Rosenthal, P. A. (1982). Koro in an adolescent: Hypochondriasis as a stress response. In S. C. Feinstein, et al. (Eds.), Adolescent psychiatry: Developmental and clinical studies (Vol. 10, pp. 523-531). Chicago: University of Chicago Press.

Schwarz, J. C., & Getter, H. (1980). Parental conflict and dominance in late adolescent maladjustment: A triple interaction model. Journal of Abnormal Psychology 89, 573-580.

Silver, L. B. (1982). Conversion disorder with pseudoseizures in adolescence: A stress reaction to unrecognized and untreated learning disabilities. Journal of the American Academy of Child Psychiatry 21, 508-512.

Slavin, M. O. (1985-1986). A developmental disorder of late adolescence. International Journal of Psychoanalytic Psychotherapy 11, 219-241.

Sorosky, A. D., & Sticher, M. B. (1980). Trichotillomania in adolescence. In S. C. Feinstein, et al. (Eds.), Adolescent psychiatry: Developmental and clinical studies (Vol. 8, pp. 437-545). Chicago: University of Chicago Press.

Targum, S. D., & Capodanno, A. E. (1983). The dexamethasone suppression test in adolescent psychiatric inpatients. American Journal of Psychiatry 140, 589-591.

5. Sexual Identity, Personality, and Aggressive Behavior Disorders

Gibbons, T. C. N. (1957). The sexual behavior of young criminals. Journal of Mental Science (now British Journal of Psychiatry) 103, 527-540.

Gilpin, D. C., & Maltz, P. (1980). The oppositional personality in childhood. Child Psychiatry and Human Development 11, 79-86.

Glaser, K. (1967). Masked depression in children and adolescents. American Journal of Psychotherapy 21, 565-574.

Golomeier, H. (1975). Vandalism: The effects of unmanageable confrontations. Adolescence 9, 49.

Green, R. (1971). Diagnosis and treatment of gender identity disorders during childhood. Archives of Sexual Behavior 1, 167-173.

Green, R. (1974). Sexual identity conflict in children and adults. New York: Basic Books.
Green, R., & Fuller, M. (1973). Family doll play and female identity in pre-adolescent males. American Journal of Orthopsychiatry 43, 123-127.
Green, R., & Money, J. (1966). Stage-acting, role-taking, and effeminate impersonation during boyhood. Archives of General Psychiatry 15, 535-538.
Green, R., Newman, D. E., & Stoller, R. J. (1972). Treatment of boyhood "transsexualism": An interim report of four years' experience. Archives of General Psychiatry 26, 213-217.
Greenson, R. R. (1966). A transvestite boy and a hypothesis. International Journal of Psycho-Analysis 47, 396-403.
Greenspan, S., & Lourie, R. S. (1981). Developmental structuralist approach to the classification of adaptive and pathologic personality organizations: Infancy and early childhood. American Journal of Psychiatry 138, 725-735.
Groves, J. E. (1981). Current concepts in psychiatry: Borderline personality disorder. New England Journal of Medicine 305, 259-262.
Gunderson, J. G., & Englund, D. W. (1981). Characterizing the families of borderlines. A review of the literature. Psychiatric Clinics of North America 4, 159-168.
Harrison, S. I. (1970). Reared in the wrong sex. Journal of the American Academy of Child Psychiatry 9, 44-102.
Harrison, S. I., Cain, A. C., & Benedek, E. (1968). The childhood of a transsexual. Archives of General Psychiatry 19, 28-37.
Holemon, R. E., & Winokur, G. (1965). Effeminate homosexuality: A disease of childhood. American Journal of Orthopsychiatry 35, 48-56.
Horton, P. C. (1976). The psychological treatment of personality disorder. American Journal of Psychiatry 133, 262-265.
Johnson, A. M., & Szurek, S. A. (1952). The genesis of antisocial acting out in children and adults. Psychoanalytic Quarterly 21, 323.
Kaufman, I., Heims, L. W., & Reiser, D. E. (1961). A re-evaluation of the psychodynamics of firesetting. American Journal of Orthopsychiatry 31, 123-136.
Kaufman, I., Makkay, E. S., & Zilbach, J. (1959). The impact of adolescence on girls with delinquent character formation. American Journal of Orthopsychiatry 29, 130-143.
Knight, R. P. (1942). Intimidation of others as a defence against anxiety. Bulletin of the Menninger Clinic 6, 4-14.
Lapouse, R., & Monk, M. A. (1964). Behavior deviations in a representative sample of children: Variation by sex, age, race, social class and family size. American Journal of Orthopsychiatry 34, 436-446.
Lebovitz, P. S. (1972). Feminine behavior in boys: Aspects of its outcome. American Journal of Psychiatry 128, 1283-1289.
Lehrman, P. R. (1939). Some unconscious determinants in homicide. Psychiatric Quarterly 13, 605-621.
Leicester, J. (1982). Temper tantrums, epilepsy and episodic dyscontrol. British Journal of Psychiatry 141, 262-266.

Lewis, M., & Sarrel, P. M. (1969). Some psychological aspects of seduction, incest, and rape in childhood. Journal of the American Academy of Child Psychiatry 8, 609-619.

Makkay, E. S., & Schwaab, E. H. (1962). Some problems in the differential diagnosis of antisocial character disorders in early latency. Journal of the American Academy of Child Psychiatry 1, 414-430.

Marohn, R. C. (1974). Trauma and the delinquent. In S. C. Feinstein, et al. (Eds.), Adolescent psychiatry: Developmental and clinical studies (Vol. 3, pp. 354-361). Chicago: University of Chicago Press.

Marohn, R. C. (1977). The juvenile imposter: Some thoughts on narcissism and the delinquent. In S. C. Feinstein, et al. (Eds.), Adolescent psychiatry: Developmental and clinical studies (Vol. 5, pp. 186-212). Chicago: University of Chicago Press.

Marohn, R. C. (1979). A psychiatric overview of juvenile delinquency. In S. C. Feinstein, et al. (Eds.), Adolescent psychiatry: Developmental and clinical studies (Vol. 7, pp. 425-432). Chicago: University of Chicago Press.

Marohn, R. C. (1980). The psychiatric response to delinquency. In M. Sugar (Ed.), Responding to adolescent needs. New York: Spectrum Publications.

Marohn, R. C. (1981a). The negative transference in the treatment of juvenile delinquents. Annual Psychoanalysis 9, 21-42.

Marohn, R. C. (1981b). Personality disorders and adolescence. In J. R. Lion (Ed.), Personality disorders, diagnosis and management. Baltimore: Williams and Wilkins.

Marohn, R. C., Locke, E., Rosenthal, R., & Curtiss, G. (1982). Juvenile delinquents and violent death. In S. C. Feinstein, et al. (Eds.), Adolescent psychiatry: Developmental and clinical studies (Vol. 10, pp. 147-170). Chicago: University of Chicago Press.

Marohn, R. C., Offer, D., Ostrov, E., & Trujillo, J. (1979). Psychodynamic types of hospitalized juvenile delinquents. In S. C. Feinstein, et al. (Eds.), Adolescent psychiatry: Developmental and clinical studies (Vol. 7, pp. 466-483). Chicago: University of Chicago Press.

Meeks, J. E. (1979). Behavioral and antisocial disorders. In J. D. Noshpitz (Ed.), Basic handbook of child psychiatry (pp. 482-530). New York: Basic Books.

Meissner, W. W. (1978). Theoretical assumptions of concepts of the borderline personality. Journal of the American Psychoanalytic Association 26, 559-598.

Meissner, W. W. (1985). The case of phallic narcissistic personality. Journal of the American Psychoanalytic Association 33, 437-469.

Menaker, E. (1939). A contribution to the study of the neurotic stealing symptom. American Journal of Orthopsychiatry 9, 368-377.

Michaels, J. J. (1941). Parallels between persistent enuresis and delinquency in the psychopathic personality. American Journal of Orthopsychiatry 11, 260.

Money, J. W., & Ehrhardt, A. A. (1972). Man and woman, boy and girl. Baltimore: Johns Hopkins University Press.

Monopolis, S., & Lion, J. R. (1983). Problems in the diagnosis of the intermittent explosive disorder. American Journal of Psychiatry 140, 1200-1202.

Morris, H. H., Jr., Escoll, P. J., & Wekler, R. (1956). Aggressive behavior disorders of childhood: A follow-up study. American Journal of Psychiatry 112, 991-997.

Morrison, J. R., & Minkoff, K. (1975). Explosive personality as a sequel to the hyperactive-child syndrome. Comprehensive Psychiatry 16, 343-348.

Nagera, H. (1964). On arrest in development, fixation, and regression. In R. S. Eissler, et al. (Eds.), Psychoanalytic study of the child (Vol. 19, pp. 222-239). New York: International Universities Press.

Nagera, H. (1970). Children's reactions to the death of important objects: A developmental approach. In R. S. Eissler, et al. (Eds.), Psychoanalytic study of the child (Vol. 25, pp. 360-400). New York: International Universities Press.

Neubauer, P. B. (1960). The one-parent child and his oedipal development. In R. S. Eissler, et al. (Eds.), Psychoanalytic study of the child (Vol. 15, pp. 286-309). New York: International Universities Press.

Newman, L. E., & Stoller, R. J. (1971). The oedipal situation in male transsexualism. British Journal of Medical Psychology 44, 295-303.

Ornstein, A., Gropper, C., & Bogner, J. Z. (1983). Shoplifting: An expression of revenge and restitution. Annual Psychoanalysis 11, 311-331.

Perry, J. C. (1985). Depression in borderline personality disorder: Lifetime prevalence at interview and longitudinal course of symptoms. American Journal of Psychiatry 142, 15-21.

Petti, T. A., & Law, W. (1982). Borderline psychotic behavior in hospitalized children: Approaches to assessment and treatment. Journal of the American Academy of Child Psychiatry 21, 197-202.

Poznanski, E. O. (1973). Children with excessive fears. American Journal of Orthopsychiatry 43, 428-438.

Pringle, M. L. K., & Bossio, V. (1960). Early, prolonged separation and emotional maladjustment. Journal of Child Psychology and Psychiatry and Allied Disciplines 1, 37-48.

Rainer, J. D. (1979). Heredity and character disorders. American Journal of Psychotherapy 33, 6-16.

Rexford, E. N., & van Amerongen, S. T. (1957). The influence of unsolved maternal oral conflicts upon impulsive acting out in young children. American Journal of Orthopsychiatry 27, 75-87.

Rinsley, D. B. (1981). Dynamic and developmental issues in borderline and related "spectrum" disorders. Psychiatric Clinics of North America 4, 117-132.

Robbins, M. (1983). Toward a new mind model for the primitive personalities. International Journal of Psycho-Analysis 64, 127-148.

Robbins, M. D. (1976). Borderline personality organization: The need for a new theory. Journal of the American Psychoanalytic Association 24, 831-853.

Robbins, L. N. (1966). Deviant children grown up. Baltimore: Williams and Wilkins.

Sandler, A., Daunton, E., & Schnurmann, A. (1957). Inconsistency in the mother as a factor in character development: A comparative study of three cases. In R. S. Eissler, et al. (Eds.), Psychoanalytic study of the child (Vol. 12, pp. 209-225). New York: International Universities Press.

Schmideberg, M. (1935). The psychoanalysis of asocial children and adolescents. International Journal of Psychiatry 16, 22-48.

Sendi, I. B., & Blombren, P. G. (1975). A comparative study of predictive criteria in the predisposition of homicidal adolescents. American Journal of Psychiatry 132, 423.

Settlage, C. F. (1977). The psychoanalytic understanding of narcissistic and borderline personality disorders: Advances in developmental theory. Journal of the American Psychoanalytic Association 25, 805-833.

Singer, M. (1974). Family structure, disciplinary configurations and adolescent psychopathology. In S. C. Feinstein, et al. (Eds.), Adolescent psychiatry: Developmental and clinical studies (Vol. 3, p. 372). Chicago: University of Chicago Press.

Smith, H. F., Bemporad, J. R., & Hanson, G. (1982). Aspects of the treatment of borderline children. American Journal of Psychotherapy 36, 181-197.

Spitz, R. A. (1951). The psychogenic diseases in infancy. An attempt at their etiologic classification. In R. S. Eissler, et al. (Eds.), Psychoanalytic study of the child (Vol. 6, pp. 255-275). New York: International Universities Press.

Stierlin, H. (1973). A family perspective on adolescent runaways. Archives of General Psychiatry 29, 56.

Stoller, R. J. (1966a). The mother's contribution to infantile transvestic behaviour. International Journal of Psycho-Analysis 47, 384-395.

Stoller, R. J. (1966b). The treatment of transvestism and transsexualism. Current Psychiatric Therapies 6, 92-104.

Stoller, R. J. (1974). Symbiosis, anxiety and the development of masculinity. Archives of General Psychiatry 30, 164-172.

Stone, M. H. (1981). Borderline syndromes: A consideration of subtypes and an overview, directions for research. Psychiatric Clinics of North America 4, 3-24.

Thomas, A., Chess, S., & Birch, H. G. (1968). Temperament and behavior disorders in children. New York: New York University Press.

van Ophuijsen, J. H. W. (1929). The sexual aim of sadism as manifested in acts of violence. International Journal of Psychiatry 10, 139-144.

Winnicott, D. W. (1958). The antisocial tendency. In D. W. Winnicott (Ed.), Collected papers. New York: Basic Books.

Winnicott, D. W. (1961). Delinquency as a sign of hope. Journal of Child Psychology and Psychiatry and Allied Disciplines 2, 269-276.

Wolff, S. (1967). The contribution of obstetric complications to the etiology of behaviour disorders in childhood. Journal of Child Psychology and Psychiatry and Allied Disciplines 8, 57-66.

Wolff, S. (1984). The concept of personality disorder in childhood. Journal of Child Psychology and Psychiatry and Allied Disciplines 25, 5-13.

Woodside, M., Harrow, A., Basson, J. V., & Affleck, J. W. (1976). Experiment in managing sociopathic behaviour disorders. British Medical Journal 2, 1056-1059.

Zander, A. (1984). "The fragile princess." Midway on the borderline-narcissistic personality continuum. Perspectives in Psychiatric Care 22, 77-84.

Zuger, B. (1974). Effeminate behavior in boys. Archives of General Psychiatry 30, 173-177.

6. Affective Disorders in Adolescents

Akiskal, H. S., Downs, J., Jordan, P., Watson, S., Daugherty, D., & Pruitt, D. B. (1985). Affective disorders in referred children and younger siblings of manic-depressives. Mode of onset and prospective course. Archives of General Psychiatry 42, 996-1003.

Anthony, E. J. (1983). Depression in adolescents: A psychodynamic approach to nosology. In H. Golombek & B. D. Garfinkel (Eds.), The adolescent and mood disturbances (pp. 151-165). New York: International Universities Press.

Ballenger, J. C., Reus, V. I., & Post, R. M. (1982). The "atypical" clinical picture of adolescent mania. American Journal of Psychiatry 139, 602-606.

Brumback, R. A., Staton, R. D., & Wilson, H. (1980). Neuropsychological study of children during and after remission of endogenous depressive episodes. Perceptual and Motor Skills 50, 1163-1167.

Cantwell, D. P. (1985). Depressive disorders in children. Validation of clinical syndromes. Psychiatric Clinics of North America 8, 779-792.

Cantwell, D. P., & Carlson, G. A. (1983). Affective disorders in childhood and adolescents: An update. New York: Spectrum Publications.

Carlson, G. A. (1984). Classification issues of bipolar disorders in childhood. Psychiatric Developments 2, 273-285.

Chambers, W. J., Puig-Antich, J., Hirsch, M., Paez, P., Ambrosini, P. J., Tabrizi, M. A., & Davies, M. (1985). The assessment of affective disorders in children and adolescents by semistructured interview. Archives of General Psychiatry 42, 696-702.

DeLong, G. R., & Neiman, G. W. (1983). Lithium-induced behavior changes in children with symptoms suggesting manic-depressive illness. Psychopharmacology Bulletin 19, 258-265.

Emery, G., Bedrosian, R., & Garber, J. (1983). Cognitive therapy with depressed children and adolescents. In D. P. Cantwell & G. A. Carlson (Eds.), Affective disorders in childhood and adolescence: An update. New York: Spectrum Publications.

Feinstein, S. C. (1982). Manic-depressive disorder in children and adolescents. In S. C. Feinstein, et al. (Eds.), Adolescent psychiatry: Developmental and clinical studies (Vol. 10, pp. 256-272). Chicago: University of Chicago Press.

Fine, S., Moretti, M., Haley, G., & Marriage, K. (1985). Affective disorders in children and adolescents: The dysthymic disorder dilemma. Canadian Journal of Psychiatry 30, 173-177.

French, A., & Berlin, I. (Eds.). (1979). Depression in children and adolescents. New York: Human Sciences Press.

Geller, B., Chestnut, E. C., Miller, M. D., Price, D. T., & Yates, E. (1985). Preliminary data on DSM-III associated features of major depressive disorder in children and adolescents. American Journal of Psychiatry 142, 643-644.

Geller, B., Cooper, T. B., & Chestnut, E. C. (1985). Serial monitoring and achievement of steady state nortriptyline plasma levels in depressed children and adolescents: Preliminary data. Journal of Clinical Psychopharmacology 5, 213-216.

Glaser, K. (1978). The treatment of depressed and suicidal adolescents. American Journal of Psychotherapy 32, 252-269.

Glaser, K. (1981). Psychopathic patterns in depressed adolescents. American Journal of Psychotherapy 35, 368-382.

Guttman, H. A. (1983). Family therapy in the treatment of mood disturbance in adolescents. In H. Golombek & B. D. Garfinkel (Eds.), The adolescent and mood disturbances (pp. 263-272). New York: International Universities Press.

Harmon, R. J., Wagonfeld, S., & Emde, R. N. (1982). Anaclitic depression. A follow-up from infancy to puberty. In A. Solnit, et al. (Eds.), Psychoanalytic study of the child (Vol. 37, pp. 67-94). New Haven: Yale University Press.

Kandel, D. B., & Davies, M. (1982). Epidemiology of depressive mood in adolescents. Archives of General Psychiatry 39, 1205-1216.

Kashani, J. H. (1982). Epidemiology of childhood depression. In L. Grinspoon (Ed.), Psychiatry 1982: The American Psychiatric Association's annual review of psychiatry (pp. 281-288). Washington, D.C.: American Psychiatric Association.

Kaplan, S. L., Hong, G. K., & Weinhold, C. (1984). Epidemiology of depressive symptomatology in adolescents. Journal of the American Academy of Child Psychiatry 23, 91-98.

Orvaschel, H., Puig-Antich, J., Chambers, W., Tabrizi, M. A., & Johnson, R. (1982). Retrospective assessment of prepubertal major depression with the Kiddie-SADS-E. American Journal of Child Psychology 21, 392-397.

Poznanski, E. O., Grossman, J. A., Buchsbaum, Y., Banegas, M., Freeman, L., & Gibbons, R. (1984). Preliminary studies of the reliability and validity of the children's depression rating scale. Journal of the American Academy of Child Psychiatry 23, 191-197.

Puig-Antich, J. (1982). Major depression and conduct disorder in prepuberty. Journal of the American Academy of Child Psychiatry 21, 118-128.

Puig-Antich, J. (1986). Effects of age and puberty in psychobiological markers of depressive illness. In M. Rutter, C. E. Izard, & P. B. Read (Eds.), Depression in young people: Developmental and clinical perspectives (pp. 341-381). New York: Guilford Press.

Robins, D. R., Alessi, N. E., Yanchyshyn, G. W., & Colfer, M. (1983). Psychodynamic and characterological heterogeneity among adolescents with major depressive disorders. Journal of the American Academy of Child Psychiatry 22, 487-491.

Strober, M., & Carlson, G. (1982). Bipolar illness in adolescents with major depression: Clinical, genetic, and psychopharmacological predictors in a 3-4 prospective follow-up investigation. Archives of General Psychiatry 39, 549-555.

7. Biologic Factors in Adolescent Disorders

Brickman, A. S., McManus, M., Grapentine, W. L., & Alessi, N. (1984). Neuropsychological assessment of seriously delinquent adolescents. Journal of the American Academy of Child Psychiatry 23, 453-457.

Dye, O. A., Saxon, S. A., & Milby, J. B. (1981). Long-term neuropsychological deficits after traumatic head injury with comatosis. Journal of Clinical Psychology 37, 472-477.

Fabian, J. J., & Jacobs, U. W. (1981). Discrimination of neurological impairment in the learning disabled adolescent. Journal of Learning Disabilities 14, 594-596.

Goldings, A. S., & Stewart, R. M. (1982). Organic lead encephalopathy: Behavioral change and movement disorder following gasoline inhalation. Journal of Clinical Psychiatry 43, 70-72.

Greenwood, R., Bhalla, A., Gordon, A., & Roberts, J. (1983). Behaviour disturbances during recovery from herpes simplex encephalitis. Journal of Neurology, Neurosurgery and Psychiatry 46, 809-817.

Korman, M., Matthews, R. W., & Lovitt, R. (1981). Neuropsychological effects of abuse of inhalants. Perceptual and Motor Skills 53, 547-553.

Kupke, T., & Lewis, R. (1985). WAIS and neuropsychological tests: Common and unique variance within an epileptic population. Journal of Clinical and Experimental Neuropsychology 7, 353-366.

Lewis, D. O., Pincus, J. H., Shanok, S. S., & Glaser, G. H. (1982). Psychomotor epilepsy and violence in a group of incarcerated adolescent boys. American Journal of Psychiatry 139, 882-887.

Wolff, P. H., Waber, D., Bauermeister, M., Cohen, C., & Ferber, R. (1982). The neuropsychological status of adolescent delinquent boys. Journal of Child Psychology and Psychiatry and Allied Disciplines 23, 267-279.

Yeudall, L. T., Fromm-Auch, D., & Davies, P. (1982). Neuropsychological impairment of persistent delinquency. Journal of Nervous and Mental Disease 170, 257-265.

8. Adolescents and Their Families: Psychopathology and Treatment

Abelsohn, D. (1983). Dealing with the abdication dynamic in the post divorce family: A context for adolescent crisis. Family Process 22, 359-383.

Anolik, S. A. (1983). Family influences upon delinquency: Biosocial and psychosocial perspectives. Adolescence 18, 489-498.

Asarnow, J. R., Lewis, J. M., Doane, J. A., Goldstein, M. J., & Rodnick, E. H. (1982). Family interaction and the course of adolescent psychopathology: An analysis of adolescent and parent effects. Journal of Abnormal Child Psychology 10, 427-441.

Barnes, G. M. (1977). The development of adolescent drinking behavior: An evaluative review of the impact of the socialization process within the family. Adolescence 12, 571-591.

Baumrind, D. (1985). Familial antecedents of adolescent drug use: A developmental perspective. National Institute on Drug Abuse Research Monograph Series 56, 13-44.

Berg, I., Butler, A., Fairbairn, I., & McGuire, R. (1981). The parents of school phobic adolescents: A preliminary investigation of family life variables. Psychological Medicine 11, 79-83.

Berkowitz, D. A. (1979). The disturbed adolescent and his family: Problems of individuation. Journal of Adolescence 2, 27-39.

Berman, S. (1980). The response of parents to adolescent depression. In S. C. Feinstein, et al. (Eds.), Adolescent psychiatry: Developmental and clinical studies (Vol. 8, pp. 367-378). Chicago: University of Chicago Press.

Blos, P. (1976). The split parental imago in adolescent social relations. An inquiry into group psychology. In R. S. Eissler, et al. (Eds.), Psychoanalytic study of the child (Vol. 31, pp. 7-33). New York: International Universities Press.

Blos, P. (1984). Son and father. Journal of the American Psychoanalytic Association 32, 301-324.

Blotcky, M. J., Looney, J. C., & Grace, K. D. (1982). Treatment of the adopted adolescent: Involvement of the biologic mother. Journal of the American Academy of Child Psychiatry 21, 281-285.

Borgman, R. (1986). Don't come home again: Parental banishment of delinquent youths. Child Welfare 65, 295-304.

Braconnier, A., & Marcelli, D. (1979). The adolescent and his parents: The parental crisis. Journal of Adolescence 2, 325-336.

Bright, P. D., & Robin, A. L. (1981). Ameliorating parent-adolescent conflict with problem-solving communication training. Journal of Behavior Therapy and Experimental Psychiatry 12, 275-280.

Cleveland, M. (1981). Families and adolescent drug abuse: Structural analysis of children's roles. Family Process 20, 295-304.

Cohen, M., Adler, N., Beck, A., & Irwin, C. E. (1986). Parental reactions to the onset of adolescence. Journal of Adolescent Health Care 7, 101-106.

Doane, J. A., West, K. L., Goldstein, M. J., Rodnick, E. H., & Jones, J. E. (1981). Parental communication deviance and affective style. Predictors of subsequent schizophrenia spectrum disorders in vulnerable adolescents. Archives of General Psychiatry 38, 679-685.

Earls, F., & Siegel, B. (1980). Precocious fathers. American Journal of Orthopsychiatry 50, 469-480.

Elizur, A., Gaoni, B., & Davidson, S. (1981). The treatment of adolescents and their parents in group settings in a psychiatric hospital. International Journal of Social Psychiatry 27, 83-91.

Farber, S. S., Felner, R. D., & Primavera, J. (1985). Parental separation/divorce and adolescents: An examination of factors mediating adaptation. American Journal of Community Psychology 13, 171-185.

Feinsilver, D. B. (1985). The family meeting as a darkroom: Countertransference issues with severely disturbed adolescents. In S. C. Feinstein, et al. (Eds.),

Adolescent psychiatry: Developmental and clinical studies (Vol. 12, pp. 509-523). Chicago: University of Chicago Press.

Frey, J. (1984). A family/systems approach to illness: Maintaining behaviors in chronically ill adolescents. Family Process 23, 251-260.

Garbarino, J., Sebes, J., & Schellenbach, C. (1984). Families at risk for destructive parent-child relations in adolescents. Child Development 55, 174-183.

Gunderson, J. G., Kerr, J., & Englund, D. W. (1980). The families of borderlines. A comparative study. Archives of General Psychiatry 37, 27-33.

Harbin, H. T., & Madden, D. J. (1983). Assaultive adolescents: Family decision-making parameters. Family Process 22, 109-118.

Hauser, S. T., Powers, S. I., Noam, G. G., Jacobson, A. M., Weiss, B., & Follansbee, D. J. (1984). Familial contexts of adolescent ego development. Child Development 55, 195-213.

Hickey, B. A. (1984). Bowen's family projection process and Tennessee William's "The Glass Menagerie." Perspectives in Psychiatric Care 22, 26-32.

Hill, J. P. (1985). Family relations in adolescence: Myths, realities, and new directions. Genetic, Social, and General Psychology Monographs 111, 233-248.

Kalter, N. (1984). Conjoint mother-daughter treatment: A beginning phase of psychotherapy with adolescent daughters of divorce. American Journal of Orthopsychiatry 54, 490-497.

Kelly, J. B. (1981). Observations on adolescent relationships five years after divorce. In S. C. Feinstein, et al. (Eds.), Adolescent psychiatry: Developmental and clinical studies (Vol. 9, pp. 133-141). Chicago: University of Chicago Press.

Kerfoot, M. (1980). The family context of adolescent suicidal behaviour. Journal of Adolescence 3, 335-346.

Klein, H., & Erlich, H. S. (1978). Some psychoanalytic structural aspects of family function and growth. In S. C. Feinstein, et al. (Eds.), Adolescent psychiatry: Developmental and clinical studies (Vol. 6, pp. 171-194). Chicago: University of Chicago Press.

Levine, E. M. (1984). The middle-class family and middle-class adolescents in a state of disarray: A social-psychiatric analysis. Psychiatry 47, 152-161.

Lewis, J. M. (1978). The adolescent and the healthy family. In S. C. Feinstein, et al. (Eds.), Adolescent psychiatry: Developmental and clinical studies (Vol. 6, pp. 156-170). Chicago: University of Chicago Press.

Matthews, S. H., & Sprey, J. (1985). Adolescents' relationships with grandparents: An empirical contribution to conceptual clarification. Journal of Gerontology 40, 621-626.

McDermott, J. F., Robillard, A. B., Char, W. F., Hsu, J., Tseng, W. S., & Ashton, G. C. (1983). Reexamining the concept of adolescence: Differences between adolescent boys and girls in the context of their families. American Journal of Psychiatry 140, 1318-1322.

Miller, T. W. (1984). Paternal absence and its effect on adolescent self-esteem. International Journal of Social Psychiatry 30, 293-296.

Newton, B. (1985). Tough love: Help for parents with troubled teenagers--reorganizing the hierarchy in disorganized families. Pediatrics 76, 691-694.

Noller, P., & Callan, V. J. (1986). Adolescent and parent perceptions of family cohesion and adaptability. Journal of Adolescence 9, 97-106.

O'Connor, J. J., & Horowitz, A. N. (1984). The Bogeyman cometh: A strategic approach for difficult adolescents. Family Process 23, 237-249.

Patterson, G. R., & Stouthamer-Loeber, M. (1984). The correlation of family management practices and delinquency. Child Development 55, 1299-1307.

Pelcovitz, D., Kaplan, S., Samit, C., Krieger, R., & Cornelius, D. (1984). Adolescent abuse: Family structure and implications for treatment. Journal of the American Academy of Child Psychiatry 23, 85-90.

Post, S. (1982). Adolescent parricide in abusive families. Child Welfare 61, 445-455.

Prosen, H., Toews, J., & Martin, R. (1981). The life cycle of the family: Parental midlife crisis and adolescent rebellion. In S. C. Feinstein, et al. (Eds.), Adolescent psychiatry: Developmental and clinical studies (Vol. 9, pp. 170-179). Chicago: University of Chicago Press.

Reposa, R. E. (1979). Adolescent and family abandonment: A family systems approach to treatment. International Journal of Group Psychotherapy 29, 359-368.

Rossman, P. G., & Freedman, J. A. (1982). Hospital treatment for disturbed adolescents: The role of parent counseling groups. In S. C. Feinstein, et al. (Eds.), Adolescent psychiatry: Developmental and clinical studies (Vol. 10, pp. 391-406). Chicago: University of Chicago Press.

Shapiro, E. R. (1978). Research on family dynamics: Clinical implications for the family of the borderline adolescent. In S. C. Feinstein, et al. (Eds.), Adolescent psychiatry: Developmental and clinical studies (Vol. 6, pp. 360-376). Chicago: University of Chicago Press.

Shapiro, R. L. (1978). The adolescent, the therapist and the family: The management of external resistances to psychoanalytic therapy of adolescents. Journal of Adolescence 1, 3-10.

Spillane-Grieco, E. (1984). Characteristics of a helpful relationship: A study of empathic understanding and positive regard between runaways and their parents. Adolescence 19, 63-75.

Wallerstein, J. S. (1985). Children of divorce: Preliminary report of a ten-year follow-up of older children and adolescents. Journal of the American Academy of Child Psychiatry 24, 545-553.

Weissman, S., & Cohen, R. S. (1985). The parenting alliance and adolescence. In S. C. Feinstein, et al. (Eds.), Adolescent psychiatry: Developmental and clinical studies (Vol. 12, pp. 24-45). Chicago: University of Chicago Press.

9. Behavior Disorders and Delinquency: Etiology and Treatment

Arbuthnot, J., & Gordon, D. A. (1986). Behavioral and cognitive effects of a moral reasoning development intervention for high-risk behavior-disordered adolescents. Journal of Consulting and Clinical Psychology 54, 208-216.

Armstrong, H., Morris, R. M., Amerongen, M., & Kernaghan, P. (1983). Group therapy for parents of delinquent children. International Journal of Group Psychotherapy 33, 85-97.

Awad, G. A. (1981). The early phase of psychotherapy with antisocial early adolescents. Canadian Journal of Psychiatry 26, 38-42.

Bartollas, C., & Sieverdes, C. M. (1983). Institutional games played by confined juveniles. Adolescence 18, 609-617.

Bastien, R. T., & Adelman, H. S. (1984). Noncompulsory versus legally mandated placement, perceived choice, and response to treatment among adolescents. Journal of Consulting and Clinical Psychology 52, 171-179.

Beck, S. J., & Ollendick, T. H. (1976). Personal space, sex of experimenter, and locus of control in normal and delinquent adolescents. Psychological Reports 38, 383-387.

Berman, T., & Paisey, T. (1984). Personality in assaultive and non-assaultive juvenile male offenders. Psychological Reports 54, 527-530.

Biggs, S. J., Bender, M. P., & Foreman, J. (1983). Are there psychological differences between persistent solvent-abusing delinquents and delinquents who do not abuse solvents? Journal of Adolescence 6, 71-86.

Braukmann, C. J., Bedlington, M. M., Belden, B. D., Braukmann, P. D., Husted, J. J., Ramp, K. K., & Wolf, M. M. (1985). Effects of community-based group-home treatment programs on male juvenile offenders' use and abuse of drugs and alcohol. American Journal of Drug and Alcohol Abuse 11, 249-278.

Brooks, B. (1985). Sexually abused children and adolescent identity development. American Journal of Psychotherapy 39, 401-410.

Brown, B. (1985). An application of social learning methods in a residential programme for young offenders. Journal of Adolescence 8, 321-331.

Bruhn, A. R., & Davidow, S. (1983). Earliest memories and the dynamics of delinquency. Journal of Personality Assessment 47, 476-482.

Bry, B. H. (1982). Reducing the incidence of adolescent problems through preventive intervention: One- and five-year follow-up. American Journal of Community Psychology 10, 265-276.

Byles, J. A. (1980). Adolescent girls in need of protection. American Journal of Orthopsychiatry 50, 264-278.

Cadoret, R. J., & Cain, C. (1980). Sex differences in predictors of antisocial behavior in adoptees. Archives of General Psychiatry 37, 1171-1175.

Calhoun, G., Connley, S., & Bolton, J. A. (1984). Comparison of delinquents and nondelinquents in ethnicity, ordinal position, and self-perception. Journal of Clinical Psychology 40, 323-328.

Callan, V. J., & Jackson, D. (1986). Children of alcoholic fathers and recovered alcoholic fathers: Personal and family functioning. Journal of Studies on Alcohol 47, 180-182.

Carpenter, P., & Sandberg, S. (1985). Further psychodrama with delinquent adolescents. Adolescence 20, 599-604.

Cauce, A. M., Felner, R. D., & Primavera, J. (1982). Social support in high-risk adolescents: Structural components and adaptive impact. American Journal of Community Psychology 10, 417-428.

Chassin, L., Presson, C. C., Young, R. D., & Light, R. (1981). Self-concepts of institutionalized adolescents: A framework for conceptualizing labeling effects. Journal of Abnormal Psychology 90, 143-151.

Coleman, J. C. (1980). Central issues in the residential care of young people. Journal of Adolescence 3, 175-186.

Cormier, B. M., & Markus, B. (1980). A longitudinal study of adolescent murders. Bulletin of the American Academy of Psychiatry and the Law 8, 240-260.

Crabtree, L. H. (1982). Hospitalized adolescent who act out: A treatment approach. Psychiatry 45, 147-158.

Crabtree, L. H. (1983). Treatment of acting-out adolescents. Current Psychiatric Therapies 22, 215-220.

Curtiss, G., Rosenthal, R. H., Marohn, R. C., Ostrov, E., Offer, D., & Trujillo, J. (1983). Measuring delinquent behavior in inpatient treatment settings: Revision and validation of the adolescent antisocial behavior checklist. Journal of the American Academy of Child Psychiatry 22, 459-466.

Dattilio, F. M. (1981). The Carkhuff systematic human relations training model in a short-term treatment program for adolescent offenders. Adolescence 16, 865-869.

Daum, J. M. (1983). Emotional indicators in drawings of aggressive or withdrawn male delinquents. Journal of Personality Assessment 47, 243-249.

Daum, J. M., & Bieliauskas, V. J. (1983). Fathers' absence and moral development of male delinquents. Psychological Reports 53, 223-228.

Degrave, G., Riordan, B., & Mathias, R. (1976). Sex education for delinquent boys--unveiling the taboo. Nursing 6, 22-25.

Denkowski, G. C., Denkowski, K. M., & Mabli, J. (1984). A residential treatment model for MR adolescent offenders. Hospital and Community Psychiatry 35, 279-281.

Dickerson, P. S., & Ouellette, M. D. (1982). Prenatal education for adolescents in a delinquent youth facility. Journal of Obstetric, Gynecologic, and Neonatal Nursing 11, 39-44.

Dishion, T. J., Loeber, R., Stouthamer-Loeber, M., & Patterson, G. R. (1984). Skill deficits and male adolescent delinquency. Journal of Abnormal Child Psychology 12, 37-54.

Dornbusch, S. M., Carlsmith, J. M., Bushwall, S. J., Ritter, P. L., Leiderman, H., Hastorf, A. H., & Gross, R. T. (1985). Single parents, extended households, and the control of adolescents. Child Development 56, 326-351.

Downes, C. (1982). How endings are experienced in time limited family placement of difficult adolescents. Journal of Adolescence 5, 379-394.

Duke, M. P., & Fenhagen, E. (1975). Self-parental alienation and locus of control in delinquent girls. Journal of Genetic Psychology 127, 103-107.

Dumas, J. E., & Albin, J. B. (1986). Parent training outcome: Does active parental involvement matter? Behavior Research and Therapy 24, 227-230.

Eth, S. (1983). Adolescent separation-individuation and the court. Bulletin of the American Academy of Psychiatry and the Law 11, 231-238.

Fleetwood, R. S., & Parish, T. S. (1976). Relationship between moral development test scores of juvenile delinquents and their inclusion in a moral dilemma discussion group. Psychological Reports 39, 1075-1080.

Friesen, W. J., & Wright, P. G. (1985). The validity of the Carlson Psychological Survey with adolescents. Journal of Personality Assessment 49, 422-426.

Furnham, A. (1984). Personality, social skills, anomie and delinquency: A self-report study of a group of normal non-delinquent adolescents. Journal of Child Psychology and Psychiatry and Allied Disciplines 25, 409-420.

Gaffney, L. R., & McFall, R. M. (1981). A comparison of social skills in delinquent and nondelinquent adolescent girls using a behavioral role-playing inventory. Journal of Consulting and Clinical Psychology 49, 959-967.

Gavaghan, M. P., Arnold, K. D., & Gibbs, J. C. (1983). Moral judgment in delinquents and nondelinquents: Recognition versus production measures. Journal of Psychology 114, 267-274.

Gibbs, J. C., Arnold, K. D., Ahlborn, H. H., & Cheesman, F. L. (1984). Facilitation of sociomoral reasoning in delinquents. Journal of Consulting and Clinical Psychology 52, 37-45.

Gibbs, J. T. (1982). Personality patterns of delinquent females: Ethnic and sociocultural variations. Journal of Clinical Psychology 38, 198-206.

Gibbs, J. T. (1984). Black adolescents and youth: An endangered species. American Journal of Orthopsychiatry 54, 6-21.

Goldstein, H. S. (1984). Parental composition, supervision, and conduct problems in youths 12 to 17 years old. Journal of the American Academy of Child Psychiatry 23, 679-684.

Griffith, R. (1975). A philosophy os psychotherapy of juvenile delinquency. Psychotherapy and Psychosomatics 25, 134-137.

Hanson, C. L., Henggeler, S. W., Haefele, W. F., & Rodick, J. D. (1984). Demographic, individual, and family relationship correlates of serious and repeated crime among adolescents and their siblings. Journal of Consulting and Clinical Psychology 52, 528-538.

Hanson, R. A., & Mullis. R. L. (1984). Moral reasoning in offender and nonoffender youth. Journal of Genetic Psychology 144, 295-296.

Harbin, H. T., & Madden, D. J. (1983). Assaultive adolescents: Family decision-making parameters. Family Process 22, 109-118.

Hartstone, E., & Cocozza, J. (1983). Violent youth: The impact of mental health treatment. International Journal of Law and Psychiatry 6, 207-224.

Hechtman, L., Weiss, G., & Perlman, T. (1984). Hyperactives as young adults: Past and current substance abuse and antisocial behavior. American Journal of Orthopsychiatry 54, 415-425.

Henggeler, S. W., Hanson, C. L., Borduin, C. M., Watson, S. M., & Brunk, M. A. (1985). Mother-son relationships of juvenile felons. Journal of Consulting and Clinical Psychology 53, 942-943.

Henn, F. A., Bardwell, R., & Jenkins, R. L. (1980). Juvenile delinquents revisited. Adult criminal activity. Archives of General Psychiatry 37, 1160-1163.

Hollander, H. E., & Turner, F. D. (1985). Characteristics of incarcerated delinquents: Relationship between developmental disorders, environmental and family factors, and patterns of offence and recidivism. Journal of the American Academy of Child Psychiatry 24, 221-226.

Inamdar, S. C., Lewis, D. O., Siomopoulos, G., Shanok, S. S., & Lamela, M. (1982). Violent and suicidal behavior in psychotic adolescents. American Journal of Psychiatry 139, 932-935.

Jenkins, R. L. (1980). Child psychiatry perspectives: Status offenders. Journal of the American Academy of Child Psychiatry 19, 320-325.

Karoly, P. (1975). Comparison of "psychological styles" in delinquent and nondelinquent females. Psychological Reports 36, 567-570.

Kifer, R. E., Lewis, M. A., Green, D. R., & Phillips, E. L. (1974). Training predelinquent youths and their parents to negotiate conflict situations. Journal of Applied Behavior Analysis 7, 357-364.

Kraft, S. P., & DeMaio, T. J. (1982). An ecological intervention with adolescent in low-income families. American Journal of Orthopsychiatry 52, 131-140.

Krebs, H. (1980). On the biology of juvenile delinquency: Comments on the essay by Felton Earls, "The social reconstruction of adolescence: Toward an explanation for increasing rates of violence in youth." Perspectives in Biology and Medicine 23, 179-190.

Levine, M. D., Karniski, W. M., Palfrey, J. S., Meltzer, L. J., & Fenton, T. (1985). A study of risk factor complexes in early adolescent delinquency. American Journal of Diseases of Children 139, 50-56.

Lewis, D. O., Feldman, M., & Barrengos, A. (1985). Race, health, and delinquency. Journal of the American Academy of Child Psychiatry 24, 161-167.

Lewis, D. O., & Shanok, S. S. (1980). The use of a correctional setting for follow-up care of psychiatrically disturbed adolescents. American Journal of Psychiatry 137, 953-955.

Marohn, R. C. (1982). Adolescent violence: Causes and treatment. Journal of the American Academy of Child Psychiatry 21, 354-360.

Marvit, R. C., Lind, J., & McLaughlin, D. G. (1974). Use of videotapes to induce attitude change in delinquent adolescents. American Journal of Psychiatry 131, 996-999.

Maskin, M. B., & Flescher, B. E. (1975). Change in self-concept in work-oriented versus communication-oriented juvenile correction programs. Psychological Reports 36, 460-462.

McManus, M., Alessi, N. E., Grapentine, W. L., & Brickman, A. (1984). Psychiatric disturbance in serious delinquents. Journal of the American Academy of Child Psychiatry 23, 602-615.

McManus, M., Brickman, A., Alessi, N. E., & Grapentine, W. L. (1984). Borderline personality in serious delinquents. Comprehensive Psychiatry 25, 446-454.

McManus, M., Brickman, A., Alessi, N. E., & Grapentine, W. L. (1985). Neurological dysfunction in serious delinquents. Journal of the American Academy of Child Psychiatry 24, 481-486.

Meltzer, L. J., Levine, M. D., Karniski, W., Palfrey, J. S., & Clarke, S. (1984). An analysis of the learning styles of adolescent delinquents. Journal of Learning Disabilities 17, 600-608.

Mio, J. S., Nanjundappa, G., Verleur, D. E., & de Rios, M. D. (1986). Drug abuse and the adolescent sex offender: A preliminary analysis. Journal of Psychoactive Drugs 18, 65-72.

Mitchell, C. M., Davidson, W. S., Chodakowski, J. A., & McVeigh, J. (1985). Intervention orientation: Quantification of "person-blame" versus "situation-blame" intervention philosophies. American Journal of Community Psychology 13, 543-552.

Moffitt, T. E., Gabrielli, W. F., Mednick, S. A., & Schulsinger, F. (1981). Socioeconomic status, IQ, and delinquency. Journal of Abnormal Psychology 90, 152-156.

Morash, M. (1982). Relationships of legal reasoning to social class, closeness to parents, and exposure to a high level of reasoning among adolescent varying in seriousness of delinquency. Psychological Reports 50, 755-760.

Mullis, R. L, & Hanson, R. A. (1984). Adult judgments of delinquent and non-delinquent adolescent moral reasoning. Child Psychiatry and Human Development 14, 261-268.

Mulvey, E. P., & LaRosa, J. F. (1986). Delinquency cessation and adolescent development: Preliminary data. American Journal of Orthopsychiatry 56, 212-224.

Offer, D., Marohn, R. C., & Ostrov, E. (1975). Violence among hospitalized delinquents. Archives of General Psychiatry 32, 1180-1186.

Olczak, P. V., Parcell, S. R., & Stott, M. W. (1983). Defining juvenile delinquency: Specificity of the research sample and the right to treatment. Journal of Clinical Psychology 39, 1007-1012.

Paley, M. G. (1981). Accentuating the positive in adolescent patients. American Journal of Psychoanalysis 41, 51-55.

Parrott, C. A., & Strongman, K. T. (1984). Locus of control and delinquency. Adolescence 19, 459-471.

Patterson, G. R., & Stouthamer-Loeber, M. (1984). The correlation of family management practices and delinquency. Child Development 55, 1299-1307.

Riemer, J. W. (1981). Deviance as fun. Adolescence 16, 39-43.

Ritvo, E., Shanok, S. S., & Lewis, D. O. (1983). Firesetting and nonfiresetting delinquents. A comparison of neuropsychiatric, psychoeducational, experiential, and behavioral characteristics. Child Psychiatry and Human Development 13, 259-267.

Robbins, D. M., Beck, J. C., Pries, R., Jacobs, B., & Smith, C. (1983). Learning disability and neuropsychological impairment in adjudicated, unincarcerated male delinquents. Journal of the American Academy of Child Psychiatry 22, 40-46.

Roff, J. D. (1986). Identification of boys at high risk for delinquency. Psychological Reports 58, 615-618.

Roff, J. D., & Wirt, R. D. (1984). Childhood aggression and social adjustment as antecedents of delinquency. Journal of Abnormal Child Psychology 12, 111-126.

Rosenthal, P. A., & Doherty, M. B. (1985). Psychodynamics of delinquent girls' rage and violence directed toward mother. In S. C. Feinstein, et al. (Eds.), Adolescent psychiatry: Developmental and clinical studies (Vol. 12, pp. 281-289). Chicago: University of Chicago Press.

Rotenberg, M. (1974). Conceptual and methodological notes on affective and cognitive role taking (sympathy and empathy): An illustrative experiment with delinquent and nondelinquent boys. Journal of Genetic Psychology 125, 177-185.

Russell, D. H., & Hardman, G. L. (1980). Juvenile delinquency and the quality of life: The 17-year depression. Journal of Forensic Sciences 25, 908-911.

Satterfield, J. H., Hoppe, C. M., & Schell, A. M. (1982). A prospective study of delinquency in 110 adolescent boys with attention deficit disorder and 88 normal adolescent boys. American Journal of Psychiatry 139, 795-798.).

Schaughency, E. A., & Lahey, B. B. (1985). Mothers' and fathers' perceptions of child deviance: Roles of child behavior, parental depression, and marital satisfaction. Journal of Consulting and Clinical Psychology 53, 718-723.

Seeman, L., Tittler, B. I., & Friedman, S. (1985). Early interactional change and its relationship to family therapy outcome. Family Process 24, 59-68.

Shanok, S. S. (1980). On protecting the status offender from the juvenile justice system. Journal of the American Academy of Child Psychiatry 19, 326-327.

Singh, N. (1982). Notes and observations on the practice of multiple family therapy in an adolescent unit. Journal of Adolescence 5, 319-332.

Spellacy, F. J., & Brown, W. G. (1984). Prediction of recidivism in young offenders after brief institutionalization. Journal of Clinical Psychology 40, 1070-1074.

Spence, S. H., & Marzillier, J. S. (1981). Social skills training with adolescent male offenders. II. Short-term, long-term and generalized effects. Behavior Research and Therapy 19, 349-368.

Stolberg, A. L., & Garrison, K. M. (1985). Evaluating a primary prevention program for children of divorce. American Journal of Community Psychology 13, 111-124.

Stuck, M. F., & Glassner, B. (1985). The transition from drug use and crime to noninvolvement: A case study. Adolescence 20, 669-679.

Tarter, R. E., Hegedus, A. M., Winsten, N. E., & Alterman, A. I. (1985). Intellectual profiles and violent behavior in juvenile delinquents. Journal of Psychology 119, 125-128.

Valasquez, J. S., & Lyle, C. G. (1985). Day versus residential treatment for juvenile offenders: The impact of program evaluation. Child Welfare 64, 145-156.

Voorhees, J. (1981). Neuropsychological differences between juvenile delinquents and functional adolescents: A preliminary study. Adolescence 16, 66-76.

Welch, G. J. (1985). Contingency contracting with a delinquent and his family. Journal of Behavior Therapy and Experimental Psychiatry 16, 253-259.

Wells, L. E., & Rankin, J. H. (1983). Self-concept as a mediating factor in delinquency. Social Psychology Quarterly 46, 11-22.
Woolf, A., & Funk, S. G. (1985). Epidemiology of trauma in a population of incarcerated youth. Pediatrics 75, 463-468.

10. Substance Abuse and Antisocial Behavior

Adlaf, E. M., & Smart, R. G. (1983). Risk-taking and drug-use behaviour: An examination. Drug and Alcohol Dependency 11, 287-296.
Adler, I., & Kandel, D. B. (1981). Cross-cultural perspectives on developmental stages in adolescent drug use. Journal of Studies on Alcohol 42, 701-715.
Amini, F., Zilberg, N. J., Burke, E. L., & Salasnek, S. (1982). A controlled study of inpatient vs. outpatient treatment of delinquent drug abusing adolescents: One year results. Comprehensive Psychiatry 23, 436-444.
Bachman, J. G., Johnston, L. D., & O'Malley, P. M. (1981). Smoking, drinking, and drug use among American high school students: Correlates and trends, 1975-1979. American Journal of Public Health 71, 59-69.
Bean, M. (1982). Identifying and managing alcohol problems of adolescents. Psychosomatics 23, 389-396.
Blaine, J. D., Renault, P. F., & Julius, D. A. (1981). A comprehensive psychiatric approach to drug dependence. Hillside Journal of Clinical Psychiatry 3, 3-25.
Botvin, G. J. (1983). Prevention of adolescent substance abuse through the development of personal and social competence. National Institute on Drug Abuse Research Monograph Series 47, 115-140.
Bowers, A. J., & Sage, L. R. (1983). Solvent abuse in adolescents: The who? what? and why? Child: Care, Health and Development 9, 169-178.
Brook, J. S., Lukoff, I. F., & Whiteman, M. (1980). Initiation into adolescent marijuana use. Journal of Genetic Psychology 137, 133-142.
Bry, B. (1983). Empirical foundations of family-based approaches to adolescent substance abuse. National Institute on Drug Abuse Research Monograph Series 47, 154-171.
Bumpass, E. R., Brix, R. J., & Preston, D. (1985). A community-based program for juvenile firesetters. Hospital and Community Psychiatry 36, 529-533.
Burke, E. L., Zilberg, N. J., Amini, F., Salasnek, S., & Forkin, D. (1978). Some empirical evidence for Erikson's concept of negative identity in delinquent adolescent drug abusers. Comprehensive Psychiatry 19, 141-152.
Cadoret, R. J., Cain, C. A., & Crowe, R. R. (1983). Evidence for gene-environment interaction in the development of adolescent antisocial behavior. Behavior Genetics 13, 301-310.
Carman, R. S. (1979). Motivations for drug use and problematic outcomes among rural junior high school students. Addictive Behavior 4, 91-93.
Channer, K. S., & Stanley, S. (1983). Persistent visual hallucinations secondary to chronic solvent encephalopathy: Case report and review of the literature. Journal Neruology, Neurosurgery and Psychiatry 46, 83-86.

Dembo, R., Pilaro, L., Burgos, W., Des Jarlais, D. C., & Schmeidler, J. (1979). Self-concept and drug involvement among urban junior high school youths. International Journal of the Addictions 14, 1125-1144.

Dembo, R., Schmeidler, J., & Burgos, W. (1980). Life-style and drug involvement among youths in an inner city junior high school. International Journal of the Addictions 15, 171-188.

Donovan, J. E., Jessor, R., & Jessor, L. (1983). Problem drinking in adolescence and young adulthood. A follow-up study. Journal of Studies on Alcohol 44, 109-137.

Duncan, J. W. (1974). Persisting psychotic states in adolescent drug uses. Child Psychiatry and Human Development 5, 51-62.

Gersick, K. E., Grady, K., Sexton, E., & Lyons, M. (1980). Personality and sociodemographic factors in adolescent drug use. National Institute on Drug Abuse Research Monograph Series 38, 39-56.

Gibbs, J. T. (1982a). Personality patterns of delinquent females: Ethnic and sociocultural variations. Journal of Clinical Psychology 38, 198-206.

Gibbs, J. T. (1982b). Psychosocial factors related to substance abuse among delinquent females: Implications for prevention and treatment. American Journal of Orthopsychiatry 52, 261-271.

Goodman, J. D. (1976). The behavior of hypersexual delinquent girls. American Journal of Psychiatry 133, 662-668.

Lewis, D. O., & Balla, D. A. (1975). "Sociopathy" and its synonyms: Inappropriate diagnoses in child psychiatry. American Journal of Psychiatry 132, 720-722.

Russe, B. R., McCoy, C. B., & Barton, J. E. (1980). Recent findings concerning inhalant use. Chemical Dependency 4, 113-126.

Setffenhagen, R. A., Polich, J. M., & Lash, S. (1978). Alienation, delinquency and patterns of drug use. International Journal of Social Psychiatry 24, 125-137.

Simonds, J. F., & Kashani, J. (1980). Specific drug use and violence in delinquent boys. American Journal of Drug and Alcohol Abuse 7, 305-322.

Teicher, J. D., Sinay, R. D., & Stumphauzer, J. S. (1976). Training community-based paraprofessionals as behavior therapists with families of alcohol-abusing adolescents. American Journal of Psychiatry 133, 847-850.

11. Adolescent Suicide: Brief Overview

Berlin, I. N. (1985). Prevention of adolescent suicide among some native American tribes. In S. C. Feinstein, et al. (Eds.), Adolescent psychiatry: Developmental and clinical studies (Vol. 12, pp. 77-93). Chicago: University of Chicago Press.

Corder, B. F., Shorr, W., & Corder, R. F. (1974). A study of social and psychological characteristics of adolescent suicide attempters in an urban, disadvantaged area. Adolescence 9, 1-16.

Crumley, F. E. (1979). Adolescent suicide attempts. Journal of the American Medical Association 241, 2404-2407.

Deykin, E. Y., Perlow, R., & McNamarra, J. (1985). Non-fatal suicidal and life-threatening behavior among 13- to 17-year-old adolescents seeking emergency medical care. American Journal of Public Health 75, 90-92.

Eisenberg, L. (1984). The epidemiology of suicide in adolescents. Pediatric Annals 13, 47-54.

Erlich, H. S. (1978). Adolescent suicide: Maternal longing and cognitive development. In A. Solnit, et al. (Eds.), Psychoanalytic study of the child (Vol. 33, pp. 261-277). New Haven: Yale University Press.

Gispert, M., Wheeler, K., Marsh, L., & Davis, M. S. (1985). Suicidal adolescents: Factors in evaluation. Adolescence 20, 753-762.

Greene, J. W., & Keown, M. (1986). Depression and suicide in children and adolescents. Comprehensive Therapy 12, 38-43.

Hamlin, W. T. (1982). Adolescent suicide. Journal of the National Medical Association 74, 25-28.

Hatton, C. L., & Valente, S. M. (1981). Bereavement group for parents who suffered a suicidal loss of a child. Suicide and Life-Threatening Behavior 11, 141-150.

Hawton, A., Osborn, M., O'Grady, J., & Cole, D. (1982). Classification of adolescents who take overdoses. British Journal of Psychiatry 140, 125-131.

Hendin, H. (1986). Suicide: A review of new directions in research. Hospital and Community Psychiatry 37, 148-154.

Hese, R. T., Szwed, A., & Kret-Plucinska, K. (1982). Incidence of suicide and attempted suicide among patients of an open psychiatric department. Psychiatria Polska 16, 53-58.

Holinger, P. C. (1977). Suicide in adolescence. American Journal of Psychiatry 134, 1433-1434.

Holinger, P. C. (1978). Adolescent suicide: An epidemiological study of recent trends. American Journal of Psychiatry 135, 754-756.

Inamdar, S. C., Lewis, D. O., Siomopoulos, G., Shanok, S. S., & Lamela, M. (1982). Violent and suicidal behavior in psychotic adolescents. American Journal of Psychiatry 139, 932-935.

Johnson, R. (1978). Youth in crisis: Dimensions of self-destructive conduct among adolescent prisoners. Adolescence 13, 461-482.

Keidel, G. C. (1983). Adolescent suicide. Nursing Clinics of North America 18, 323-332.

Klosinski, G. (1979). Self mutilation in adolescence. Acta Paedopsychiatrica 44, 311-323.

Konopka, G. (1983). Adolescent suicide. Exceptional Children 49, 390-394.

Korpi, E. R., Kleinman, J. E., Goodman, S. I., Phillips, I., DeLisi, L. E., Linnoila, M., & Wyatt, R. J. (1986). Serotonin and 5-hydroxyindoleacetic acid in brains of suicide victims. Comparison in chronic schizophrenic patients with suicide as cause of death. Archives of General Psychiatry 43, 594-600.

Ladame, F., & Jeanneret, O. (1982). Suicide in adolescence: Some comments on epidemiology and prevention. Journal of Adolescence 5, 355-366.

Linkowski, P., de Maertelaer, V., & Mendlewicz, J. (1985). Suicidal behaviour in major depressive illness. Acta Psychiatrica Scandinavica 72, 233-238.

Looney, J. G., Oldham, D. G., Claman, C., Crumley, F. E., & Waller, D. A. (1985). Suicide by adolescents. Texas Medicine 81, 45-49.

McIntire, M. S., Angle, C. R., Wikoff, R. L., & Schlicht, M. L. (1977). Recurrent adolescent suicidal behavior. Pediatrics 60, 605-608.

McIntosh, J. L., & Santos, J. F. (1985-1986). Methods of suicide by age: Sex and race differences among the young and old. International Journal of Aging and Human Development 22, 123-139.

McKenry, P. C., Tishler, C. L., & Kelley, C. (1982). Adolescent suicide. A comparison of attempters and nonattempters in an emergency room population. Clinical Pediatrics 21, 266-270.

Mehr, M., Zeltzer, L. K., & Robinson, R. (1981). Continued self-destructive behaviors in adolescent suicide attempters: Part I. Journal of Adolescent Health Care 1, 269-274.

Miller, M. L., Chiles, J. A., & Barnes, V. E. (1982). Suicide attempters within a delinquent population. Journal of Consulting and Clinical Psychology 50, 491-498.

Mintz, T. (1981). Clinical experience with suicidal adolescents. In S. C. Feinstein, et al. (Eds.), Adolescent psychiatry: Developmental and clinical studies (Vol. 9, pp. 493-496). Chicago: University of Chicago Press.

Nardini-Maillard, D., & Ladame, F. G. (1980). The results of a follow-up study of suicidal adolescents. Journal of Adolescence 3, 253-260.

Parker, A. (1981). The meaning of attempted suicide to young parasuicides: A repertory grid study. British Journal of Psychiatry 139, 306-312.

Petzel, S. V., & Cline, D. W. (1978). Adolescent suicide: Epidemiological and biological aspects. In S. C. Feinstein, et al. (Eds.), Adolescent psychiatry: Developmental and clinical studies (Vol. 6, pp. 239-266). Chicago: University of Chicago Press.

Reynolds, P. & Eaton, P. (1986). Multiple attempters of suicide presenting at an emergency department. Canadian Journal of Psychiatry 31, 328-330.

Rich, C. L., Young, D., & Fowler, R. C. (1986). San Diego suicide study. I. Young versus old subjects. Archives of General Psychiatry 43, 577-582.

Robbins, D., & Conroy, R. C. (1983). A cluster of adolescent suicide attempts: Is suicide contagious? Journal of Adolescent Health Care 3, 253-255.

Rosenthal, M. J. (1981). Sexual differences in the suicidal behavior of young people. In S. C. Feinstein, et al. (Eds.), Adolescent psychiatry: Developmental and clinical studies (Vol. 9, pp. 422-442). Chicago: University of Chicago Press.

Schreiber, T. J., & Johnson, R. L. (1986). The evaluation and treatment of adolescent overdoses in an adolescent medical service. Journal of the National Medical Association 78, 101-108.

Shafii, M., Carrigan, S., Whittinghill, J. R., & Derrick, A. (1985). Psychological autopsy of completed suicide in children and adolescents. American Journal of Psychiatry 142, 1061-1064.

Steele, R. E. (1977). Clinical comparison of black and white suicide attempters. Journal of Consulting and Clinical Psychology 45, 982-986.

Stonddard, F. J., & Cahners, S. S. (1985). Suicide attempted by self-immolation during adolescence. II. Psychiatric treatment and outcome. In S. C. Feinstein, et al. (Eds.), Adolescent psychiatry: Developmental and clinical studies (Vol. 12, pp. 266-280). Chicago: University of Chicago Press.

Tishler, C. L. (1981). Adolescent suicide attempts following elective abortion: A special case of anniversary reaction. Pediatrics 68, 670-671.

Tishler, C. L., McKenry, P. C., & Morgan, K. C. (1981). Adolescent suicide attempts: Some significant factors. Suicide and Life-Threatening Behavior 11, 86-92.

Waltzer, H. (1984). Suicide risk in young schizophrenics. General Hospital Psychiatry 6, 219-225.

Welner, A., Welner, Z., & Fishman, R. (1979). Psychiatric adolescent inpatients: Eight- to ten-year follow-up. Archives of General Psychiatry 36, 698-700.

Wenz, F. V. (1979a). Self-injury behavior, economic status and the family anomie syndrome among adolescents. Adolescence 14, 387-398.

Wenz, F. V. (1979b). Sociological correlates of alienation among adolescent suicide attempts. Adolescence 14, 19-30.

12. Treatment of Psychiatric Disorders

Abelsohn, D. (1983). Dealing with the abdication dynamic in the post divorce family: A context for adolescent crisis. Family Process 22, 359-383.

Akister, J., & Canever, N. (1980). A year in the life of an adolescent group. Journal of Adolescence 3, 155-163.

Allchin, W. H. (1978). Passion and commitment in therapy. Journal of Adolescence 1, 385-391.

Altman, K. P. (1985). The role-taking interview: An assessment technique for adolescents. Adolescence 20, 845-851.

Amanat, E. (1979). Paradoxical treatment of adolescent resistance. Adolescence 14, 851-862.

Anthony, E. J. (1981). The paranoid adolescent as viewed through psychoanalysis. Journal of the American Psychoanalysis Association 29, 754-787.

Arbuthnot, J., & Gordon, D. A. (1986). Behavioral and cognitive effects of a moral reasoning developmental intervention for high-risk behavior-disordered adolescents. Journal of Consulting and Clinical Psychology 54, 208-216.

Awad, G. A. (1985). Responsiveness in psychotherapy with antisocial adolescents. American Journal of Psychotherapy 39, 490-498.

Barcai, A., & Rabkin, L. Y. (1975). Family therapy for the "incorrigible" adolescent. Current Psychiatric Therapies 15, 65-70.

Bastien, R. T., & Adelman, H. S. (1984). Noncompulsory versus legally mandated placement, perceived choice, and response to treatment among adolescents. Journal of Consulting and Clinical Psychology 52, 171-179.

Berkowitz, D. A., Shapiro, R. L., Zinner, J., & Shapiro, E. R. (1974). Concurrent family treatment of narcissistic disorders in adolescence. International Journal of Psychoanalytic Psychotherapy 3, 379-396.

Berlin, I. N. (1981). Familial treatment of severe adolescent problems. Current Psychiatric Therapies 20, 61-69.

Bernfeld, G., Clark, L., & Parker, G. (1984). The process of adolescent group psychotherapy. International Journal of Group Psychotherapy 34, 111-126.

Blos, P. (1983). The contribution of psychoanalysis to the psychotherapy of adolescents. In S. C. Feinstein, et al. (Eds.), Adolescent psychiatry: Developmental and clinical studies (Vol. 11, pp. 104-124). Chicago: University of Chicago Press.

Blotcky, M. J., Grace, K. D., & Looney, J. G. (1984). Treatment of adolescents in family therapy after divorce. Journal of the American Academy of Child Psychiatry 23, 222-225.

Bonham, H. E., Armstrong, T. D., & Bonham, G. M. (1981). Group psychotherapy with deaf adolescents. American Annals of the Deaf 126, 806-809.

Braden, E. (1984). Supportive containment in the hospital care of treatment-resistant borderline adolescents. Psychiatry 47, 315-322.

Bright, P. D., & Robin, A. L. (1981). Ameliorating parent-adolescent conflict with problem-solving communication training. Journal of Behavior Therapy and Experimental Psychiatry 12, 275-280.

Brown, B. (1985). An application of social learning methods in a residential programme for young offenders. Journal of Adolescence 8, 321-331.

Cahill, A. J. (1981). Aggression revisited: The value of anger in therapy and other close relationships. In S. C. Feinstein, et al. (Eds.), Adolescent psychiatry: Developmental and clinical studies (Vol. 9, pp. 539-549). Chicago: University of Chicago Press.

Caldwell, T. A., & Stewart, R. S. (1981). Hysterical seizures and hypnotherapy. American Journal of Clinical Hypnosis 23, 294-298.

Canever, N., & Walduck, J. (1979). Programmes and contracts: Their uses and abuses in the treatment of adolescent disorders. Journal of Adolescence 2, 251-254.

Carpenter, P., & Sandberg, S. (1985). Further psychodrama with delinquent adolescents. Adolescence 20, 599-604.

Carsky, M. (1985-1986). The resolution of impasses in long-term intensive, inpatient psychotherapy. International Journal of Psychoanalytic Psychotherapy 11, 435-458.

Chwast, J. (1977). Psychotherapy of disadvantaged acting-out adolescents. American Journal of Psychotherapy 31, 216-226.

Colarusso, C. A. (1980). Psychoanalysis of a severe neurotic learning disturbance in a gifted adolescent boy. Bulletin of the Menninger Clinic 44, 585-602.

Coleman, J. C. (1980). Central issues in the residential care of young people. Journal of Adolescence 3, 175-186.

Cooper, L. (1979). Clinical and administrative synthesis in adolescent treatment: Search for a sane integration of thought and action. Adolescence 14, 81-92.

Crabtree, L. H. (1982). Hospitalized adolescents who act out: A treatment approach. Psychiatry 45, 147-158.

Davidson, W. S., & Wolfred, T. R. (1977). Evaluation of a community-based behavior modification program for prevention of delinquency: The failure of success. Community Mental Health Journal 13, 296-306.

Downey, T. W. (1978). Transitional phenomena in the analysis of early adolescent males. In A. Solnit, et al. (Eds.), Psychoanalytic study of the child (Vol. 33, pp. 19-46). New Haven: Yale University Press.

Dunne, C., Bruggen, P., & O'Brian, C. (1982). Tough and action in group therapy of younger adolescents. Journal of Adolescence 5, 31-38.

Eitzen, D. S. (1974). Impact of behavior modification techniques on locus of control of delinquent boys. Psychological Reports 35, 1317-1318.

Eitzen, D. S. (1975). The effects of behavior modification on the attitudes of delinquents. Behavior Research and Therapy 13, 295-299.

Eitzen, D. S. (1976). The self-concept of delinquents in a behavior modification treatment. Journal of Social Psychology 99, 203-206.

Ekstein, R. (1978). The process of termination and its relation to outcome in the treatment of psychotic disorders in adolescence. In S. C. Feinstein, et al. (Eds.), Adolescent psychiatry: Developmental and clinical studies (Vol. 6, pp. 448-460). Chicago: University of Chicago Press.

Elizur, A., Gaoni, B., & Davidson, S. (1981). The treatment of adolescents and their parents in group settings in a psychiatric hospital. International Journal of Social Psychiatry 27, 83-91.

Evans, J. (1980). Ambivalence and how to turn it to your advantage: Adolescence and paradoxical intervention. Journal of Adolescence 3, 273-284.

Evans, R. (1976). Development of the treatment alliance in the analysis of an adolescent boy. In R. S. Eissler, et al. (Eds.), Psychoanalytic study of the child (Vol. 31, pp. 193-224). New York: International Universities Press.

Feinsilver, D. B. (1985). The family meeting as a darkroom: Countertransference issues with severely disturbed adolescents. In S. C. Feinstein, et al. (Eds.), Adolescent psychiatry: Developmental and clinical studies (Vol. 12, pp. 509-523). Chicago: University of Chicago Press.

Fineberg, B. L., Sowards, S. K., & Kettlewell, P. W. (1980). Adolescent inpatient treatment: A literature review: Adolescence 15, 913-925.

Fraiberg, S. (1982). The adolescent mother and her infant. In S. C. Feinstein, et al. (Eds.), Adolescent psychiatry: Developmental and clinical studies (Vol. 10, pp. 7-23). Chicago: University of Chicago Press.

Framrose, R. (1982). Adolescent enmeshment: A case for brief strategic therapy. Journal of Adolescence 5, 149-157.

Frey, J. (1984). A family/systems approach to illness: Maintaining behaviors in chronically ill adolescents. Family Process 23, 251-260.

Friedman, R., Schlise, S., & Selgman, S. (1975). Issues involved in the treatment of an adolescent group. Adolescence 10, 357-368.

Galatzer-Levy, R. M. (1985). The analysis of an adolescent boy. In S. C. Feinstein, et al. (Eds.), Adolescent psychiatry: Developmental and clinical studies (Vol. 12, pp. 336-360). Chicago: University of Chicago Press.

Giovacchini, P. L. (1985). Countertransference and the severely disturbed adolescent. In S. C. Feinstein, et al. (Eds.), Adolescent psychiatry: Developmental and clinical studies (Vol. 12, pp. 449-467). Chicago: University of Chicago Press.

Glenn, T. J., & Simonds, J. F. (1977). Hypnotherapy of a psychogenic seizure disorder in an adolescent. American Journal of Clinical Hypnosis 19, 245-249.

Godenne, G. D. (1982). The adolescent girl and her female therapist. Adolescence 17, 225-242.

Goudsmit, W., & Reicher, J. W. (1978). Experience with psychotherapeutic treatment of delinquents with a serious social risk: Indication, methods, result. International Journal of Law and Psychiatry 1, 309-318.

Graafsma, T., & Anbeek, M. (1984). Resistance in psychotherapy with adolescents. Journal of Adolescence 7, 1-16.

Green, D. (1980). A behavioural approach to the treatment of obsessional rituals: An adolescent case study. Journal of Adolescence 3, 297-306.

Hoffer, A., Goettsche, R., & Linden, F. (1980). A psychoanalytic approach to a therapeutic impasse with an impulsive adolescent: Permission to speak the unspeakable. American Journal of Psychiatry 137, 1404-1409.

Schimel, J. L. (1986). Psychotherapy with adolescents: The art of interpretation. In S. C. Feinstein, et al. (Eds.), Adolescent psychiatry: Developmental and clinical studies (Vol. 13, pp. 178-187). Chicago: University of Chicago Press.

Schulman, G. L. (1985). Treatment of the disturbed adolescent: A family approach. International Journal of Family Therapy 7, 11-24.

Shapiro, E. R., Shapiro, R. L., Zinner, J., & Berkowitz, D. A. (1977). The borderline ego and the working alliance: Indications for family and individual treatment in adolescence. International Journal of Psycho-Analysis 58, 77-87.

13. Recent Books

Golembek, H., & Garfinkel, B. D. (Eds.). (1983). The adolescent and mood disturbance. New York: International Universities Press.

Petti, T. A. (Ed.). (1983). Childhood depression. New York: Hawthorne Press.

Rutter, M., Izard, C. E., & Rad, P. B. (Eds.). (1986). Depression in young people: Developmental and clinical perspectives. New York: Guilford Press.

P. Antisocial-Violent-Delinquent and Substance Abusing Behavior

Charles Keith, M.D., Section Editor

Marc Amaya, M.D., Sidney Berman, M.D., Thomas Haslip, M.D., John Looney, M.D., Richard C. Marohn, M.D., and Cynthia Pfeffer, M.D., Associate Editors

Psychopathology: Disease and Disorder

1. Recent Books

Golembek, H., & Garfinkel, B. D. (Eds.). (1983). The adolescent and mood disturbances. New York: International Universities Press.

Petti, T. A. (Ed.). (1983). Childhood depression. New York: Hawthorne Press.

Rutter, M., Izard, C. E., & Rad, P. B. (Eds.). (1986). Depression in young people: Developmental and clinical perspectives. New York: Guilford Press.

2. History of Antisocial Behavior

Aichhorn, A. (1935). Wayward youth. New York: Viking Press.

Aichhorn, A. (1964). Delinquency and child guidance--selected papers. New York: International Universities Press.

Berman, S. (1959). Antisocial character disorder: Its etiology and relationship to delinquency. American Journal of Orthopsychiatry 29, 612-621.

Bettelheim, B. (1955). Truants from life. Glencoe, Ill.: The Free Press.

Bowlby, J. (1944). Forty-four juvenile thieves: Their characters and home life. International Journal of Psycho-Analysis 25, 19-52.

Eissler, K. R. (Ed.). (1949). Searchlights on delinquency. New York: International Universities Press.

Friedlander, K. (1947). The psychoanalytical approach to juvenile delinquency. London: Kegal Paul, Trench, Turbner.

Glover, E. (1950). On the desirability of isolating a functional (psychosomatic) group of delinquent disorders. British Journal of Delinquency 1, 104-112.

Glover, E. (1960). The roots of crime. Selected papers on psychoanalysis. New York: International Universities Press.

Glueck, S. (1959). The problem of delinquency. Boston: Houghton Mifflin.

Healy, W., & Bronner, A. F. (1936). New light on delinquency and its treatment. New York: Yale University Press.

Johnson, A. M. (1959). Juvenile delinquency. In S. Arieti (Ed.), American handbook of psychiatry (pp. 848-856). New York: Basic Books.

Redl, F., & Wineman, D. (1957). The aggressive child. Glencoe, Ill.: The Free Press.

Whitaker, C. A. (1946). Ormsby Village: An experiment with forced psychotherapy in the rehabilitation of the delinquent adolescent. Psychiatry 9, 239-250.

Winnicott, D. W. (1958). The antisocial tendency. Collected papers. New York: Basic Books.

3. Biological Factors in Antisocial Behavior

Brown, G. L., & Goodwin, F. K. (1984). Aggression, adolescence and psychobiology. In C. R. Keith (Ed.), The aggressive adolescent. New York: The Free Press.

Delga, I., Heinssen, R., Fritsch, R., Goodrich, W., & Yates, B. (1989). Psychosis, aggression, & self-destructive behavior in hospitalized adolescents. American Journal of Psychiatry 14(4), 521-525.

Herzberg, J. L., & Fenwick, P. B. C. (1988). The aetiology of aggression in temporal-lobe epilepsy. British Journal of Psychiatry 153, 50-55.

Kashani, J. H., Daniel, A. E., Reid, J. C., & Sirinek, A. J. (1984). Comparison of delinquent boys and girls in group homes and factors associated with the outcome. British Journal of Psychiatry 144, 156-160.

Kashani, J. H., Husain, A., Robins, A. J., Reid, J. C., & Wooderson, P. C. (1980). Patterns of delinquency in girls and boys. Journal of the American Academy of Child Psychiatry 19, 300-310.

Lewis, D. O. (Ed.). (1981). Psychobiologic vulnerabilities to delinquency. New York: S.P. Medical and Scientific Books.

Lewis, D. O., Shanok, S. S., Grant, M., & Ritvo, E. (1983). Homicidally aggressive young children: Neuropsychiatric and experiential correlates. American Journal of Psychiatry 140(2), 148-153.

Maccoby, E. E., & Jacklin, C. N. (1980). Sex differences in aggression: A rejoinder and reprise. Child Development 51(4), 964-980.

McGee, R., Williams, S., & Silva, P. A. (1984). Behavioral and developmental characteristics of aggressive, hyperactive and aggressive-hyperactive boys. Journal of the American Academy of Child Psychiatry 23, 270-279.

Mednick, S., & Kandel, E. (1988). Congenital determinants of violence. Bulletin of the American Academy of Psychiatry and the Law 16(2), 101-109.

Mednick, S. A., & Hutchings, B. (1978). Genetic and psychophysiological factors in asocial behavior. Journal of the American Academy of Child Psychiatry 17(2), 209-223.

Olweus, D., Mattsson, A., Schalling, D., & Low, H. (1988). Circulating testosterone levels and aggression in adolescent males: A causal analysis. Psychosomatic Medicine 50, 261-272.

Pfeffer, C. R., Plutchik, R., & Mizruchi, M. S. (1983). Predictors of assaultiveness in latency age children. American Journal of Psychiatry 140(1), 31-35.

Puig-Antich, J. (1982). Major depression and conduct disorder in prepuberty. Journal of the American Academy of Child Psychiatry 21(2), 118-128.

Reitsma-Street, M., Offords, D. R., & Finch, T. (1985). Pairs of same-sexed siblings discordant for antisocial behaviour. British Journal of Psychiatry 146, 415-423.

Rogeness, G. A., Hernandez, J. M., Macedo, C. A., Amrung, S. A., & Hoppe, S. K. (1986). Near-zero plasma dopamine-b-hydroxylase and conduct disorder in emotionally disturbed boys. Journal of the American Academy of Child Psychiatry 25, 521-527.

Schmidt, K., Solant, M. V., & Bridger, W. H. (1985). Electrodermal activity of undersocialized aggressive children: A pilot study. Journal of Child Psychology and Psychiatry and Allied Disciplines 26, 653-660.

Shaffer, D., Meyer-Bahlburg, H. F. L., & Stokman, C. L. J. (1981). The development of aggression. In M. Rutter (Ed.), Scientific foundations of developmental psychiatry. Baltimore: University Park Press.

Sigvardsson, S., Cloninger, C. R., Bohman, M., & von Knorring, A. L. (1982). Predisposition to petty criminality in Swedish adoptees. III. Sex differences and validation of the male typology. Archives of General Psychiatry 39, 1248-1253.
Stewart, M. A., & deBlois, S. (1983). Father-son resemblances in aggressive and antisocial behavior. British Journal of Psychiatry 142, 78-84.
Stewart, M. A., & deBlois, S. (1985). Diagnostic criteria for aggressive conduct disorder. Psychopathology 18, 11-17.

4. Sociologic Factors in Delinquency

Gadow, K., & Sprafkin, J. (1989). Field experiments of television violence with children: Evidence for an environmental hazard? Pediatrics 38(3), 399-405.
Heath, L., Bresolin, L., & Rinaldi, R. (1989). Effects of media violence on children. Archives of General Psychiatry 46, 376-379.
Jenkins, R. L. (1980). Status offenders. Journal of the American Academy of Child Psychiatry 19, 320-325.
Malmquist, C. P. (1967). Dilemmas of the juvenile court. Journal of the American Academy of Child Psychiatry 7, 723-748.
Short, J. R., & Strodtbeck, F. L. (1965). Group process and gang delinquency. Chicago: University of Chicago Press.
West, D. J. (1982). Delinquency. London: Heinemann.
Wilson, J. Q., & Hernstein, R. J. (1985). Crime and human nature. New York: Simon & Schuster.
Wizner, S. (1980). Punishing the innocent: Juvenile court jurisdiction over "status offenders." Journal of the American Academy of Child Psychiatry 19, 328-333.
Wolfgang, M. E. (1967). The culture of youth. Task Force report: Juvenile delinquency and youth crime. Washington, D.C.: Committee on Law Enforcement & the Administration of Justice.

5. Predictors of Antisocial Behavior

Farrington, D. P. (1985). Delinquency prevention in the 1980s. Journal of Adolescence 8, 3-16.
Kelso, J., & Stewart, M. A. (1986). Factors which predict the persistence of aggressive conduct disorder. Journal of Child Psychology and Psychiatry and Allied Disciplines 27, 77-86.
Limentani, A. (1981). From denial to self awareness: A twenty-year study of a case of childhood delinquency evolving into adult neurosis. British Journal of Medical Psychology 54(2), 175-186.
Loeber, R., & Dishion, T. (1983). Early predictors of male delinquency: A review. Psychological Bulletin 94, 68-99.
Monahan, J. (1984). The prediction of violent behavior: Toward a second generation of theory and policy. American Journal of Psychiatry 141(1), 10-15.
Marohn, R. C., Locke, E., Rosenthal, R., & Curtiss, G. (1982). Juvenile delinquents and violent death. In S. C. Feinstein, et al. (Eds.), Adolescent psychiatry:

Developmental and clinical studies (Vol. 10, pp. 147-170). Chicago: University of Chicago Press.

Robins, L. N. (1981). Epidemiological approaches to natural history research: Antisocial disorders in children. Journal of the American Academy of Child Psychiatry 20, 556-580.

Shore, M. F., & Massimo, J. L. (1979). Fifteen years after treatment: A follow up study of comprehensive vocationally-oriented psychotherapy. American Journal of Orthopsychiatry 49(2), 240-245.

6. Psychodynamic Issues in Antisocial Behavior

Benedek, E. (1979). Female delinquency: Fantasies, facts, and future. In S. C. Feinstein, et al. (Eds.), Adolescent psychiatry: Developmental and clinical studies (Vol. 7, pp. 424-437). Chicago: University of Chicago Press.

Beres, D. (1958). Vicissitudes of superego functions and superego precursors in childhood. In R. S. Eissler, et al. (Eds.), Psychoanalytic study of the child (Vol. 13, pp. 324-351). New York: International Universities Press.

Bernabeu, E. P. (1958). Underlying ego mechanisms in delinquency. Psychoanalytic Quarterly 27, 393-396.

Blos, P. (1963). The concept of acting out in relation to the adolescent process. In E. N. Rexford (Ed.), A developmental approach to problems of acting out (pp. 118-143). New York: International Universities Press.

Carpenter, P. (1984). "Green stamp therapy" revisited: The evolution of 12 years of behavior modification and psychoeducational techniques with young delinquent boys. Psychological Reports 54, 99-111.

Falstein, E. I. (1958). The psychodynamics of male adolescent delinquency. American Journal of Orthopsychiatry 28, 613-626.

Haizlip, T. M., Corder, B. F., & Ball, B. C. (1984). The adolescent murderer. In C. R. Keith (Ed.), The aggressive adolescent. New York: The Free Press.

Josselyn, I. M. (1958). A type of predelinquent behavior. American Journal of Orthopsychiatry 28, 606-612.

Johnson, A. M. (1949). Sanctions for superego lacunae of adolescents. In K. R. Eissler (Ed.), Searchlights on delinquency (pp. 225-245). New York: International Universities Press.

Johnson, A. M., & Szurek, S. A. (1952). The genesis of antisocial acting out in children and adults. Psychoanalytic Quarterly 21, 323-343.

Kaufman, I., Heims, L. W., & Reiser, D. E (1961). A re-evaluation of the psychodynamics of fire-setting. American Journal of Orthopsychiatry 31, 123-136.

Lochman, J. E., Lampron, L. B., & Rabiner, D. L. (1989). Format differences and salience effects in the social problem-solving assessment of aggressive and nonaggressive boys. Journal of Clinical Child Psychology 18(3), 230-236.

Malmquist, C. P. (1968). Conscience development. In R. S. Eissler, et al. (Eds.), Psychoanalytic study of the child (Vol. 23, pp. 301-331). New York: International Universities Press.

Marohn, R. (1982). Adolescent violence: Causes and treatment. Journal of the American Academy of Child Psychiatry 21, 354-360.
McCarthy, J. B (1978). Narcissism and the self in homicidal adolescents. American Journal of Psychoanalysis 38, 19-29.
Offer, D., Marohn, R. C., & Ostov, E. (1979). The psychological world of the juvenile delinquent. New York: Basic Books.
Pfeffer, C. R., Solomon, G., Plutchik, R., Mizruchi, M. S., & Weinter, A. (1985). Variables that predict assaultiveness in child psychiatric inpatients. Journal of the American Academy of Child Psychiatry 24, 775-780.
Reiser, D. E. (1963). Observations of delinquent behavior in very young children. Journal of the American Academy of Child Psychiatry 2, 50-71.
Rexford, E. N. (1978). A selective review of the literature. In E. N. Rexford (Ed.), A developmental approach to problems of acting out (pp. 249-326). New York: International Universities Press.
Rosenberg, R. M., & Mueller, B. C. (1968). Preschool antisocial children: Psychodynamic considerations and implications for treatment. Journal of the American Academy of Child Psychiatry 7, 421-441.
Rosenthal, P. A., & Doherty, M. B. (1984). Serious sibling abuse by preschool children. Journal of the American Academy of Child Psychiatry 23, 186-190.
Sendl, I. B., & Blomgren, P. G. (1975). A comparative study of predictive criteria in the predisposition of homicidal adolescents. American Journal of Psychiatry 132, 423-427.
Winnicott, D. W. (1973). Delinquency as a sign of hope. In S. C. Feinstein, et al. (Eds.), Adolescent psychiatry: Developmental and clinical studies (Vol. 2, pp. 364-371). Chicago: University of Chicago Press.

7. Delinquency Prevention

Farrington, D. P. (1985). Delinquency prevention in the 1980s. Journal of Adolescence 8, 3-16.

8. Treatment of Aggressive Behavior with Psychoactive Drugs

Amery, B., Minichiello, M. D., & Brown, G. L. (1984). Aggression in hyperactive boys: Response to a d-amphetamine. Journal of the American Academy of Child Psychiatry 23, 291-294.
Campbell, M., Cohen, M., Cohen, I. L., & Small, A. M. (1982). Drugs in aggressive behavior. Journal of the American Academy of Child Psychiatry 21(2), 107-117.
Campbell, M., Small, A. M., Green, W. H., Jennings, S. J., Perry, R., Bennett, W. G., & Anderson, L. (1984). Behavioral efficacy of haloperidol and lithium carbonate--a comparison in hospitalized aggressive children with conduct disorder. Archives of General Psychiatry 41, 650-656.

Leventhal, B. L. (1984). The neuropharmacology of violent and aggressive behavior in children and adolescents. In C. R. Keith (Ed.), The aggressive adolescent (pp. 299-358). New York: The Free Press.

9. Treatment of Delinquents

Averill, S. C., Cadman, W. H., Craig, L. P., & Linden, R. E. (1973). Group psychotherapy with young delinquents. Report from a residential treatment center. Bulletin of the Menninger Clinic 37, 1-70.

Franklin, G., & Nottage, W. (1969). Psychoanalytic treatment of severely disturbed juvenile delinquents in group therapy. International Journal of Group Psychotherapy 19, 165-175.

Julian, A., & Kilmann, P. (1979). Group treatment of juvenile delinquents: A review of the outcome literature. International Journal of Group Psychotherapy 29, 3-37.

Keith, C. R. (1988). Community treatment of violent youth: Seven years of experience with a class action suit. Journal of the American Academy of Child and Adolescent Psychiatry 27(5), 600-604.

Saunders, E., & Awad, G. (1988). Assessment, management, and treatment planning for male adolescent sexual offenders. American Journal of Orthopsychiatry 58, 571-579.

Slavson, S. R. (1965). Reclaiming the delinquent by para-analytic group psychotherapy and the inversion technique. New York: The Free Press.

10. Family Therapy and Antisocial Behavior

Bowlby, J. (1984). Violence in the family as a disorder of the attachment and caregiving systems. American Journal of Psychoanalysis 44, 9-27, 29-31.

Fischer, B. J., & Bersani, C. A. (1979). Self-esteem and institutionalized delinquent offenders: The role of background characteristics. Adolescence 14, 197-214.

Harbin, H. T. (1983). Assaultive adolescents: Family decision-making parameters. Family Process 22(1), 109-118.

Hetherington, E. M., & Martin, B. (1979). Family interaction. In H. C. Quay & J. S. Werry (Eds.), Psychopathological disorders in childhood (pp. 257-276). New York: Wiley.

Klein, N., Alexander, J., & Parsons, B. (1977). Impact of family systems intervention on recidivism and sibling delinquency: A model of primary prevention and program evaluation. Journal of Consulting and Clinical Psychology 45, 469-474.

Malone, C. A. (1963). Some observations on children of disorganized families and problems of acting out. Journal of the American Academy of Child Psychiatry 2, 22-49.

Rosenthal, P., Moestetler, S., Wells, J. & Rolland, R. (1974). Family therapy with multiproblem, multichildren families in a court clinic setting. Journal of the American Academy of Child Psychiatry 13, 126-142.

Szurek, S. A., & Berlin, I. N. (1969). The antisocial child: His family and his community. Palo Alto, Calif.: Science and Behavior Books.

Wells, K. C., & Egan, J. (1988). Social learning and systems family therapy for childhood oppositional disorder: Comapaative treatment outcome. Comprehensive Psychiatry 29(2), 138-146.

Youngerman, J. K. (1983). Violent kids, violent parents: Family pharmacotherapy. American Journal of Orthopsychiatry 53(1), 152-156.

11. Behavioral Treatment of Antisocial Behavior

Carpenter, P. (1984). "Green stamp therapy" revisited: The evolution of 12 years of behavior modification and psychoeducational techniques with young delinquent boys. Psychological Reports 54, 99-111.

Frankel, F., & Simmons, J. Q., III (1985). Behavioral treatment approaches to pathological unsocialized physical aggression in young children. Journal of Child Psychology and Psychiatry and Allied Disciplines 26, 525-551.

Kazdin, A. E., Bass, D., Siegel, T., & Thomas, C. (1989). Cognitive-behavioral therapy and relationship therapy in the treatment of children referred for antisocial behavior. Journal of Consulting and Clinical Psychology 54(4), 522-535.

Moss, G. R., & Rick, G. R. (1981). Overview: Applications of operant technology to behavioral disorders of adolescents. American Journal of Psychiatry 138, 1161-1169.

12. Secure Treatment of Antisocial Adolescents

Agee, V. (1979). Treatment of the violent, incorrigible adolescent. Lexington, Mass.: Lexington Books.

Baittle, B., & Kobrin, S. (1964). On the relationship of a characterological type of delinquent to the milieu. Psychiatry 27, 6-16.

Berman, S. (1964). Techniques of treatment of a form of juvenile delinquency. Journal of the American Academy of Child Psychiatry 3, 24-52.

Brinich, P. M. (1984). Aggression in early childhood. In A. Solnit, et al. (Eds.), Psychoanalytic study of the child (Vol. 39, pp. 493-508). New Haven: Yale University Press.

Crocker, D. (1955). A study of a problem of aggression. In R. S. Eissler, et al. (Eds.), Psychoanalytic study of the child (Vol. 10, pp. 300-335). New York: International Universities Press.

Ekstein, R., & Friedman, S. W. (1957). The function of acting out, play action and play acting in the therapeutic process. Journal of the American Psychoanalytic Association 5, 581-629.

Garrison, W. T. (1984). Aggressive behavior, seclusion and physical restraint in an inpatient child population. Journal of the American Academy of Child Psychiatry 23, 448-452.

Gordon, S. (1960). A psychotherapeutic approach to adolescents with character disorders. American Journal of Orthopsychiatry 30, 757-766.

Jones, J. D. (1984). Principles of hospital treatment of the aggressive adolescent. In C. R. Keith (Ed.), The aggressive adolescent (pp. 359-400). New York: The Free Press.

King, C. H. (1976). Counter-transference and counter-experience in the treatment of violence-prone youth. American Journal of Orthopsychiatry 46(1), 43-52.

Marohn, R. C., Dalle-Molle, D., McCarter, E., & Linn, D. (1980). Juvenile delinquents: Psychodynamic assessment and hospital treatment. New York: Brunner/Mazel.

Noshpitz, J. (1957). The opening phase in the psychotherapy of adolescent character disorder. Bulletin of the Menninger Clinic 21, 153-164.

Paluszny, M., & McNabb, M. (1975). Therapy of a six-year-old who committed fratricide. Journal of the American Academy of Child Psychiatry 14(2), 319-336.

Pfeffer, C. R. (1982). Acute psychiatric hospital treatment of assaultive and homicidal children. In B. L. Danto, J. Bruhns, & A. H. Kutscher (Eds.), The human side of homicide (pp. 175-189). New York: Columbia University Press.

Tooley, K. (1975). The small assassins: Clinical notes in a sub-group of murderous children. Journal of the American Academy of Child Psychiatry 14, 306-318.

13. Overview of Aggression in Adolescents

Hamburg, D. A., & Trudeau, M. D. (Eds.) (1981). Biobehavioral aspects of aggression. New York: Adam R. Liss, Inc.

Hersov, L. A., Berger, M., & Shaffer, D. (Eds.). (1978). Aggression and antisocial behavior in childhood and adolescence (pp. 143-159). Oxford: Pergamon Press.

Keith, C. R. (Ed.). (1984). The aggressive adolescent. New York: The Free Press.

Lewis, D. O., Lovely, R., Yeager, C., & Femina, D. D. (1989). Toward a theory of the genesis of violence: A follow-up study of delinquents. Journal of the American Academy of Child and Adolescent Psychiatry 28(3), 431-436.

Malmquist, C. P. (1981). Handbook of adolescence. New York: Jason Aronson.

Parens, H. (1979). The development of aggression in early childhood. New York: Jason Aronson.

Parke, R. D., & Slaby, R. G. (1983). The development of aggression, IV. Socialization, personality, and social development. In P. H. Mussen (Ed.), Handbook of child psychology (pp. 547-642). New York: Wiley.

Rutter, M., & Giller, H. (1983). Juvenile delinquency: Trends and perspectives. Harmondsworth, England: Penguin Press.

14. Drug Abuse

Brook, J. S., Gordon, A. S., & Brook, D. W. (1980). Perceived paternal relationships, adolescent personality, and female marijuana use. Journal of Psychology 105, 277-285.

Dewinne, R., & Johnson, R. W. (1976). Extraversion-introversion: The personality characteristics of drug abusers. Journal of Clinical Psychology 32, 744-746.

Hendren, R. L. (1986). Adolescent alcoholism and substance abuse. In A. J. Frances & R. E. Hales (Eds.), Psychiatry update: American Psychiatric Association annual review (pp. 468-479). Washington, D.C.: American Psychiatric Association.

a. Prevention

Bailey, G. (1989). Current perspectives on substance abuse in youth. Journal of the American Academy on Child and Adolescent Psychiatry 28(2), 151-162.

Battjes, R. J. (1985). Prevention of adolescent drug abuse. International Journal of the Addictions 20(6 & 7), 1112-1134.

Bukstein, O. G., Brent, D. A., & Kaminer, Y. (1989). Comorbidity of substance abuse and other psychiatric disorders in adolescents. American Journal of Psychiatry 146(9), 1131-1141.

Czechowicz, D. (1988). Adolescent alcohol and drug abuse and its consequences--an overview. American Journal of Drug and Alcohol Abuse 14(2), 189-197.

Glynn, T. J., Leukefeld, C. G., & Ludford, J. P. (Eds). (1983). Preventing adolescent drug abuse. National Institute on Drug Abuse Research Monograph Series, No. 47.

Meeks, J. E. (1988). Adolescent chemical dependency. In S. C. Feinstein, et al. (Eds.), Adolescent psychiatry: Developmental and clinical studies (Vol. 15, pp. 509-521). Chicago: University of Chicago Press.

Murray, D. J., & Perry, D. L. (1985). The prevention of adolescent drug abuse: Implications of etiological, developmental, behavioral and environmental models. National Institute on Drug Abuse Research Monograph Series, No. 56.

b. Epidemiology and Genetics

Cadoret, R. S., Troughton, E., O'Gorman, T. W., & Heywood, E. (1986). An adoptive study of genetic and environmental factors in drug abuse. Archives of General Psychiatry 43, 1131-1136.

Kandel, D. (1982). Epidemiological and psychosocial perspectives on adolescent drug abuse. Journal of the American Academy of Child Psychiatry 21(4), 328-347.

Kandell, D. B., Davies, M., Karns, D., & Yamaguchi, K. (1986). The consequences in young adulthood of adolescent drug involvement. Archives of General Psychiatry 43, 746-754.

Kellam, S. G., Stevenson, D. L., & Rubin, B. R. (1983). How specific are the early predictors of teenage drug use? National Institute on Drug Abuse Research Monograph Series, No. 52 (pp. 329-334).

Kraus, J. (1981). Juvenile drug abuse and delinquency: Some differential associations. British Journal of Psychiatry 43, 746-754.

Simonds, J. F., & Kashani, J. (1979). Drug abuse and criminal behavior in delinquent boys committed to a training school. American Journal of Psychiatry 136(11), 1444-1448.

c. Dynamics

Berman, S. (1982). Psychic structure reorganization in drug dependent adolescents. Psychoanalytic Inquiry 2. Hillsdale, N.J.: Analytic Press.
Hartman, D. (1969). A study of drug-taking adolescents. In R. S. Eissler, et al. (Eds.), Psychoanalytic study of the child (Vol. 24, pp. 24-31). New York: International Universities Press.
Hendin, H., Pollinger, A., Ullman, R., & Carr, A. C. (1981). Adolescent marihuana abusers and their families. National Institute on Drug Abuse Research Monograph Series, No. 40.
Hendin, H., Pollinger, A., Ullman, R. B., & Carr, A. C. (1981-1982). The functions of marihuana abuse for adolescents. American Journal of Drug and Alcohol Abuse 8(4), 441-456.
Lichtenberg, J. (1982). Adolescent addiction: Varieties and vicissitudes. Psychoanalytic Inquiry 2. Hillsdale, N.J.: Analytic Press.
Lidz, R., Lidz, R., & Rubenstein, R. (1976). An anaclitic syndrome in adolescent amphetamine addicts. In R. S. Eissler, et al. (Eds.), Psychoanalytic study of the child (Vol. 31, pp. 317-348). New York: International Universities Press.
Nichtern, S. (1973). The child of drug users. Journal of the American Academy of Child Psychiatry 12, 24-31.
Watson, J. J. (1980). Solvent abuse by children and young adults: A review. British Journal of Addiction 75, 27-36.
Wieder, H., & Kaplan, E. H. (1969). Drug use in adolescents: Psychodynamic meaning and pharmocogenic effect. In R. S. Eissler, et al. (Eds.), Psychoanalytic study of the child (Vol. 24, pp. 399-431). New York: International Universities Press.
Wiener, J. M., & Egan, J. H. (1973). Heroin addiction in an adolescent population. Journal of the American Academy of Child Psychiatry 12, 48-58.

d. Treatment

Amini, R., Zilberg, N. J., Burke, E. L., & Salasnek, S. (1982). A controlled study of inpatient vs. outpatient treatment of delinquent drug abusing adolescents: One year results. Comprehensive Psychiatry 5(4), 399-414.
Berthelsdorf, S. (1976). Survey of the successful analysis of a young man addicted to heroin. In R. S. Eissler, et al. (Eds.), Psychoanalytic study of the child (Vol. 31, pp. 165-191). New York: International Universities Press.
Beschner, G. M., & Friedman, A. S. (1985). Treatment of adolescent drug abusers. International Journal of the Addictions 20(6 & 7), 971-993.
De Angelis, G. G., & Goldstein, E. (1978). Treatment of adolescent phencyclidine (PCP) abusers. American Journal of Drug and Alcohol Abuse 5(4), 399-414.

Kaufman, E. (1985). Adolescent substance abusers and family therapy. In M. P. Mirkin & S. L. Koman (Eds.), Handbook of adolescent and family therapy. (Vol. 51, pp. 245-254). New York: Garden Press.

Niven, R. G. (1986). Adolescent drug abuse. Hospital and Community Psychiatry 37(6), 596-607.

Prouskauer, S., & Rolland, R. S. (1973). Youth who use drugs: Psychodynamic diagnosis and treatment planning. Journal of the American Academy of Child Psychiatry 12, 32-47.

Rosenthal, M. S. (1984). Therapeutic communities: A treatment alternative for many but not all. Journal of Substance Abuse Treatment 1, 55-58.

Stanton, M. D., Todd, T. C., et al. (1982). The family therapy of drug abuse and addiction. New York: Guilford Press.

Suffet, F., & Brotman, R. (1984). A comprehensive care program for pregnant addicts: Obstetrical, neonatal and child development outcomes. International Journal of the Addictions 19(2), 199-219.

Weidman, A. A. (1985). Engaging the families of substance abusing adolescents in family therapy. Journal of Substance Abuse Treatment 2, 97-105.

e. General Issues in Drug Abuse

Peterson, R. C., & Stillman, R. C. (1978). Phencyclidine (PCP) abuse: An appraisal. National Institute on Drug Abuse Research Monograph Series, No. 21.

Rahdert, E. R., & Grabowski, J. (1988). Adolescent drug abuse: Analyses of treatment research. National Institute on Drug Abuse Research Monograph Series, No. 77.

Sharp, C. W., & Carroll, L. T. (Eds.). (1978). Voluntary inhalation of industrial solvents. Rockville, Md.: U.S. Department of Health, Education and Welfare.

15. Alcohol Abuse

a. Epidemiology

Nylander, I., & Rydelius, P. A. (1982). A comparison between children of alcoholic fathers from excellent vs. poor social conditions. Acta Paediatrica Scandinavica 71, 809-813.

Schulsinger, F., Knop, J., Goodwin, D. W., Teasdale, T. W., & Kkelsen, U. M. (1986). A prospective study of young men at high risk for alcoholism. Archives of General Psychiatry 43, 755-760.

Vaillant, G. E. (1983). The natural history of alcoholism. Cambridge: Harvard University Press.

Winokur, G. (1976). Alcoholism in adoptees raised apart from biological alcoholic parents. In M. Greenblatt & M. A. Schuckit (Eds.), Alcoholism problems in women and children (pp. 239-250). New York: Grune & Stratton.

b. Effects on Children

Fetal effects of maternal alcohol use. (1975). Council on Scientific Affairs. Journal of the American Medical Association 249(18), 2517-2521.

Shaywitz, S. E., Cohen, J., & Shaywitz, B. A. (1980). Behavior and learning difficulties in children of normal intelligence born to alcoholic mothers. Journal of Pediatrics 96(6), 978-982.

Steinhausen, H. C., & Spohr, H. L. (1986). Fetal alcohol syndrome. In B. B. Lahey & A. E. Kazdin (Eds.), Advances in clinical child psychology (pp. 217-243). New York: Plenum Press.

Streissguth, A. P. (1976). Maternal alcoholism and the outcome of pregnancy: Review of the fetal alcohol syndrome. In M. Greenblatt & M. A. Schuckit (Eds.), Alcoholism problems in women and children (pp. 251-276). New York: Grune & Stratton.

Zucker, R. (1976). Parental influences upon drinking patterns of their children. In M. Greenblatt & M. A. Schuckit (Eds.), Alcoholism problems in women and children (pp. 211-238). New York: Grune & Stratton.

c. Background of Alcohol Abuse

Maisto, S. A., & Carey, K. B. (1986). Origins of alcohol abuse in children and adolescents. In B. B. Lahey & A. E. Kazdin (Eds.), Advances in clinical child psychology (pp. 149-195). New York: Plenum Press.

Q. Mental Health Issues in Divorce and Custody

Harry H. Wright, M.D., M.B.A., Section Editor

1. Effects of Divorce on Children and Family

Abelsohn, D. (1983). Dealing with the abdication dynamic in the post divorce family: A context for adolescent crisis. Family Process 22, 359-383.

Anthony, E. J. (1974). Children at risk from divorce: A review. In E. J. Anthony & C. Koupernik (Eds.), The child in his family: Children at psychiatric risk (pp. 461-577). New York: Wiley .

Atwell, A. E., Moore, U. S., & Nowell, C. S. (1982). The role of stepparents in child custody disputes. Bulletin of the American Academy of Psychiatry and the Law 10, 211-217.

Bowlby, J., & Parkes, C. M. (1970). Separation and loss within the family. In E. J. Anthony & C. Koupernik (Eds.), The child in his family (p. 208). New York: Wiley.

Caplan, G. (1986). Preventing psychological disorders in children of divorce: Guidelines for the general practitioner. British Medical Journal 292, 1563-1566.

Chess, S., Thomas, A., Korn, S., Mittelman, M., & Cohen, J. (1983). Early parental attitudes, divorce and separation, and young adult outcome: Findings of a longitudinal study. Journal of the American Academy of Child Psychiatry 22, 47-51.

Clingempeel, W. G., Ievoli, R., & Brand, E. (1984). Structural complexity and the quality of stepfather-stepchild relationships. Family Process 23, 547-560.

Critchley, D. L. (1981). The child as patient: Assessing the effects of family stress and disruption on the mental health of the child. Perspectives in Psychiatric Care 19, 144-155.

Crossman, S. M., & Adams, G. R. (1980). Divorce, single parenting, and child development. Journal of Psychology 106, 205-217.

Ellison, E. S. (1983). Issues concerning parental harmony and children's psychosocial adjustment. American Journal of Orthopsychiatry 53, 73-80.

Farber, S. S., Felner, R. D., & Primavera, J. (1985). Parental separation/divorce and adolescents: An examination of factors mediating adaptation. American Journal of Community Psychology 13, 171-185.

Friedman, H. J. (1980). The father's parenting experience in divorce. American Journal of Psychiatry 137, 1177-1182.

Friedman, H. J. (1982). The challenge of divorce to adequate fathering: The peripheral father in marriage and divorce. Psychiatric Clinics of North America 5, 565-580.

Futterman, E. H. (1980). Child psychiatry perspectives. After the "civilized" divorce. Journal of the American Academy of Child Psychiatry 19, 525-530.

Gardner, R. A. (1978). Social, legal, and therapeutic changes that should lessen the traumatic effects of divorce on children. Journal of the American Academy of Psychoanalysis 6, 231-247.

Goldstein, J., Freud, A., Solnit, A. J. (1979). Beyond the best interests of the child. New York: The Free Press.

Guidubaldi, J., & Perry, J. D. (1984). Divorce, socioeconomic status, and children's cognitive-social competence at school entry. American Journal of Orthopsychiatry 54, 459-468.

Guidubaldi, J., & Perry, J. D. (1985). Divorce and mental health sequelae for children: A two-year follow up of a nationwide sample. Journal of the American Academy of Child Psychiatry 24, 531-537.

Halperin, D. A. (1980). The issue of custody in psychotherapy: Its changing therapeutic and legal parameters. Bulletin of the American Academy of Psychiatry and the Law 8, 62-71.

Hetherington, E. M., Cox, M., & Cox, R. (1985). Long-term effects of divorce and remarriage on the adjustment of children. Journal of the American Academy of Child Psychiatry 24, 518-530.

Horne, A. M. (1981). Aggressive behavior in normal and deviant members of intact versus mother-only families. Journal of Abnormal Child Psychology 9, 283-290.

Huntington, D. S. (1985). Theory and method: The use of psychological tests in research on divorce. Journal of the American Academy of Child Psychiatry 24, 583-589.

Johnston, J. R., Campbell, L. E., & Mayers, S. S. (1985). Latency children in post-separation and divorce disputes. Journal of the American Academy of Child Psychiatry 24, 563-574.

Johnston, J. R., Campbell, L. E., & Tall, M. C. (1985). Impasses to the resolution of custody and visitation disputes. American Journal of Orthopsychiatry 55, 112-129.

Kalter, N. (1977). Children of divorce in an outpatient psychiatric population. American Journal of Orthopsychiatry 47, 40-51.

Kalter, N. (1984). Conjoint mother-daughter treatment: A beginning phase of psychotherapy with adolescent daughters of divorce. American Journal of Orthopsychiatry 54, 490-497.

Kalter, N., Alpern, D., Spence, R., & Plunkett, J. W. (1984). Locus of control in children of divorce. Journal of Personality Assessment 48, 410-414.

Kalter, N., Pickar, J., & Lesowitz, M. (1984). School-based developmental facilitation groups for children of divorce: A preventive intervention. American Journal of Orthopsychiatry 54, 613-623.

Kalter, N., & Plunkett, J. W. (1984). Children's perceptions of the causes and consequences of divorce. Journal of the American Academy of Child Psychiatry 23, 326-334.

Kalter, N., & Rembar, J. (1981). The significance of a child's age at the time of parental divorce. American Journal of Orthopsychiatry 51, 85-100.

Kalter, N., Riemer, B., Brickman, A., & Chen, J. W. (1985). Implications of parental divorce for female development. Journal of the American Academy of Child Psychiatry 24, 538-544.

Kaplan, S. L. (1977). Structural family therapy for children of divorce: Case reports. Family Process 16, 75-83.

Kelly, J. B. (1981). Observations on adolescent relationships five years after divorce. In S. C. Feinstein, et al. (Eds.), Adolescent psychiatry: Developmental and clinical studies (Vol. 9, pp. 131-141). Chicago: University of Chicago Press.

Kelly, J. B., & Wallerstein, J. S. (1976). The effects of parental divorce: Experiences of the child in early latency. American Journal of Orthopsychiatry 46, 20-32.

Kelly, J. B., & Wallerstein, J. S. (1977). Brief interventions with children in divorcing families. American Journal of Orthopsychiatry 47, 23-39.

Kohen, J. A. (1981). From wife to family head: Transitions in self-identity. Psychiatry 44, 230-240.

Lansky, S. B., Cairns, N. U., Hassanein, R., Wehr, J., & Lowman, J. T. (1978). Childhood cancer: Parental discord and divorce. Pediatrics 62, 184-188.

Messinger, L., & Walker, K. N. (1981). From marriage breakdown to remarriage: Parental tasks and therapeutic guidelines. American Journal of Orthopsychiatry 51, 429-438.

Offord, D. R., Abrams, N., Allen, N., & Poushinsky, M. (1979). Broken homes, parental psychiatric illness, and female delinquency. American Journal of Orthopsychiatry 49, 252-264.

Parish, T. S., & Wigle, S. E. (1985). A longitudinal study of the impact of parental divorce on adolescents' evaluations of self and parents. Adolescence 20, 239-244.

Pedro-Carroll, J. L., & Cowen, E. L. (1985). The Children of Divorce Intervention Program: An investigation of the efficacy of a school-based prevention program. Journal of Consulting and Clinical Psychology 53, 603-611.

Perkins, T. F., & Kahan, J. P. (1979). An empirical comparison of natural-father and stepfathers family systems. Family Process 18, 175-183.

Plunkett, J. W., & Kalter, N. (1984). Children's beliefs about reactions to parental divorce. Journal of the American Academy of Child Psychiatry 23, 616-621.

Plunkett, J. W., Riemer, B., Kalter, N., & Alpern, D. (1985). Parents' beliefs about children's reactions to divorce: The development of an assessment instrument. Journal of the American Academy of Child Psychiatry 24, 334-337.

Plunkett, J. W., Schaefer, M., Kalter, N., Okla, K., & Schreier, S. (1986). Perceptions of quality of life following divorce: A study of children's prognostic thinking. Psychiatry 49, 1-12.

Psychological parenthood as the controlling factor in determining the best interests of the child. (1973). Rutgers Law Review 26, 693-713.

Ransom, J. W., Schlesinger, S., & Derdeyn, A. P. (1979). A stepfamily in formation. American Journal of Orthopsychiatry 49, 36-43.

Rembar, J., Novick, J., & Kalter, N. (1982). Attrition among families of divorce: Patterns in an outpatient psychiatric population. Journal of the American Academy of Child Psychiatry 21, 409-413.

Rickel, A. U., & Langner, T. S. (1985). Short- and long-term effects of marital disruption on children. American Journal of Community Psychology 13, 599-611.

Rothberg, B. (1983). Joint custody: Parental problems and satisfactions. Family Process 22, 43-52.

Rozendal, F. G. (1983). Halos vs. stigmas: Long-term effects of parents' death or divorce on college students' concepts of the family. Adolescence 18, 947-955.

Rutter, M. (1971). Parent-child separation: Psychological effects on the children. Journal of Child Psychology and Psychiatry and Allied Disciplines 12, 233-260.

Saucier, J. F., & Ambert, A. M. (1983). Adolescents' self-perceived health and parental marital status. Canadian Journal of Public Health 74, 396-400.

Schoettle, U. C., & Cantwell, D. P. (1980). Children of divorce. Demographic variables, symptoms, and diagnoses. Journal of the American Academy of Child Psychiatry 19, 453-475.

Slater, E. J., Stewart, K. J., & Linn, M. W. (1983). The effects of family disruption on adolescent males and females. Adolescence 18, 931-942.

Small, G. W., & Nicholi, A. M. (1982). Mass hysteria among schoolchildren. Early loss as a predisposing factor. Archives of General Psychiatry 39, 721-724.

Snyder, A. A., Minnick, K., & Anderson, D. E. (1980). Children from broken homes: Visits to the school nurse. Journal of School Health 50, 189-194.

Steinman, S. (1981). The experience of children in a joint-custody arrangement: A report of a study. American Journal of Orthopsychiatry 51, 403-414.

Steinman, S. B., Zemmelman, S. E., & Knoblauch, T. M. (1985). A study of parents who sought joint custody following divorce: Who reaches agreement and sustains joint custody and who returns to court. Journal of the American Academy of Child Psychiatry 24, 554-562.

Stern, H. P., & Casey, P. H. (1984). Judicial failure to thrive. Journal of Developmental and Behavioral Pediatrics 5, 139-141.

Stolberg, A. L., & Garrison, K. M. (1985). Evaluating a primary prevention program for children of divorce. American Journal of Community Psychology 13, 111-124.

Tepp, A. V. (1983). Divorced fathers: Predictors of continued paternal involvement. American Journal of Psychiatry 140, 1465-1469.

Terr, L. C. (1983). Child snatching: A new epidemic of an ancient malady. Journal of Pediatrics 103, 151-156.

Tooley, K. (1976). Antisocial behavior and social alienation post divorce: The "man of the house" and his mother. American Journal of Orthopsychiatry 46, 33-42.

Turner, J. R. (1984). Divorced fathers who win contested custody of their children: An exploratory study. American Journal of Orthopsychiatry 54, 498-501.

Visher, E. B., & Visher, J. S. (1978). Common problems of stepparents and their spouses. American Journal of Orthopsychiatry 48, 252-262.

Walker, K. N., & Messinger, L. (1979). Remarriage after divorce: Dissolution and reconstruction of family boundaries. Family Process 18, 185-192.

Walker, L., Brown, H., Crohn, H., Rodstein, E., Zeisel, E., & Sager, C. J. (1979). An annotated bibliography of the remarried, the living together, and their children. Family Process 18, 193-212.

Wallerstein, J. S. (1985a). Children of divorce. Emerging trends. Psychiatric Clinics of North America 8, 837-855.

Wallerstein, J. S. (1985b). Children of divorce: Preliminary report of a ten-year follow-up of older children and adolescents. Journal of the American Academy of Child Psychiatry 24, 545-553.

Wallerstein, J. S., & Kelly, J. B. (1974). The effects of parental divorce: The adolescent experience. In E. J. Anthony & C. J. Koupernik (Eds.), The child in his family. New York: Wiley.

Wallerstein, J. S., & Kelly, J. B. (1975). The effects of parental divorce: Experiences of the preschool child. Journal of the American Academy of Child Psychiatry 14, 600-616.

Wallerstein, J. S., & Kelly, J. B. (1976). The effects of parental influence: Experiences of the child in later latency. American Journal of Orthopsychiatry 46, 256-269.

Wallerstein, J. S., & Kelly, J. B. (1980a). Effects of divorce on the visiting father-child relationship. American Journal of Psychiatry 137, 1534-1539.

Wallerstein, J. S., & Kelly, J. B. (1980b). Surviving the breakup: How children and parents cope with divorce. New York: Basic Books.

Weiner, B. A. (1985). An overview of child custody laws. Hospital and Community Psychiatry 36, 838-843.

Weisfeld, D., & Laser, M. S. (1977). Divorced parents in family therapy in a residential treatment setting. Family Process 16, 229-236.

Welch, G. J., & Granvold, D. K. (1977). Seminars for separated/divorced: An educational approach to postdivorce adjustment. Journal of Sex and Marital Therapy 3, 31-39.

Westman, J. C., & Lord, G. R. (1981). Model for a child psychiatry custody study. Journal of Psychiatry and the Law 8, 253-269.

Wise, M. J. (1980). The aftermath of divorce. American Journal of Psychoanalysis 40, 148-149.

Wolchik, S. A., Sandler, I. N., Braver, S. L., & Fogas, B. S. (1986). Events of parental divorce: Stressfulness ratings by children, parents, and clinicians. American Journal of Community Psychology 14, 59-74.

Wolfenstein, M. (1973). The image of the lost parent. In R. S. Eissler, et al. (Eds.), Psychoanalytic study of the child (Vol. 28, pp. 433-456). New York: International Universities Press.

Young, D. M. (1980). A court-mandated workshop for adolescent children of divorcing parents: A program evaluation. Adolescence 15, 763-774.

Zager, R. P. (1981). Children and divorce: A review of real world factors. Journal of the American Medical Women's Association 36, 204-207.

2. Custody Issues--Effects on Children and Family

Abarbanel, A. (1979). Shared parenting after separation and divorce: A study of joint custody. American Journal of Orthopsychiatry 49, 320-329.

Ahrons, C. R. (1981). The continuing coparental relationship between divorced spouses. American Journal of Orthopsychiatry 51, 415-428.

Ahrons, C. R., & Arnn, S. (1981). When children from divorced families are hospitalized: Issues for staff. Health and Social Work 6, 21-28.

Ash, P., & Guyer, M. (1984). Court implementation of mental health professionals' recommendations in contested child custody and visitation cases. Bulletin of the American Academy of Psychiatry and the Law 12, 137-147.

Atwell, A. E., Moore, U. S., Nielsen, E., & Levite, Z. (1984). Effects of joint custody on children. Bulletin of the American Academy of Psychiatry and the Law 12, 149-157.

Awad, G. A. (1983). Joint custody: Preliminary impressions. Canadian Journal of Psychiatry 25, 357-365.

Awad, G. A., & Parry, R. (1980). Access following marital separation. Canadian Journal of Psychiatry 25, 357-365.

Ball, D. W., Newman, J. M., & Scheuren, W. J. (1984). Teachers' generalized expectations of children of divorces. Psychological Reports 54, 347-353.

Benedek, E. P., & Benedek, R. S. (1979). Joint custody: Solution or illusion? American Journal of Psychiatry 136, 1540-1544.

Benedek, E. P., & Schetky, D. H. (1985). Custody and visitation. Problems and perspectives. Psychiatric Clinics of North America 8, 857-873.

Benedek, R. S., & Benedek, E. P. (1977). Postdivorce visitation. A child's right. Journal of the American Academy of Child Psychiatry 16, 256-271.

Berkman, C. F. (1984). Psychodynamic and family issues in post-divorce child custody litigation. Journal of the American Academy of Child Psychiatry 23, 708-712.

Blotcky, M. J., Grace, K. D., & Looney, J. G. (1984). Treatment of adolescents in family therapy after divorce. Journal of the American Academy of Child Psychiatry 23, 222-225.

Chethik, M., & Kalter, N. (1980). Developmental arrest following divorce: The role of therapist as a developmental facilitator. Journal of the American Academy of Child Psychiatry 19, 281-288.

Clingempeel, W. G., & Reppucci, N. D. (1982). Joint custody after divorce: Major issues and goals for research. Psychological Bulletin 91, 102-127.

Derdeyn, A. P. (1976). Child custody contests in historical perspective. American Journal of Psychiatry 133, 1369-1376.

Derdeyn, A. P. (1977). Children in divorce: Intervention in the phase of separation. Pediatrics 60, 20-27.

Derdeyn, A. P. (1980). Divorce and children: Clinical interventions. Psychiatric Annals 10, 145-159.

Derdeyn, A. P. (1983). The family in divorce: Issues of parental anger. Journal of the American Academy of Child Psychiatry 22, 385-391.

Derdeyn, A. P., & Scott, E. (1984). Joint custody: A critical analysis and appraisal. American Journal of Orthopsychiatry 54, 199-209.

Farber, S. S., Felner, R. D., & Primavera, J. (1985). Parental separation/divorce and adolescents: An examination of factors mediating adaptation. American Journal of Community Psychology 13, 171-185.

Farson, R. (1978). Parental divorce: A growth experience for children? American Journal of Orthopsychiatry 48, 183-185.

Fine, S. (1980). Children in divorce, custody and access situations: The contribution of the mental health professional. Journal of Child Psychology and Psychiatry and Allied Disciplines 21, 353-361.

Foster, H. H. (1983). Child custody and divorce: A lawyers's view. Journal of the American Academy of Child Psychiatry 22, 392-398.

Frankel, S. A. (1985). Joint custody awards and children: A theoretical framework and some practical considerations. Psychiatry 48, 318-328.

Friedman, H. J. (1982). The challenge of divorce to adequate fathering: The peripheral father in marriage and divorce. Psychiatric Clinics of North America 5, 565-580.

Futterman, E. H. (1980). Child psychiatry perspectives. After the "civilized" divorce. Journal of the American Academy of Child Psychiatry 19, 525-530.

Gardner, R. A. (1970). The boys and girls books about divorce. New York: Science House.

Gardner, R. A. (1976). Psychotherapy with children of divorce. New York: Jason Aronson.

Gardner, R. A. (1977). The parents book about divorce. New York: Doubleday.

Gardner, R. A. (1978). Social, legal, and therapeutic changes that should lessen the traumatic effects of divorce on children. Journal of the American Academy of Psychoanalysis 6, 231-247.

Gardner, R. A. (1982). Family evaluation in child custody litigation. Creskill, N.J.: Creative Therapeutics.

Glaser, R. D., & Borduin, C. M. (1986). Models of divorce therapy: An overview. American Journal of Psychotherapy 40, 233-242.

Goldman, J., & Coane, J. (1977). Family therapy after the divorce: Developing a strategy. Family Process 16, 357-362.

Goldstein, J., Freud, A., & Solnit, A. J. (1979). Beyond the best interests of the child. New York: The Free Press.

Granvold, D. K., & Welch, G. J. (1977). Intervention for post-divorce adjustment problems: The treatment seminar. Journal of Divorce 1, 81-91.

Greif, J. B. (1979). Fathers, children, and joint custody. American Journal of Orthopsychiatry 49, 311-319.

Guidubaldi, J., & Perry, J. D. (1984). Divorce, socioeconomic status, and children's cognitive-social competence at school entry. American Journal of Orthopsychiatry 54, 459-468.

Guidubaldi, J., & Perry, J. D. (1985). Divorce and mental health sequelae for children: A two-year follow-up of a nationwide sample. Journal of the American Academy of Child Psychiatry 24, 531-537.

Haller, L. H. (1981). Before the judge: The child-custody evaluation. In S. C. Feinstein, et al. (Eds.), Adolescent psychiatry: Developmental and clinical studies (Vol. 9, pp. 142-164). Chicago: University of Chicago Press.

Hauser, B. B. (1985). Custody in dispute: Legal and psychological profiles of contesting families. Journal of the American Academy of Child Psychiatry 24, 575-582.

Haynes, J. M. (1981). Divorce mediation: A practical guide for therapists and counselors. New York: Springer.

Hetherington, E. M. (1979). Divorce: A child's perspective. American Psychologist 34, 851-858.

Hetherington, E. M., Cox, M., & Cox, R. (1985). Long-term effects of divorce and remarriage on the adjustment of children. Journal of the American Academy of Child Psychiatry 24, 518-530.

Huntington, D. S. (1985). Theory and method: The use of psychological tests in research on divorce. Journal of the American Academy of Child Psychiatry 24, 583-589.

Ilfeld, F. W., Ilfeld, H. Z., & Alexander, J. R. (1982). Does joint custody work? A first look at outcome data of relitigation. American Journal of Psychiatry 139, 62-66.

Irving, H. H., Benjamin, M., & Trocme, N. (1984). Shared parenting: An empirical analysis utilizing a large data base. Family Process 23, 561-569.

Jacobs, J. W. (1982). The effect of divorce on fathers: An overview of the literature. American Journal of Psychiatry 139, 1235-1241.

Jacobs, J. W. (1983). The effect of divorce on fathers: Social and psychotherapeutic considerations. American Journal of Psychiatry 140, 1294-1299.

Jacobs, J. W. (1986). Divorce and child custody resolution: Conflicting legal and psychological paradigms. American Journal of Psychiatry 143, 192-197.

Jacobson, D. S. (1978). The impact of marital separation/divorce on children: II. Interparent hostility and child adjustment. Journal of Divorce 2, 3-20.

Johnston, J. R., Campbell, L. E., & Mayes, S. S. (1985). Latency children in post-separation and divorce disputes. Journal of the American Academy of Child Psychiatry 24, 563-574.

Johnston, J. R., Campbell, L. E., & Tall, M. C. (1985). Impasses to the resolution of custody and visitation disputes. American Journal of Orthopsychiatry 55, 112-129.

Kalter, N. (1977). Children of divorce in an outpatient psychiatric population. American Journal of Orthopsychiatry 47, 40-51.

Kalter, N. (1984). Conjoint mother-daughter treatment: A beginning phase of psychotherapy with adolescent daughters of divorce. American Journal of Orthopsychiatry 54, 490-497.

Kalter, N., Alpern, D., Spence, R., & Plunkett, J. W. (1984). Locus of control in children of divorce. Journal of Personality Assessment 48, 410-414.

Kalter, N., Pickar, J., & Lesowitz, M. (1984). School-based developmental facilitation groups for children of divorce: A preventive intervention. American Journal of Orthopsychiatry 54, 613-623.

Kalter, N., & Plunkett, J. W. (1984). Children's perceptions of the causes and consequences of divorces. Journal of the American Academy of Child Psychiatry 23, 326-334.

Kalter, N., & Rembar, J. (1981). The significance of a child's age at the time of parental divorce. American Journal of Orthopsychiatry 51, 85-100.

Kalter, N., Riemer, B., Brickman, A., & Chen, J. W. (1985). Implications of parental divorce for female development. Journal of the American Academy of Child Psychiatry 24, 538-544.

Kelly, J. B. (1981). Observations on adolescent relationships five years after divorce. In S. C. Feinstein, et al. (Eds.), Adolescent psychiatry: Developmental and clinical studies (Vol. 9, pp. 133-141). Chicago: University of Chicago Press.

Kelly, J. B., & Wallerstein, J. S. (1976). The effects of parental divorce: Experiences of the child in early latency. American Journal of Orthopsychiatry 46, 20-32.

Kelly, J. B., & Wallerstein, J. S. (1977). Brief interventions with children in divorcing families. American Journal of Orthopsychiatry 47, 23-39.

Kitson, G. C., Moir, R. N., & Mason, P. R. (1982). Family social support in crises: The special case of divorce. American Journal of Orthopsychiatry 52, 161-165.

Kressel, K., Jaffee, N., Tuchman, B., Watson, C., & Deutsch, M. (1980). A typology of divorcing couples: Implications for mediation and the divorce process. Family Process 19, 101-116.

Kurdek, L. A. (1981). An integrative perspective on children's divorce adjustment. American Psychologist 36, 856-866.

Lansky, S. B., Cairns, N. U., Hassanein, R., Wehr, J., & Lowman, J. T. (1978). Childhood cancer: Parental discord and divorce. Pediatrics 62, 184-188.

Lassers, E., & Lassers, W. J. (1985). Children and parents in the divorce court. American Journal of Psychoanalysis 45, 77-91.

Leahey, M. (1984). Findings from research on divorce: Implications for professionals' skill development. American Journal of Orthopsychiatry 54, 298-317.

Lewis, M. (1974). The latency child in a custody conflict. Journal of the American Academy of Child Psychiatry 13, 635-647.

McDermott, J. F., Tseng, W. S., Char, W. F., & Fukunaga, C. S. (1978). Child custody decision making. The search for improvement. Journal of the American Academy of Child Psychiatry 17, 104-116.

McLoughlin, D., & Whitfield, R. (1984). Adolescents and their experience of parental divorce. Journal of Adolescence 7, 155-170.

Miller, E. (1976). Psychotherapy of a child in a custody dispute. Journal of the American Academy of Child Psychiatry 15, 441-452.

Miller, M. J., & Soper, B. (1982). An emerging contingency, the stepfamily: Review of literature. Psychological Reports 50, 715-722.

Ollendick, D. G., & Otto, B. J. (1984). MMPI characteristics of parents referred for child-custody studies. Journal of Psychology 117, 227-232.

Parish, T. S., & Wigle, S. E. (1985). A longitudinal study of the impact of parental divorce on adolescents' evaluations of self and parents. Adolescence 20, 239-244.

Pedro-Carroll, J. L., & Cowen, E. L. (1985). The Children of Divorce Intervention Program: An investigation of the efficacy of a school-based prevention program. Journal of Consulting and Clinical Psychology 53, 603-611.

Plunkett, J. W., & Kalter, N. (1984). Children's beliefs about reactions to parental divorce. Journal of the American Academy of Child Psychiatry 23, 616-621.

Plunkett, J. W., Riemer, B., Kalter, N., & Alpern, D. (1985). Parents' beliefs about children's reactions to divorce: The development of an assessment instrument. Journal of the American Academy of Child Psychiatry 24, 334-337.

Plunkett, J. W., Schaefer, M., Kalter, N., Okla, K., & Schreier, S. (1986). Perceptions of quality of life following divorce: A study of children's prognostic thinking. Psychiatry 49, 1-12.

Rembar, J., Novick, J., & Kalter, N. (1982). Attrition among families of divorce: Patterns in an outpatient psychiatric population. Journal of the American Academy of Child Psychiatry 21, 409-413.

Rickel, A. U., & Langner, T. S. (1985). Short- and long-term effects of marital disruption on children. American Journal of Community Psychology 13, 599-611.

Stern, H. P., & Casey, P. H. (1984). Judicial failure to thrive. Journal of Developmental and Behavioral Pediatrics 5, 139-141.

Terr, L. C. (1983). Child snatching: A new epidemic of an ancient malady. Journal of Pediatrics 103, 151-156.

PART IV

Therapeutics

A. Individual Therapy with Children and Adolescents

Section Editor:

Donald J. Carek, M.D.
Professor of Psychiatry
Chief, Youth Division
Medical University of South Carolina
Charleston, South Carolina

Subsection Editor:

Irving N. Berlin, M.D.
Professor of Psychiatry and Pediatrics
University of New Mexico Medical School
Albuquerque, New Mexico

Associate Editors:

Eugene L. Arnold, M.D.
Professor of Psychiatry
Director, Division of Child-Adolescent Psychiatry
Ohio State University School of Medicine
Columbus, Ohio

Charles D. Casat, M.D.
Assistant Professor of Psychiatry
Youth Division
Medical University of South Carolina
Charleston, South Carolina

1. History of Psychological Treatment of Psychiatric Disorders of Childhood

Ayllon, T., Smith, D., & Rogers, M. (1970). Behavioral management of school phobia. Journal of Behavior Therapy and Experimental Psychiatry 1, 125-138.

Beiser, H. R. (1955). Therapeutic play techniques. Symposium,1954. 8. Play equipment for diagnosis and therapy. American Journal of Orthopsychiatry 25, 761-770.

Bennett, C. C., & Rogers, C. R. (1941). Predicting the outcomes of treatment. American Journal of Orthopsychiatry 11, 210-221.

Berkovitz, I. H. (1972). Adolescents grow in groups: Experiences in adolescent group psychotherapy. New York: Brunner/Mazel.

Berman, S. (1954). Psychotherapeutic techniques with adolescents. American Journal of Orthopsychiatry 24, 238-245.

Bixler, R. H. (1964). Limits are therapy. In M. R. Haworth (Ed.), Child psychotherapy (pp. 134-147). New York: Basic Books.

Bronner, A. F. (1944). Treatment and what happened afterward (a second report). American Journal of Orthopsychiatry 14, 28-35.

Chess, S., & Lyman, M. S. (1969). A psychiatric unit in a general hospital pediatric clinic. American Journal of Orthopsychiatry 39, 77-85.

Clement, P. W., Fazzone, R. A., & Goldstein, B. (1970). Tangible reinforcers and child group therapy. Journal of the American Academy of Child Psychiatry 9, 409-427.

Eisenberg, L. (1958). School phobia: A study in the communication of anxiety. American Journal of Psychiatry 114, 712-718.

Eissler, K. R. (1958). Notes of the problems of technique in the psychoanalytic treatment of adolescents, with some remarks on perversions. In R. S. Eissler, et al. (Eds.), Psychoanalytic study of the child (Vol. 13, pp. 223-254). New York: International Universities Press.

Ekstein, R., & Wallerstein, J. (1966). Choice of interpretation in the treatment of borderline and psychotic children. In R. Ekstein (Ed.), Children of time and space, of action and impulse (pp. 148-157). New York: Appleton-Century-Crofts.

Engel, M. (1964). Public education and the "emotionally disturbed" child. Journal of the American Academy of Child Psychiatry 3, 617-637.

Erikson, E. H. (1963). Play and cure. In E. H. Erikson (Ed.), Childhood and society (pp. 222-234). New York: Norton.

Erikson, E. H. (1964). Toys and reasons. In M. R. Haworth (Ed.), Child psychotherapy (pp. 3-11). New York: Basic Books.

Erikson, E. H. (1972). Play and actuality. In M. W. Piers (Ed.), Play and development (pp. 127-167). New York: Norton.

Eysenck, H. J., & Rachman, S. J. (1965). The application of learning theory to child psychiatry. In J. G. Howells (Ed.), Modern perspectives in child psychiatry (pp. 104-169). London: Oliver & Boyd.

Feinstein, S. C., & Wolpert, E. A. (1973). Juvenile manic-depressive illness: Clinical and therapeutic considerations. Journal of the American Academy of Child Psychiatry 12, 123-136.

Fraiberg, S. (1951). Clinical notes on the nature of transference in child analysis. In R. S. Eissler, et al. (Eds.), Psychoanalytic study of the child (Vol. 6, pp. 286-306). New York: International Universities Press.

Fraiberg, S. (1955). Some considerations in the introduction to therapy in puberty. In R. S. Eissler, et al. (Eds.), Psychoanalytic study of the child (Vol. 10, pp. 264-286). New York: International Universities Press.

Freud, A. (1945). Indications for child analysis. In R. S. Eissler, et al. (Eds.), Psychoanalytic study of the child (Vol. 1, pp. 127-149). New York: International Universities Press.

Furman, E. (1957). Treatment of under-fives by way of their parents. In R. S. Eissler, et al. (Eds.), Psychoanalytic study of the child (Vol. 12, pp. 250-262). New York: International Universities Press.

Gardner, R. A. (1974). The mutual storytelling technique in the treatment of psychogenic problems secondary to minimal brain dysfunction. Journal of Learning Disabilities 7, 135-143.

Geist, R. A. (1974). Some observations on adolescent drug use: Therapeutic implications. Journal of the American Academy of Child Psychiatry 13, 54-71.

Geleerd, E. R. (1957). Some aspects of psychoanalytic technique in adolescence. In R. S. Eissler, et al. (Eds.), Psychoanalytic study of the child (Vol. 12, pp. 263-283). New York: International Universities Press.

Gelfand, D. M. & Hartmann, D. P. (1968). Behavior therapy with children: A review and evaluation of research methodology. Psychological Bulletin 69, 204-215.

Ginott, H. G. (1958). Play group therapy: A theoretical framework. International Journal of Group Psychotherapy 8, 410-418.

Ginott, H. G. (1964a). Problems in the playroom. In M. R. Haworth (Ed.), Child psychotherapy (pp. 125-130). New York: Basic Books.

Ginott, H. G. (1964b). The theory and practice of "therapeutic intervention" in child treatment. In M. R. Haworth (Ed.), Child psychotherapy (pp. 148-158). New York: Basic Books.

Ginott, H. G. & Lebo, D. (1961). Play therapy limits and theoretical orientation. Journal of Consulting Psychology 25, 337-340.

Goldings, C. R., & Goldings, H. J. (1972). Books in the playroom: A dimension of child psychiatric technique. Journal of the American Academy of Child Psychiatry 11, 52-65.

Group for the advancement of psychiatry. (1957). Committee on child psychiatry: The diagnostic process in child psychiatry. GAP Report No. 38. New York: Group for the Advancement of Psychiatry.

Haley, J. (1973). Strategic therapy when a child is presented as the problem. Journal of the American Academy of Child Psychiatry 12, 641-659.

Hambidge, G. (1955). Therapeutic play techniques. Symposium, 1954. IV. Structured play therapy. American Journal of Orthopsychiatry 25, 601-617.

Haworth, M. R., & Keller, M. J. (1962). The use of food in the diagnosis and therapy of emotionally disturbed children. Journal of the American Academy of Child Psychiatry 1, 548-563.

Heinicke, C. M. (1965). Frequency of psychotherapeutic session as a factor affecting the child's developmental status. In R. S. Eissler, et al. (Eds.), Psychoanalytic study of the child (Vol. 20, pp. 42-98). New York: International Universities Press.

Heinicke, C. M. (1969). Frequency of psychotherapeutic session as a factor affecting outcome: Analysis of clinical ratings and test results. Journal of Abnormal Psychology 74, 553-560.

Hobbs, N. (1966). Helping disturbed children: Psychological and ecological strategies. American Psychologist 21, 1105-1115.

Kaplan, S. L., & Escoll, P. (1973). Treatment of two silent adolescent girls. Journal of the American Academy of Child Psychiatry 12, 59-72.

Kennedy, W. A. (1965). School phobia: Rapid treatment of fifty cases. Journal of Abnormal Psychology 70, 285-289.

Khan, M. M. R. (1963). The concept of cumulative trauma. In R. S. Eissler, et al. (Eds.), Psychoanalytic study of the child (Vol. 18, pp. 286-306). New York: International Universities Press.

Klein, M. (1955). The psychoanalytic play technique. American Journal of Orthopsychiatry 25, 223-237.

Kramer, S., & Settlage, C. F. (1962). On the concepts and technique of child analysis. Journal of the American Academy of Child Psychiatry 1, 509-535.

Lazarus, A. A., Davison, G. C., & Polefka, D. A. (1965). Classical and operant factors in the treatment of a school phobia. Journal of Abnormal Psychology 70, 225-229.

Levin, S., & Wermer, H. (1966). The significance of giving gifts to children in therapy. Journal of the American Academy of Child Psychiatry 5, 630-652.

Lewis, M. (1974). Interpretation in child analysis: Developmental considerations. Journal of the American Academy of Child Psychiatry 13, 32-53.

Lorenz, K. (1972). The enmity between generations and its probable ethological causes. In M. W. Piers (Ed.), Play and development (pp. 64-118). New York: Norton.

Maenchen, A. (1970). On the technique of child analysis in relation to stages of development. In R. S. Eissler, et al. (Eds.), Psychoanalytic study of the child (Vol. 25, pp. 175-208). New York: International Universities Press.

Marcus, J. (1963). Borderline states in childhood. Journal of Child Psychology and Psychiatry and Allied Disciplines 4, 207-218.

Markowitz, I. (1966). Family therapy in a child guidance clinic. Psychiatric Quarterly 40, 308-318.

Mattsson, A., Hawkins, J. W., & Seese, L. R. (1967). Child psychiatric emergencies: Clinical characteristics and follow-up results. Archives of General Psychiatry 17, 584-592.

Meeks, J. E. (1970). Children who cheat at games. Journal of the American Academy of Child Psychiatry 9, 157-170.

Minuchin, S. (1965). Conflict-resolution family therapy. Psychiatry 28, 278-286.

Minuchin, S., & Montalvo, B. (1967). Techniques for working with disorganized low socioeconomic families. American Journal of Orthopsychiatry 37, 880-887.

Morrison, G. C. (1969). Therapeutic intervention in a child psychiatry emergency service. Journal of the American Academy of Child Psychiatry 8, 542-558.

Morrison, G. C., & Collier, J. G. (1969). Family treatment approaches to suicidal children and adolescents. Journal of the American Academy of Child Psychiatry 8, 140-153.

Mowrer, O. H., & Mowrer, W. M. (1938). Enuresis--a method for its study and treatment. American Journal of Orthopsychiatry 8, 436-459.

Therapeutics

Phillips, E. L., & Johnston, M. S. H. (1954). Theoretical and clinical aspects of short-term parent-child psychotherapy. Psychiatry 17, 267-275.

Piaget, J. (1972). Some aspects of operations. In M. W. Piers (Ed.), Play and development (pp. 15-27). New York: Norton.

Piers, M. W. (Ed.). (1972). Play and development. New York: Norton.

Poznanski, E., & Zrull, J. P. (1970). Childhood depression: Clinical characteristics of overtly depressed children. Archives of General Psychiatry 23, 8-15.

Proskauer, S. (1969). Some technical issues in time-limited psychotherapy with children. Journal of the American Academy of Child Psychiatry 8, 154-169.

Proskauer, S. (1971). Focused time-limited psychotherapy with children. Journal of the American Academy of Child Psychiatry 10, 619-639.

Rabinovitch, R. D. (1964). An evaluation of present trends in psychotherapy with children. In M. R. Haworth (Ed.), Child psychotherapy (pp. 39-45). New York: Basic Books.

Radin, N. (1972). Three degrees of maternal involvement in a preschool program: Impact on mothers and children. Child Development 43, 1355-1364.

Rexford, E. N., Schleifer, M., & Van Amerongen, S. T. (1956). A follow-up of a psychiatric study of 57 antisocial young children. Mental Hygiene 40, 196-214.

Rosenthal, A. J., & Levine, S. V. (1971). Brief psychotherapy with children: Process of therapy. American Journal of Psychiatry 128, 141-146.

Ross, A. O. (1964). Techniques of therapy. In M. R. Haworth (Ed.), Child psychotherapy (pp. 121-125). New York: Basic Books.

Sandler, J., & Nagera, H. (1963). Aspects of the metapsychology of fantasy. In R. S. Eissler, et al. (Eds.), Psychoanalytic study of the child (Vol. 18, pp. 159-194). New York: International Universities Press.

Solomon, J. C. (1938). Active play therapy. American Journal of Orthopsychiatry 8, 479-498.

Spitz, R. A. (1972). Fundamental education. In M. W. Piers (Ed.), Play and development (pp. 43-64). New York: Norton.

Subotnik, L. (1971). Transference toward the child therapist and other parent surrogates. Journal of Genetic Psychology 119, 215-231.

Szurek, S. A. (1959). Playfulness, creativity and schisis. American Journal of Orthopsychiatry 29, 667-683.

Szurek, S. A., & Berlin, I. N. (1956). Elements of psychotherapeutics with the schizophrenic child and his parents. Psychiatry 19, 1-9.

Wenar, C. (1957). The therapeutic value of setting limits with inhibited children. Journal of Nervous and Mental Disease 125, 390-395.

Werry, J. S., & Wollersheim, J. P. (1967). Behavior therapy with children: A broad overview. Journal of the American Academy of Child Psychiatry 6, 346-370.

Wimberger, H. C., & Kogan, K. L. (1974). A direct approach to altering mother-child interaction in disturbed children. Archives of General Psychiatry 30, 636-639.

Wolff, P. H. (1972). Operational thought and social adaptation. In M. W. Piers (Ed.), Play and development (pp. 28-42). New York: Norton.

Woltmann, A. G. (1964). Concepts of play therapy techniques. In M. R. Haworth (Ed.), Child psychotherapy (pp. 20-32). New York: Basic Books.

2. Psychoanalytic Base of Psychotherapy with Children and Adolescents

Anthony, E. J. (1976). The treatment of the latency child. Canadian Psychiatric Association Journal 21, 199-209.

Anthony, E. J. (1982). The comparable experience of a child and adult analyst. In A. Solnit, et al. (Eds.), Psychoanalytic study of the child (Vol. 37, pp. 339-366). New Haven: Yale University Press.

Berlin, I. N. (1987). Some transference and countertransference issues in the playroom. Journal of the American Academy of Child and Adolescent Psychiatry 26(1), 101-107.

Brenner, C. (1985). Some contributions of adult analysis to child analysis. In A. Solnit, et al. (Eds.), Psychoanalytic study of the child (Vol. 40, pp. 221-233). New Haven: Yale University Press.

Carek, D. J. (1979). Individual psychodynamically oriented therapy. In J. D. Noshpitz (Ed.), Handbook of child psychiatry (pp. 35-37). New York: Basic Books.

Domash, L. (1975). The use of with and the comic by a borderline psychotic child in psychotherapy. American Journal of Psychotherapy 29, 261-270.

Domash, L. (1976). The therapeutic use of writing in the service of the ego. Journal of the American Academy of Psychoanalysis 4, 261-269.

Ekstein, R. (1979). Psychoanalysis. In J. D. Noshpitz (Ed.), Handbook of child psychiatry (pp. 21-35). New York: Basic Books.

Ekstein, R. (1983). The adolescent self during the process of termination of treatment: Termination, interruption, or intermission? In S. C. Feinstein, et al. (Eds.), Adolescent psychiatry: Developmental and clinical studies (Vol. 11, pp. 125-146). Chicago: University of Chicago Press.

Fraiberg, S., Adelson, E., & Shapiro, V. (1975). Ghosts in the nursery. A psychoanalytic approach to the problems of impaired infant-mother relationships. Journal of the American Academy of Child Psychiatry 14, 387-421.

Friedman, R. M. (1982). Therapeutic techniques for the treatment of certain infantile personality disorders in ego disturbed children. Psychoanalytic Review 69, 191-206.

Furman, E. (1985). On fusion, integration, and feeling good. In A. Solnit, et al. (Eds.), Psychoanalytic study of the child (Vol. 40, pp. 81-110). New Haven: Yale University Press.

Jansma, P., & French, R. (1979). Transactional analysis: An alternative approach to managing inappropriate behavior. American Therapeutics Journal 33, 155-162.

Kernberg, P. F. (1985-1986). Child analysis with a severely disturbed adopted child. International Journal of Psychoanalytic Psychotherapy 11, 277-313.

King, C. H. (1976). Counter-transference and counter-experience in the treatment of violence prone youth. American Journal of Orthopsychiatry 46, 43-52.

Kliman, G. W. (1975). Analyst in the nursery. Experimental application of child analytic techniques in a therapeutic nursery: The cornerstone method. In R. S. Eissler, et al. (Eds.), Psychoanalytic study of the child (Vol. 30, pp. 477-510). New York: International Universities Press.

Meissner, W. W. (1974). Portrait of a rebel as a young man. International Journal of Psychoanalytic Psychotherapy 3, 456-482.

Plank, E. N., & Plank, R. (1978). Children and death: As seen through art and autobiographies. In A. Solnit, et al. (Eds.), Psychoanalytic study of the child (Vol. 33, pp. 593-620). New Haven: Yale University Press.

Prentice, N. M., Goldenberg, G. M., & McDevitt, S. C. (1977). Issues in the transfer of children in dynamic psychotherapy. Journal of the American Academy of Child Psychiatry 16, 693-702.

Rees, K. (1978). The child's understanding of his past: Cognitive factors in reconstruction with children. In A. Solnit, et al. (Eds.), Psychoanalytic study of the child (Vol. 33, pp. 237-259). New Haven: Yale University Press.

Ritvo, S. (1978). The psychoanalytic process in childhood. In A. Solnit, et al. (Eds.), Psychoanalytic study of the child (Vol. 33, pp. 295-305). New Haven: Yale University Press.

Roskin, G., & Rabiner, C. J. (1976). Psychotherapists' passivity--a major training problem. International Journal of Psychoanalytic Psychotherapy 5, 319-331.

Ross, J. M. (1985-1986). The darker side of fatherhood: Clinical and developmental ramifications of the "Laius motif." International Journal of Psychoanalytic Psychotherapy 11, 117-154.

Sandler, J., Kennedy, H., & Tyson, R. L. (1975). Discussions on transference. The treatment situation and technique in child psychoanalysis. In R. S. Eissler, et al. (Eds.), Psychoanalytic study of the child (Vol. 30, pp. 409-441). New York: International Universities Press.

Sarnoff, C. A. (1978-1979). Developmental considerations in the psychotherapy of latency-age children. International Journal of Psychoanalytic Psychotherapy 7, 283-304.

Schowalter, J. E. (1976). Therapeutic alliance and the role of speech in child analysis. In R. S. Eissler, et al. (Eds.), Psychoanalytic study of the child (Vol. 31, pp. 415-436). New York: International Universities Press.

Schowalter, J. E. (1986). Countertransference in work with children: Review of a neglected concept. Journal of the American Academy of Child Psychiatry 25, 40-45.

Slipp, S. (1982). Interface between psychoanalysis and family therapy. American Journal of Psychoanalysis 42, 221-228.

Tyson, P. (1978). Transference and developmental issues in the analysis of a prelatency child. In A. Solnit, et al. (Eds.), Psychoanalytic study of the child (Vol. 33, pp. 213-236). New Haven: Yale University Press.

Tyson, R. L., & Tyson, P. (1986). The concept of transference in child psychoanalysis. Journal of the American Academy of Child Psychiatry 25, 30-39.

Van Dam, H., Heinicke, C. M., & Shane, M. (1975). On termination in child analysis. In R. S. Eissler, et al. (Eds.), Psychoanalytic study of the child (Vol. 30, pp. 443-474). New York: International Universities Press.

3. Play Therapy

a. History of Play Therapy

Allen, F. H. (1942). Psychotherapy with children. New York: Norton.
Axline, V. M. (1964). Dibs. New York: Ballentine Books.
Dorfman, E. (1951). Play therapy. In C. R. Rogers (Ed.), Client-centered therapy (pp. 235-277). Boston: Houghton Mifflin.
Erikson, E. H. (1964). Toys and reason. In M. R. Haworth (Ed.), Child psychotherapy (pp. 3-11). New York: Basic Books.
Freud, A. (1946). The psychoanalytical treatment of children. London: Imago.
Klein, M. (1955). Psychoanalytic play technique. American Journal of Orthopsychiatry 25, 223-237.
Lebo, D. (1955). The expressive value of toys recommended for nondirective play therapy. Journal of Clinical Psychology 11, 144-145.
Lebo, D. (1958). A theoretical framework for nondirective play therapy: Concepts from psychoanalysis and learning theory. Journal of Consulting Psychology 22, 275-279.
Lowenfeld, M. (1969). Play in childhood. Portway Bath, England: Cedric Chivers Ltd.
Taft, J. J. (1962). The dynamics of therapy in a controlled relationship. New York: Dover.
Witmer, H. L. (Ed.). (1946). Psychiatric interviews with children. Cambridge: Harvard University Press.
Wolfman, A. G. (1964). Concepts of play therapy techniques. In M. R. Haworth (Ed.), Child psychotherapy (pp. 20-32). New York: Basic Books.

b. Some Theoretical Aspects

Anthony, E. J. (1964). Communicating therapeutically with the child. Journal of the American Academy of Child Psychiatry 3, 106-125.
Bateson, G. (1972). A theory of play and fantasy. In G. Bateson (Ed.), Steps to an ecology of mind. New York: Basic Books.
Bishop, J. (1986). Change lives in the poetry of its meaning. Canadian Journal of Counseling 20(1), 21-32.
Bretherton, I. (Ed.). (1984). Symbolic play: The development of social understanding. New York: Academic Press.
Freud, A. (1963). The role of regression in mental development. In A. J. Solnit & S. A. Provence (Eds.), Modern perspectives in child development (pp. 97-106). New York: International Universities Press.

Kohut, H. (1972). Thoughts on narcissism and narcissistic rage. In R. S. Eissler, et al. (Eds.), Psychoanalytic study of the child (Vol. 27, pp. 360-400). New York: International Universities Press.

Kordas, E., & Peto, A. (1956). Contributions to the theory of play. British Journal of Medical Psychology 29, 100-112.

Lanyado, M. (1987). Asymbolic and symbolic play: Developmental perspectives in the treatment of disturbed children. Journal of Child Psychotherapy 13(2), 33-44.

Lowenstein, R. M. (1966). On the theory of the super ego: A discussion. In R. M. Lowenstein, et al. (Eds.), Psychoanalysis: A general psychology (pp. 298-306). New York: International Universities Press.

Moore, T. (1964). Realism and fantasy in children's play. Journal of Child Psychology and Psychiatry and Allied Disciplines 5, 15-36.

Murphy, L. (1970). The problem of defence and the concept of coping. In E. J. Anthony & C. J. Koupernik (Eds.), The child and his family (pp. 65-85). New York: Wiley-Interscience.

Orenstein, A. (1981). Self pathology in childhood: Developmental and clinical considerations. Psychiatric Clinics of North America 4(8), 435-453.

Piaget, J. (1962). Play, dreams and imitation in child abuse. New York: Norton.

Piaget, J. (1972). Some aspects of operations. In M. W. Piers (Ed.), Play and development (pp. 15-27). New York: Norton.

Sutton-Smith, B. (1985). Toys as culture. New York: Gardner Press.

Tolpin, M. (1978). Self objects and oedipal objects: A crucial developmental distinction. In A. Solnit, et al. (Eds.), Psychoanalytic study of the child (Vol. 33, pp. 187-189). New Haven: Yale University Press.

Vandenberg, B. (1980). Play, problem solving and creativity. In K. H. Rubin (Ed.), New directions for child development: Children's play. (pp. 84-99). San Francisco: Jossey-Bass.

Waelder, R. (1933). The psychoanalytic theory of play. Psychoanalytic Quarterly 2, 208-224.

West, J. (1984). Ending or beginning? A discussion of theory and practice of termination procedures in play therapy. Journal of Social Work Practice 1(2), 49-65.

Winnicott, D. W. (1965). The maturational process and the facilitating enviornment. New York: International Universities Press.

Wolff, D. H. (1972). Operational thought and social adaptation. In M. W. Piers (Ed.), Play and development (pp. 28-42). New York: Norton.

c. Transference and Countertransference

Berlin, I. N. (1987). Some transference and countertransference issues in the playroom. Journal of the American Academy of Child Psychiatry 26(1), 101-104.

Bornstein, B. (1948). Emotional barriers in the understanding and treatment of young children. American Journal of Orthopsychiatry 18, 691-697.

Brody, S. (1961). Transference resistance in prepuberty. In R. S. Eissler, et al. (Eds.), Psychoanalytic study of the child (Vol. 16, pp. 251-274). New York: International Universities Press.

Colm, H. (1955). A field theory approach to transference and its particular application to children. Psychiatry 18, 329-352.

Fraiberg, S. (1951). Clinical notes on the nature of transference in child analysis. In R. S. Eissler, et al. (Eds.), Psychoanalytic study of the child (Vol. 6, pp. 286-306. New York: International Universities Press.

Fraiberg, S. (1962). Transference aspects of the analysis of a child with a severe behavior disorder. Journal of the American Psychoanalytic Association 10, 338-367.

Furman, E. (1981). Transference and externalization in latency. In A. Solnit, et al. (Eds.), Psychoanalytic study of the child (Vol. 35, pp. 267-284). New Haven: Yale University Press.

Habermas, T. (1987). Social cognitive aspects of therapeutic interactions. Journal of the American Academy of Child Psychiatry 26(5), 770-773.

Kabcenell, R. (1974). On countertransference. In R. S. Eissler, et al. (Eds.), Psychoanalytic study of the child (Vol. 29, pp. 22-33). New York: International Universities Press.

Marcus, I. M. (1980). Countertransference and the psychoanalytic process in children and adolescents. In A. Solnit, et al. (Eds.), Psychoanalytic study of the child (Vol. 35, pp. 285-298). New Haven: Yale University Press.

Markowitz, J. (1964). The nature of the child's initial resistance to psychotherapy. In M. R. Haworth (Ed.), Child psychotherapy (pp. 186-193). New York: Basic Books.

Marshall, R. J. (1979). Countertransference in the psychotherapy of children and adolescence. Contemporary Psychoanalysis 15, 595-629.

Rubenstein, B. O., & Levitt, M. (1964). Countertransference. In M. R. Haworth (Ed.), Child psychotherapy (pp. 256-268). New York: Basic Books.

Schowalter, J. E. (1986). Countertransference in work with children: Review of a neglected concept. Journal of the American Academy of Child Psychiatry 25(1), 40-45.

Tyson, R. L., & Tyson, P. (1986). The concept of transference in child psychoanalysis. Journal of the American Academy of Child Psychiatry 25(1), 30-39.

Winnicott, D. W. (1949). Hate in the countertransference. International Journal of Psycho-Analysis 30, 69-77.

d. Play Therapy Methods and Techniques

Adams-Tucker, C. (1984). Early treatment of child incest victims. American Journal of Psychotherapy 38(4), 505-516.

Allan, J., & Berry, P. (1981). Sandplay. Elementary School Guidance and Counseling 21(4), 300-306.

Therapeutics

Allen, F. H. (1964). The beginning phase of therapy. In M. R. Haworth (Ed.), Child psychotherapy (pp. 101-105). New York: Basic Books.

Axline, V. M. (1955). Play therapy procedures and results. American Journal of Orthopsychiatry 25, 574-584.

Axline, V. M. (1964a). The eight basic principles. In M. R. Haworth (Ed.), Child psychotherapy (pp. 161-174). New York: Basic Books.

Axline, V. M. (1964b). Establishing rapport. In M. R. Haworth (Ed.), Child psychotherapy (pp. 95-101). New York: Basic Books.

Beiser, H. R. (1955). Play therapy techniques symposium 1954: Play equipment for diagnosis and therapy. American Journal of Orthopsychiatry 25, 761-770.

Berlin, I. N. (1977). Play therapy: Checkers as a means of communication with children and adolescents. In P. F. Ostwald (Ed.), Communication and social interaction (pp. 227-236). New York: Grune & Stratton.

Berlin, I. N. (1986). The use of competitive games in play therapy. In C. Schaefer & S. Reid (Eds.), Home play: therapeutic uses of childhood games (pp. 197-214). New York: Wiley.

Bixler, R. H. (1964). Limits are therapy. In M. R. Haworth (Ed.), Child psychotherapy (pp. 134-147). New York: Basic Books.

Davidson, D. (1988). Playing and the growth of imagination, In M. Sidoli & M. Davies (Eds.), Jungian child psychotherapy (pp. 73-92). London: Karnac Books.

Dulcan, M. K. (1984). Brief psychotherapy with children and their families: State of the art. Journal of the American Academy of Child Psychiatry 23(5), 552-567.

Erikson, E. H. (1963). Play and cure. In E. H. Erikson (Ed.), Childhood and society (pp. 222-234). New York: Norton.

Federation, S. (1986). Sexual abuse: Treatment modalities for the younger child. Journal of Psychosocial Nursing and Mental Health Services 24(7), 26-29.

Fordham, M. (1988). Acting out. In M. Sidoli & M. Davies (Eds.), Jungian child psychotherapy (pp. 131-140). London: Karnac Books.

Gabriellini, F., & Nissins, S. (1988). Sand play therapy with a psychotic child. In M. Sidoli & M. Davies (Eds.), Jungian child psychotherapy (pp. 221-232). London: Karnac Books.

Gardner, R. A. (1975a). The alphabet soup game. In R. A. Gardner (Ed.), Psychotherapeutic approach to the resistant child (pp. 351-373). New York: Jason Aronson.

Gardner, R. A. (1975b). Bag of words game. In R. A. Gardner (Ed.), Psychotherapeutic approach to the resistant child (pp. 86-123). New York: Jason Aronson.

Gardner, R. A. (1975c). Dramatization of the therapeutic communications. In R. A. Gardner (Ed.), Psychotherapeutic approach to the resistant child (pp. 141-180). New York: Jason Aronson.

Gardner, R. A. (1975d). Mutual storytelling technique. In R. A. Gardner (Ed.), Psychotherapeutic approach to the resistant child (pp. 240-256). New York: Jason Aronson.

Gardner, R. A. (1975e). The talking, feeling, doing game. In R. A. Gardner (Ed.), Psychotherapeutic approach to the resistant child (pp. 181-227). New York: Jason Aronson.

Gillman, R. D. (1987). A child analyzes a dream. In A. Solnit, et al. (Eds.), Psychoanalytic study of the child (Vol. 42, pp. 263-273). New Haven: Yale University Press.

Ginott, H. (1964). Problems in the play room. In M. R. Haworth (Ed.), Child psychotherapy (pp 125-130). New York: Basic Books.

Golden, D. B. (1983). Play therapy for hospitalized children. In C. E. Shaeffer & K. J. O'Connor (Eds.), Handbook of play therapy (pp. 101-130). New York: Wiley.

Golden, L. B. (1985). A critical case study of play therapy. Journal of Child and Adolescent Psychotherapy 2(4), 286-290.

Golding, C. R. (1972). Books in the play room: A dimension of child psychiatric technique. Journal of the American Academy of Child Psychiatry 11, 52-65.

Hambridge, G. J. (1955). Structured play therapy. American Journal of Orthopsychiatry 25(3), 601-617.

Heiniche, C. M., & Ramsey-Klee, D. M. (1986). Outcome of child psychotherapy as a function of frequency of session. Journal of the American Academy of Child Psychiatry 25(2), 247-253.

Irwin, E. C. (1983). Puppets in therapy: An assessment procedure. American Journal of Psychotherapy 39(3), 389-400.

Jeffrey, L. D. (1984). Developmental play therapy: An assessment and therapeutic technique in child psychiatry. Journal of Occupational Therapy 47(3), 70-74.

Kuhli, L. (1979). The use of two houses in play therapy. American Journal of Orthopsychiatry 49(3), 431-435.

Levin, S., & Wermer, H. (1966). The significance of giving gifts to children in therapy. Journal of the American Academy of Child Psychiatry 6, 630-632.

Levy, D. (1976). Release therapy. In C. Schaefer (Ed.), The therapeutic use of child's play (pp. 138-152). New York: Jason Aronson.

Levy, D. M. (1939). Release therapy. American Journal of Orthopsychiatry 9(4), 713-736.

Loomis, E. A. (1957). The use of checkers in handling certain resistances in child therapy and child analysis. Journal of the American Psychoanalytic Association 5, 130-135.

Looney, J. G. (1984). Treatment planning in child psychiatry. Journal of the American Academy of Child Psychiatry 23(15), 529-536.

Maenchen, A. (1984). The handling of overt aggression in child analysis. In A. Solnit, et al. (Eds.), Psychoanalytic study of the child (Vol. 39, pp. 393-405). New Haven: Yale University Press.

Marcus, I. D. (1966). Costume play therapy. Journal of the American Academy of Child Psychiatry 5(3), 441-452.

McDermott, D. F., & Char, W. F. (1984). Stage related models of psychotherapy with children. Journal of the American Academy of Child Psychiatry 23(5), 537-543.

Meeks, J. E. (1970). Children who cheat at games. Journal of the American Academy of Child Psychiatry 9, 157-170.

Modarressi, T., & McClaney, M. (1978). Psychiatric evaluation of the child: The psychiatric foundation of medicine. In G. Balis (Ed.), A psychiatry handbook (pp. 420-433). Woodlawn, Mass.: Medical Handbook Publishers

Noshpitz, G. D., & Loughman, S. (1983). A narcissistic reaction in a six year old girl with a seizure disorder. American Journal of Psychotherapy 37(4), 533-543.

O'Connor, K. (1986). The interaction of hostile and depressive behaviors: A case study of a depressed boy. Journal of Child and Adolescent Psychotherapy 3(2), 105-108.

Ornstein, A. (1976). Making contact with the inner world of the child. Comprehensive Psychiatry 17, 3-36.

Peterlin, K., & Sloves, R. (1985). Time limited psychotherapy with children: Central theme and time as major tools. Journal of the American Academy of Child Psychiatry 24(6), 788-792.

Reams, R. (1987). Darkness in play therapy: Anonymity and a sense of control as facilitators of disclosure. Journal of Child and Adolescent Psychotherapy 4, 112-115.

Sloves, R., & Peterlin, K. B. (1986). The process of time limited psychotherapy with latency aged children. Journal of the American Academy of Child Psychiatry 25(6), 847-851.

Smith, H. F. (1986). The elephant on the fence: Approaches to the psychotherapy of attention deficit disorder. American Journal of Psychotherapy 4(22), 252-264.

Stirtzinger, R. M. (1983). Storytelling: A creative therapeutic technique. Canadian Journal of Psychiatry 28(7), 561-565.

Susselman, S. (1973). The use of physical restraints and its relation to other formal psychotherapeutic intervention. In S. A. Szurek & I. N. Berlin (Eds.), Clinical studies in childhood psychoses (pp. 522-528). New York: Brunner/Mazel.

West, J. (1983). Play therapy with Rosy. British Journal of Social Work 13(6), 645-661.

Wolfman, A. G. (1972). Puppetry as a tool in child psychotherapy. International Journal of Child Psychiatry 1(1), 84-96.

Zelman, A. B., Samuels, S., & Abrams, D. (1985). IQ changes in young children following intensive long-term psychotherapy. American Journal of Psychotherapy 39(2), 215-227.

e. Books

Coppolillo, H. P. (1987). Psychodynamic psychotherapy of children. Madison, Conn.: International Universities Press.

Jernberg, A. M. (1979). Theraplay. San Francisco: Jossey-Bass.

Haworth, M. (1989). A child's therapy: Hour by hour. New York: International Universities Press.

Schaefer, C. E., & O'Connor, K. J. (1983). Handbook of play therapy. New York: Wiley.

4. Dynamic Psychotherapy with Children and Adolescents

Bauer, R., & Modarressi, T. (1977). Strategies of therapeutic contact: Working with children with severe object relationship disturbance. American Journal of Psychotherapy 31, 605-617.

Beratis, S., Miller, R., & Galenson, E. (1982-1983). Separation-individuation and transitional objects in a four-year-old psychotic child. International Journal of Psychoanalytic Psychotherapy 9, 561-582.

Blum, H. P. (1978). Reconstruction in a case of postpartum depression. In A. Solnit, et al. (Eds.), Psychoanalytic study of the child (Vol. 33, pp. 335-362). New Haven: Yale University Press.

Cohen, D. J. (1980). constructive and reconstructive activities in the analysis of a depressed child. In A. Solnit, et al. (Eds.), Psychoanalytic study of the child (Vol. 35, pp. 237-266). New Haven: Yale University Press.

Conceptualizing the nature of the therapeutic action of child analysis. (1980). Journal of the American Psychoanalytic Association 28, 161-179.

de Saussure, J. (1982). Dreams and dreaming in relation to trauma in childhood. International Journal of Psycho-Analysis 63, 167-175.

Edington, G. (1985). Hand puppets and dolls in psychotherapy with children. Perceptual and Motor Skills 61, 691-696.

Ekstein, R. (1981). Some thoughts concerning the clinical use of children's dreams. Bulletin of the Menninger Clinic 45, 115-124.

Esman, A. H. (1985). A developmental approach to the psychotherapy of adolescents. In S. C. Feinstein, et al. (Eds.), Adolescent psychiatry: Developmental and clinical studies (Vol. 12, pp. 119-133). Chicago: University of Chicago Press.

Fisher, S. (1981). Some observations of psychotherapy and creativity. In S. C. Feinstein, et al. (Eds.), Adolescent psychiatry: Developmental and clinical studies (Vol. 9, pp. 528-538). Chicago: University of Chicago Press.

Fraiberg, S. (1982). The adolescent mother and her infant. In S. C. Feinstein, et al. (Eds.), Adolescent psychiatry: Developmental and clinical studies (Vol. 10, pp. 7-23). Chicago: University of Chicago Press.

Frankel, S. (1977). The management aspect of psychotherapy with aggressive children. Child Psychiatry and Human Development 7, 169-185.

Friedman, R. M. (1982). Therapeutic techniques for the treatment of certain infantile personality disorders in ego disturbed children. Psychoanalytic Review 69, 191-206.

Friedman, T. L. (1978). Piaget and psychotherapy. Journal of the American Academy of Psychoanalysis 6, 175-192.

Gair, D. S., Hersch, C., & Wiesenfeld, S. (1980). Successful psychotherapy of severe emotional disturbance in a young retarded boy. Journal of the American Academy of Child Psychiatry 19, 257-269.

Garza-Guerrero, A. C. (1981-1982). The superego concept. II. Superego development, superego pathology summary. Psychoanalytic Review 68, 513-546.

Geist, R. A. (1979). Onset of chronic illness in children and adolescents: Psychotherapeutic and consultative intervention. American Journal of Orthopsychiatry 49, 4-23.

Green, A. H. (1978). Psychiatric treatment of abused children. Journal of the American Academy of Child Psychiatry 17, 356-371.

Greenspan, S. I. (1980). Analysis of a five-and-a-half-year-old girl: Indications for a dyadicphallic phase of development. Journal of the American Psychoanalytic Association 28, 575-603.

Kazdin, A. E., & Wilson, G. T. (1978). Criteria for evaluating psychotherapy. Archives of General Psychiatry 35, 407-416.

Kelley, S. J. (1984). The use of art therapy with sexually abused children. Journal of Psychiatric Nursing and Mental Health Services 22, 12-18.

Kernberg, P. F. (1985-1986). Child analysis with a severely disturbed adopted child. International Journal of Psychoanalytic Psychotherapy 11, 277-313.

Kestenbaum, C. J. (1985). The creative process in child psychotherapy. American Journal of Psychotherapy 39, 479-489.

Kliman, G. W. (1975). Analyst in the nursery. Experimental application of child analytic techniques in a therapeutic nursery: The cornerstone method. In R. S. Eissler, et al. (Eds.), Psychoanalytic study of the child (Vol. 30, pp. 477-510). New York: International Universities Press.

Kris, A. O. (1981). On giving advice to parents in analysis. In A. Solnit, et al. (Eds.), Psychoanalytic study of the child (Vol. 36, pp. 151-162). New Haven: Yale University Press.

Kris, K. (1978). The school consultant as an object for externalization. In A. Solnit, et al. (Eds.), Psychoanalytic study of the child (Vol. 33, pp. 641-651). New Haven: Yale University Press.

Kuhli, L. (1979). The use of two houses in play therapy. American Journal of Orthopsychiatry 49, 431-435.

Levinson, L. (1979). The world of disguises: Unusual defenses in a latency girl. In A. Solnit, et al. (Eds.), Psychoanalytic study of the child (Vol. 34, pp. 273-306). New Haven: Yale University Press.

Lindenbaum, S., & Clark, D. (1983). Toward an integrative approach to psychotherapy with children. American Journal of Orthopsychiatry 53, 449-459.

Lopez, T., & Kliman, G. W. (1979). Memory, reconstruction, and mourning in the analysis of a 4-year-old child: Maternal bereavement in the second year of life. In A. Solnit, et al. (Eds.), Psychoanalytic study of the child (Vol. 34, pp. 235-271). New Haven: Yale University Press.

Lopez, T., & Kliman, G. W. (1980). The cornerstone treatment of a preschool boy form an extremely impoverished environment. In A. Solnit, et al. (Eds.), Psychoanalytic study of the child (Vol. 35, pp. 341-375). New Haven: Yale University Press.

MacVicar, K. (1979). Psychotherapeutic issues in the treatment of sexually abused girls. Journal of the American Academy of Child Psychiatry 18, 342-353.
McConville, B. J. (1976). Opening moves and sequential strategies in child psychotherapy. Canadian Psychiatric Association Journal 21, 295-301.
McDermott, J. F., & Char, W. F. (1984). Stage-related models of psychotherapy with children. Journal of the American Academy of Child Psychiatry 23, 537-543.
McDonald, M. (1981). Alternative treatment of a young boy with a traumatic psychosis: The rediscovery and reconstitution of the self. Psychiatric Clinics of North America 4, 509-532.
Meeks, J. E. (1980-1981). What did the therapists say? What did the therapists do? International Journal of Psychoanalytic Psychotherapy 8, 233-241.
Menahem, S., Lipton, G. L., & Caplan, G. (1981). The psychologically orientated pediatrician and the provision of psychoanalytic psychotherapy. Child Psychiatry and Human Development 12, 67-81.
Milos, M. E., & Reiss, S. (1982). Effects of three play conditions on separation anxiety in young children. Journal of Consulting and Clinical Psychology 50, 389-395.
Minde, K. K., & Minde, R. (1981). Psychiatric intervention in infancy: A review. Journal of the American Academy of Child Psychiatry 20, 217-238.
Nicol, A. R., & Eccles, M. (1985). Psychotherapy for Munchausen syndrome by proxy. Archives of Disease in Childhood 60, 344-348.
Noshpitz, J. D. (1981). Psychotherapy with children: Basic principles. Current Psychiatric Therapies 20, 47-59.
Noshpitz, J. D., & Loughman, S. (1983). A narcissistic reaction in a six-year-old girl with a seizure disorder. American Journal of Psychotherapy 37, 533-543.
Novick, J. (1980). Negative therapeutic motivation and negative therapeutic alliance. In A. Solnit, et al. (Eds.), Psychoanalytic study of the child (Vol. 35, pp. 299-320). New Haven: Yale University Press.
Paul, H. A. (1984). Horneyan developmental psychoanalytic theory and its application to the treatment of the young. American Journal of Psychoanalysis 44, 59-71, 73-78.
Pfeffer, C. R. (1980). Psychiatric hospital treatment of assaultive homicidal children. American Journal of Psychotherapy 34, 197-207.
Pfeffer, C. R. (1984). Modalities of treatment for suicidal children: An overview of the literature on current practice. American Journal of Psychotherapy 38, 364-372.
Pfeffer, C. R., & Plutchik, R. (1982). Psychopathology of latency age children. Relation to treatment planning. Journal of Nervous and Mental Disease 170, 193-197.Pfefferbaum, B., & Lucas, R. H. (1979). Management of acute psychologic problems in pediatric oncology. General Hospital Psychiatry 1, 214-219.
Post, S. L. (1980). Origins, elements, and functions of therapeutic empathy. International Journal of Psycho-Analysis 61, 277-293.
Pruett, K. D. (1979). Home treatment for two infants who witnessed their mother's murder. Journal of the American Academy of Child Psychiatry 18, 647-657.

5. Various Treatment Modalities

Abrams, S. (1980). Therapeutic action and ways of knowing. Journal of the American Psychoanalytic Association 28, 291-307.

Abramson, R. M., Hoffman, L., & Johns, C. A. (1979). Play group psychotherapy for early latency-age children on an inpatient psychiatric unit. International Journal of Group Psychotherapy 29, 383-392.

Anthony, E. J. (1980). The family and the psychoanalytic process in children. In A. Solnit, et al. (Eds.), Psychoanalytic study of the child (Vol. 35, pp. 3-34). New Haven: Yale University Press.

Anthony, E. J. (1981). Treatment of the paranoid adolescent. In S. C. Feinstein, et al. (Eds.), Adolescent psychiatry: Developmental and clinical studies (Vol. 9, pp. 501-527). Chicago: University of Chicago Press.

Anthony, E. J. (1982). The comparable experience of a child and adult analyst. In A. Solnit, et al. (Eds.), Psychoanalytic study of the child (Vol. 37, pp. 339-366). New Haven: Yale University Press.

Ascher, M. (1985-1986). Conjoint treatment of a mother and her 16-month-old toddler. International Journal of Psychoanalytic Psychotherapy 11, 315-337.

6. Behavioral Therapies

Awad, G. A. (1983). The middle phase of psychotherapy with antisocial adolescents. American Journal of Psychotherapy 37, 190-201.

Ayllon, T., Garber, S. W., & Allison, M. G. (1977). Behavioral treatment of childhood neurosis. Psychiatry 40, 315-322.

Azrin, N. H., Nunn, R. G., & Frantz-Renshaw, S. E. (1982). Habit reversal vs. negative practice treatment of self-destructive oral habits (biting, chewing or licking of the lips, cheeks, tongue or palate). Journal of Behavior Therapy and Experimental Psychiatry 13, 49-54.

Ballard, K. D., & Crooks, T. J. (1984). Videotape modeling for preschool children with low levels of social interaction and low peer involvement in play. Journal of Abnormal Child Psychology 12, 95-109.

Bean, A. W., & Roberts, M. W. (1981). The effect of time-out release contingencies on changes in child noncompliance. Journal of Abnormal Child Psychology 9, 95-105.

Bernal, M. E., Klinnert, M. D., & Schultz, L. A. (1980). Outcome evaluation of behavioral parent training and client-centered parent counseling for children with conduct problems. Journal of Applied Behavior Analysis 13, 677-691.

Blotcky, M. J., Sheinbein, M., Wiggins, K. M., & Forgotson, J. H. (1980-1981). A verbal group technique for ego-disturbed children: Action to words. International Journal of Psychoanalytic Psychotherapy 8, 203-232.

Blount, R. L., & Stokes, T. F. (1984). Self-reinforcement by children. Progress in Behavior Modification 18, 195-225.

Blumberg, M. L. (1979). Collateral therapy for the abused child and the problem parent. American Journal of Psychotherapy 33, 339-353.

Bollard, J. (1982). A 2-year follow-up of bedwetters treated by dry-bed training and standard conditioning. Journal of Behavior Research in Therapy 20, 571-580.

Bornstein, P. H., Balleweg, B. J., McLellarn, R. W., Wilson, G. L., Sturm, C. A., Andre, J. C., & van den Pol, R. A. (1983). The "bathroom game": A systematic program for the elimination of encopretic behavior. Journal of Behavior Therapy and Experimental Psychiatry 14, 67-71.

Bornstein, P. H., & Knapp, M. (1981). Self-control desensitization with a multi-phobic boy: A multiple baseline design. Journal of Behavior Therapy and Experimental Psychiatry 12, 281-285.

Botvin, G. J., & Wills, T. A. (1985). Personal and social skills training: Cognitive-behavioral approaches to substance abuse prevention. National Institute on Drug Abuse Research Monograph Series 63, 8-49.

Braswell, L., Kendall, P. C., & Urbain, E. S. (1982). A multistudy analysis of socioeconomic states (SES) and the measures and outcome of cognitive-behavioral treatment with children. Journal of Abnormal Child Psychology 10, 443-449.

Brightman, R. P., Baker, B. L., Clark, D. B., & Ambrose, S. A. (1982). Effectiveness of alternative parent training formats. Journal of Behavior Therapy and Experimental Psychiatry 13, 113-117.

Brinich, P. M. (1984). Aggression in early childhood. Joint treatment of children and parents. In A. Solnit, et al. (Eds.), Psychoanalytic study of the child (Vol. 39, pp. 493-508). New Haven: Yale University Press.

Brown, B. J. (1979). A behavioral approach to adolescents in trouble. Journal of Adolescence 2, 77-87.

Brown, R. T., & Alford, N. (1984). Ameliorating attentional deficits and concomitant academic deficiencies in learning disabled children through cognitive training. Journal of Learning Disabilities 17, 20-26.

Brownell, K. D. (1982). Obesity: Understanding and treating a serious, prevalent, and refractory disorder. Journal of Consulting and Clinical Psychology 50, 820-840.

Cade, B. (1984). Paradoxical techniques in therapy. Journal of Child Psychology and Psychiatry and Allied Disciplines 25, 509-516.

Campbell, M., Anderson, L. T., Meier, M., Cohen, I. L., Small, A. M., Samit, C., & Sachar, E. J. (1978). A comparison of haloperidol and behavior therapy and their interaction in autistic children. Journal of the American Academy of Child Psychiatry 17, 640-655.

Cautela, J. R. (1983). The self-control triad. Description and clinical applications. Behavior Modification 7, 299-315.

Christophersen, E. R. (1982). Incorporating behavioral pediatrics into primary care. Pediatric Clinics of North America 29, 261-296.

Clement, P. W., Roberts, P. V., & Lantz, C. E. (1976). Mothers and peers as child behavior therapists. International Journal of Group Psychotherapy 26, 335-359.

Conger, J. C., & Keane, S. P. (1981). Social skills intervention in the treatment of isolated or withdrawn children. Psychological Bulletin 90, 478-495.

Therapeutics

Cunningham, C. E., & Peltz, L. (1982). In vivo desensitization in the management of self-injurious behavior. Journal of Behavior Therapy and Experimental Psychiatry 13, 135-140.

Dahlquist, L. M., Gil, K. M., Armstrong, F. D., Ginsberg, A., & Jones, B. (1985). Behavioral management of children's distress during chemotherapy. Journal of Behavior Therapy and Experimental Psychiatry 16, 325-329.

Dash, J. (1981). Rapid hypno-behavioral treatment of a needle phobia in a five-year-old cardiac patient. Journal of Pediatric Psychology 6, 37-42.

Delamater, A. M., Conners, C. K., & Wells, K. C. (1984). A comparison of staff training procedures. Behavioral applications in the child psychiatric inpatient setting. Behavior Modification 8, 39-58.

Delamater, A. M., Rosenbloom, N., Conners, C. K., & Hertweck, L. (1983). The behavioral treatment of hysterical paralysis in a ten-year-old boy. A case study. Journal of the American Academy of Child Psychiatry 22, 73-79.

Doke, L., Wolery, M., & Sumberg, C. (1983). Treating chronic aggression. Effects and side effects of response-contingent ammonia spirits. Behavior Modification 7, 531-556.

Dorsey, M. F., Iwata, B. A., Ong, P., & McSween, T. E. (1980). Treatment of self-injurious behavior using a water mist: Initial response suppression and generalization. Journal of Applied Behavior Analysis 13, 343-353.

Dubey, D. R., O'Leary, S. G., & Kaufman, K. F. (1983). Training parents of hyperactive children in child management: A comparative outcome study. Journal of Abnormal Child Psychology 11, 229-245.

Epstein, L. H., Wing, R. R., & Valoski, A. (1985). Childhood obesity. Pediatric Clinics of North America 32, 363-379.

Epstein, Y. M., & Borduin, C. M. (1984). "The children's feedback game": An approach for modifying disruptive group behavior. American Journal of Psychotherapy 38, 63-72.

Esveldt-Dawson, K., Wisner, K. L., Unis, A. S., Matson, J. L., & Kazdin, A. E. (1982). Treatment of phobias in a hospitalized child. Journal of Behavior Therapy and Experimental Psychiatry 13, 77-83.

Fine, P. (1982). Play and family therapy as core skills for child psychiatry: Some implications of Piaget's theory for integrations in training and practice. Child Psychiatry and Human Development 13, 79-96.

Firestone, P., & Witt, J. E. (1982). Characteristics of families completing and prematurely discontinuing a behavioral parent-training program. Journal of Pediatric Psychology 7, 209-222.

Fisher, D. C., & Wollersheim, J. P. (1986). Social reinforcement: A treatment component in verbal self-instructional training. Journal of Abnormal Child Psychology 14, 41-48.

Fisher, L., Anderson, A., & Jones, J. E. (1981). Types of paradoxical intervention and indications/contraindications for use in clinical practice. Family Process 20, 25-35.

Foreyt, J. P., & Kondo, A. T. (1984). Advances in behavioral treatment of obesity. Progress in Behavior Modification 16, 231-261.

Fraiberg, S., Adelson, E., & Shapiro, V. (1983). Ghosts in the nursery. A psychoanalytic approach to problems which affect the mother-infant relations. Psychiatrie de l'Enfant 26, 57-98.

Frankel, F., & Simmons, J. Q. (1985). Behavioral treatment approaches to pathological unsocialized physical aggression in young children. Journal of Child Psychology and Psychiatry and Allied Disciplines 26, 525-551.

Friedman, S. (1980). Self-control in the treatment of Gilles de la Tourette's syndrome: Case study with 18-month follow-up. Journal of Consulting and Clinical Psychology 48, 400-402.

Fundudis, T. (1986). Anorexia nervosa in a pre-adolescent girl: A multimodal behavior therapy approach. Journal of Child Psychology and Psychiatry and Allied Disciplines 27, 261-273.

Furniss, T. (1984). Organizing a therapeutic approach to intra-familial child sexual abuse. Journal of Adolescence 7, 309-317.

Gambrill, E. D. (1983). Behavioral intervention with child abuse and neglect. Progress in Behavior Modification 15, 1-56.

Garrison, S. R., & Stolberg, A. L. (1983). Modification of anger in children by affective imagery training. Journal of Abnormal Child Psychology 11, 115-129.

Glasgow, R. E., & Rosen, G. M. (1978). Behavioral bibliotherapy: A review of self-help behavior therapy manuals. Psychological Bulletin 85, 1-23.

Graziano, A. M., & Mooney, K. C. (1982). Behavioral treatment of "nightfears" in children: Maintenance of improvement at 2 1/2- to 3-year follow-up. Journal of Consulting and Clinical Psychology 50, 598-599.

Gresham, F. M. (1985). Utility of cognitive-behavioral procedures for social skills training with children: A critical review. Journal of Abnormal Child Psychology 13, 411-423.

Harris, K. R. (1985). Conceptual, methodological, and clinical issues in cognitive-behavioral assessment. Journal of Abnormal Child Psychology 13, 373-390.

Hinshaw, S. P., Henker, B., & Whalen, C. K. (1984a). Cognitive-behavioral and pharmacologic interventions for hyperactive boys: Comparative and combined effects. Journal of Consulting and Clinical Psychology 52, 739-749.

Hinshaw, S. P., Henker, B., & Whalen, C. K. (1984b). Self-control in hyperactive boys in anger-inducing situations: Effects of cognitive-behavioral training and of methylphenidate. Journal of Abnormal Child Psychology 12, 55-77.

Hobbs, S. A., Walle, D. L., & Caldwell, H. S. (1984). Maternal evaluation of social reinforcement and time-out: Effects of brief parent training. Journal of Consulting and Clinical Psychology 52, 135-136.

Horn, W. F., Chatoor, I., & Conners, C. K. (1983). Addictive effects of dexedrine and self-control training. A multiple assessment. Behavior Modification 7, 383-402.

Howe, P. A., & Silvern, L. E. (1981). Behavioral observation of children during play therapy: Preliminary development of a research instrument. Journal of Personality Assessment 45, 168-182.

Hug-Hellmuth, H. (1975). Technics of child psychoanalysis. Psychiatrie de l'Enfant 18, 191-210.

Irwin, E. C. (1985). Puppets in therapy: An assessment procedure. American Journal of Psychotherapy 39, 389-400.

Jay, S. M., Elliott, C. H., Ozolins, M., Olson, R. A., & Pruitt, S. D. (1985). Behavioral management of children's distress during painful medical procedures. Behavior Research and Therapy 23, 513-520.

Jessee, E. H., Jurkovic, G. J., Wilkie, J., & Chiglinsky, M. (1982). Positive reframing with children: conceptual and clinical considerations. American Journal of Orthopsychiatry 52, 314-322.

Kaplan, S. L. (1979). Behavior modification as a limit-setting task in the family psychotherapy of a disruptive boy. Journal of the American Academy of Child Psychiatry 18, 492-504.

Kavanagh, C. (1983). Psychological intervention with the severely burned child: Report of an experimental comparison of two approaches and their effects on psychological sequelae. Journal of the American Academy of Child Psychiatry 22, 145-156.

Kazdin, A. E. (1982). The token economy: A decade later. Journal of Applied Behavior Analysis 15, 431-445.

Kazdin, A. E. (1984). Acceptability of aversive procedures and medication as treatment alternatives for deviant child behavior. Journal of Abnormal Child Psychology 12, 289-301.

Kazdin, A. E., French, N. H., & Sherick, R. B. (1981). Acceptability of alternative treatments for children: Evaluations by inpatient children, parents, and staff. Journal of Consulting and Clinical Psychology 49, 900-907.

Kellerman, J. (1979). Behavioral treatment of night terrors in a child with acute leukemia. Journal of Nervous and Mental Disease 167, 182-185.

Kendall, P. C. (1985). Toward a cognitive-behavioral model of child psychopathology and a critique of related interventions. Journal of Abnormal Child Psychology 13, 357-372.

Kendall, P. C., Lerner, R. M., & Craighead, W. E. (1984). Human development and intervention in childhood psychopathology. Child Development 55, 71-82.

Kettlewell, P. W., & Kausch, D. F. (1983). The generalization of the effects of a cognitive-behavioral treatment program for aggressive children. Journal of Abnormal Child Psychology 11, 101-114.

Koles, M. R., & Jenson, W. R. (1985). Comprehensive treatment of chronic fire setting in a severely disordered boy. Journal of Behavior Therapy and Experimental Psychiatry 16, 81-85.

Koverola, C., Manion, I., & Wolfe, D. (1985). A microanalysis of factors associated with child-abusive families: Identifying individual treatment priorities. Behavior Research and Therapy 23, 499-506.

La Greca, A. M. (1981). Social behavior and social perception in learning-disabled children: A review with implications for social skills training. Journal of Pediatric Psychology 6, 395-416.

La Greca, A. M., & Santogrossi, D. A. (1980). Social skills training with elementary school students: A behavioral group approach. Journal of Consulting and Clinical Psychology 48, 220-227.

Land, H. M. (1986). Child abuse: Differential diagnosis, differential treatment. Child Welfare 65, 33-44.

Lebaron, S., & Zeltzer, L. (1984). Behavioral intervention for reducing chemotherapy-related nausea and vomiting in adolescents with cancer. Journal of Adolescent Health Care 5, 178-182.

Lester, E. P., & LaRoche, C. (1978). Schizophreniform psychosis of childhood: Therapeutic considerations. Comprehensive Psychiatry 19, 153-159.

Levin, S., Rubenstein, J. S., & Streiner, D. L. (1976). The parent-therapist program: An innovative approach to treating emotionally disturbed children. Hospital and Community Psychiatry 27, 407-410.

Lewis, M., & Brown, T. E. (1979). Psychotherapy in the residential treatment of the borderline child. Child Psychiatry and Human Development 9, 181-188.

Lim, M. H., & Bottomley, V. (1983). A combined approach to the treatment of effeminate behavior in a boy: A case study. Journal of Child Psychology and Psychiatry and Allied Disciplines 24, 469-479.

Looney, J. G. (1984). Treatment planning in child psychiatry. Journal of the American Academy of Child Psychiatry 23, 529-536.

Lothstein, L. M., & Levine, S. B. (1981). Expressive psychotherapy with gender dysphoric patients. Archives of General Psychiatry 38, 924-929.

Luiselli, J. K., & Slocumb, P. R. (1983). Management of multiple aggressive behaviors by differential reinforcement. Journal of Behavior Therapy and Experimental Psychiatry 14, 343-347.

Mahoney, M. J., & Nezworski, M. T. (1985). Cognitive-behavioral approaches to children's problems. Journal of Abnormal Child Psychology 13, 467-476.

Marshall, R. J. (1976). "Joining techniques" in the treatment of resistant children and adolescents. American Journal of Psychotherapy 30, 73-84.

Matson, J. L., Kazdin, A. E., & Esveldt-Dawson, K. (1980). Training interpersonal skills among mentally retarded and socially dysfunctional children. Behavior Research and Therapy 18, 419-427.

McCarthy, W. J. (1985). The cognitive developmental model and other alternatives to the social skills deficit model of smoking onset. National Institute on Drug Abuse Research Monograph Series 63, 153-169.

McDonnell, L. (1979). Paraverbal therapy in pediatric cases with emotional complications. American Journal of Orthopsychiatry 49, 44-52.

McLoughlin, C. S. (1985). Utility and efficacy of knowledge of behavioral principles as applied to children. Psychological Reports 56, 463-467.

Michelson, L. (1981). Psychotherapeutic outcome for children in a community mental health center: Psychological, demographic, and treatment predictors. Psychological Reports 48, 323-326.

Michelson, L., Mannarino, A. P., Marchione, K. E., Stern, M., Figueroa, J., & Beck, S. (1983). A comparative outcome study of behavioral social-skills training, interpersonal-problem-solving and non-directive control treatments with child psychiatric outpatients. Behavior Research and Therapy 21, 545-556.

Miller, N. B., & Cantwell, D. P. (1976). Siblings as therapists: A behavioral approach. American Journal of Psychiatry 133, 447-450.

Therapeutics

Moskowitz, J. A. (1979). The "wish book" in child psychotherapy. American Journal of Psychiatry 136, 848-849.

Murphy, H. A., Hutchison, J. M., & Bailey, J. S. (1983). Behavioral school psychology goes outdoors: The effects of organized games on playground aggression. Journal of Applied Behavior Analysis 16, 29-35.

Nadler, J. H. (1983). Effecting change in stepfamilies: A psychodynamic/behavioral group approach. American Journal of Psychotherapy 37, 100-112.

Noland, S. A., Arnold, J., & Clement, P. W. (1980). Self-reinforcement by under-achieving, under-controlled girls. Psychological Reports 47, 671-678.

O'Dell, S. L. (1985). Progress in parent training. Progress in Behavior Modification 19, 57-108.

Odom, S. L., & Strain, P. S. (1984). Peer-mediated approaches to promoting children's social interaction: A review. American Journal of Orthopsychiatry 54, 544-557.

Overholser, J., & Beck, S. (1985). Assessing generalization of treatment effects and self-efficacy in the modification of eating styles in obese children. Addictive Behavior 10, 145-152.

Parker, L. H., & Cinciripini, P. M. (1984). Behavioral medicine with children: Applications in chronic disease. Progress in Behavior Modification 17, 135-165.

Parrish, V., & Hester, P. (1980). Controlling behavioral techniques in an early intervention program. Community Mental Health Journal 16, 169-175.

Pearl, R. (1985). Cognitive-behavioral interventions for increasing motivation. Journal of Abnormal Child Psychology 13, 443-453.

Petti, T. A., Bornstein, M., Delamater, A., & Conners, C. K. (1980). Evaluation and multimodality treatment of a depressed prepubertal girl. Journal of the American Academy of Child Psychiatry 19, 690-702.

Pevsner, R. (1982). Group parent training versus individual family therapy: An outcome study. Journal of Behavior Therapy and Experimental Psychiatry 13, 119-122.

Phillips, D., & Wolpe, S. (1981). Multiple behavioral techniques in severe separation anxiety of a twelve-year-old. Journal of Behavior Therapy and Experimental Psychiatry 12, 329-332.

Pruett, K. D., & Dahl, E. K. (1982). Psychotherapy of gender identity conflict in young boys. Journal of the American Academy of Child Psychiatry 21, 65-70.

Queiroz, L. O., Motta, M. A., Madi, M. B., Sossai, D. L., & Boren, J. J. (1981). A functional analysis of obsessive-compulsive problems with related therapeutic procedures. Behavior Research and Therapy 19, 377-388.

Rakos, R. F., Grodek, M. V., & Mack, K. K. (1985). The impact of a self-administered behavioral intervention program on pediatric asthma. Journal of Psychosomatic Research 29, 101-108.

Ramer, J. C., Tinker, D. E., & Domoto, M. (1986). Short-term admission for behavior modification. American Journal of Diseases of Children 140, 242-244.

Raue, J., & Spence, S. H. (1985). Group versus individual applications of reciprocity training for parent-youth conflict. Behavior Research and Therapy 23, 177-186.

7. Behavioral Treatment of Pediatric Disorders

Alexander, A. B., Cropp, G. J., & Chai, H. (1979). Effects of relaxation training on pulmonary mechanics in children with asthma. Journal of Applied Behavior Analysis 12, 27-35.

Altman, K., Grahs, C., & Friman, P. (1982). Treatment of unobserved trichotillomania by attention-reflection and punishment of an apparent covariant. Journal of Behavior Therapy and Experimental Psychiatry 13, 337-340.

Altman, K., Haavik, S., & Higgins, S. T. (1983). Modifying the self-injurious behavior of an infant with spina bifida and diminished pain sensitivity. Journal of Behavior Therapy and Experimental Psychiatry 14, 165-168.

Anderson, L., Dancis, J., & Alpert, M. (1978). Behavioral contingencies and self-mutilation in Lesch-Nyhan disease. Journal of Consulting and Clinical Psychology 46, 529-536.

Ayllon, T., Garber, S. W., & Allison, M. G. (1977). Behavioral treatment of childhood neurosis. Psychiatry 40, 315-322.

Azrin, N. H., Nunn, R. G., & Frantz-Renshaw, S. E. (1982). Habit reversal vs. negative practice treatment of self-destructive oral habits (biting, chewing or licking of the lips, cheeks, tongue or palate). Journal of Behavior Therapy and Experimental Psychiatry 13, 49-54.

Barmann, B. C., Croyle-Barmann, C., & McLain, B. (1980). The use of contingent-interrupted music in the treatment of disruptive bus-riding behavior. Journal of Applied Behavior Analysis 13, 693-698.

Barrett, T. E. (1985). Clinical application of behavioral social skills training with children. Psychological Reports 57, 1183-1186.

Baumeister, A. A., & Baumeister, C. F. (1978). Suppression of repetitive self-injurious behavior by contingent inhalation of aromatic ammonia. Journal of Autism and Childhood Schizophrenia 8, 71-77.

Bean, A. W., & Roberts, M. W. (1981). The effect of time-out release contingencies on changes in child noncompliance. Journal of Abnormal Child Psychology 9, 95-105.

Belcastro, F. P. (1979). Use of behavior modification with hearing impaired subjects. American Annals of the Deaf 124, 820-824.

Blagg, N. R., & Yule, W. (1984). The behavioral treatment of school refusal--a comparative study. Behavior Research and Therapy 22, 119-127.

Blanchard, E. B., & Andrasik, F. (1982). Psychological assessment and treatment of headache: Recent developments and emerging issues. Journal of Consulting and Clinical Psychology 50, 795-796.

Blechman, E. A., Taylor, C. J., & Schrader, S. M. (1981). Family problem solving versus home notes as early intervention with high-risk children. Journal of Consulting and Clinical Psychology 49, 919-926.

Bogdanov, O. V., Smetankin, A. A., Inin, Y. S., & Khakhan, Y. V. (1983). Voluntary control of heart rate by external feedback in normal children and children with infantile cerebral palsy. Human Physiology 9, 319-322.

Bollard, J. (1982). A 2-year follow-up of bedwetters treated by dry-bed training and standard condition. Behavior Research and Therapy 20, 571-580.

Bornstein, M. R., Bellack, A. S., & Hersen, M. (1977). Social-skills training for unassertive children: A multiple-baseline analysis. Journal of Applied Behavior Analysis 10, 183-195.

Bornstein, P. H., Balleweg, B. J., McLellarn, R. W., Wilson, G. L., Sturm, C. A., Andre, J. C., & van den Pol, R. A. (1983). The "bathroom game": A systematic program for the elimination of encopretic behavior. Journal of Behavior Therapy and Experimental Psychiatry 14, 67-71.

Bornstein, P. H., Sturm, C. A., Retzlaff, P. D., Kirby, K. L., & Chong, H. (1981). Paradoxical instruction in the treatment of encopresis and chronic constipation: An experimental analysis. Journal of Behavior Therapy and Experimental Psychiatry 12, 167-170.

Brown, R. T., Wynne, M. E., & Medenis, R. (1985). Methylphenidate and cognitive therapy: A comparison of treatment approaches with hyperactive boys. Journal of Abnormal Child Psychology 13, 69-87.

Brownell, K. D., & Stunkard, A. J. (1978). Behavioral treatment of obesity in children. American Journal of Diseases of Children 132, 403-412.

Bryant, L. E., & Budd, K. S. (1984). Teaching behaviorally handicapped preschool children to share. Journal of Applied Behavior Analysis 17, 45-46.

Buell, G., & Snyder, J. (1981). Assertiveness training with children. Psychological Reports 49, 71-80.

Bull, M., & LaVecchio, F. (1978). Behavior therapy for a child with Lesch Nyhan syndrome. Developmental Medicine and Child Neurology 20, 368-375.

Bull, R. W., Lindquist, B. E., & Schroeder, D. H. (1980). Television puppet skits as a tool for modeling children's behavior. Hospital and Community Psychiatry 31, 706-707.

Camp, B. W., Blom, G. E., Hebert, F., & van Doorninck, W. J. (1977). "Think aloud": A program for developing self-control in young aggressive boys. Journal of Abnormal Child Psychology 5, 157-169.

Carr, E. G., & Newsom, C. (1985). Demand-related tantrums. Conceptualization and treatment. Behavior Modification 9, 403-426.

Carstens, C. (1982). Behavioral treatment of functional dysphagia in a 12 year old boy. Psychosomatics 23, 195-196.

Christie, D. J., Dewitt, R. A., Kaltenbach, P., & Reed, D. (1984). Using EMg biofeedback to signal hyperactive children when to relax. Exceptional Children 50, 547-548.

Clement, P. W., Anderson, E., Arnold, J., Butman, R., Fantuzzo, J., & Mays, R. (1978). Self-observation and self-reinforcement as sources of self-control in children. Biofeedback and Self Regulation 3, 247-267.

Conners, C. K. (1979). Application of biofeedback to treatment of children. Journal of the American Academy of Child Psychiatry 18, 143-153.

Corral-Romero, M. A., & Bustamante-Balcarcel, A. (1982). Biofeedback rehabilitation in seventh nerve paralysis. Annals of Otology, Rhinology and Laryngology 91, 166-168.

Cracco, A., Belloli, G. P., & Ronconi, G. F. (1984). Sound alarms and conditioning therapy in hte treatment of childhood enuresis: A study of 180 cases. Pediatria Medica e Chirurgica 6, 681-689.

Cullinan, D., Epstein, M. H., & Silver, L. (1977). Modification of impulsive tempo in learning disabled pupils. Journal of Abnormal Child Psychology 5, 437-444.

Czyzewski, M. J., Barrera, R. D., & Sulzer-Azaroff, B. (1982). An abbreviated overcorrection program to reeuce self-stimulatory behaviors. Journal of Behavior Therapy and Experimental Psychiatry 13, 55-62.

Dahl, J., Melin, L., Brorson, L. O., & Schollin, J. (1985). Effects of a broad-spectrum behavior modification treatment program on children with refractory epileptic deizures. Eplipesia 26, 303-339.

Dahlquist, L. M., Gil, K. M., Armstrong, F. D., Ginsberg, A., & Jones, B. (1985). Behavioral management of children's diseases during chemotherapy. Journal of Behavior Therapy and Experimental Psychiatry 16, 325-329.

Daniel, W. J. (1982). Management of chronic rumination with a contingent exercies procedure employing topographically dissimilar behavior. Journal of Behavior Therapy and Experimental Psychiatry 13, 149-152.

Dash, J. (1981). Rapid hypno-behavioral treatment of a needle phobia in a five-year-old cardiac paticnt. Journal of Pediatric Psychology 6, 37-42.

De Vriendt, X., & Ruel, J. M. (1980). Simultaneous use of psychotherapy based on the analytic and behavioral schools. Neuropsychiatrie de l'Enfance et de l'Adolescence 28, 243-246.

Delamater, A. M., Rosenbloom, N., Conners, C. K., & Hertweck, L. (1983). The behavioral treatment of hysterical paralysis in a ten-year-old boy. A case study. Journal of the American Academy of Child Psychiatry 22, 73-79.

Diamond, S., & Montrose, D. (1984). The value of biofeedback in the treatment of chronic headache: A four-year retrospective study. Headache 24, 5-18.

Dorsey, M. F., Iwata, B. A., Ong, P., & McSween, T. E. (1980). Treatment of self-injurious behavior using a water mist: Initial response suppression and generalization. Journal of Applied Behavior Analysis 13, 343-353.

Duker, P. C. (1981). Treatment of food refusal by the overcorrective functional movement training method. Journal of Behavior Therapy and Experimental Psychiatry 12, 337-340.

Egel, A. L. (1981). Reinforcer variation: Implications for motivating developmentally disabled children. Journal of Applied Behavior Analysis 14, 345-350.

Epstein, L. H., Wing, R. R., Steranchak, L., Dickson, B., & Michelson, J. (1980). Comparison of family-based behavior modification and nutrition education for childhood obesity. Journal of Pediatric Psychology 5, 25-36.

Epstein, Y. M., & Borduin, C. M. (1984). "The children's feedback game": An approach for modifying disruptive group behavior. American Journal of Psychotherapy 38, 63-72.

Fielding, D. (1980). The response of day and night wetting children and children who wet only at night to retention control training and the enuresis alarm. Behavior Research and Therapy 18, 305-317.

Finley, W. W., Rainwater, A. J., & Johnson, G. (1982). Effect of varying alarm schedules on acquisition and relapse parameters in the conditioning treatment of enuresis. Behavior Research and Therapy 20, 69-80.

Finney, J. W., Russo, D. C., & Cataldo, M. F. (1982). Reduction of pica in young children with lead poisoning. Journal of Pediatric Psychology 7, 197-207.

Forehand, R., Rogers, T., McMahon, R. J., Wells, K. C., & Griest, D. L. (1981). Teaching parents to modify child behavior problems: An examination of some follow-up data. Journal of Pediatric Psychology 6, 313-322.

Fox, J. E., & Houston, B. K. (1981). Efficacy of self-instructional training for reducing children's anxiety in an evaluative situation. Behavior Research and Therapy 19, 509-515.

Frankel, F., & Simmons, J. Q. (1985). Behavioral treatment approaches to pathological unsocialized physical aggression in young children. Journal of Child Psychology and Psychiatry and Allied Disciplines 26, 525-551.

Freschi, D. F., & DiLeo, P. D. (1982). Treatment of self-abusive behaviors using positive intervention with an autistic boy. Exceptional Children 49, 77-78.

Friedling, C., & O'Leary, S. G. (1979). Effects of self-instructional training on second and third grade hyperactive children: A failure to replicate. Journal of Applied Behavior Analysis 12, 211-219.

Friedman, S. (1980). Self-control in the treatment of Gilles de la Tourette's syndrome: Case study with 18-month follow-up. Journal of Consulting and Clinical Psychology 48, 400-402.

Gittleman-Klein, R., Klein, D. F., Abikoff, H., Katz, S., Gloisten, A. C., & Kates, W. (1976). Relative efficacy of methylphenidate and behavior modification in hyperkinetic children: An interim report. Journal of Abnormal Child Psychology 4, 361-379.

Griffiths, P., Meldrum, C., & McWilliam, R. (1982). Dry-bed training in the treatment of nocturnal enuresis in childhood: A research report. Journal of Child Psychology and Psychiatry and Allied Disciplines 23, 485-495.

Hall, M. D. (1983). Using relaxation imagery with children with malignancies: A developmental perspective. American Journal of Clinical Hypnosis 25, 143-149.

Haynes, S. N., Wilson, C. C., Jaffe, P. G., & Britton, B. T. (1979). Biofeedback treatment of atopic dermatitis: Controlled case studies of eight cases. Biofeedback and Self Regulation 4, 195-209.

Hill, L. D. (1985). Contributions of behavior modification to cerebral palsy habilitation. Physical Therapy 65, 341-345.

Hinshaw, S. P., Henker, B., & Whalen, C. K. (1984). Self-control in hyperactive boys in anger-inducing situations: Effects of cognitive-behavioral training and of methylphenidate. Journal of Abnormal Child Psychology 12, 55-77.

Hock, R. A., Rodgers, C. H., Reddi, C., & Kennard, D. W. (1978). Medico-psychological interventions in male asthmatic children: An evaluation of physiological change. Psychosomatic Medicine 40, 210-215.

Horn, W. F., Chatoor, I., & Conners, C. K. (1983). Addictive effects of dexedrine and self-control training. A multiple assessment. Behavior Modification 7, 383-402.

Jackson, H. J., & King, N. J. (1981). The emotive imagery treatment of a child's trauma-induced phobia. Journal of Behavior Therapy and Experimental Psychiatry 12, 325-328.

Jay, S. M., Elliott, C. H., Ozolins, M., Olson, R. A., & Pruitt, S. D. (1985). Behavioral management of children's distress during painful medical procedures. Behavior Research and Therapy 23, 513-520.

Jones, D. P., & Verduyn, C. M. (1983). Behavioral management of sleep problems. Archives of Disease in Childhood 58, 442-444.

Kauffman, J., Hallahan, D. P., & Ianna, S. (1977). Suppression of a retardate's tongue protrusion by contingent imitation: A case study. Behavior Research and Therapy 15, 196-197.

Keating, J. C., Butz, R. A., Burke, E., & Heimberg, R. G. (1983). Dry bed training without a urine alarm: Lack of effect of setting and therapist contact with child. Journal of Behavior Therapy and Experimental Psychiatry 14, 109-115.

Kellerman, J. (1979). Behavioral treatment of night terrors in a child with acute leukemia. Journal of Nervous and Mental Disease 167, 182-185.

Kelley, M. L., Jarvie, G. J., Middlebrook, J. L., McNeer, M. F., & Drabman, R. S. (1984). Decreasing burned children's pain behavior: Impacting the trauma of hydrotherapy. Journal of Applied Behavior Analysis 17, 147-158.

Kelton, A., & Belar, C. D. (1983). The relative efficacy of autogenic phrases and autogenic-feedback training in teaching and warming to children. Biofeedback and Self Regulation 8, 461-475.

King, N. J. (1980). The behavioral management of asthma and asthma-related problems in children: A critical review of the literature. Behavior Research and Therapy 3, 169-189.

Klesges, R. C., Malott, J. M., & Ugland, M. (1984). The effects of graded exposure and parental modeling on the dental phobias of a four year old girl and her mother. Journal of Behavior Therapy and Experimental Psychiatry 15, 161-164.

Koepke, J. M., & Thyer, B. A. (1985). Behavioral treatment of failure to thrive in a two year old. Child Welfare 64, 511-516.

Kohen, D. P., Olness, K. N., Colwell, S. O., & Heimel, A. (1984). The use of relaxation-mental imagery (self-hypnosis) in the management of 505 pediatric behavioral encounters. Journal of Developmental and Behavioral Pediatrics 5, 21-25.

Koles, M. R., & Jenson, W. R. (1985). Comprehensive treatment of chronic fire setting in a severely disordered boy. Journal of Behavior Therapy and Experimental Psychiatry 16, 81-85.

Kotses, H., & Glaus, K. D. (1981). Applications of biofeedback to the treatment of asthma: A critical review. Biofeedback and Self Regulation 6, 573-593

Labbe, E. L., & Williamson, D. A. (1984). Treatment of childhood migraine using autogenic feedback training. Journal of Consulting and Clinical Psychology 52, 968-976.

Ladouceur, R., & Martineau, G. (1982). Evaluation of regulated-breathing method with and without parental assistance in the treatment of child stutterers. Journal of Behavior Therapy and Experimental Psychiatry 13, 301-306.

LaVecchio, F. (1980). Behavioral treatment of Lesch-Nyhan syndrome. Developmental Medicine and Child Neurology 22, 405-407.

Masek, B. J., Russo, D. C., & Varni, J. W. (1984). Behavioral approaches to the management of chronic pain in children. Pediatric Clinics of North America 31, 1113-1131.

McAuley, R. (1982). Training parents to modify conduct problems in their children. Journal of Child Psychology and Psychiatry and Allied Disciplines 23, 335-342.

Minderaa, R. B., & Wit, J. M. (1983). Behavior therapy of obese children and results 21 months after treatment. International Journal of Obesity 7, 143-152.

Nakanishi, D. A., & Anderson, D. R. (1982). Behavior therapy of obese children and results 21 months after treatment. Journal of Psychosocial Nursing and Mental Health Services 20, 17-20.

Olness, K., & MacDonald, J. (1981). Self-hypnosis and biofeedback in the management of juvenile migraine. Journal of Developmental and Behavioral Pediatrics 2, 168-170.

Overholser, J., & Beck, S. (1985). Assessing generalization of treatment effects and self-efficacy in the modification of eating styles in obese children. Addictive Behavior 10, 145-152.

Page, T. J., Finney, J. W., Parrish, J. M., & Iwata, B. A. (1983). Assessment and reduction of food stealing in Prader-Willi children. Applied Research in Mental Retardation 4, 219-228.

Parker, L. H., & Cinciripini, P. M. (1984). Behavioral medicine with children: Applications in chronic disease. Progress in Behavior Modification 17, 135-165.

Peterson, L. (1984). The "safe at home" game. Training comprehensive prevention skills in latchkey children. Behavior Modification 8, 474-494.

Poster, E. C., & Betz, C. L. (1983). Allaying the anxiety of hospitalized children using stress immunization techniques. Issues in Comprehensive Pediatric Nursing 6, 227-233.

Prytula, R. E., Joyner, K. B., & Schnelle, J. F. (1981). Utilizing the school to control head-banging behavior of a child at home. Psychological Reports 48, 887-894.

Rekers, G. A., & Mead, S. (1979). Early intervention for female sexual identity disturbance: Self monitoring of play behavior. Journal of Abnormal Child Psychology 7, 405-423.

Richman, N., Douglas, J., Hunt, H., Lansdown, R., & Levere, R. (1985). Behavioral methods in the treatment of sleep disorders--a pilot study. Journal of Child Psychology and Psychiatry and Allied Disciplines 26, 581-589.

Rinchuse, D. J. (1986). Overcoming fingersucking habits. Journal of Clinical Orthodontics 20, 46-47.

Rolider, A., & Van Houten, R. (1985). Treatment of constipation-caused encopresis by a negative reinforcement procedure. Journal of Behavior Therapy and Experimental Psychiatry 16, 67-70.

Rubin, R. M. (1983). Behavior modification for orthodontic cooperation. Journal of Clinical Orthodontics 17, 321-325.

Schroeder, S. R., Kanoy, R. C., Mulick, J. A., Rojahn, J., Thios, S. J., Stephens, M., & Hawk, B. (1982). Environmental antecedents which affect management and maintenance of programs for self-injurious behavior. Monographs of the American Association on Mental Deficiency 87, 105-159.

Scott, E. A. (1977). Treatment of encopresis in a classroom setting: A case study. British Journal of Educational Psychology 47, 199-202.

Sellick, K. J., & Peck, C. L. (1981). Behavioral treatment of fear in a child with cerebral palsy using a flooding procedure. Archives of Physical Medicine and Rehabilitation 62, 398-400.

Shapiro, S. R. (1985). Enuresis: Treatment and overtreatment. Pediatric Nursing 11, 203-207, 214.

Slifer, K. J., Iwata, B. A., & Dorsey, M. F. (1984). Reduction of eye-gouging using a response interruption procedure. Journal of Behavior Therapy and Experimental Psychiatry 15, 369-375.

Smeets, P. M., Lancioni, G. E., Ball, T. S., & Oliva, D. S. (1985). Shaping self-initiated toileting in infants. Journal of Applied Behavior Analysis 18, 303-308.

Sreenivasan, U., Manocha, S. N., & Jain, V. K. (1979). Treatment of severe dog phobia in childhood by flooding: A case report. Journal of Child Psychology and Psychiatry and Allied Disciplines 20, 255-260.

Suter, S., & Loughry-Machado, G. (1981). Skin temperature biofeedback in children and adults. Journal of Experimental Child Psychology 32, 77-87.

Talbott, M. L., & Junkala, J. (1981). The effects of auditorially augmented feedback on the eye-hand coordination of students with cerebral palsy. American Journal of Occupational Therapy 35, 525-528.

Tansey, M. A. (1985). Brainwave signatures--an index reflective of the brain's functional neuroanatomy: Further findings on the effect of EEG sensorimotor rhythm biofeedback training on the neurologic precursors of learning disabilities. International Journal of Psychophysiology 3, 85-99.

Tharp, R. G., & Gallimore, R. (1985). The logical status of metacognitive training. Journal of Abnormal Child Psychology 13, 455-466.

Thompson, G. A., Iwata, B. A., & Poynter, H. (1979). Operant control of pathological tongue thrust in spastic cerebral palsy. Journal of Applied Behavior Analysis 12, 325-333.

Varni, J. W., & Banis, H. T. (1985). Behavior therapy techniques applied to eating, exercise, and diet modification in childhood obesity. Journal of Developmental and Behavioral Pediatrics 6, 367-372.

Varni, J. W., Bessman, C. A., Russo, D. C., & Cataldo, M. F. (1980). Behavioral management of chronic pain in children: Case study. Archives of Physical Medicine and Rehabilitation 61, 375-379.

8. Brief Therapy

Austin, L, & Inderbitzin, L. B. (1983). Brief psychotherapy in late adolescence: A psychodynamic and developmental approach. American Journal of Psychotherapy 37, 202-209.

Bennett, M. J. (1983). Focal psychotherapy--terminable and interminable. American Journal of Psychotherapy 37, 365-375.
Bentovim, A., & Kinston, W. (1978). Brief focal family therapy when the child is the referred patient. I. Clinical. Journal of Child Psychology and Psychiatry and Allied Disciplines 19, 1-12.
Charach, R. (1983). Brief interpretive group psychotherapy with early latency-age children. International Journal of Group Psychotherapy 33, 349-364.
Dies, R. R. (1985). Leadership in short-term group therapy: Manipulation of facilitation? International Journal of Group Psychotherapy 35, 435-455.
Dulcan, M. K. (1984). Brief psychotherapy with children and their families: The state of the art. Journal of the American Academy of Child Psychiatry 23, 544-551.
Gustafson, J. P. (1984). An integration of brief dynamic psychotherapy. American Journal of Psychiatry 141, 935-944.
Kelly, J. B., & Wallerstein, J. S. (1977). Brief interventions with children in divorcing families. American Journal of Orthopsychiatry 47, 23-39.
Koss, M. P., Butcher, J. N., & Strupp, H. H. (1986). Brief psychotherapy methods in clinical research. Journal of Consulting and Clinical Psychology 54, 60-67.
MacLean, G., MacIntosh, B. A., Taylor, E., & Gerber, M. (1982). A clinical approach to brief dynamic psychotherapies in child psychiatry. Canadian Journal of Psychiatry 27, 113-118.
Peterlin, K., & Sloves, R. (1985). Time-limited psychotherapy with children: Central theme and time as major tools. Journal of the American Academy of Child Psychiatry 24, 788-792.
Poey, K. (1985). Guidelines for the practice of brief, dynamic group therapy. International Journal of Group Psychotherapy 35, 331-354.
Raubolt, R. R. (1983). Brief, problem-focused group psychotherapy with adolescents. American Journal of Orthopsychiatry 53, 157-165.
Sachs, J. S. (1983). Negative factors in brief psychotherapy: An empirical assessment. Journal of Consulting and Clinical Psychology 51, 557-564.
Scheidlinger, S. (1984). Short-term group psychotherapy for children: An overview. International Journal of Group Psychotherapy 34, 573-586.
Shafii, M., McCue, A., Ice, J. F., & Schwab, J. J. (1979). The development of an acute short-term inpatient child psychiatry setting: A pediatric-psychiatric model. American Journal of Psychiatry 136, 427-429.

B. Family Therapy

Section Editor:

Pirooz Sholevar, M.D.
Professor of Psychiatry
Director, Division of Child and Adolescent Psychiatry
Jefferson Medical College
Jefferson University
Philadelphia, Pennsylvania

1. Classic Literature in Family Therapy

Ackerman, N. W. (1958). The psychodynamics of family life. New York: Basic Books.

Ackerman, N. W. (1966). Treating the troubled family. New York: Basic Books.

Beavers, W. R. (1982). Health, midrange and severely dysfunctional families. In M. Walsh (Ed.), Normal family process (pp. 45-66). New York: Guilford Press.

Bell, N. W., & Vogel, E. F. (1968). The emotionally disturbed child as the family scapegoat. In N. W. Bell & E. F. Vogel (Eds.), A modern introduction to the family (pp. 412-427). New York: The Free Press.

Boszormenyi-Nagy, I., & Framo, J. L. (1965). Intensive family therapy: Theoretical and practical aspects. New York: Harper and Row.

Bowen, M. (1966). The use of family theory in clinical practice. Comprehensive Psychiatry 7, 345-374.

Bowen, M. (1978). Family therapy in clinical practice. New York: Jason Aronson.

Dicks, H. V. (1967). Marital tensions: Clinical studies towards a psychological theory of interaction. London: Routledge & Kegan Paul.

Friedman, A. S. (1965). Psychotherapy for the whole family. New York: Springer.

Gurman, A. S., & Kniskern, D. P. (Eds.). (1981). Handbook of family therapy. New York: Brunner/Mazel.

Jackson, D. D. (1959). Family interaction, family homeostasis and some implications for conjoint family psychotherapy. Science and Psychoanalysis 2, 122-141.

Lewis, J. M. (1976). No single thread: Psychological health in family systems. New York: Brunner/Mazel.

Lewis, J. M., & Looney, J. G. (1983). The long struggle: Well-functioning working class black families. New York: Brunner/Mazel.

MacGregor, R. (1964). Multiple impact therapy with families. New York: McGraw-Hill.

Minuchin, S. (1967). Families of the slums: An exploration of their structure and treatment. New York: Basic Books.

Nichols, M. (1984). Family therapy concepts & methods. New York: Gardner Press.

Parsons, T., & Bales, R. F. (1954). Family socialization and interaction process. Glencoe, Ill.: The Free Press.

Walsh, F. (1982). Conceptualization of normal family functioning. In F. Walsh (Ed.), Normal family process (pp. 3-42). New York: Guilford Press.

Watzlawick, P., Beavin, J. H., & Jackson, D. D. (1967). Pragmatics of human communication. New York: Norton.

Zuk, G. H., & Boszormenyi-Nagy, I. (Eds.). (1967). Family therapy and disturbed families. Palo Alto: Science and Behavior Books.

2. Assessment for Family Therapy

Cromwell, R. E., Olson, D. H., & Fournier, D. G. (1976). Tools and techniques for diagnosis and evaluation in marital and family therapy. Family Process 15, 1-49.

Cromwell, R. E., & Peterson, G. W. (1983). Multisystem-multimethod family assessment in clinical contexts. Family Process 22, 147-163.

Feldman, L. B. (1976). Strategies and techniques of family therapy. American Journal of Psychotherapy 30, 14-28.

Haley, J. (1976). Conducting the first interview. In J. Haley (Ed.), Problem solving therapy (pp. 9-47). San Francisco: Jossey-Bass.

Haley, J., & Hoffman, L. (1967). Techniques of family therapy. New York: Basic Books.

Papp, P. (1980). The Greek chorus and other techniques of paradoxical therapy. Family Process 19, 45-57.

Penn, P. (1985). Feed-forward: Future questions, future maps. Family Process 24, 299-310.

Pittman, F. S. (1984). Wet cocker spaniel theory: An essay on techniques in family therapy. Family Process 23, 1-9.

Tseng, W., Arensdorf, A. M., McDermott, J. F., Hansen, J. J., & Fukunaga, C. S. (1976). Family diagnosis and classification. Journal of the American Academy of Child Psychiatry 15, 15-33.

Tseng, W. S., & McDermott, J. F. (1979). Triaxial family classification: A proposal. Journal of the American Academy of Child Psychiatry 18, 22-43.

Will, D. (1983). Some techniques for working with resistant families of adolescents. Journal of Adolescence 6, 13-26.

3. Family Therapy with Adolescents

Ackerman, N. J. (1982). Adolescence. In D. Block & R. Simon (Eds.), The strength of family therapy (pp 232-247). New York: Brunner/Mazel.

Berkowitz, D., Shapiro, R., Zinner, J., & Shapiro, E. (1974). Concurrent family treatment in narcissistic disorders in adolescence. International Journal of Psychoanalytic Psychotherapy 3, 379-396.

Foodman, A., & Estrada, C. (1977). Adolescents who commit accidental homicide. The emotional consequences to the individual, family, and community. Journal of the American Academy of Child Psychiatry 16, 314-326.

Haley, J. (1980). Leaving home: Therapy with disturbed young people. New York: McGraw-Hill.

Loeber, R., Weissman, W., & Reid, J. B. (1983). Family interactions of assaultive adolescents, stealers, and nondelinquents. Journal of Abnormal Child Psychology 11, 1-14.

Minuchin, S., Auerswald, E., King, C., & Rabinowitz, C. (1964). The study and treatment of families that produce multiple acting-out boys. American Journal of Orthopsychiatry 34, 125-134.

O'Connor, J. J., & Hoorwitz, A. N. (1984). The bogeyman cometh: A strategic approach for difficult adolescents. Family Process 23, 237-249.

Ravenscroft, K. (1974). Normal family regression at adolescence. American Journal of Psychiatry 131, 31-55.

Stierlin, H. (1976). The dynamics of owning and disowning: Psychoanalytic and family perspectives. Family Process 15, 277-288.

Tyerman, A., & Humphrey, M. (1983). Life stress, family support and adolescent disturbance. Journal of Adolescence 6, 1-12.

Walker, B. A., & Mehr, M. (1983). Adolescent suicide--a family crisis: A model for effective intervention by family therapists. Adolescence 18, 285-292.

Zinner, J. (1978). Combined individual and family therapy of borderline adolescents: Rationale and management of the early phase. In S. C. Feinstein, et al. (Eds.), Adolescent psychiatry: Developmental and clinical studies (Vol. 6, pp. 420-433). Chicago: University of Chicago Press.

4. Children in Family Therapy

Berlin, I. N. (1979). A developmental approach to work with disorganized families. Journal of the American Academy of Child Psychiatry 18, 354-365.

Guttman, H. (1975). The child's participation in conjoint family therapy. Journal of the American Academy of Child Psychiatry 14, 490-499.

Haley, J. (1973). Strategic therapy when a child is presented as a problem. Journal of the American Academy of Child Psychiatry 12, 641-659.

Kriechman, A. M. (1985). A school-based program of mental health services. Hospital and Community Psychiatry 36, 876-878.

Montalvo, B., & Haley, J. (1973). In defense of child therapy. Family Process 12, 227-244.

Rollins, N., Lord, J. P., Walsh, E., & Weil, G. (1973). Some roles children play in their families: Scapegoat, baby, pet, and peacemaker. Journal of the American Academy of Child Psychiatry 12, 511-530.

Serrano, A. C. (1979). A child-centered family diagnostic interview. In J. Call (Ed.), Basic handbook of child psychiatry (Vol. 1, pp. 624-630.) New York: Basic Books.

Villeneuve, C. (1979). The specific participation of the child in family therapy. Journal of the American Academy of Child Psychiatry 18, 44-53.

Zilbach, J. (1986). Young children in family therapy. New York: Brunner/Mazel.

5. Family Versus Individual Therapy

Boszormenyi-Nagy, I., & Spark, G. M. (1973). Invisible loyalties: Reciprocity in intergenerational family therapy. Hagerstown, Md.: Harper and Row.

Sander, F. M. (1985). Family of individual therapy: The determinants of modality choice. Hillside Journal of Clinical Psychiatry 7, 63-70.

Shapiro, R. (1980). Psychodynamic family therapy. In G. P. Sholevar (Ed.), Emotional disorders in children and adolescents: Medical and psychological approaches to treatment (pp. 145-158). Jamaica, N.Y.: SP Medical and Scientific Books.

Slipp, S. (1984). Object relations: A dynamic bridge between individual and family treatment. New York: Jason Aronson.

Solomon, M. L. (1975). Family psychiatry, transactional systems, and the frontiers of child psychiatry. Canadian Psychiatric Association Journal 20, 151-155.

Zinner, J., & Shapiro, R. (1972). Projective identification as a mode of perception and behavior in families of adolescents. International Journal of Psycho-Analysis 53, 523.

6. Family Life Cycle and Family Therapy

Brown, S. L. (1980). The developmental cycle of families: Clinical implications. Clinics of North America 3, 369-381.

Combrinck-Graham, L. (1985). A developmental model for family systems. Family Process 24, 139-150.

Karpel, M. A., & Strauss, E. S. (1983). The family life cycle. In G. P. Sholivar (Ed.), Family evaluation (pp. 49-77). New York: Gardner Press.

McGoldrick, M., & Carter, E. A. (1982). The family life cycle. In F. Walsh (Ed.), Normal family process (pp. 167-195). New York: Guilford Press.

7. Family Therapy with Hospitalized Children and Adolescents

Combrinck-Graham, L., Gursky, E. J., & Brendler, J. (1982). Hospitalization of single parent families of disturbed children. Family Process 21, 141-152.

Dydyk, B., French, G., Gertsman, C., & Morrison, N. (1982). Admission of whole families. Canadian Journal of Psychiatry 27, 640-643.

Glick, I. D., Clarkin, J. F., Spencer, J. H., Hass, G. L., Lewis, A. B., Peyser, J., DeMane, N., & Good-Ellis, M. (1985). A controlled evaluation of inpatient family intervention. I. Preliminary results of the six-month follow-up. Archives of General Psychiatry 42, 882-886.

Looney, J. G., Blotchky, M. J., Carson, D. I., & Gossett, J. T. (1980). A family-systems model for inpatient treatment of adolescents. In S. C. Feinstein, et al. (Eds.), Adolescent psychiatry: Developmental and clinical studies (Vol. 8, pp. 499-511). Chicago: University of Chicago Press.

Lynch, M., Steinberg, D., & Ounsted, C. (1975). Family unit in a children's psychiatric hospital. British Medical Journal 2, 127-129.

Rosenfeld, A. H. (1982). Closing the revolving door through family therapy. Hospital and Community Psychiatry 33, 893-894.

Sholevar, G. P. (1980). Families of institutionalized children. In G. P. Sholevar (Ed.), Emotional disorders of children and adolescents: Medical and psychological approaches to treatment (pp. 181-190). Jamaica, N.Y.: SP Medical and Scientific Books.

Sholevar, G. P. (1983). Family therapy with hospitalized and disabled patients. In M. R. Textor (Ed.), Helping families with special problems (pp. 15-34). New York: Jason Aronson.

Singh, N. (1982). Notes and observations on the practice of multiple family therapy in an adolescent unit. Journal of Adolescence 5, 319-331.

Tovey, R., & Morton, J. (1985). Adapting multiple impact therapy for day treatment intake. Child Welfare 64, 421-426.

Whitley, M. J., & Zankowski, G. L. (1986). Family therapy in a hospital setting: A model for time-limited treatment. Journal of Psychoactive Drugs 18, 61-64.

8. A Family Therapy Approach to Learning Disorders

Amerikaner, M. J., & Omizo, M. M. (1984). Family interaction and learning disabilities. Journal of Learning Disabilities 17, 540-543.

Byrne, E. A., & Cunningham, C. C. (1985). The effects of mentally handicapped children on families--a conceptual review. Journal of Child Psychology and Psychiatry 26, 847-864.

Goodyer, I. M. (1986). Family therapy and the handicapped child. Developmental Medicine and Child Neurology 28, 247-250.

Gordon, N. (1978). Hyperkinesis: The overactive child makes the whole family suffer. Nursing Mirror 147, 35-36.

Idol-Maestas, L. (1981). Behavior patterns in families of boys with learning and behavioral problems. Journal of Learning Disabilities 14, 347-349.

Margalit, M. (1982). Learning disabled children and their families: Strategies of extension and adaptation of family therapy. Journal of Learning Disabilities 15, 594-595.

9. Family Therapy in Physical and Sexual Abuse

Alexander, P. C. (1985). A systems theory conceptualization of incest. Family Process 24, 79-88.

Barnhill, L. R. (1980a). Basic interventions for violence in families. Hospital and Community Psychiatry 31, 547-551.

Barnhill, L. R. (1980b). Clinical assessment of intrafamilial violence. Hospital and Community Psychiatry 31, 543-547.

Canepa, G., & Bandini, T. (1980). Incest and family dynamics: A clinical study. International Journal of Law and Psychiatry 3, 453-460.

Lewis, M., & Sarrel, P. M. (1969). Some psychological aspects of seduction, incest, and rape in childhood. Journal of the American Academy of Child Psychiatry 8, 606-619.

Lutz, S. E., & Medway, J. P. (1984). Contextual family therapy with the victims of incest. Journal of Adolescence 7, 319-327.

Sholevar, G. P. (1975). A family therapist looks at the problem of incest. Bulletin of the American Academy of Psychiatry and the Law 3, 25-31.

Will, D. (1983). Approaching the incestuous and sexually abusive family. Journal of Adolescence 6, 229-246.

10. Divorce and Family Therapy

Blotcky, M. J., Grace, K. D. & Looney, J. G. (1984). Treatment of adolescents in family therapy after divorce. Journal of the American Academy of Child

Psychiatry 23, 222-225.

Blotcky, M. J., Looney, J. G., & Grace, K. D. (1982). Treatment of the adopted adolescent: Involvement of the biologic mother. Journal of the American Academy of Child Psychiatry 21, 281-285.

Hauser, B. B. (1985). Custody in dispute: Legal and psychological profiles of contesting families. Journal of the American Academy of Child Psychiatry 24, 275-282.

Isaacs, M. B. (1982). Helping mom fail: A case of a stalemated divorcing process. Family Process 21, 225-234.

Kaplan, S. L. (1977). Structural family therapy for children of divorce: Case reports. Family Process 16, 75-83.

Kelly, J. B. (1981). Observations on adolescent relationships five years after divorce. In S. C. Feinstein, et al. (Eds.), Adolescent psychiatry: Developmental and clinical studies (Vol. 9, pp. 133-134). Chicago: University of Chicago Press.

Schechter, M., & Holter, F. R. (1975). Adopted children in their adoptive families. Pediatric Clinics of North America 22, 661-663.

11. Drug Abuse and Family Therapy

Byram, O. W., & Fly, J. W. (1984). Family structure, race, and adolescent's alcohol use: A research note. American Journal of Drug and Alcohol Abuse 10, 467-478.

Kaufman, E. (1985). Family systems and family therapy of substance abuse: An overview of two decades of research and clinical experience. International Journal of the Addictions 20, 897-916.

Kaufman, E. (1986). The family of the alcoholic parent. Psychosomatics 27, 347-349, 352, 356-360.

Weidman, A. A. (1985). Enlarging the families of substance abusing adolescents in family therapy. Journal of Substance Abuse Treatment 2, 97-105.

12. Family Therapy with Psychiatric Disorders

Byassee, J. E., & Murrell, S. A. (1975). Interaction patterns in families of autistic, disturbed, and normal children. American Journal of Orthopsychiatry 45, 473-478.

Callagan, A. R. (1981). Gender role and family relationships in adolescent children of chronic schizophrenic mothers: Findings from a longitudinal study of whole families. American Journal of Orthopsychiatry 51, 521-535.

Callan, V. J., & Jackson, D. (1986). Children of alcoholic fathers and recovered alcoholic fathers: Personal and family functioning. Journal of Studies on Alcohol 47, 180-182.

Martino, M. S., & Newman, M. B. (1975). Intrapsychic conflict, interpersonal relationship, and family mythology. Journal of the American Academy of Child Psychiatry 14, 422-435.

Moos, R. H., & Billings, A. G. (1982). Children of alcoholics during the recovery process: Alcoholic and matched control families. Addictive Behavior 7, 155-163.

Pfeffer, C. R. (1982). Interventions for suicidal children and their parents. Suicide and Life-Threatening Behavior 12, 240-248.

Richman, J. (1979). The family therapy of attempted suicide. Family Process 18, 131-142.

Shapiro, E. R., Shapiro, R. L., Zinner, J., & Berkowitz, D. A. (1977). The borderline ego and the working alliance: Indications for family and individual treatment in adolescence. International Journal of Psycho-Analysis 58, 77-87.

Zinner, J. (1978). Combined individual and family therapy of borderline adolescents: Rationale and management of the early phase. In S. C. Feinstein, et al. (Eds.), Adolescent psychiatry: Developmental and clinical studies (Vol. 6, pp. 420-433). Chicago: University of Chicago Press.

13. Family Therapy with Psychosomatic Conditions

Minuchin, S., & Fishman, H. C. (1979). The psychosomatic family in child psychiatry. Journal of the American Academy of Child Psychiatry 18, 76-90.

Minuchin, S., Rosman, B., & Baker, L. (1978). Psychosomatic families: Anorexia nervosa in context. Cambridge: Harvard University Press.

Sholevar, G. P. (1980). Family therapy in psychosomatic disorders. In G. P. Sholevar (Ed.), Emotional disorders of children and adolescents: Medical and psychological approaches to treatment. Jamaica, N.Y.: SP Medical and Scientific Books.

Weakland, J. H. (1977). Family somatics--a neglect shape. Family Process 16, 263-271.

White, M. (1979). Structural and strategic approaches to psychosomatic families. Family Process 18, 314-330.

14. Family Therapy of Miscellaneous Conditions

Borduin, C. M., Henggler, S. W., & Pruitt, J. A. (1985). The relationship between juvenile delinquency and personality dimensions of family members. Journal of Genetic Psychology 146, 563-565.

Goll, K. (1979). Role structure and subculture in families of elective mutists. Family Process 18, 55-68.

Malone, C. A. (1963). Some observations on children of disorganized families of acting out. Journal of the American Academy of Child Psychiatry 2, 22-49.

Rosenberg, J. B., & Lindblad, M. B. (1978). Behavior therapy in a family context: Creating elective mutism. Family Process 17, 77-82.

Tittler, J. W. (1978). Brief family therapy for childhood tic syndrome. Family Process 17, 217-223.

Venn, J. (1984). Family etiology and remission in a case of psychogenic fugue. Family Process 23, 429-435.

15. Family Reactions to Various Somatic Diseases

Apponte, H., & Hoffman, L. (1973). The open door: A structural approach to a family with an anorectic child. Family Process 12(1), 1-44.

Baird, M. (1974). Characteristic interaction patterns in families of encopretic children. Bulletin of the Menninger Clinic 38, 133-153.

Copeland, E. T., & Baucom-Copeland, S. (1981). Childhood obesity: A family systems view. American Family Physician 24, 153-157.

Cowen, L., Corey, M., Keennan, R., Simmons, R., Arndt, E., & Levison, H. (1985). Family adaptation and psychosocial adjustment to cystic fibrosis in the preschool child. Social Science and Medicine 20, 553-560.

Ferrari, M., Mathews, W. S., & Barabas, G. (1983). The family and the child with epilepsy. Family Process 22, 53-59.

Fife, B. L. (1980). Childhood cancer is a family crisis: A review. Journal of Psychiatric Nursing and Mental Health Services 18, 29-34.

Hilliard, J. P., Fritz, G. K., & Lewiston, N. J. (1985). Levels of aspiration of parents for their asthmatic, diabetic, and healthy children. Journal of Clinical Psychology 41, 587-597.

Humphrey, L. L., Apple, R. F., & Kirchenbaum, D. S. (1986). Differentiating bulimic-anorexic from normal families. National Academy of Science--United States of America 78, 2665-2668.

Kalnins, I. V., Churchill, M. P., & Terry, G. E. (1980). Concurrent stresses in families with a leukemic child. Journal of Pediatric Psychology 5, 81-92.

Kaplan, S. L. (1977). Structural family therapy for children of divorce: Case reports. Family Process 16, 75-83.

Kotelchuck, M., & Newberger, E. H. (1983). Failure to thrive: A controlled study of familial characteristics. Journal of the American Academy of Child Psychiatry 22, 322-328.

Kupst, M. J., Schulman, J. L., Honig, G., Maurer, H., Morgan, E., & Fochtman, D. (1982). Family coping with childhood leukemia: One year after diagnosis. Journal of Pediatric Psychology 7, 157-174.

Levenberg, S. B., Jenkins, C., & Wendorf, D. J. (1978-1979). Studies in family-oriented crisis intervention with hemodialysis patients. International Journal of Psychiatry and Medicine 9, 83-92.

Lewis, B. L., & Khaw, K. T. (1982). Family functioning as a mediating variable affecting psychosocial adjustment of children with cystic fibrosis. Journal of Pediatrics 101, 636-640.

Liebman, R., Minuchin, S., & Baker, L. (1974). The use of structural family therapy in the treatment of intractable asthma. American Journal of Psychiatry 131, 535-540.

Liebman, R., Sargent, J., & Silver, M. (1983). A family systems orientation to the treatment of anorexia nervosa. Journal of the American Academy of Child Psychiatry 22, 128-133.

Masterson, J. (1985). Family assessment of the child with intractable asthma. Journal of Developmental and Behavioral Pediatrics 6, 244-251.

McCowen, C., Hackett, A. F., Court, S., & Parkin, J. M. (1986). Are families of diabetic children adequately taught? British Medical Journal 292, 1361.

McGowan, M. P. (1980). Tailored advice and practical rehabilitation for families with a disabled child: An experiment. Lancet 2, 1018-1019.

Meijer, A. (1975). Psychological factors in maternal grandparents of asthmatic children. Child Psychiatry and Human Development 6, 15-25.

Mulder, H. C., & Suurmeijer, T. P. (1977). Families with a child with epilepsy: A sociological contribution. Journal of Biosocial Science 9, 13-24.

Newbrough, J. R., Simkins, C. G., & Maurer, H. (1985). A family development approach to studying factors in the management and control of childhood diabetes. Diabetes Care 8, 83-92.

O'Connor, J. J. (1984). The resurrection of a magical reality: Treatment of functional migraine in a child. Family Process 23, 501-509.

Richman, N. (1981). A community survey of characteristics of one-to two-year-olds with sleep disruptions. Journal of the American Academy of Child Psychiatry 20, 281-292.

Ritchie, K. (1981). Research note: Interaction in the families of epileptic children. Journal of Child Psychology and Psychiatry and Allied Disciplines 22, 65-71.

Sampson, T. F. (1975). The child in renal failure, emotional impact of treatment on the child and his family. Journal of the American Academy of Child Psychiatry 14, 462-476.

Sayed, A. J., & Leaverton, D. R. (1974). Kinetic-family drawings of children with diabetes. Child Psychiatry and Human Development 5, 40-50.

Simon, R. (1984). Hemophilia and the family system. Psychosomatics 25, 845-849.

Sokoloff, B. (1979). Adoptive families. Clinical Pediatrics 18, 188-190.

Tousley, M. M. (1982). The use of family therapy in terminal illness and death. Journal of Psychosocial Nursing and Mental Health Services 20, 17-22.

Vandvik, I. H., & Storhaug, K. (1985). Family focused services for children with rare disorders, exemplified by bladder exstrophy. Clinical Pediatrics 24, 97-100.

White, M. (1983). Anorexia nervosa: A transgenerational system perspective. Family Process 22, 255-273.

16. Family Interrelationships

Brody, S. (1981). The concepts of attachment and bonding. Journal of the American Psychoanalytic Association 29, 815-829.

Cameron, J. R. (1978). Parental treatment, children's temperament, and the risk of childhood behavioral problems. II. Initial temperament, parental attitudes, and the incidence and form of behavioral problems. American Journal of Orthopsychiatry 48, 140-147.

Dell, P. F., & Appelbaum, A. S. (1977). Trigenerational enmeshment: Unresolved ties of single-parents to family of origin. American Journal of Orthopsychiatry 47, 52-59.

Earls, F. (1976). The fathers (not the mothers): Their importance and influence with infants and young children. Psychiatry 39, 209-226.

Fraibeg, S., Adelson, E., & Shapiro, V. (1975). Ghosts in the nursery. A psychoanalytic approach to the problems of impaired infant-mother relationships. Journal of the American Academy of Child Psychiatry 14, 387-421.

Gauthier, Y., Fortin, C., Drapeau, P., Breton, J. J., Gosselin, J., Quintal, L., Weisnagel, J., & Tetreault, L. (1977). The mother-child relationship and the development of autonomy and self-assertion in young (14-30 months) asthmatic children. Correlating allergic and psychological factors. Journal of the American Academy of Child Psychiatry 16, 109-131.

Klein, H., & Last, U. (1978). Attitudes toward persecutor representations in children of traumatized and nontraumatized parents--cross-cultural comparison. In S. C. Feinstein, et al. (Eds.), Adolescent psychiatry: Developmental and clinical studies (Vol. 6, pp. 224-238). Chicago: University of Chicago Press.

Ross, J. M. (1979). Fathering: A review of some psychoanalytic contributions on paternity. International Journal of Psycho-Analysis 60, 317-327.

Tronick, E., Als, H., Adamson, L., Wise, S., & Brazelton, T. B. (1978). The infant's response to entrapment between contradictory messages in face-to-face interaction. Journal of the American Academy of Child Psychiatry 17, 1-13.

17. Social Networks as Related to Family Therapy

Attneave, C. L. (1976). Social networks as the unit of intervention. In P. J. Guerin (Ed.), Family therapy: Theory and practice (pp. 220-231). New York: Gardner Press.

Henderson, S. (1977). The social network, support and neurosis. The function of attachment in adult life. British Journal of Psychiatry 131, 185-191.

Schoenfeld, P., Halevy, J., Hemley-Van de Velden, E., & Ruhf, L. (1986). Longterm outcome of network therapy. Hospital and Community Psychiatry 37, 373-376.

Speck, J. L., & Speck, R. V. (1985). Social network intervention with adolescents. In M. P. Mirkin & A. L. Koman (Eds.), Handbook of adolescence and family therapy. New York: Gardner Press.

Speck, R. V., & Speck, J. L. (1984). Family networking in the 1980's. International Journal of Family Therapy, Special Issue, 34, 136-137.

18. Training in Family Therapy

Feldman, R. B., & Feldman, S. (1982). Resident training systems and family systems training: Limits of compatibility. Canadian Journal of Psychiatry 27, 559-560.

Flomenhaft, K., & Carter, R. E. (1977). Family therapy training: Program and outcome. Family Process 16, 211-218.

Harbin, H. T. (1980). Family therapy training for psychiatric residents. American Journal of Psychiatry 137, 1595-1598.

Malone, C. A. (1974). Observations on the role of family therapy in child psychiatric training. Journal of the American Academy of Child Psychiatry 13, 437-458.

Malone, C. A. (1979). Child psychiatry and family therapy: An overview. Journal of the American Academy of Child Psychiatry 18, 4-21.

McDermott, J. F. (1979). Family therapy in child psychiatry: Introduction. Journal of the American Academy of Child Psychiatry 18, 1-3.

McDermott, J. F., & Char, W. F. (1974). The undeclared war between child and family therapy. Journal of the American Academy of Child Psychiatry 13, 422-436.

Sander, F. M., & Beels, C. C. (1970). A didactic course for family therapy trainees. Family Process 9, 411-423.

Sugarman, S. (1984). Integrating family therapy training into psychiatry residency programs: Policy issues and alternatives. Family Process 23, 23-32.

Tomm, K. M., & Wright, L. M. (1979). Training in family therapy: Perceptual, conceptual and executive skills. Family Process 18, 227-250.

Tucker, S. J., & Pinsof, W. M. (1984). The empirical evaluation of family therapy training. Family Process 23, 437-456.

19. Evaluation of Family Therapy

DeWitt, K. N. (1978). The effectiveness of family therapy: A review of outcome research. Archives of General Psychiatry 35, 549-561.

Gurman, A. S., & Kniskern, D. P. (1981). Family therapy outcome research: Knowns and unknowns. In A. S. Gurman & D. P. Kniskern (Eds.), Handbook of family therapy (pp. 741-776). New York: Brunner/Mazel.

Harris, J., & Mills, G. I. (1980). Current practice in a child and family psychiatric service: Analysis of 200 consecutive new referrals. Public Health 94, 316-323.

20. Books and Special Papers on Family Therapy

Haley, J. (1963). Strategies of psychotherapy. New York: Grune & Stratton.

Hoffman, L. (1981). Foundations of family therapy. New York: Basic Books.

Madanes, C. (1981). Strategic family therapy. San Francisco: Jossey-Bass.

Madanes, C., & Haley, J. (1977). Dimensions of family therapy. Journal of Nervous and Mental Disease 165, 88-98.

Minuchin, S. (1974). Families and family therapy: A structural approach. Cambridge: Harvard University Press.

Musliner, P. (1980). Strategic therapy with families and children. Journal of the American Academy of Child Psychiatry 19, 101-117.

Stanton, D. M. (1980). Systems approach to family therapy. In G. P. Sholevar (Ed.), Emotional disorders of children and adolescents: Medical and psychological approaches to treatment (pp. 159-179). Jamaica, N.Y.: SP Medical and Scientific Books.

Werry, J. S. (1979). Family therapy: Behavioral approaches. Journal of the American Academy of Child Psychiatry 18, 91-102.

C. Group Psychotherapy of Children and Adolescents

Section Editor:

Irvin A. Kraft, M.D.
Professor of Psychiatry and Public Health
University of Texas Health Science Center
Houston, Texas

1. History of Group Psychotherapy

Abramowitz, S. I., & Abramowitz, C. V. (1974). Psychological-mindedness and benefit from insight-oriented group therapy. Archives of General Psychiatry 30, 610-615.

Andronico, M. P., Fidler, J., Guerney, B. J. R., & Guerney, L. F. (1967). The combination of didactic and dynamic elements in filial therapy. International Journal of Group Psychotherapy 17, 10-17.

Anthony, E. J. (1968). Reflections on twenty-five years of group psychotherapy. International Journal of Group Psychotherapy 18, 277-301.

Berkovitz, I. H. (1972). Adolescents grow in groups: Experiences in adolescent group psychotherapy. New York: Brunner/Mazel.

Boll, T. J. (1971). Systematic observation of behavior change with children in group therapy. Psychological Reports 28, 26.

Boulanger, J. B. (1961). Group psychoanalytic therapy in child psychiatry. Canadian Psychiatric Association Journal 6, 272-275.

Brandt, D. E. (1973). A descriptive analysis of selective aspect of group therapy with severely delinquent boys. Journal of the American Academy of Child Psychiatry 12, 473-481.

Christmas, J. J. (1966). Group therapy with the disadvantaged. Psychiatric Therapies 6, 163-171.

Churchill, S. R. (1965). Social group work: A diagnostic tool in guidance. American Journal of Orthopsychiatry 35, 581-588.

Duffy, J. H., & Kraft, I. A. (1966-1967). Beginning and middle phase characteristics of group psychotherapy of early adolescent boys and girls. Journal of Psychoanalysis in Groups 2(1), 23-29.

Fried, E. (1956). Ego emancipation of adolescents through group psychotherapy. International Journal of Group Psychotherapy 6, 358-373.

Ginott, H. G. (1961). Group psychotherapy with children: The theory and practice of play-therapy. New York: McGraw-Hill.

Godenne, G. D. (1964). Outpatient adolescent group psychotherapy. I. Review of the literature on use of co-therapists, psychodrama, and parent group therapy. American Journal of Psychotherapy 18, 584-593.

Godenne, G. D. (1965). Outpatient adolescent group psychotherapy. II. Use of co-therapists, psychodrama, and parent group therapy. American Journal of Psychotherapy 19, 40-53.

Herrick, R. H., & Binger, C. M. (1974). Group psychotherapy for early adolescent: An adjunct to a comprehensive treatment program. Journal of the American Academy of Child Psychiatry 13, 110-125.

Kassoff, A. I. (1958). Advantages of multiple therapists in a group of severely acting-out adolescent boys. International Journal of Group Psychotherapy 8, 70-75.

Kaufmann, P. N., & Deutsch, A. L. (1967). Group therapy for pregnant unwed adolescents in the prenatal clinic of a general hospital. International Journal of Group Psychotherapy 17, 302-309.

Kraft, I. A. (1960). The nature of sociodynamics and psychodynamics in a therapy group of adolescents. International Journal of Group Psychotherapy 10, 218-223.

Kraft, I. A. (1966). Multiple impact therapy as a teaching device. Psychiatric Research Reports of the American Psychiatric Association 20, 218-223.

Kraft, I. A. (1968). An overview of group therapy with adolescents. International Journal of Group Psychotherapy 18, 461-480.

Kraft, I. A. (1971). Child and adolescent group psychotherapy. In H. I. Kaplan & B. J. Sadock (Eds.), Comprehensive group psychotherapy (pp. 534-565). Baltimore: Williams and Wilkins.

Lebovici, S. (1961). Psychodrama as applied to adolescents. Journal of Child Psychology and Psychiatry and Allied Disciplines 1, 298-305.

Novick, J. I. (1965). Comparison between short-term group and individual psychotherapy in effecting change in nondesirable behavior in children. International Journal of Group Psychotherapy 15, 366-373.

Patterson, G. R., & Anderson, D. (1964). Peers as social reinforcers. Child Development 35, 951-960.

Richmond, A. H., & Schecter, S. (1964). A spontaneous request for treatment by a group of adolescents. International Journal of Group Psychotherapy 14, 97-106.

Rosenbaum, M., & Kraft, I. A. (1972). Group psychotherapy for children. In B. B. Wolman (Ed.), Manual of child psychopathology (pp. 935-950). New York: McGraw-Hill.

Sadock, B., & Gould, R. E. (1964). A preliminary report on short-term group psychotherapy on an acute adolescent male service. International Journal of Group Psychotherapy 14, 465-473.

Scheidlinger, S. (1960). Experiential group treatment of severely deprived latency-age children. American Journal of Orthopsychiatry 30, 356-368.

Schiffer, M. (1969). The therapeutic play group. New York: Grune & Stratton.

Schulman, I. (1959). Transference, resistance and communication problems in adolescent psychotherapy groups. International Journal of Group Psychotherapy 9, 496-503.

Speers, R. W., & Lansing, C. (1965). Group therapy in childhood psychosis. Chapel Hill, N.C.: University of North Carolina Press.

Spruiell, V. (1967). Countertransference and an adolescent group crisis. International Journal of Group Psychotherapy 17, 298-308.

Straight, B., & Werkman, S. L. (1958). Control problems in group therapy with aggressive adolescent boys in a mental hospital. American Journal of Psychiatry 114, 998-1001.

2. Applications of Group Psychotherapy

Abramowitz, C. V. (1976). The effectiveness of group psychotherapy with children. Archives of General Psychiatry 33, 320-326.

Abramson, R. M., Hoffman, L., & Johns, C. A. (1979). Play group psychotherapy for early latency-age children on an inpatient psychiatric unit. International Journal of Group Psychotherapy 29, 383-392.

Ackerman, N. W. (1955). Group psychotherapy with a mixed group of adolescents. International Journal of Group Psychotherapy 5, 244-260.

Anderson, N., & Marrone, R. T. (1977). Group therapy for emotionally disturbed children: A key to affective education. American Journal of Orthopsychiatry 47, 97-103.

Azima, F. (1973). Transference-countertransference in adolescent group psychotherapy. In N. Brander & M. Gardner (Eds.), Group therapy for the adolescent (pp. 101-126). New York: Jason Aronson.

Azima, F. J. (1976). Group psychotherapy for latency-age children. Canadian Psychiatric Association Journal 21, 210-211.

Baider, L., & De Nour, A. K. (1989). Group therapy with adolescent cancer patients. Journal of Adolescent Health Care 10(1), 35-38.

Baract, A., & Robinson, E. H. (1969). Conventional group therapy with preadolescent children. International Journal of Group Psychotherapy 19, 34-45.

Barcai, A. (1973). A comparison of three group approaches to understanding children. American Journal of Orthopsychiatry 43, 133-141.

Bardill, D. R. (1977). A behavior-contracting program of group treatment for early adolescents in a residential treatment setting. International Journal of Group Psychotherapy 27, 389-400.

Barsky, M., & Mozenter, G. (1976). The use of creative drama in a children's group. International Journal of Group Psychotherapy 26, 105-114.

Bell, S., & Letford, T. (1978). The effects of sociodrama on the behaviors and attitudes of elementary school boys. Psychodrama and Sociometry 31, 117-135.

Bernet, W. (1982). The technique of verbal games in group therapy with early adolescents. Journal of the American Academy of Child Psychiatry 21, 496-501.

Bernfeld, G., Clark, L., & Parker, G. (1984). The process of adolesçent group psychotherapy. International Journal of Group Psychotherapy 34, 111-126.

Bingham, A., & Bargar, J. (1985). Children of alcoholic families: A group treatment approach for latency age children. Journal of Psychosocial Nursing and Mental Health Services 23, 13-15.

Blick, I. C., & Porter, F. S. (1982). Group therapy with female adolescent incest victims. In S. M. Sgroi (Ed.), Handbook of clinical intervention in child sexual abuse. Lexington, Mass.: Lexington Books.

Bonham, H. E., Armstrong, T. D., & Bonham, G. M. (1981). Group psychotherapy with deaf adolescents. American Annals of the Deaf 126, 806-809.

Brandes, M. S. (1977). Group therapy is not for every adolescent: Two case illustrations. International Journal of Group Psychotherapy 27, 229-237.

Bromfield, R., & Pfeifer, G. (1988). Combining group and individual psychotherapy: Impact on the individual treatment experience. Journal of the American Academy of Child and Adolescent Psychiatry 27(2), 220-225.
Charach, R. (1983). Brief interpretive group psychotherapy with early latency-age children. International Journal of Group Psychotherapy 33, 349-364.
Chen, C. C. (1984). Group therapy with Chinese schoolchildren. International Journal of Group Psychotherapy 34, 485-501.
Clement, P. W., Roberts, P. V., & Lantz, C. E. (1976). Mothers and peers as child behavior therapists. International Journal of Group Psychotherapy 26, 335-359.
Clifford, M., & Cross, T. (1980). Group therapy for seriously disturbed boys in residential treatment. Child Welfare 59, 560-565.
Coche, E., & Douglas, A. A. (1977). Therapeutic effects of problem-siblings training and play-reading groups. Journal of Clinical Psychology 33(3), 820-882.
Colman, M. D., Dougher, C. A., & Tanner, M. R. (1976). Group therapy for physically handicapped toddlers with delayed speech and language development. Journal of the American Academy of Child Psychiatry 15, 395-413.
Corder, B. (1981). An experimental study of structured videotape on adolescent group psychotherapy process. Journal of Youth and Adolescence 10, 255-262.
Cunningham, J. M., & Matthews, K. L. (1982). Impact of multiple-family therapy approach on a parallel latency-age/parent group. International Journal of Group Psychotherapy 32, 91-102.
Dannefer, E., Brown, R., & Epstein, N. (1975). Experience in developing a combined activity and verbal group therapy program with latency-age boys. International Journal of Group Psychotherapy 25, 331-337.
Davis, L, Geikie, G., & Schamess, G. (1988). The use of genograms in a group for latency age children. International Journal of Group Psychotherapy 38(2), 189-210.
Deter, H. C., & Allert, G. (1983). Group therapy for asthma patients: A concept for the psychosomatic treatment of patients in a medical clinic--a controlled study. Psychotherapy and Psychosomatics 40, 95-105.
Duffy, J., & Kraft, I. (1966). Beginning and middle phase characteristics of group psychotherapy of early adolescent boys and girls. Journal of Psychoanalysis in Groups 11, 23-29.
DuPlessis, J. M., & Lochner, L. M. (1981). The effects of group psychotherapy on the adjustment of four 12-year-old boys with learning and behavior problems. Journal of Learning Disabilities 14, 209-212.
Fielding, J., Guy, L., Harry, M., & Hook, R. H. (1971). A therapy group observed by medical students. International Journal of Group Psychotherapy 2(4), 456-469.
Fieldsteel, N. D. (1980). Therapist or leader: Group and family therapy experience. Journal of the Eastern Group Psychotherapy Society 4(3), 40-42.
Fine, S., Gilbert, M., Schmidt, L., Haley, G., Maxwell, A., & Forth, A. (1989). Short-term group therapy with depressed adolescent outpatients. Canadian Journal of Psychiatry 34(2), 97-102.
Fineberg, B. L. (1984). Bean bag chairs as versatile play objects in boys' latency groups. International Journal of Group Psychotherapy 34, 503-509.

Fluet, N. R., Holmes, G. R., & Gordon, L. C. (1980). Adolescent group psychotherapy: A modified fishbowl format. Adolescence 15, 75-82.

Frances, A., & Schiff, M. (1976). Popular music as a catalyst in the induction of therapy groups for teenagers. International Journal of Group Psychotherapy 26, 393-398.

Frank, J. D. (1979). Thirty years of group therapy: A personal perspective. International Journal of Group Psychotherapy 29(4), 439-452.

Freedman, H., & King, C. (1975). The role of visitors in group therapy. International Journal of Group Psychotherapy 6, 321-337.

Gatz, M., Tyler, F. B., & Pargament, K. I. (1978). Goal attainment, locus of control, and coping style in adolescent group counseling. Journal of Counseling Psychology 25, 310.

Gilder, R., Buschman, P. R., Sitarz, A. L., & Wolff, J. A. (1978). Group therapy with parents of children with leukemia. American Journal of Psychotherapy 32, 276-287.

Goldman, A. S., Murphy, R. J., & Babikian, H. M. (1973). Group therapy in obstetric management of pregnant teen-agers. New York Journal of Medicine 73, 407-411.

Goodwin, J. M., & Talwar, N. (1989). Group psychotherapy for victims of incest. Psychiatric Clinics of North America 12(2), 279-293.

Grant, D. (1988). Support groups for youth with the AIDS virus. International Journal of Group Psychotherapy 38(2), 237-251.

Granvold, D. K., & Welch, G. J. (1979). Structured, short-term group treatment of post-divorce adjustment. International Journal of Group Psychotherapy 29(4), 347-358.

Gratton, L., Lafontaine, C., & Gurbeautt, J. (1966). Group psychoanalytic work with children. Canadian Psychiatric Journal(Suppl.) 11, 430-442.

Green, R., & Fuller, M. (1973). Group therapy with feminine boys and their parents. International Journal of Group Psychotherapy 23, 54-68.

Grunebaum, H., & Solomon, L. (1980). Toward a peer theory of group psychotherapy. I. On the developmental significance of peers and play. International Journal of Group Psychotherapy 30(4), 23-46.

Haizlip, T., McRee, C., & Corder, B. F. (1975). Issues in developing psychotherapy groups for preschool children in outpatient clinics. American Journal of Psychiatry 132, 1061-1063.

Hardwick, P. J., Pounds, A. B., & Brown, M. (1985). Preventative adolescent psychiatry? Practical problems in running social skills groups for the younger adolescents. Journal of Adolescence 8, 357-367.

Hardy-Fanta, C., & Montana, P. (1982). The Hispanic female adolescent: A group therapy model. International Journal of Group Psychotherapy 32, 351-366.

Hoffman, T. E., Byrne, K. M., Belnap, K. L., & Steward, M. S. (1981).

Simultaneous semipermeable groups for mothers and their early latency-age boys. International Journal of Group Psychotherapy 31, 83-98.

Holmes, P. (1983). "Dropping out" from an adolescent therapeutic group: A study of factors in the patients and their parents which may influence this process. Journal of Adolescence 6, 333-346.

Horwitz, L. (1980). Group therapy for borderline and narcissistic patients. Bulletin of the Menninger Clinics 44(2), 181-200.

Hurvitz, N. (1970). Peer self-help psychotherapy groups and their implications for psychotherapy. Psychotherapy: Theory, Research and Practice 7(1), 41-49.

Johnson, D. L., & Gold, S. R. (1971). An empirical approach to issues of selection and evaluation in group therapy. International Journal of Group Psychotherapy 21(4), 456-469.

Kaplan, H. I., & Sadock, B. J. (1983). Comprehensive group psychotherapy. Baltimore: Williams and Wilkins.

Kartha, M., & Ertel, I. J. (1976). Short-term group therapy for mothers of leukemic children. What professional staff can do to help parents cope with chronic illness. Clinical Pediatrics 15, 803-806.

Kellerman, H. (1979). The group therapist: Role functions and countertransference. In H. Kellerman (Ed.), Group psychotherapy and personality: Intersecting structures (pp. 268-286). New York: Grune & Stratton.

Kernberg, P. F. (1978). Use of latency-age groups in the training of child psychiatrists. International Journal of Group Psychotherapy 28, 95-108.

Kernberg, P. F., & Ware, L. M. (1975). Understanding child development through group techniques and play. Bulletin of the Menninger Clinic 39, 409-419.

Kessein, M. (1981). Exploring general systems processes in group settings. Psychotherapy: Theory, Research and Practice 18(4), 424-430.

Kraft, I., & Jody, V. W. (1973). Flexibility and variability of group psychotherapy with adolescent girls. In M. S. Schwartz & H. D. Holberg (Eds.), Group therapy 1973. An overview (pp. 71-91). New York: Intercontinental Medical Book Corp.

Kraft, I. A. (1968). An overview of group therapy with adolescents. International Journal of Group Psychotherapy 18(4), 461-480.

Levin, S. (1982). The adolescent group as transitional object. International Journal of Group Psychotherapy 32, 217-232.

Lewis, J. M. (1970). Development of a protreatment group process among hospitalized adolescents. Timberlawn Foundation Report 40, 1-22.

Lilleskov, R. K., Harris, S., Hughron, H., & Willig, C. (1969). A therapeutic club for severely disturbed prepubertal boys. American Journal of Orthopsychiatry 39(2), 262-263.

Lothstein, L. (1985). Group therapy for latency age black males: Unplanned interventions, setting, and racial transferences as catalysts for change. International Journal of Group Psychotherapy 35, 603-623.

Lubin, B., & Lubin, A. W. (1986). Comprehensive index of group psychotherapy writings. New York: International Universities Press.

Lubin, B., Reddy, W. B., Stansberry, C., & Lubin, A. W. (1977). The group psychotherapy literature: 1976. International Journal of Group Psychotherapy 27, 521-552.

Maclennan, B. W. (1977). Modifications of activity group therapy for children. International Journal of Group Psychotherapy 27, 85-96.

Mallery, B., & Navas, M. (1982). Engagement of preadolescent boys in group therapy: Videotape as a tool. International Journal of Group Psychotherapy 32, 453-467.

Marwitt, R. C., Lind, J., & McLaughlin, D. G. (1974). Use of video tape to induce attitude change in delinquent adolescents. American Journal of Psychiatry 131(9), 996-999.

McGuire, T. J. (1988). A time-limited dynamic approach to adolescent inpatient group psychotherapy. Adolescence 23(90), 373-382.

Melville, K. (1973). Changing the family game. Sciences 13, 17-19.

Miller, A. N. (1973). The spontaneous use of poetry in an adolescent girl's group. International Journal of Group Psychotherapy 23, 224-227.

Oberfield, R., & Ciliotta, C. (1983). A school-age boys/single mothers group. Journal of the American Academy of Child Psychiatry 22, 375-381.

Olsson, P. A., & Myers, I. (1972). Non-verbal techniques in an adolescent group. International Journal of Group Psychotherapy 22, 186-192.

Parloff, H., & Dies, R. (1977). Group psychotherapy outcome research, 1966-1975. International Journal of Group Psychotherapy 27, 281-319.

Pasnau, R. O., Meyer, M., Davis, L. J., Lloyd, R., & Kline, G. (1976). Coordinated group psychotherapy of children and parents. International Journal of Group Psychotherapy 26, 89-103.

Phelan, J. R. (1974). Parent, teacher, or analyst: The adolescent group therapist's trilemma. International Journal of Group Psychotherapy 24(2), 238-244.

Pickar, D. B. (1988). Group psychotherapy and the learning disabled adolescents. Adolescence 23(92), 761-772.

Piper, W., Debbane, E., & Garant, J. (1977). Group psychotherapy outcome research: Problems and prospects of a first year project. International Journal of Group Psychotherapy 27, 321-340.

Porter, K. (1980). Combined individual and group psychotherapy: A review of the literature. International Journal of Group Psychotherapy 30(1), 107-114.

Rachman, A. W., & Heller, M. E. (1976). Peer group psychotherapy with adolescent drug abusers. International Journal of Group Psychotherapy 26, 373-384.

Raubolt, R. R., & Rachman, A. W. (1980). A therapeutic group experience for fathers. International Journal of Group Psychotherapy 30, 229-239.

Reister, A., & Kraft, I. A. (1986). Group psychotherapy for children. New York: International Universities Press.

Richmond, L. H. (1974). Observations on private practice and community clinic adolescent psychotherapy groups. Group Process 6, 57-62.

Rose, S. D. (1972). Treating children in groups. San Francisco: Jossey-Bass.
Schamess, G. (1976). Group treatment modalities for latency-age children. International Journal of Group Psychotherapy 26, 455-473.
Scheidlinger, S. (1974). On the concept of the "mother group." International Journal of Group Psychotherapy 24, 417-428.
Scheidlinger, S. (1984). Short-term group psychotherapy for children: An overview. International Journal of Group Psychotherapy 34, 573-586.
Scheidlinger, S. (1985). Group treatment of adolescents: An overview. American Journal of Orthopsychiatry 55, 102-111.
Schiffer, M. (1977). Activity-interview group psychotherapy: Theory, principles, and practice. International Journal of Group Psychotherapy 27, 377-388.
Shapiro, Z., & Berkowitz, I. (1975). The impact of group experiences on adolescent development. In M. Sugar (Ed.), The adolescent in group and family therapy (pp. 87-103). New York: Brunner/Mazel.
Slavson, S. R. (1974). The practice of group therapy. New York: International Universities Press.
Smith, J. D., Walsh, R. T., & Richardson, M. A. (1985). The clown club: A structured fantasy approach to group therapy with the latency-age child. International Journal of Group Psychotherapy 35, 49-64.
Soo, E. (1974). The impact of activity group therapy upon a highly constricted child. International Journal of Group Psychotherapy 24(2), 207-216.
Soo, E. S. (1979). Premature terminations in activity group therapy. International Journal of Group Psychotherapy 29, 115-118.
Soo, E. S. (1985). Applications of object relations concepts to children's group psychotherapy. International Journal of Group Psychotherapy 35, 37-47.
Stewart, M., Farquhar, L. C., Dicharry, D. C., Glick, D. R., & Martin, P. W. (1986). Group therapy: A treatment of choice for young victims of child abuse. International Journal of Group Psychotherapy 36(2), 261-277.
Strunk, C. S., & Witkin, L. J. (1974). The transformation of a latency-age girls' group from unstructured play to problem-focused discussion. International Journal of Group Psychotherapy 24, 460-470.
Sugar, M. (1967). Group therapy for pubescent boys with absent fathers. International Journal of Group Psychotherapy 6, 478-498.
Sugar, M. (1974). Interpretive group psychotherapy with latency children. Journal of the American Academy of Child Psychiatry 13, 648-666.
Trafimow, E., & Pattak, S. I. (1981). Group psychotherapy and objectal development in children. International Journal of Group Psychotherapy 31, 193-204.
Tramentara, M. G. (1980). Critical review of research on psychotherapy outcome with adolescents: 1967-1977. Psychological Bulletin 88, 429-450.
Weber, L. A. (1980). The effect of videotape and playback on an in-patient adolescent group. International Journal of Group Psychotherapy 30, 213-227.
Yalom, I. (1975). Theory and practice of group psychotherapy. New York: Basic Books.

D. Pharmacotherapy

Section Editor:

Magda Campbell, M.D.
Professor of Psychiatry
Division of Child Psychiatry
and
Director
Children's Psychopharmacology Unit, Bellevue Hospital
New York University School of Medicine
New York, New York

Associate Editors:

Richard Perry, M.D.
Clinical Associate Professor of Psychiatry
New York University School of Medicine
New York, New York

Arthur M. Small, M.D.
Clinical Professor of Psychiatry
New York University School of Medicine
New York, New York

1. Overview of Pharmacotherapy

Achenbach, T. M., & Edelbrock, C. S. (1979). The child behavior profile: II. Boys aged 12-16 and girls aged 6-11 and 12-16. Journal of Consulting and Clinical Psychology 47, 223-233.

Aman, M. G., & Singh, N. N. (1980). The usefulness of thioridazine for treating childhood disorders--fact or folklore. American Journal of Mental Deficiency 84, 331-338.

Aman, M. G., & Werry, J. S. (1982). Methylphenidate and diazepam in severe reading retardation. Journal of the American Academy of Child Psychiatry 21(1), 31-37.

Ambrosini, P. J. (1987). Pharmacotherapy in child and adolescent major depressive disorder. In H. Y. Meltzer (Ed.), Psychopharmacology: The third generation of progress (pp. 1247-1254). New York: Raven Press.

Anderson, L. T., Campbell, M., Adams, P., Small, A. M., Perry, R., & Shell, J. (1989). The effects of haloperidol on discrimination learning and behavioral symptoms in autistic children. Journal of Autism and Developmental Disorders 19, 227-239.

Ballinger, C. T., Varley, C. K., & Nolan, P. A. (1984). Effects of methylphenidate on reading in children with attention deficit disorder. American Journal of Psychiatry 141, 1590-1593

Bradley, C. (1937). The behavior of children receiving benzedrine. American Journal of Psychiatry 94, 577-585.

Bradley, C., & Bowen, M. (1940). School performance of children receiving amphetamine (benzedrine) sulfate. American Journal of Orthopsychiatry 10, 782-788.

Campbell, M. (1979). Psychopharmacology for children and adolescents. In J. D. Noshpitz (Ed.), Basic handbook of child psychiatry. New York: Basic Books.

Campbell, M. (1985a). On the use of neuroleptics in children and adolescents. Psychiatric Annals 15, 101-107.

Campbell, M. (1985b). Pervasive development disorders: Autistic and schizophrenic disorders. In J. M. Wiener (Ed.), Diagnosis and psychopharmacology of childhood and adolescent disorders. New York: Wiley.

Campbell, M. (1987a). Consent issues with disturbed and/or retarded children. Psychopharmacology Bulletin 23(3), 379-381.

Campbell, M. (1987b). Drug treatment of infantile autism: The past decade. In H. Y. Meltzer (Ed.), Psychopharmacology: The third generation of progress (pp. 1225-1231). New York: Raven Press.

Campbell, M. (1988). Fenfluramine treatment of autism. Annotation. Journal of Child Psychology and Psychiatry and Allied Disciplines 29(1), 1-10.

Campbell, M., Adams, P., Perry, R., Spencer, E. K., & Overall, J. E. (1988). Tardive and withdrawal dyskinesia in autistic children: A prospective study. Psychopharmacology Bulletin 24(2), 251-255.

Campbell, M., Adams, P., Small, A. M., Curren, E. L., Overall, J. E., Anderson, L. T., Lynch, N., & Perry, R. (1988). Efficacy and safety of fenfluramine in autistic children. Journal of the American Academy of Child and Adolescent Psychiatry 27(4), 434-439.

Campbell, M., Anderson, L. T., Small, A. M., Locascio, J. J., Lynch, N. S., & Choroco, M. C. (1990). Naltrexone in autistic children: A double-blind and placebo controlled study. Psychopharmacology Bulletin 26(1), 130-136.

Campbell, M., Green, W. H., & Deutsch, S. I. (1985). Child and adolescent psychopharmacology. Beverly Hills: Sage Publications.

Campbell, M., Locascio, J. J., Choroco, M. C., Spencer, E. K., Malone, R. P., Kafantaris, V., & Overall, J. E. (1990). Stereotypes and tardive dyskinesia: Abnormal movements in autistic children. Psychopharmacology Bulletin 26(1), 180-187.

Campbell, M., Overall, J. E., Small, A. M., Sokol, M. S., Spencer, E. K., Adams, P., Foltz, R. L., Monti, K., Perry, R., Nobler, M., & Roberts, E. (1989). Naltrexone in autistic children: An acute dose range tolerance trial. Journal of the American Academy of Child and Adolescent Psychiatry 28(2), 200-206.

Campbell, M., & Spencer, E. K. (1988). Psychopharmacology in child and adolescent psychiatry: A review of the last five years. Journal of the American Academy of Child and Adolescent Psychiatry 27, 269-279.

Coffey, B., Shader, R. I., & Greenblatt, D. J. (1983). Pharmacokinetics of benzadiazepines and psychostimulants in children. Journal of Clinical Psychopharmacology 3(4), 217-225.

Conners, C. K., Rothschild, G., Eisenberg, L., Schwartz, L. S., & Robinson, E. (1969). Dextroamphetamine sulfate in children with learning disorders: Effects on perception, learning, and achievement. Archives of General Psychiatry 21, 182-190.

Conners, C. K., & Taylor, E. (1980). Pemoline, methylphenidate, and placebo in children with minimal brain dysfunction. Archives of General Psychiatry 37, 922-930.

Cunningham, M. A., Pillai, V., & Rogers, W. J. B. (1968). Haloperidol in the treatment of children with severe behavior disorders. British Journal of Psychiatry 114, 845-854.

DeLong, G. R., & Aldershof, A. L. (1987). Long-term experience with lithium treatment in childhood: Correlation with clinical diagnosis. Journal of the American Academy of Child and Adolescent Psychiatry 26, 389-394.

Deutsch, S. I. (1986). Rationale for the administration of opiate antagonists in treating infantile autism. American Journal of Mental Deficiency 90, 631-635.

Farber, J. M (1987). Psychopharmacology of self-injurious behavior in the mentally retarded. Journal of the American Academy of Child and Adolescent Psychiatry 26, 296-302.

Fish, B. (1968). Drug use in psychiatric disorders in children. American Journal of Psychiatry 124, 31-36.

Frommer, E. A. (1967). Treatment of childhood depression with anti-depressant drugs. British Medical Journal 1, 729-732.

Geller, B., Cooper, T. B., Graham, D., Marsteller, F. A., & Bryant, M. (1990). Double-blind placebo controlled study of nortriptyline in depressed adolescents using a "fixed plasma level" design. Psychopharmacology Bulletin 26, 85-90.

Geller, B., Cooper, T. B., McCombs, H. G., Graham, D., & Wells, J. (1989). Double-blind placebo controlled study of nortriptyline in depressed children using a "fixed plasma level" design. Psychopharmacology Bulletin 25, 101-108.

Geller, B., Perel, J. M., Knitter, E. F., Lycaki, H., & Farooki, Z. Q. (1983). Nortriptyline in major depressive disorder in children: Response, steady-state plasma levels, predictive kinetics, and pharmacokinetics. Psychopharmacology Bulletin 19, 62-65.

Gittelman-Klein, R. (1987). Pharmacotherapy of childhood hyperactivity: An update. In H. Y. Meltzer (Ed.), Psychopharmacology: The third generation of progress (pp. 1215-1224). New York: Raven Press.

Gittelman-Klein, R., & Klein, D. F. (1973). School phobia: Diagnostic consideration in the light of imipramine effects. Journal of Nervous and Mental Disease 156, 199-215.

Gittelman-Klein, R., Spitzer, R., & Cantwell, D. P. (1978). Diagnostic classifications and psychopharmacological indications. In J. S. Werry (Ed.), Pediatric psychopharmacology: The use of behavior modifying drugs in children. New York: Brunner/Mazel.

Golden, R. R., Campbell, M., & Perry, R. (1987). A taxometric method for diagnosis of tardive dyskinesias. Journal of Psychiatric Research 21(3), 233-241.

Gualtieri, C. T., Golden, R., Evans, R. W., & Hicks, R. E. (1984). Blood level measurement of psychoactive drugs in pediatric psychiatry. Therapeutic Drug Monitoring 6, 127-141.

Herjanic, B., & Campbell, W. (1977). Differentiating psychiatrically disturbed children on the basis of a structured interview. Journal of Abnormal Child Psychology 5, 127-134.

Law, W., Petti, T. A., & Kazdin, A. E. (1981). Withdrawal symptoms after graduated cessation of imipramine in children. American Journal of Psychiatry 138, 647-650.

Leckman, J. F., Detlor, J., Harcherik, D., Ort, S., & Cohen, D. J. (1985). Short- and long-term treatment of Tourette's syndrome with clonidine: A clinical perspective. Neurology 35, 343-351.

Leckman, J. F., Walkup, J. T., Riddle, M. A., Towbin, K. E., & Cohen, D. J. (1987). Tic disorders. In H. Y. Meltzer (Ed.), Psychopharmacology: The third generation of progress (pp. 1239-1246). New York: Raven Press.

Lucas, A. R., & Pasley, F. C. (1969). Psychoactive drugs in treatment of emotionally disturbed children: Haloperidol and diazepam. Comprehensive Psychiatry 10(5), 376-386.

Mattes, J., & Gittelman, R. (1983). Growth of hyperactive children on maintenance methylphenidate. Archives of General Psychiatry 40, 317-321.

Meiselas, K., Spencer, E. K., Oberfield, R., Peselow, E. D., Angrist, B., & Campbell, M. (1989). Differentiation of stereotypes from neuroleptic-related dyskinesias in autistic children. Journal of Clinical Psychopharmacology 9(3), 207-209.

Nino-Murcia, G., & Dement, W. C. (1987). Psychophysiological and pharmacological aspects of somnambulism and night terrors in children. In H. Y. Meltzer (Ed.), Psychopharmacology: The third generation of progress (pp. 873-879). New York: Raven Press.

Perry, R., Campbell, M., Adams, P., Lynch, N., Spencer, E. K., Curren, E. L., & Overall, J. E. (1989). Long-term efficacy of haloperidol in autistic children: Continuous vs. discontinuous drug administration. Journal of the American Academy of Child Psychiatry 28, 87-92.

Perry, R., Nobler, M. S., & Campbell, M. (1989). Case report: Tourette-like symptoms associated with chronic neuroleptic therapy in an autistic child. Journal of the American Academy of Child and Adolescent Psychiatry 28, 93-96.

Petti, T. A., & Law, W. (1981). Abrupt cessation of high-dose imipramine treatment in children. Journal of the American Medical Association 246, 768-769.

Pliszka, S. R. (1987). Tricyclic antidepressants in the treatment of children with attention deficit disorders. Journal of the American Academy of Child and Adolescent Psychiatry 26, 127-132.

Polakoff, S. A., Sorgi, P. J., & Ratey, J. J. (1986). The treatment of impulsive and aggressive behavior with nadolol. Journal of Clinical Psychopharmacology 6, 125-126.

Poussaint, A. F., & Ditman, K. S. (1965). A controlled study of imipramine (trofranil) in the treatment of childhood enuresis. Journal of Pediatrics 67, 283-290.

Preskorn, S. H., Weller, E. B., Weller, R. A., & Glotzbach, E. (1983). Plasma levels of imipramine and adverse effects in children. American Journal of Psychiatry 140, 1332-1335.

Puig-Antich, J. (1980). Affective disorders in childhood: A review and perspective. Psychiatric Clinics of North America 3(3), 403-424.

Puig-Antich, J., Greenhill, L. L., Sassin, J., & Sacher, E. J. (1978). Growth hormone, prolactin and cortisol responses and growth patterns in hyperkinetic children treated with dextro-amphetamine. Journal of the American Academy of Child Psychiatry 17, 457-475.

Puig-Antich, J., Perel, J. M., Lupatkin, W., Chambers, W. J., Tabrizi, M. A., King, J., Goetz, R., Davies, M., & Stiller, R. L. (1987). Imipramine in prepubertal major depressive disorders. Archives of General Psychiatry 44, 81-89.

Rapoport, J. L., Mikkelsen, E. J., Zavadil, A., Nee, L., Gruenau, C., Mendelson, W., Gillin, J. C. (1980). Childhood enuresis. II. Psychopathology, tricyclic concentration in plasma, and antienuretic effects. Archives of General Psychiatry 37, 1146-1152.

Ratey, J. J., Mikkelsen, F. J., Smith, G. B., et al. (1986). B-blockers in the severely and profoundly mentally retarded. Journal of Clinical Psychopharmacology 6, 103-107.

Realmuto, G. M., Jensen, J., Klykylo, W., et al. (1986). Untoward effects of fenfluramine in autistic children. Journal of Clinical Psychopharmacology 6, 350-355.

Rosenthal, N. E., Carpenter, C. J., James, S. P., Parry, B. L., Rogers, S. L. B., & Wehr, T. A. (1986). Seasonal affective disorder in children and adolescents. American Journal of Psychiatry 143, 356-358.

Ryan, N. D., Puig-Antich, J., Cooper, T., et al. (1986). Imipramine in adolescent major depression: Plasma level and clinical response. Acta Psychiatrica Scandinavica 73, 275-288.

Sandman, C. A., Datta, P. C., Barron, J., Hoehler, F. K., Williams, C., & Swanson, J. M. (1983). Naloxone attenuates self-abusive behavior in developmentally disabled children. Applied Research in Mental Retardation 4, 5-11.

Saraf, K. R., Klein, D. F., Gittelman-Klein, R., Gottman, N., & Greenhill, P. (1978). EKG effects of imipramine treatment in children. Journal of the American Academy of Child Psychiatry 17, 60-69.

Satterfield, J. H., Cantwell, D. P., Schell, A., & Blaschke, T. (1979). Growth of hyperactive children treated with methylphenidate. Archives of General Psychiatry 36, 212-217.

Shapiro, E., Shapiro, A. K., Fulop, G., Hubbard, M., Mandeli, J., Nordlie, J., & Phillips, R. A. (1989). Controlled study of haloperidol, pimozide, and placebo for the treatment of Gilles de la Tourette's syndrome.

Sokol, M. S., Campbell, M., Goldstein, M., & Kriechman, A. M. (1987). Attention deficit disorder with hyperactivity and the dopamine hypothesis: A case presentation with theoretical background. Journal of the American Academy of Child Psychiatry 26, 428-433.

Sonis, W. A., Yellin, A. M., Garfinkel, B. D., & Hoberman, H. H. (1987). The antidepressant effect of light in seasonal affective disorder of childhood and adolescence. Psychopharmacology Bulletin 23, 360-363.

Special feature: Rating scales and assessment instruments for use in pediatric psychopharmacology research. (1985). Psychopharmacology Bulletin 21(4), 12-24.

Spencer, E. K., Campbell, M., Adams, P., Perry, R., Choroco, M. C., Padron-Gayol, M., & Small, A. M. (1990). Saliva and serum lithium monitoring in hospitalized children. Psychopharmacology Bulletin 26(1), 36-49.

Spitzer, R. L., & Cantwell, D. P. (1980). The DSM-III classification of the psychiatric disorders of infancy, childhood, and adolescence. Journal of the American Academy of Child Psychiatry 19, 356-370.

Stores, G. (1978). Antiepileptics (anticonvulsants). In J. S. Werry (Ed.), Pediatric psychopharmacology: The use of behavior modifying drugs in children. New York: Brunner/Mazel.

Walsh, B. T. (1987). Psychopharmacology of bulimia. In H. Y. Meltzer (Ed.), Psychopharmacology: The third generation of progress (pp. 1277-1280). New York: Raven Press.

Werry, J. S., Aman, M. G., & Diamond, E. (1980). Imipramine and methylphenidate in hyperactive children. Journal of Child Psychology and Psychiatry and Allied Disciplines 21, 27-35.

Werry, J. S., Aman, M. G., & Lampen, E. (1975). Haloperidol and methylphenidate in hyperactive children. Acta Paedopsychiatrica 42, 26-40.

Wiener, J. M. (Ed.). (1985). Diagnosis and psychopharmacology of childhood and adolescent disorders. New York: Wiley.

Winsberg, B. G., Goldstein, S., Yepes, L. E., & Perel, J. M. (1975). Imipramine and electrocardiographic abnormalities in hyperactive children. American Journal of Psychiatry 132, 542-545.

Winsberg, B. G., Kupietz, S. S., Sverd, J., Hungund, B. L., & Young, N. L. (1982). Methylphenidate oral dose plasma concentrations and behavioral response in children. Psychopharmacology 76, 329-332.

Youngerman, J. K., & Canino, I. A. (1983). Violent kids, violent parents: Family, pharmacotherapy. American Journal of Orthopsychiatry 53(1), 152-156.

Zametkin, A. J., & Rapoport, J. L. (1987). Noradrenergic hypothesis of attention deficit disorder with hyperactivity: A critical review. In H. Y. Meltzer (Ed.), Psychopharmacology: The third generation of progress (pp. 837-842). New York: Raven Press.

2. Tardive Dyskinesia

Campbell, M., & Palij, M. (1985). Measurement of untoward effects including tardive dyskinesia. Psychopharmacology Bulletin 21(4), 1063-1082.

Gualtieri, C. T., Barnhill, J., McGimsey, J., & Schell, D. (1980). Tardive dyskinesia and other movement disorders in children treated with psychotropic drugs. Journal of the American Academy of Child Psychiatry 19(3), 491-510.

Gualtieri, C. T., Quade, D., Hicks, R. E., Mayo, J. P., & Schroeder, S. R. (1984). Tardive dyskinesia and other clinical consequences of neuroleptic treatment in children and adolescents. American Journal of Psychiatry 141(1), 20-23.

Gualtieri, C. T., Schroeder, S. R., Hicks, R. E., & Quade, D. (1986). Tardive dyskinesia in young mentally retarded individuals. Archives of General Psychiatry 43, 335-340.

3. Use of Lithium--Children and Adolescents

Bennett, W. G., Korein, J., Kalmijn, M., Grega, D. M., & Campbell, M. (1983). EEG and treatment of hospitalized aggressive children with haloperidol or lithium. Biological Psychiatry 18(12), 1427-1440.

Campbell, M., Perry, R., & Green, W. H. (1984). Use of lithium in children and adolescents. Psychosomatics 25(2), 95-106.

Campbell, M., Small, A. M., Green, W. H., Jennings, S. J., Perry, R., Bennett, W. G., & Anderson, L. (1984). Behavioral efficacy of haloperidol and lithium carbonate: A comparison of hospitalized aggressive children. with conduct disorder. Archives of General Psychiatry 41(7), 650-656.

DeLong, G. R. (1978). Lithium carbonate treatment of select behavior disorders in children suggesting manic-depressive illness. Journal of Pediatrics 93(4), 689-694.

DeLong, G. R., & Nieman, G. W. (1983). Lithium-induced behavior changes in children with symptoms suggesting manic-depressive illness. Psychopharmacology Bulletin 19(2), 258-265.

Jefferson, J. W. (1982). The use of lithium in childhood and adolescence: An overview. Journal of Clinical Psychiatry 43(5), 174-177.

Lena, B., Surtees, S. J., & Maggs, R. (1978). The efficacy of lithium in the treatment of emotional disturbance in children and adolescence. In F. N. Johnson & S. Johnson (Eds.), Lithium in medical practice. Baltimore, Md.: University Park Press.

McKnew, D. H., Cytryn, L., Buchsbaum, M. S., Hamovit, J., Lamour, M., Rapoport, J. L., & Gershon, E. S. (1981). Lithium in children of lithium-responding parents. Psychiatry Research 4, 171-180.

Platt, J. E., Campbell, M., Green, W. H., & Grega, D. M. (1984). Cognitive effects of lithium carbonate and haloperidol in treatment-resistant aggressive children. Archives of General Psychiatry 41, 657-662.

Siassi, I. (1982). Lithium treatment of impulsive behavior in children. Journal of Clinical Psychiatry 43(12), 482-484.

4. Pharmacotherapy with Retarded Children and Adolescents

Donaldson, J. Y. (1984). Specific psychopharmacological approaches and rationale for mentally ill-mentally retarded children. In F. J. Menolascino & J. A. Stark (Eds.), Handbook of mental illness in the mentally retarded (pp. 171-187). New York: Plenum Press.

Varley, C. K., & Trupin, E. W. (1982). Double-blind administration of methylphenidate to mentally retarded children with attention deficit disorder: A preliminary study. American Journal of Mental Deficiency 86, 560-566.

Williams, D. T., Mehl, R., Yudofsky, S., Adams, D., & Roseman, B. (1982). The effects of propranolol on uncontrolled rage outbursts in children and adolescents with organic brain dysfunction. Journal of the American Academy of Child Psychiatry 21, 129-135.

5. Treatment of Affective Disorders

Kashani, J. H., Shekim, W. O., & Reid, J. C. (1984). Amitriptyline in children with minor depressive disorder: A double-blind crossover pilot study. Journal of the American Academy of Child Psychiatry 23, 348-351.

Kazdin, A. E. (1981). Assessment techniques for childhood depression. A critical appraisal. Journal of the American Academy of Child Psychiatry 20, 358-375.

Kazdin, A. E., French, N. H., Unis, A. S., & Esveldt-Dawson, K. (1983). Assessment of childhood depression: Correspondence of child and parent ratings. Journal of the American Academy of Child Psychiatry 22, 157-164.

Kazdin, A. E., & Petti, T. A. (1982). Self-report and interview measures of childhood and adolescent depression. Journal of Child Psychology and Psychiatry and Allied Disciplines 23, 437-457.

Petti, T. A. (1978). Depression in hospitalized child psychiatry patients: Approaches to measuring depression. Journal of the American Academy of Child Psychiatry 17, 49-59.

Petti, T. A., & Law, W. (1982). Imipramine treatment of depressed children: A double-blind pilot study. Journal of Clinical Psychopharmacology 2, 107-110.

Poznanski, E. O., Cook, S. C., & Carroll, B. J. (1979). A depression rating scale for children. Pediatrics 46, 442-450.

Preskorn, S. H., Weller, E. B., & Weller, R. A. (1982). Depression in children: Relationship between plasma imipramine levels and response. Journal of Clinical Psychiatry 43, 450-453.

Puig-Antich, J., Perel, J., Lupatkin, W., Chambers, W. J., Tabrizi, M. A., King, J., Davies, M., & Stiller, R. (1987). Imipramine effectiveness in prepubertal major depressive disorders. I. Relationship of plasma levels to clinical response of the depressive syndrome. Archives of General Psychiatry 44, 81-89.

Puig-Antich, J., Perel, J. M., Lupatkin, W., Chambers, W. J., Shea, C., Tabrizi, M. A., & Stiller, R. L. (1979). Plasma levels of imipramine (IMI) and desmethylimipramine (DMI) and clinical response in prepubertal major depressive disorder. A preliminary report. Journal of the American Academy of Child Psychiatry 18, 616-627.

Weller, E. B., Preskorn, S. H., Weller, R. A., & Croskell, M. (1983). Childhood depression: Imipramine levels and response. Psychopharmacology Bulletin 19(1), 56-62.

Weller, E. B., Weller, R. A., Preskorn, S. H., & Glotzbach, R. (1982). Steady-state plasma imipramine levels in prepubertal depressed children. American Journal of Psychiatry 139, 506-508.

White, J. W., & O'Shanick, G. (1977). Juvenile manic-depressive illness. American Journal of Psychiatry 134(9), 1035-1036.

6. Treatment of Autism and Schizophrenia

Anderson, L. T., Campbell, M., Grega, D. M., Perry, R., Small, A. M., & Green, W. H. (1984). Haloperidol in infantile autism: Effects on learning and behavioral symptoms. American Journal of Psychiatry 141(10), 1195-1201.

Campbell, M., Cohen, I. L., & Anderson, L. T. (1981). Pharmacotherapy for autistic children: A summary of research. Canadian Journal of Psychiatry 26, 265-273.

Campbell, M., Deutsch, S. I., Perry, R., Wolsky, B. B., & Palij, M. (1986). Short-term efficacy and safety of fenfluramine in hospitalized preschool-age autistic children: An open study. Psychopharmacology Bulletin 22(1), 141-147.

Campbell, M., & Palij, M. (1985). Behavioral and cognitive measures in psychopharmacological studies of infantile autism. Psychopharmacology Bulletin 21(4), 1047-1053.

Campbell, M., Perry, R., Polonsky, B. B., Deutsch, S. I., Palij, M., & Lukashok, D. (1986). Brief report: Fenfluramine in hospitalized young autistic children: An open study. Journal of Autism and Developmental Disorders 16, 495-501.

Campbell, M., Perry, R., Small, A. M., & Green, W. H. (1986). Overview of drug treatment in autism. In E. Schopler (Ed.), Neurobiological issues in autism. New York: Plenum Press.

Campbell, M., Small, A. M., Palij, M., Perry, R., Polonsky, B. B., Lukashok, D., & Anderson, L. T. (1987). The efficacy and safety of fenfluramine in autistic children: Preliminary analysis of a double-blind study. Psychopharmacology Bulletin 23(1), 123-127.

Deutsch, S. I., & Campbell, M. (1986). Relative affinities for different classes of neurotransmitter receptors predict neuroleptic efficacy in infantile autism: A hypothesis. Neuropsychobiology 15, 3-4.

Lowe, T. L., Cohen, D. J., Miller, S., & Young, J. G. (1981). Folic acid and B12 in autism and neuropsychiatric disturbances of childhood. Journal of the American Academy of Child Psychiatry 20, 104-111.

Perry, R., Campbell, M., Green, W. H., Small, A. M., Die Trill, M. L., Meiselas, R. R., Golden, R. R., & Deutsch, S. I. (1985). Neurologic-related dyskinesias in autistic children: A prospective study. Psychopharmacology Bulletin 21(1), 140-143.

Ritvo, E. J., Freeman, B. J., Geller, E., & Yuwiler, A. (1983). Effects of fenfluramine on 14 outpatients with the syndrome of autism. Journal of the American Academy of Child Psychiatry 22, 549-558.

Ritvo, E. R., Freeman, B. J., Yuwiler, A., Geller, E., Schroth, P., Yokota, A., Mason-Brothers, A., & Leventhal, B. (1986). Fenfluramine treatment of autism: UCLA Collaborative study of 81 patients at nine medical centers. Psychopharmacology Bulletin 22(1), 133-140.

7. Miscellaneous References on Schizophrenia

Campbell, M., Fish, B., Shapiro, T., & Floyd, A. (1972). Acute responses of schizophrenic children to a sedative and "stimulating" neuroleptic: A pharmacologic yardstick. Current Therapeutic Research 14(12), 759-766.

Pool, D., Bloom, W., Mielke, D. H., Roniger, J. J., & Gallant, D. M. (1976). A controlled evaluation of loxitane in seventy-five adolescent schizophrenic patients. Current Therapeutic Research 19, 99-104.

Realmuto, G. M., Erickson, W. D., Yellin, A. M., Hopwood, J. H., & Greenberg, L. M. (1984). Clinical comparison of thiothixene and thioridazine in schizophrenic adolescents. American Journal of Psychiatry 141(3), 440-442.

8. Evaluation of Clinical Effectiveness and Side Effects of Psychopharmacological Drugs

Campbell, M., Cohen, I. L., & Small, A. M. (1982). Drugs on aggressive behavior. Journal of the American Academy of Child Psychiatry 21, 107-117.

Campbell, M., Green, W. H., Perry, R., & Anderson, L. T. (1983). Pharmacotherapy. In C. E. Walker & M. C. Roberts (Eds.), Handbook on clinical child psychology. New York: Wiley.

Campbell, M., Grega, D. J., Green, W. H., & Bennett, W. G. (1983). Neuroleptic-induced dyskinesias in children. Clinical Neuropharmacology 6, 207-222.

Campbell, M., & Palij, M. (1985). Documentation of demographic data and family history of psychiatric illness. Psychopharmacology Bulletin 21(4), 719-733.

Cantwell, D. P. (1980). The diagnostic process and diagnostic classification in child psychiatry--DSM-III. Journal of the American Academy of Child Psychiatry 19, 345-355.

Carroll, B. J. (1978). Neuroendocrine function in psychiatric disorders. In M. A. Lipton, A. DiMascio, & K. F. Killam (Eds.), Psychopharmacology: A generation of progress. New York: Raven Press.

Casey, D. E. (1985). Spontaneous and tardive dyskinesias: Clinical and laboratory studies. Journal of Clinical Psychiatry 46, 42-47.

Charney, D. S., Menkes, D. B., & Heninger, G. R. (1981). Receptor sensitivity and the mechanism of action of antidepressant treatment: Implications for the etiology and therapy of depression. Archives of General Psychiatry 38, 1160-1180.

Chouinard, G., & Jones, B. D. (1980). Neuroleptic-induced super-sensitivity psychosis: Clinical and pharmacological characteristics. American Journal of Psychiatry 137, 16-21.

Comings, D. E., & Comings, B. G. (1984). Tourette's syndrome and attention deficit with hyperactivity: Are they genetically related? Journal of the American Academy of Child Psychiatry 23, 138-146.

Conners, C. K. (1969). A teacher rating scale for use in drug studies with children. American Journal of Psychiatry 126, 152-156.

Conners, C. K. (1985). Methodological and assessment issues in pediatric psychopharmacology. In J. M. Wiener (Ed.), Diagnosis and psychopharmacology of childhood and adolescent disorders. New York: Wiley.

Denckla, M. B., Bemporad, J. R., & MacKay, M. C. (1976). Tics following methylphenidate administration: A report of 20 cases. Journal of the American Medical Association 235(13), 1349-1351.

Forsythe, W. I., & Redmond, A. (1974). Enuresis and spontaneous cure rate. Archives of Disease in Childhood 49, 259-263.

Friedhoff, A. J., & Chase, T. N. (1982). Advances in neurology. Vol. 35. Gilles de la Tourette syndrome. New York: Raven Press.

Geller, B., & Greydanus, B. E. (1979). Haloperidol-induced comatose state with hyperthermia and rigidity in adolescence. Two case reports and a literature review. Journal of Clinical Psychiatry 40, 102-103.

Gualtieri, C. T., Wafgin, W., Kanoy, R., Patrick, K., Shen, D., Youngblood, W., Mueller, R., & Breese, G. (1982). Clinical studies of methylphenidate serum levels in children and adults. Journal of the American Academy of Child Psychiatry 21, 19-26.

Hardesty, A. S. (1982). Behavioral assessment of children and adolescents. In E. I. Burdock, A. Sudilovsky, & S. Gershon (Eds.), The behavior of psychiatric patients. Quantitative techniques for evaluation. New York: Marcel Dekker.

Klawans, H. L., Nausieda, P. A., Goetz, C. G., Tanner, C. M., & Weiner, W. J. (1982). Tourette-like symptoms following chronic neuroleptic therapy. In A. J. Friedhoff & T. N. Chase (Eds.), Gilles de la Tourette syndrome. New York: Raven Press.

Levenson, J. L. (1985). Neuroleptic malignant syndrome. American Journal of Psychiatry 142, 1137-1145.

Lowe, T. L., Cohen, D. J., Detlor, J., Kremenitzer, M. W., & Shaywitz, B. A. (1982). Stimulant medications precipitate Tourette's syndrome. Journal of the American Medical Association 247(12), 1729-1731.

MacLeod, C. M., Dekeban, A. S., & Hunt, E. (1978). Memory impairment in epileptic patients: Selective effects of phenobarbital concentration. Science 202, 1102-1104.

Mikkelsen, E. J., Detlor, J., & Cohen, D. J. (1981). School avoidance and social phobia triggered by haloperidol in patients with Tourette's disorder. American Journal of Psychiatry 138(12), 1572-1576.

Mikkelsen, E. J., Rapoport, J. L., Nee, L., Gruenau, C., Mendelson, W., & Gillin, J. C. (1980). Childhood enuresis. I. Sleep patterns and psychopathology. Archives of General Psychiatry 37, 1139-1144.

Rapoport, J. L., Buchsbaum, M. S., Weingartner, H., Zahn, T. P., Ludlow, C., & Mikkelsen, E. J. (1980). Dextroamphetamine: Its cognitive and behavioral effects in normal and hyperactive boys and normal men. Archives of General Psychiatry 37, 933-943.

Richardson, J. S., & Zaleski, W. A. (1983). Naloxone and self-mutilation. Biological Psychiatry 18, 99-101.

Shapiro, A. K., & Shapiro, E. (1984). Controlled study of pimozide vs. placebo in Tourette's syndrome. Journal of the American Academy of Child Psychiatry 23, 161-173.

Shaywitz, S. E., Hunt, R. D., Jatlow, P., Cohen, D. J., Young, J. G., Pierce, R. N., Andersen, G. M., & Shaywitz, B. A. (1982). Psychopharmacology of attention deficit disorders: Pharmacokinetic, neuroendocrine, and behavioral measures following acute and chronic treatment with methylphenidate. Pediatrics 69, 688-694.

Weiss, G., Hechtman, L., Perlman, T., Hopkins, J., & Wenar, A. (1979). Hyperactives as young adults: A controlled prospective ten-year follow-up of 75 children. Archives of General Psychiatry 36, 675-681.

E. Evaluation of the Effectiveness of Various Therapies with Children and Adolescents

Section Editor:

David Shaffer, M.D.
Professor of Child Psychiatry
Director of Child and Adolescent Psychiatry
Columbia University School of Medicine
New York, New York

1. Classic Description of Therapies

a. Designed Specifically for Children

Axline, V. (1969). Play therapy. New York: Ballantine Books.

Bixler, R. (1949). Limits are therapy. Journal of Consulting Psychology 13, 1-11.

Freud, A. (1928). Introduction to the technique of child analysis (L. P. Clark, Trans.). New York: Nervous and Mental Disease Publishing.

Ginott, H. (1961). Group psychotherapy with children. New York: McGraw-Hill.

Hambridge, G. (1955). Structured play therapy. American Journal of Orthopsychiatry 25, 601-617.

Klein, M. (1932). The psycho-analysis of children. London: Hogarth Press.

Levy, D. (1938). Release therapy. American Journal of Orthopsychiatry 9, 713-736.

Moustakas, C. (1973). Children in play therapy (rev. ed.). New York: Jason Aronson.

b. Designed for Parents/Families and Children

Guerney, B. G., Jr. (1964). Filial therapy. Description and rationale. Journal of Clinical Child Psychology 9, 242-244.

Patterson, G. R. (1975). Families--applications of social learning to family life. Champaign, Ill.: Research Press.

Safer, D. (1965). Conjoint play therapy for the young child and his parent. Archives of General Psychiatry 13, 320-326.

2. Evaluating Psychotherapy

Fiske, D. W., et al. (1970). Planning of research on effectiveness of psychotherapy. Archives of General Psychiatry 22, 22-32.

Harter, S. (1983). Cognitive developmental considerations in the conduct of play therapy. In C. Shaefer & A. E. O'Connor (Eds.), Handbook of play therapy. New York: Wiley.

Kazdin, A. E. (Ed.). (1982). Single-case research designs: Methods for clinical and applied settings. New York: Oxford University Press.

Levinson, D. G., & Kitchener, H. (1966). Treatment of delinquents. Journal of Consulting and Clinical Psychology 30, 364.

Mintz, J., et al. (1980). Predicting the outcome of psychotherapy. Archives of General Psychiatry 37, 471-481.

Parloff, M. B., et al. (1979). Research on therapist variables in relation to progress and outcome. In S. L. Garfield & A. E. Bergin (Eds.), Handbook of psychotherapy and behavior change: An empirical analysis (2nd ed.). New York: Wiley.

Ricks, D. F. (1974). Supershrink: Methods of a therapist judged successful on the basis of adult outcomes of adolescent patients. In M. Roff & D. F. Ricks (Eds.), Life history research in psychopathology (Vol. 3). Minneapolis: University of Minnesota Press.

Shaffer, D., et al. (1983). A children's global assessment scale (CGAS). Archives of General Psychiatry 40, 1228-1231

Strupp, H. H., & Bergin, A. E. (1969). Some empirical and conceptual bases for coordinated research in psychotherapy: A critical review of issues, trends and evidence. International Journal of Psychiatry 7, 18-90.

Weissman, M., et al. (1984). Families--applications of social learning to family life. New York: Whitehead.

3. Reviews of Evaluations of Child Psychotherapy

Barrett, C. L., et al. (1978). Research on child psychotherapy. In S. L. Garfield &

A. E. Bergin (Eds.), Handbook of psychotherapy and behavior change (2nd ed.). New York: Wiley.

Gossett, J. T., et al. (1973). Follow-up of adolescents treated in a psychiatric hospital: I. A review of studies. American Journal of Orthopsychiatry 43, 602-610.

Hartman, E., et al. (1977). An evaluation of alternative modes of child psychotherapy. In B. B. Lahey & A. E. Kazdin (Eds.), Advances in clinical child psychology (Vol. 1). New York: Plenum Press.

Levitt, E. E. (1971). Research on psychotherapy with children. In S. L. Garfield & A. E. Bergin (Eds.), Handbook of psychotherapy and behavior change: An empirical analysis (2nd ed.). New York: Wiley.

Luborsky, L., et al. (1980). Predicting the outcome of psychotherapy. Archives of General Psychiatry 37, 471-481.

Rutter, M. (1972). Critical notice. Journal of Child Psychology and Psychiatry and Allied Disciplines 139, 219-222.

Rutter, M. (1982). Psychological therapies in child psychiatry. Psychological Medicine 12, 723-740.

Rutter, M., & Giller, H. (1982). Juvenile delinquency: Trends and perspective. Harmondsworth, England: Penguin.

Shaffer, D., et al. (1984). Behavior and bladder disturbance in enuretics: The rational classification of a common disorder. Unpublished manuscript.

Tramontana, M. G. (1980). Critical review of research on psychotherapy outcome with adolescents: 1967-1977. Psychological Bulletin 88, 429-450.

Wright, D. M., et al. (1976). The outcome of individual child psychotherapy: Increments at follow-up. Journal of Child Psychology and Psychiatry and Allied Disciplines 17, 275-285.

4. Well-Evaluated Outcomes of Different Treatments

a. Behavior Therapy

Gelfand, D. M. (1978). Behavior treatment of avoidance, social withdrawal and negative emotional states. In B. B. Wolman, J. Egan, & A. O. Ross (Eds.), Handbook of mental disorders in childhood and adolescence. Englewood Cliffs, N.J.: Prentice Hall.

Graziano, A. M., et al. (1979). Behavior treatment of children's fears: A review. Psychological Bulletin 86, 804-830.

Kolvin, I., et al. (1981). Help starts here: The maladjusted child in the ordinary school. London: Tavistock.

Mash, E. J., & Dalby, J. T. (1979). Behavioral interventions for hyperactivity. In R. L. Trites (Ed.), Hyperactivity in children (pp. 161-216). Baltimore: University Park Press.

Miller, L. V., et al. (1972). Comparison of reciprocal inhibition, psychotherapy and waiting list control for phobic children. Journal of Abnormal Psychology 49, 269-279.

O'Leary, K. D., & O'Leary, S. G. (1977). Classroom management. The successful use of behavior modification. New York: Pergamon.

Ross, A. O. (1981). Child behavior therapy: Principles, procedures and empirical basis. New York: Wiley.

b. Cognitive Therapy

Beck, A. (1976). Cognitive therapy and the emotional disorders. New York: International Universities Press.

Blackburn, I. M., et al. (1981). The efficacy of cognitive therapy in depression: A treatment trial using cognitive therapy and pharmacotherapy, each alone and in combination. British Journal of Psychiatry 139, 181-189.

Hinshaw, S.P., et al. (1984). Self-control in hyperactive boys in anger-inducing situations: Effects of cognitive-behavioral training and of methylphenidate. Journal of Abnormal Child Psychology 12, 55-77.

Hobbs, S. A., et al. (1980). Cognitive behavior therapy with children: Has clinical utility been demonstrated? Psychological Bulletin 87, 147-165.

Kendall, P. C. (1984). Annotation: Cognitive-behavioral self-control therapy for children. Journal of Child Psychology and Psychiatry and Allied Disciplines 25, 173-179.

Urbain, E. S., & Kendall, P. C. (1980). Review of social-cognitive problem-solving interventions with children. Psychological Bulletin 88, 109-143.

c. Family Therapy

Lebow, J. (1981). Issues in the assessment of outcome in family therapy. Family Process 20, 167-188.

Wells, R. A., & Dezen, A. E. (1978). The results of family therapy revisited: The non-behavioral methods. Family Process 17, 251-274.

d. Group Therapy

Kolvin, I., et al. (1981). Help starts here: The maladjusted child in the ordinary school. London: Tavistock.

e. Mixed--Nonspecific

McCord, J. (1978). A thirty year treatment of follow-up effects. American Psychologist 33, 284-289.

Palmer, T. P. (1974). The youth authority's community treatment project. Federal Probation 38, 3-14.

Powers, E., & Witmer, H. (1951). An experiment in the prevention of delinquency. The Cambridge Somerville youth study. New York: Columbia University Press.

Shepherd, M., et al. (1971). Childhood behavior and mental health. London: University of London Press.

f. In Patient--Milieu Care

Gossett, J. T., et al. (1973). Follow-up of adolescents treated in a psychiatric hospital: I. A review of studies. American Journal of Orthopsychiatry 43, 602-610.

g. Parent as Therapist

Atkeson, B. M., & Forehand, R. (1979). Home-based reinforcement programs designed to modify classroom behavior: A review and methodological evaluation. Psychological Bulletin 86, 1298-1308.

Bernal, M. E., et al. (1980). Outcome evaluation of behavioral parent training and client-centered parent counseling for children with conduct problems. Journal of Applied Behavior Analysis 13, 677-691.

Firestone, P., et al. (1981). Differential effects of parent training and stimulant medication with hyperactives. Journal of the American Academy of Child Psychiatry 20, 135-147.

Frame, C. (1983). Treatment of aggressive behavior and conduct disorder. In R. J. Morris & T. R. Kratochwill (Eds.), The practice of child therapy. New York: Pergamon.

Griest, D. L., et al. (1982). Effects of parent enhancement therapy on the treatment outcome and generalization of parent training programs. Behavior Research and Therapy 20, 429-436.

Kazdin, A. E. (1984). Treatment of conduct disorders. In A. E. Kazdin (Ed.), Psychotherapy research: Where are we and where should we go? (pp. 3-28). New York: Guilford Press.

Kazdin, A. E., & Frame, C. (1983). Treatment of aggressive behavior and conduct disorder. In R. J. Morris & T. R. Kratochwill (Eds.), The practice of child therapy. New York: Pergamon.

Kolvin, I. (1981). Help starts here: The maladjusted child in the ordinary school. London: Tavistock.

Ollendick, T. H., & Cerny, J. A. (1981). Clinical behavior therapy with children. New York: Plenum Press.

Reid, W. J., & Shyne, A. W. (1969). Brief and extended casework. New York: Columbia University Press.

Reisinger, J. J., et al. (1976). Toddler management training: Generalization and marital status. Journal of Behavior Therapy and Experimental Psychiatry 7, 335-340.

Rekers, G. A. (1977). Assessment and treatment of childhood gender problems. In B. B. Lahey & A. E. Kazdin (Eds.), Advances in clinical child psychology (Vol. 1). New York: Plenum Press.

Strain, P. S. (1981). An examination of child and family demographic variables related to generalized behavior change during oppositional child training. Behavior Modification 5, 12-26.

h. In Various Settings

Bergin, A. E. (1963). The effects of psychotherapy: Negative results revisited. Journal of Counseling Psychology 10, 244-250.

DeLeon, G., & Mandell, W. (1966). A comparison of conditioning and psychotherapy in the treatment of functional enuresis. Journal of Clinical Psychology 22, 326-330.

Jesness, C. F. (1975). Comparative effectiveness of behavior modification and transactional analysis programs for delinquents. Journal of Consulting and Clinical Psychology 43, 758-779.

Miller, L. V. (1972). Comparison of reciprocal inhibition, psychotherapy and waiting list control for phobic children. Journal of Abnormal Psychology 79, 269-279.

Persons, R. (1961). Psychological and behavioral change in delinquents following psychotherapy. Journal of Clinical Psychology 22, 337-340.

Seeman, J., Barry, E., & Ellinwood, C. (1964). Interpersonal assessment of play therapy outcome. Psychotherapy: Theory, Research and Practice 1, 64-66.

Wright, D. M., Loelis, I., & Pollack, A. J. (1976). The outcome of individual child psychotherapy: Increments at follow-up. Journal of Child Psychology and Psychiatry and Allied Disciplines 17, 275-285.

5. Well-Evaluated Outcomes for Different Disorders

Adams, S. (1970). The PICO project. In N. Johnston, L. Savitz, & M. E. Wolfgang (Eds.), The sociology of punishment and correction (pp. 213-224). New York: Wiley.

Firestone, P., et al. (1981). Differential effects of parent training and stimulant medication with hyperactives. Journal of the American Academy of Child Psychiatry 20, 135-147.

Hinshaw, S. P. (1984). Self-control in hyperactive boys in anger-inducing situations: Effects of cognitive-behavioral training and of methylphenidate. Journal of Abnormal Child Psychology 12, 55-77.

Kendall, P. C. (1984). Annotation: Cognitive-behavioral self-control therapy for children. Journal of Child Psychology and Psychiatry and Allied Disciplines 25, 173-179.

Mash, E. J., & Dalby, J. T. (1979). Behavioral interventions for hyperactivity. In R. L. Trites (Ed.), Hyperactivity in children (pp. 161-216). Baltimore, Md.: University Park Press.

O'Leary, K. D., & O'Leary, S. G. (1977). Classroom management. The successful use of behavior modification. New York: Pergamon.

a. Antisocial/Aggressive Behavior

Adams, S. (1970). The PICO project. In N. Johnston, L. Savitz, & M. E. Wolfgang (Eds.), The sociology of punishment and correction (pp. 213-224). New York: Wiley.

Atkeson, B. M., & Forehand, R. (1979). Home-based reinforcement programs designed to modify classroom behavior: A review and methodological evaluation. Psychological Bulletin 86, 1298-1308.

Bernal, M. E., et al. (1980). Outcome evaluation of behavioral parent training and client-centered parent counseling for children with conduct problems. Journal of Applied Behavior Analysis 13, 677-691.

Jesness, C. F. (1975). Comparative effectiveness of behavior modification and transactional analysis programs for delinquents. Journal of Consulting and Clinical Psychology 43, 758-779.

Kazdin, A. E. (1984). Treatment of conduct disorders. In A. E. Kazdin (Ed.), Psychotherapy research: Where are we and where should we go? (pp. 3-28). New York: Guilford Press.

Kazdin, A. E., & Frame, C. (1983). Treatment of aggressive behavior and conduct disorder. In R. J. Morris & T. R. Kratochwill (Eds.), The practice of child therapy. New York: Pergamon.

McCord, J. (1978). A thirty year treatment of follow-up effects. American Psychologist 33, 284-289.

Palmer, T. B. (1974). The youth authority's community treatment project. Federal Probation 38, 3-14.

Persons, R. (1966). Psychological and behavioral change in delinquents following psychotherapy. Journal of Clinical Psychology 22, 337-340.

Powers, E., & Witmer, H. (1951). An experiment in the prevention of delinquency. The Cambridge Somerville youth study. New York: Columbia University Press.

Rutter, M., & Giller, H. (1982). Juvenile delinquency: Trends and perspective. Harmondsworth, England: Penguin.

b. Emotional/Affective Disorders

Blackburn, I. M., et al. (1981). The efficacy of cognitive therapy in depression: A treatment trial using cognitive therapy and pharmacotherapy, each alone and in combination. British Journal of Psychiatry 139, 131-189.

Borstein, M. R., Bellack, A. S., & Hersen, M. (1977). Social-skills training for unassertive children. A multiple-baseline analysis. Journal of Applied Behavior Analysis 19, 183-195.

Gelfand, D. M. (1978). Behavior treatment of avoidance, social withdrawal and negative emotional states. In B. B. Wolman, J. Egan, & A. O. Ross (Eds.), Handbook of mental disorders in childhood and adolescence. Englewood Cliffs, N.J.: Prentice Hall.

Graziano, A. M., et al. (1979). Behavior treatment of children's fears: A review. Psychological Bulletin 86, 804-830.

Hampe, E., et al. (1973). Phobic children one and two years posttreatment. Journal of Abnormal Psychiatry 82, 446-453.

Miller, L. V. (1972). Comparison of reciprocal inhibition, psychotherapy and waiting list control for phobic children. Journal of Abnormal Psychology 79, 269-279.

c. Learning Disorders

Moulin, E. K. (1970). The effects of client-centered group counseling play media on the intelligence, achievement and psycholinguistics of underachieving primary school children. Elementary School Guidance and Counseling 98, 170-186.

d. Very Young Children

Reisinger, J. J., et al. (1976). Toddler management training: Generalization and marital status. Journal of Behavior Therapy and Experimental Psychiatry 7, 335-340.

Strain, P. S. (1981). An examination of child and family demographic variables related to generalized behavior change during oppositional child training. Behavior Modification 5, 12-26.

F. Residential and Inpatient Treatment of Children

Section Editor:

Carl M. Pfeifer, M.D.
Professor of Clinical Child and Adolescent Psychiatry
University of Texas Health Science Center
President and Medical Director
Southwest Neuropsychiatric Institute
San Antonio, Texas

Associate Editors:

Charles Fischer, M.D.
Clinical Assistant Professor
University of Texas Health Science Center
San Antonio, Texas

William Harris, M.D.
Clinical Assistant Professor
University of Texas Health Science Center
San Antonio, Texas

Carlos Mocedo, M.D.
Clinical Assistant Professor
University of Texas Health Science Center
San Antonio, Texas

Graham Rogeness, M.D.
Clinical Professor
University of Texas Health Science Center
San Antonio, Texas

1. General Historic and Current References

Alt, H. (1961). Residential treatment for the disturbed child: Basic principles in planning and design of programs and facilities. New York: International Universities Press.

Bettelheim, B. (1955). Truants from life. Glencoe, Ill.: The Free Press

Bettelheim, B. (1967). The empty fortress: Infantile autism and the birth of the self. New York: The Free Press.

Bettelheim, B. (1974). A home for the heart. New York: Knopf.

Blotcky, M. J., Dimperio, T. L., & Gossett, J. T. (1984). Follow-up of children treated in psychiatric hospitals: A review of studies. American Journal of Psychiatry 141, 1499-1507.

Caudill, W. A. (1958). The psychiatric hospital as a small society. Cambridge: Harvard University Press.

D'Amato, G. (1969). Residential treatment for child mental health: Towards ego-social development and a community-child model. Springfield, Ill.: Charles C. Thomas.

Davis, M., & Raffe, I. (1982). The holding environment in the inpatient treatment of adolescents. In S. C. Feinstein, et al. (Eds.), Adolescent psychiatry: Developmental and clinical studies (pp. 434-443) . Chicago: University of Chicago Press.

Evangelakis, M. G. (1974). A manual for residential and day treatment of children. Springfield, Ill.: Charles C. Thomas.

Gossett, J. T., Lewis, J. M., & Barnhart, F. D. (1983). To find a way: The outcome of hospital treatment of disturbed adolescents. New York: Brunner/Mazel.

Grace, H. (1974). The development of a child psychiatric treatment program. New York: Schenkman Publishing.

Jones, M. S., et al. (1953). The therapeutic community. New York: Basic Books.

Kashani, J. H., Daniel, A. E., Reid, J. C., & Sirinek, A. J. (1984). Comparison of delinquent boys and girls in group homes and factors associated with the outcome. British Journal of Psychiatry 144, 156-160.

Kettlewell, P. W., & Kausch, D. F. (1983). The generalization of the effects of cognitive-behavioral treatment program for aggressive children. Journal of Abnormal Psychology 11, 101-114.

Lennhoff, F. G. (1966). Exceptional children: Residential treatment of emotionally disturbed boys at Shotton Hall (2nd ed.). London: Allen & Unwin.

Lewis, M. (1980). The undoing of residential treatment: A follow-up study of 51 adolescents. Journal of the American Academy of Child Psychiatry 19, 160-171.

Mansheim, P. (1982). A comparison of two models of education in residential treatment. Hospital and Community Psychiatry 33, 844-845.

Martin, L. H. (1976). The uses of residential care. Child Welfare 55, 269-278.

Montalvo, B., & Pavlin, S. (1966). Faulty staff communications in a residential treatment center. American Journal of Orthopsychiatry 36, 706-711.

Polsky, H. W. (1962). Cottage six: The social system of delinquent boys in residential treatment. New York: Russell Sage Foundation.

Rae-Grant, Q., & Moffat, P. J. (1971). Children in Canada residential care. Toronto: Leonard Crainford.

Redl, F. (1959). The concept of a "therapeutic milieu." American Journal of Orthopsychiatry 29, 731-736.

Redl, F., & Wineman, D. (1951). Children who hate. Glencoe, Ill.: The Free Press.

Redl, F., & Wineman, D. (1952). Controls from within. Glencoe, Ill.: The Free Press.

Robertson, J. (1970). Young children in hospitals (2nd ed.). London: Tavistock.

Rubenstein, J. S., Armentrout, J. A., Levin, S., & Herald, D. (1978). The parent-therapist program: Alternate care for emotionally disturbed children. American Journal of Orthopsychiatry 48, 654-662.

Stanton, A. H., & Schwartz, M. S. (1954). The mental hospital. New York: Basic Books.

Szurek, S. A., Berlin, I. N., & Boatman, M. J. (Eds.). (1971). Inpatient care for the psychotic child. Palo Alto: Science and Behavior Books.

Weber, G. H., & Haberlein, B. J. (1972). Residential treatment of emotionally disturbed children. New York: Behavioral Publications.

Zimet, S. G., & Farley, G. K. (1985). Day treatment for children in the United States. Journal of the American Academy of Child Psychiatry 224(6), 732-738.

2. Special Issues in Residential and Inpatient Treatment

Aarkrog, T., Lauritsen, S., Mortensen, K. V., & Strom, J. (1979). Adolescents in psychiatric residential treatment and 5 years later. Acta Psychiatrica Scandinavica (Supplement) 79, 214-218.

Abruzzi, W. (1975). Severe personality disorders in an institutional setting. American Journal of Psychoanalysis 35, 269-277.

Adessa, S., & Laatsch, A. (1965a). Extended residential treatment: Eighty-year anxiety. Social Work 10(4), 16-24.

Adessa, S., & Laatsch, A. (1965b). Therapeutic use of visiting in residential treatment. Child Welfare 44, 245-251.

Alderton, H. R. (1965). Communication, learning and therapeutic process in a children's psychiatric hospital. Canadian Psychiatric Association Journal 10(5), 338-349.

Alt, H. (1953). Symposium, 1953. The education of emotionally disturbed children. II. Responsibilities and qualifications of the child care worker. American Journal of Orthopsychiatry 23, 670-675.

Amanat, E., & Tryniechi, T. (1979). Therapeutic adaptive behavior in residential treatment. Child Psychiatry and Human Development 9, 238-249.

Apter, A., Bleich, A., Plutchik, R., Mendelsohn, S., & Tyano, S. (1988). Suicidal behavior, depression and conduct disorder in hospitalized adolescents. Journal of the American Academy of Child and Adolescent Psychiatry 27(6), 696-699.

Astrachan, M. (1975). The five-day week: An alternate model in residential treatment centers. Child Welfare 54, 21-26.

Astrachan, M., & Harris, D. M. (1983). Weekend only: An alternate model in residential treatment centers. Child Welfare 62, 253-261.

Bardill, D. R. (1977). A behavior-contracting program of group treatment for early adolescents in a residential treatment setting. International Journal of Group Psychotherapy 27, 389-400.

Bartelt, R. F., & Collon, I. (1982). Implementation of goal attainment scaling in residential treatment: An administrative model. Child Welfare 61, 424-434.

Baxter, M. J. (1963). House council--an integral part of residential treatment for disturbed children. Catholic Charities Review 47(5), 13-19.

Beckham, C. O., Johnston, L., & Beckham, E. (1979). Sex education for children in a residential center. Child Welfare 58, 393-402.

Behar, L., & Stephens, D. (1978). Wilderness camping: An evaluation of a residential program for emotionally disturbed children. American Journal of Orthopsychiatry 48, 644-653.

Behrens, M. L., & Goldfarb, W. (1958). A study of patterns of interaction of families of schizophrenic children in residential treatment. American Journal of Orthopsychiatry 28, 300-312.

Bell, C. R., Mundy, P., & Quay, H. C. (1983). Modifying impulsive responding in conduct-disordered institutionalized boys. Psychological Reports 52, 307-310.

Benedek, E. P., & Salguero, R. (1973). A summer day treatment service program. Journal of the American Academy of Child Psychiatry 12, 724-737.

Benjamin, A., & Weatherly, H. E. (1947). Hospital ward treatment of emotionally disturbed children. American Journal of Orthopsychiatry 17, 665-674.

Berman, S. P. (1961). Some lessons learned in developing a residential treatment center. Child Welfare 40(4), 12-18.

Bettelheim, B., & Sylvester, E. (1947). Therapeutic influence of the group on the individual. American Journal of Orthopsychiatry 17, 684-692.

Blew, P. A., Schwartz, I. S., & Luce, S. C. (1985). Teaching functional community skills to autistic children using nonhandicapped peer tutors. Journal of Applied Behavior Analysis 18, 342-373.

Blotcky, M. J., Dimperio, T. L., & Gossett, J. T. (1984). Follow-up of children treated in psychiatric hospitals. American Journal of Psychiatry 141, 499-507.

Boatman, M. J., Paynter, J., & Parsons, C. (1962). Nursing in the psychiatric treatment of children--panel, 1961. III. Nursing in hospital psychiatric therapy for psychotic children. American Journal of Orthopsychiatry 32, 808-817.

Bond, T. C., & Auger, N. (1982). Benefits of the generic milieu in adolescent hospital treatment. In S. C. Feinstein, et al. (Eds.), Adolescent psychiatry: Developmental and clinical studies (pp. 360-372). Chicago: University of Chicago Press.

Bonier, R. J. (1982). Staff countertransference in an adolescent milieu. In S. C. Feinstein, et al. (Eds.), Adolescent psychiatry: Developmental and clinical studies (pp. 382-390). Chicago: University of Chicago Press.

Bowers, S. (1957). The social worker in a children's residential treatment program. Social Casework 38, 283-288.

Burton, A. C., Wallerstein, J., & Bernard, V. W. (1949). Dosoris--an experimental study and treatment home for adolescent girls. American Journal of Orthopsychiatry 19, 683-696.

Cawson, P. (1985). Intermediate care. Journal of Child Psychology and Psychiatry 26, 675-681.

Christ, A. E., & Wagner, N. N. (1965). Residential treatment. Iatrogenic factors in residential treatment: The psychiatric team's contribution to continues psychopathology. American Journal of Orthopsychiatry 35, 253-254.

Churven, P., & Cintio, B. (1983). An application of strategic family therapy to a residential child family psychiatry services.: Redbank House. Australian and New Zealand Journal of Psychiatry 17, 191-195.

Clifford, M., & Cross, T. (1980). Group therapy for seriously disturbed boys in residential treatment. Child Welfare 59, 560-565.

Cohen, R. L., Charney, I. W., & Lembke, P. (1961). Parental expectations as a force in treatment: The identification of unconscious parental projections onto the children's psychiatric hospital. Archives of General Psychiatry 4, 471-478.

Corboz, R. J., & Merz-Ammann, D. (1978). New experiences and thoughts on in-patient psychotherapy. Acta Paedopsychiatrica 43, 101-111.

Corder, B. F., Whiteside, R., Silverstein, E. M., & Rieder, M. J. (1984). Legal issues affecting residential child care workers. Child Welfare 63, 217-224.

Crespi, T. D. (1988). Effectiveness of time-out: A comparison of psychiatric, correctional and day-treatment programs. Adolescence 23(92), 805-811.

Davids, A. (1975). Therapeutic approaches to children in residential treatment. Changes from the mid-1950s to the mid-1979s. American Psychologist 30, 809-814.

Davids, A., & Salvatore, P. D. (1976). Residential treatment of disturbed children and adequacy of their subsequent adjustment: A follow-up study. American Journal of Orthopsychiatry 46, 62-73.

Davis, M., & Raffe, I. (1985). The holding environment in the inpatient treatment of adolescents. In S. C. Feinstein, et al. (Eds.), Adolescent psychiatry: Developmental and clinical studies (pp. 434-443). Chicago: University of Chicago Press.

DeLeon, G. (1988). The therapeutic community perspective and approach for adolescent substance abuse. In S. C. Feinstein, et al. (Eds.), Adolescent psychiatry: Developmental and clinical studies (Vol. 15, pp. 535-556). Chicago: University of Chicago Press.

Delga, I., Heinssan, R. K., Fritsch, R. C., Goodrich, W., & Yates, B. T. (1989). Psychosis, aggression, and self-destructive behavior in hospitalized adolescents. American Journal of Psychiatry 146(4), 520-525.

Denkowski, G. (1984). A residential treatment model for MR adolescent offenders. Hospital and Community Psychiatry 35(3), 279-281.

Dietzsch, S. (1978). Activity of the psychologist within the inpatient psychotherapy of behavior disordered children. and adolescents. Psychiatrie, Neurologie und Medizinische Psychologie 30, 673-678.

Dinwiddie, F. W. (1975). Humanistic behaviorism: A model for rapprochement in residential treatment milieus. Child Psychiatry and Human Development 5, 254-259.

Dittmann, A. T. (1958). Problems of reliability in observing and coding social interactions. Journal of Consulting Psychology 22, 430.

Dittman, A. T., & Kitchener, H. L. (1959). The life space interview. Workshop 1957. II. Life space interviewing and individual play therapy: A comparison of techniques. American Journal of Orthopsychiatry 29, 19-26.

Douglas, K. B. (1961). The teacher's role in a children's psychiatric hospital unit. Exceptional Children 27, 246-251.

Dowling, S. (1975). Treatment in cottage programs for children. with severe development disturbances. Child Welfare 54, 395-405.

Edelman, A. M. (1953). Some observations on occupational therapy with disturbed children. in a residential program. American Journal of Occupational Therapy 7, 113-117.

Ekstein, R. (1954). Round table: Child schizophrenia. The space child's time machine: On "reconstruction" in the psychotherapeutic treatment of a schizophrenoid child. American Journal of Orthopsychiatry 24, 492-506.

Escalona, S. K. (1948). Some considerations regarding psychotherapy with psychotic children. Bulletin of the Menninger Clinic 12, 126-134.

Feldman, R. A., Wodarski, J. S., & Flax, N. (1975). Antisocial children in a summer camp environment: A time-sampling study. Community Mental Health Journal 11, 10-18.

Fenichel, C., Freedman, A. M., & Klapper, Z. (1960). A day school for schizophrenic children. American Journal of Orthopsychiatry 30, 130-143.

Fildes, L. G. (1944). Hostels for children in need of psychiatric attention. Mental Health (London) 5, 31-41.

Finkelstein, H. (1964). The use of court commitment in the residential treatment of disturbed children. Social Casework 45, 605-609.

Finkelstein, N. E. (1974). Family participation in residential treatment. Child Welfare 53, 570-575.

Fochios, S. E. (1965). The use of families and family members as therapeutic levers in the treatment of disturbed delinquent children. Child Welfare 44, 556-562.

Force, R. C., & Sebree, J. (1985). The validation of outcomes predictors used in the admission decision at the St. Francis Boys' Homes. QRB. Quality Review Bulletin 11, 266-270.

Fraiberg, S. (1956). Some aspects of residential casework with children. Social Casework 37, 159-167.

Friedman, S., Rogers, P. P., & Gettys, J. (1975). Project re-ed: Increase in self-esteem as measured by the Coopersmith inventory. Perceptual and Motor Skills 40, 165-166.

Fullerton, C., Goodrich, W., & Berman, L. (1986). Adoption predicts psychiatric treatment resistances in hospitalized adolescents. Journal of the American Academy of Child Psychiatry 25(4), 542-551.

Gair, D. S. (1980). Limit-setting and seclusion in the psychiatric hospital. Psychiatric Opinion 43, 15-19.

Garrison, W. T. (1984). Aggressive behavior, seclusion and physical restraint in an inpatient child population. Journal of the American Academy of Child Psychiatry 23(4), 448-452.

Gerard, M. W., & Overstreet, H. M. (1953). Technical modification in the treatment of a schizoid boy within a treatment institution. American Journal of Orthopsychiatry 23, 171-185.

Geraty, R. (1989). Administrative issues in inpatient child and adolescent psychiatry. Journal of the American Academy of Child and Adolescent Psychiatry 28(1), 21-25.

Ghuman, H. S., & Sarles, R. (1988). Three group psychotherapy settings with long-term adolescent inpatients: Advantages and disadvantages. Psychiatric Hospital 19(4), 161-164.

Goldfarb, W., Goldfarb, N., & Pollack, R. C. (1966). Treatment of childhood schizophrenia. Archives of General Psychiatry 14, 119-128.

Goldfine, P. E., Heath, G. A., Hardesty, V. A., Berman, H. J., Gordon, B. J., & Lind, N. W. (1985). Alternatives to psychiatric hospitalization for children. Psychiatric Clinics of North America 8, 527-535.

Goldstein, I. M., Judas, I., Sutton, H. A., & Falstein, E. I. (1957). Adjustment patterns of leadership and defenses in a disturbed child group. Archives of Neurology and Psychiatry 77, 312-317.

Goocher, B. E. (1975). Behavioral applications of an educateur model in child care. Child Care Quarterly 4(2), 84-92.

Goodman, E. O. (1975). Behavior modification as a therapeutic technique for use with parents of emotionally disturbed children in residential treatment. Child Psychiatry and Human Development 6, 38-46.

Gossett, J. T. (1982). Adolescent inpatient treatment "failures": Subtypes and treatment implications. National Association of Public Psychiatric Hospitals Journal 13(1), 5-8.

Gossett, J. T., Lewis, J. M., & Phillips, V. A. (1973). Follow-up of adolescents treated in a psychiatric hospital: I. A review of studies. American Journal of Orthopsychiatry 43(4), 602-610.

Green, W. (1986). Child psychiatric discharges against medical advice. Journal of the American Academy of Child Psychiatry 25(2), 260-265.

Greenwood, E. D. (1955). The role of residential treatment for children. Symposium, 1954. VI. The role of psychotherapy in residential treatment. American Journal of Orthopsychiatry 25, 692-698.

Grenier, C. (1985). Treatment effectiveness in an adolescent chemical dependency treatment: A quasi-experimental design. International Journal of the Addictions 20, 381-391.

Gugelmann, A. (1977). Promotion of behavior disturbed children at the home for children. Sozial und Praventivmedizin 22, 60-61.

Gula, M. (1964). Group homes--new and differentiated tools in child welfare, delinquency, and mental health. Child Welfare 43, 393-397.

Gunning, S. V., & Holmes, T. H. (1973). Dance therapy with psychotic children.: Definition and quantitative evaluation. Archives of General Psychiatry 28, 707-713.

Harper, G. (1989). Focal inpatient treatment planning. Journal of the American Academy of Child and Adolescent Psychiatry 28(1), 31-37.

Henry, J. (1957). Types of institutional structure. Psychiatry 20, 47-60.

Herstein, H. (1977). Reflections on the primacy of the one-to-one model in residential treatment. Child Welfare 56, 311-320.

Heying, K. R. (1985). Family-based, in-home services for the severely emotionally disturbed child. Child Welfare 64, 519-527.

Hirschberg, J. C., & Mandelbaum, A. (1957). Problems of administration and supervision in an inpatient treatment center for children. Bulletin of the Menninger Clinic 21, 208-219.

Hughes, H. M. (1979). Behavioral change in children at a therapeutic summer camp as a function of feedback and individual versus group contingencies. Journal of Abnormal Child Psychology 7, 211-219.

Institutions without walls for emotionally disturbed children. Chedoke Child and Family Centre, Hamilton, Ontario. (1977). Hospital and Community Psychiatry 28, 849-851.

Jemerin, J. M., & Philips, I. (1988). Changes in inpatient child psychiatry: Consequences and recommendations. Journal of the American Academy of Child Psychiatry 27(4), 397-403.

Johnson, J. L., & Rubin, E. Z. (1964). A school follow-up study of children discharged from a psychiatric hospital. Exceptional Children 31, 19-24.

Jungjohann, E. E., & Beck, B. (1984). Catamnestic results from the total group of patients in a regional child psychiatric treatment center (1975-1980). Praxis der Kinderpsychologie und Kinderpsychiatrie 33, 148-154.

Kammerer, E., Gruneberg, B., & Goebel, D. (1984). Inpatient child psychiatric therapy from the parents' viewpoint. Praxis der Kinderpsychologie und Kinderpsychiatrie 33, 141-148.

Kane, R. P., & Chambers, G. (1961). Improvement--real or apparent? A seven year follow-up of children hospitalized and discharged from a residential setting. American Journal of Psychiatry 117, 1023-1027.

Kashani, J. H., Daniel, A. E., Reid, J. C., & Sirinek, A. J. (1984). Comparison of delinquent boys and girls in group homes and factors associated with the outcome. British Journal of Psychiatry 144, 156-160.

Kazdin, A. E. (1982). The token economy: A decade later. Journal of Applied Behavior Analysis 15, 431-445.

Kazdin, A. E., Esveldt-Dawson, K., Unis, A. S., & Rancurello, M. D. (1983). Child and parent evaluations of depression and aggression in psychiatric inpatient children. Journal of Abnormal Child Psychology 11, 401-413.

Kazdin, A. E., French, N. H., & Sherick, R. B. (1981). Acceptability of alternative treatments for children: Evaluations by inpatient children, parents, and staff. Journal of Consulting and Clinical Psychology 49, 900-907.

Kettlewell, P. W., & Kausch, D. F. (1983). The generalization of the effects of a cognitive-behavioral treatment program for aggressive children. Journal of Abnormal Child Psychology 11, 101-114.

King, J. W., & Meeks, J. E. (1988). Hospital programs for psychiatrically disturbed, drug-abusing adolescents. In S. C. Feinstein, et al. (Eds.), Adolescent psychiatry: Developmental and clinical studies (Vol. 15, pp. 522-534). Chicago: University of Chicago Press.

Klicpera, C., & Heyse, I. (1981). The effect of a minor brain dysfunction on the expression and long-term development of behavior disorders in children. Acta Paedopsychiatr 47, 9-18.

Kogler, M. (1982). Integrated psychotherapy in inpatient child psychiatry--experiences with the therapeutic team. Praxis der Kinderpsychologie und Kinderpsychiatrie 31, 41-47.

Kogler, M., & Leipersberg, H. (1985). Integrated psychotherapy in inpatient child and adolescent psychiatry--the significance of group meetings. Praxis der Kinderpsychologie und Kinderpsychiatrie 34, 9-15.

Kolb, J. E., & Shapiro, E. R. (1982). Management of separation issues with the family of the hospitalized adolescent. In S. C. Feinstein, et al. (Eds.), Adolescent psychiatry: Developmental and clinical studies (pp. 343-359). Chicago: University of Chicago Press.

Koret, S. (1980). Follow-up study on residential treatment of children, ages six through twelve. National Association of Public Psychiatric Hospitals Journal 11(3), 43-47.

Krenk, C. J. (1984). Training staff for child abuse treatment. Child Welfare 63, 167-173.

Krueger, M. A. (1974). A child care treatment plan for the self-development of emotionally disturbed children. Child Care Quarterly 3(1), 31-38.

Krueger, M. A. (1977). The 'program day' as school day in residential treatment. Child Welfare 56, 271-278.

Krug, O. (1952). The application of principles of child psychotherapy in residential treatment. American Journal of Psychiatry 108, 695-700.

Labarbera, J. D., Martin, J. E., & Dozier, J. E. (1982). Residential treatment of males: The influential role of parental attitudes. Journal of the American Academy of Child Psychiatry 21, 286-290.

LaVietes, R. L., Cohen, R., Reens, R., & Ronall, R. (1965). Day treatment center and school: Seven years experience. American Journal of Orthopsychiatry 35, 160-169.

LaVietes, R. L., Hulse, W. C., & Blau, A. (1960). A psychiatric day treatment center and school for young children and their parents. American Journal of Orthopsychiatry 30, 468-482.

Laybourne, P. C., & Miller, H. C. (1962). Pediatric hospitalization of psychiatric patients: Diagnostic and therapeutic implications. American Journal of Orthopsychiatry 32, 596-603.

Levy, E. Z. (1967). The importance of the children's needs in residential treatment. Bulletin of the Menninger Clinic 31(1), 18-31.

Levy, E. Z. (1969a). Long-term follow-up of former inpatients at the Children's Hospital of the Menninger Clinic. American Journal of Psychiatry 125(12), 47-53.

Levy, E. Z. (1969b). On the residential treatment of adolescent girls. Seminars in Psychiatry 1(1), 3-14.

Levy, M. M. (1950). Outdoor group therapy with preadolescent boys. Psychiatry 13, 333-347.

Lewis, M., & Brown, T. E. (1979). Psychotherapy in the residential treatment of the borderline child. Child Psychiatry and Human Development 9, 181-188.

Lewis, M., Lewis, D. O., Shanok, E., Klatskin, E., & Osborne, J. R. (1980). The undoing of residential treatment: A follow-up study of 51 adolescents. Journal of the American Academy of Child Psychiatry 19, 160-171.

Maier, H. W. (1975). Learning to learn and living to live in residential treatment. Child Welfare 54, 405-420.

Maier, H. W., Hilgeman, L. M., Shugart, G., & Loomis, E. A. (1955). The role of residential treatment for children. Symposium, 1954. VII. Supervision of child care workers in a residential treatment service. American Journal of Orthopsychiatry 25, 699-704.

Mansheim, P. (1982). A comparison of two models of education in residential treatment. Hospital and Community Psychiatry 33, 844-845.

Margolis, J. A., McDermott, J. F., & Vaughan, W. T. (1984). Residential treatment centers: Peer review by APA and CHAMPUS. Hospital and Community Psychiatry 35, 482-486.

Marohn, R. C., Dalle-Molle, D., Offer, D., & Ostrov, E. (1973). A hospital riot: Its determinants and implications for treatment. American Journal of Psychiatry 130(6), 631-635.

Martin, L. H., Pozdnjakoff, I., & Wilding, J. (1976). The uses of residential care. Child Welfare 55, 269-278.

Matsushima, J. (1979). Outcomes of residential treatment: Designing accountability protocols. Child Welfare 58, 303-318.

McConville, B. J., & Purohit, A. P. (1973). Classifying confusion: A study of results of inpatient treatment in a multidisciplinary children's center. American Journal of Orthopsychiatry 43, 411-417.

McManus, M. (1984). Assessment of borderline symptomatology in hospitalized adolescents. Journal of the American Academy of Child Psychiatry 23(6), 685-694.

McNeil, E., & Cohler, R. (1958). Adult aggression in the management of disturbed children. Child Development 29, 451-461.

McNeil, E. B., & Morse, W. C. (1964). The institutional management of sex in emotionally disturbed children. American Journal of Orthopsychiatry 34, 115-124.

Meeks, J. (1985). Inpatient treatment of the violent adolescent.In S. C. Feinstein, et al. (Eds.), Adolescent psychiatry: Developmental and clinical studies (pp. 393-405). Chicago: University of Chicago Press.

Meeks, J. E. (1980-1981). What did the therapists say? What did the therapists do? International Journal of Psychoanalytic Psychotherapy 8, 233-241.

Middleman, R., & Seever, F. (1963). Short-term camping for boys with behavior problems. Social Work 8(2), 88-95.

Miller, D., Walker, M. C., & Friedman, D. (1989). Use of a holding technique to control the violent behavior of seriously disturbed adolescents. Hospital and Community Psychiatry 40(5), 520-524.

Millman, H. L., & Schaefer, C. E. (1975). Behavioral change: Program evaluation and staff feedback. Child Welfare 54, 692-702.

Montalvo, B., & Pavlin, S. (1966). Faulty staff communications in a residential treatment center. American Journal of Orthopsychiatry 36, 706-711.

Mordock, J. B. (1979). Evaluation in residential treatment: The conceptual dilemmas. Child Welfare 58, 293-302.

Muir, B. J. (1986). The development of personal individuality: Limited treatment goals in a psychoanalytic hospital. In S. C. Feinstein, et al. (Eds.), Adolescent psychiatry: Developmental and clinical studies (pp. 510-523). Chicago: University of Chicago Press.

Naughton, F. X. (1957). Foster home placement as an adjunct to residential treatment. Social Casework 38, 288-295.

Newman, R. (1960). The way back: Extramural schooling as a transitional phase for residential therapy. American Journal of Orthopsychiatry 30, 588-598.

Newman, R. G. (1959). The assessment of progress in the treatment of hyperaggressive children with learning disturbances within a school setting. American Journal of Orthopsychiatry 29, 633-643.

Noshpitz, J. D. (1957). Opening phase in the psychotherapy of adolescents with character disorders. Bulletin of the Menninger Clinic 21, 153-164.

Noshpitz, J. D. (1962). Notes on the theory of residential treatment. Journal of the American Academy of Child Psychiatry 1(2), 284-296.

Nurcombe, B. (1989). Goad-directed treatment planning and the principles of brief hospitalization. Journal of the American Academy of Child and Adolescent Psychiatry 28(1), 26-30.

Offer, D., & Barglow, P. (1960). Adolescent and young adult self-mutilation incidents in a general psychiatric hospital. Archives of General Psychiatry 3, 194-204.

Olds, J. (1982). The treatment of adolescents in a milieu including younger children. In S. C. Feinstein, et al. (Eds.), Adolescent psychiatry: Developmental and clinical studies (pp. 373-381). Chicago: University of Chicago Press.

Perkins, M. J., & Hornsby, L. G. (1984). Common countertransference issues related to inpatient/residential psychiatric treatment of children. The psychiatric hospital. National Association of Public Psychiatric Hospitals Journal 15(2), 65-74.

Perkowski, S. (1974). Some observations concerning black children living in a residential care agency. International Journal of Social Psychiatry 20, 89-93.

Peshkin, M. M., & Friedman, I. (1975). Residential asthma treatment centers in the United States and problems in relation to them. Journal of Asthma Research 12, 129-175.

Petti, T., & Law, W. (1982). Borderline psychiatry behavior in hospitalized children: Approaches to assessment and treatment. Journal of the American Academy of Child Psychiatry 21(2), 197-202.

Pfeffer, C. (1985). Variables that predict assaultiveness in child psychiatric inpatients. Journal of the American Academy of Child Psychiatry 24(6), 775-780.

Pfeffer, C. R., Newcorn, J., Kaplan, G., Mizruchi, M., & Plutchik, R. (1988). Suicidal behavior in adolescent psychiatric inpatients. Journal of the American Academy of Child and Adolescent Psychiatry 27(3), 357-361.

Pfeiffer, S. I. (1989). Follow-up of children and adolescents treated in psychiatric facilities: A methodology review. Psychiatric Hospital 20(1), 15-20.

Phelan, J. F. (1959). The role of the volunteer in a residential treatment school. Federal Probation 23(3), 13-20.

Pollack, M., & Goldfarb, W. (1957). Patterns of orientation in children in residential treatment for severe behavior disorders. American Journal of Orthopsychiatry 27, 538-552.

Purcell, M. (1979). Foster grandparents in a residential treatment center. Child Welfare 58, 409-411.

Rabkin, L., Weinberger, G., & Klein, A. (1966). What made Allen run? The process of communication in residential treatment. Journal of the American Academy of Child Psychiatry 5, 272-283.

Raubolt, R. R. (1983). Treating children in residential group psychotherapy. Child Welfare 62, 147-155.

Razy, V. (1961). The value of dance and percussion in the treatment of emotionally disturbed children. Social Casework 42, 501-505.

Reardon, D. F., Butler, K., & Warshaw, K. (1978). The effect of an unlocked door in adolescent runaway and aggression. Journal of the American Academy of Child Psychiatry 17, 372-382.

Redl, F. (1949). New ways of ego support in residential treatment of disturbed children. Bulletin of the Menninger Clinic 13, 60-66.

Redl, F. (1959a). The concept of a "therapeutic milieu." American Journal of Orthopsychiatry 29(4), 1-14.

Redl, F. (1959b). The concept of a "therapeutic milieu." American Journal of Orthopsychiatry 29, 721-736.

Redl, F. (1959c). The life space interview. American Journal of Orthopsychiatry 29(1), 1-18.

Reuter, J., Archer, F. M., Dunn, V., & White, C. (1980). Social milieu of a residential treatment center for severely or profoundly handicapped young children. American Journal of Mental Deficiency 84, 367-372.

Richards, W., Church, J. A., Roberts, M. J., Newman, L. J., & Garon, M. R. (1981). A self-help program for childhood asthma in a residential treatment center. Clinical Pediatrics 20, 453-457.

Rindfleisch, N., & Rabb, J. (1984). Dilemmas in planning for the protection of children and youths in residential facilities. Child Welfare 63, 205-215.

Robinson, J. F. (1949). The role of the resident professional worker. American Journal of Orthopsychiatry 19, 674-782.

Rogeness, G. A., Hoppe, S. K., Macedo, C. A., Fischer, C., & Harris, W. R. (1988). Psychopathology in hospitalized, adopted children. Journal of the American Academy of Child and Adolescent Psychiatry 27(5), 628-631.

Rogeness, G. A., & Stewart, J. T. (1978). A positive group: A therapeutic technique in the hospital treatment of adolescents. Hospital and Community Psychiatry 29(8), 520-522.

Ross, A. L. (1983). Mitigating turnover of child care staff in group care facilities. Child Welfare 62, 63-67.

Ross, A. L., & Schreiber, L. J. (1975). Bellefaire's day treatment program: An interdisciplinary approach to the emotionally disturbed child. Child Welfare 54, 183-194.

Roth, R. (1977). A transactional analysis group in residential treatment of adolescents. Child Welfare 56, 776-786.

Ro-Trock, G. K., Wellisch, D. K., & Schooler, J. C. (1977). A family therapy outcome study in an inpatient setting. American Journal of Orthopsychiatry 47(3), 514-522.

Sanders, J. (1985). Principles of residential treatment: Staff growth and therapeutic interaction. In S. C. Feinstein, et al. (Eds.), Adolescent psychiatry: Developmental and clinical studies (pp. 361-370). Chicago: University of Chicago Press.

Scallon, R. J., Vitale, J., & Eschenauer, R. (1976). Behavior modification in a residence and school for adolescent boys: A team approach. Child Welfare 55, 561-571.

Schain, R. J., Gardella, D., & Pon, J. (1982). Five year outcome of children admitted to a state mental hospital. Hospital and Community Psychiatry 33, 847-848.

Schrager, J. (1954). A focus for supervision of residential staff in a treatment institution. Bulletin of the Menninger Clinic 18, 64-71.

Scofield, J. B. (1962). Adolescent treatment in an adult hospital. American Journal of Orthopsychiatry 32, 660-668.

Seidl, F. W. (1974). Community oriented residential care: The state of the art. Child Care Quarterly 3(3), 150-163.

Shafii, M., McCue, A., Ice, J. F., & Schwab, J. J. (1979). The development of an acute short-term inpatient child psychiatric setting: A pediatric-psychiatric model. Journal of the American Psychiatric Association 136(4A), 427-429.

Shanok, S. (1983). A comparison of delinquent and nondelinquent adolescent psychiatric inpatients. American Journal of Psychiatry 140(5), 182-185.

Sheimo, S. L. (1949). Problems encountered in dealing with handicapped and emotionally disturbed children. American Journal of Occupational Therapy 3, 303-307.

Sheimo, S. L., Paynter, J., & Szurek, S. A. (1949). Problems of staff interaction with spontaneous group formations on a children's psychiatric ward. American Journal of Orthopsychiatry 19, 599-611.

Shields, J. D., & Choras, P. T. (1982). Treatment of the hospitalized adolescent: Management of regression during discharge. In S. C. Feinstein, et al. (Eds.), Adolescent psychiatry: Developmental and clinical studies (pp. 407-424). Chicago: University of Chicago Press.

Stewart, K. K., & Axelrod, P. L. (1947). Group therapy on a children's psychiatric ward: Experiment combining group therapy with individual therapy and residential treatment. American Journal of Orthopsychiatry 17, 312-325.

Sutton, H. A. (1947). Some nursing aspects of a children's psychiatric ward. American Journal of Orthopsychiatry 17, 675-683.

Szurek, S. A. (1947). Dynamics of staff interaction in hospital psychiatric treatment of children. American Journal of Orthopsychiatry 17, 652-664.

Toigo, R. (1972). The dynamics of the juvenile institution: A systems theory approach. Child Care Quarterly 1(4), 252-263.

Ware, L. M., & Levy, E. Z. (1969). "The Meeting": A step toward a therapeutic community in an adolescent unit. Bulletin of the Menninger Clinic 33(6), 352-363.

Weathers, O. D., & Bullock, S. C. (1978). Therapeutic group home care for adolescent girls: An interagency development. Journal of the National Medical Association 70, 331-334.

Weinstock, A. (1979). Group treatment of characterologically damaged, developmentally disabled adolescents in a residential treatment center. International Journal of Group Psychotherapy 29, 369-381.

Wenar, C. (1957). The therapeutic value of setting limits with inhibited children. Journal of Nervous and Mental Disease 125, 390-395.

Whiles, W. H. (1955). Treatment of maladjusted children in hostels. Journal of Mental Science 101, 404-412.

Whitaker, C. A. (1946). Ormsby Village: An experiment in forced psychotherapy in the rehabilitation of the delinquent adolescent. Psychiatry 9, 239-250.

Williams, J. M. (1961). Children who break down foster homes: A psychological study of patterns of personality growth in grossly deprived children. Journal of Child Psychology and Psychiatry and Allied Disciplines 2, 5-20.

Wilson, P. (1977). The referral of nursery school children for treatment. In A. Solnit, et al. (Eds.), Psychoanalytic study of the child (Vol. 32, pp. 479-502). New Haven: Yale University Press.

Wineman, D. (1959). The life-space interview. Social Work 4(1), 3-17.
Winnicott, D. W. (1948). Children's hostels in war and peace. Journal of Medical Psychology 21, 175-180.
Wise, L. J. (1953). Residential treatment of a ten-year-old boy: Problems in the differential diagnosis and treatment of marked destructive behavior. Workshop 1952. In G. E. Gardner (Ed.), Case studies in childhood emotional disabilities (pp. 331-368). New York: American Orthopsychiatric Association.
Woolston, J. L. (1989). Transactional risk model for short and intermediate term psychiatric inpatient treatment of children. Journal of the American Academy of Child and Adolescent Psychiatry 28(1), 38-41.
Wynne, M. E., & Rogers, J. J. (1985). Variables discriminating residential placemnt of severely handicapped children. American Journal of Mental Deficiency 89, 515-523.
Zellner, S. K. (1955). Recreational therapy experiences with mentally ill children. Mental Hospitals 6(4), 4-5.
Zinn, L. D., & Miller, D. H. (1978). Riots on adolescent inpatient units. National Association of Public Psychiatric Hospitals Journal 9(3), 43-51.

G. Pediatric Consultation and Liaison

Section Co-Editors:

Joseph Fischoff, M.D.
Professor of Psychiatry and Pediatrics
Wayne State University School of Medicine
Detroit, Michigan

Gregory Fritz, M.D.
Associate Professor, Psychiatry and Pediatrics
Division of Child Psychiatry
Brown University School of Medicine
Providence, Rhode Island

1. Pediatric Consultation and Liaison Service

Ahsanuddin, K. M., & Adams, J. E. (1982). Setting up a pediatric consultation-liaison service. Psychiatric Clinics of North America 5, 259-270.
Awad, G. A., & Poznanski, E. O. (1975). Psychiatric consultations in a pediatric hospital. American Journal of Psychiatry 132, 915-918.
Bergman, A. S., & Fritz, G. K. (1981). Psychiatric and social work collaboration in pediatric chronic illness hospital. Social Work in Health Care 7, 45-55.
Brown, A. L., Brierley, E., & Rivlin, E. (1986). General practitioner referrals to a clinical child psychologist. British Medical Journal 292, 1241-1243.
Christophersen, E. R. (1982). Incorporating behavioral pediatrics into primary care. Pediatric Clinics of North America 29, 261-296.

Friedman, S. B. (1985). Behavioral pediatrics: Interaction with other disciplines. Journal of Developmental and Behavioral Pediatrics 6, 202-214.

Froese, A. P. (1977-1978). Pediatric referrals to psychiatry: III. Is the psychiatrist's opinion heard? International Journal of Psychiatry and Medicine 8, 295-301.

Froese, A. P., Kamin, L. E., & Levine, C. A. (1976-1977). Teamwork: A multidisciplinary pediatric-liaison service. International Journal of Psychiatry and Medicine 7, 47-56.

Geist, R. A. (1977). Consultation on a pediatric surgical work: Creating an empathic climate. American Journal of Orthopsychiatry 47, 432-444.

Greenberg, L. W., & Rice, H. W. (1980). A pediatric-child-psychiatry liaison program in a community hospital. Journal of Medical Education 55, 112-119.

Jellinek, M. S., Herzog, D. B., & Selter, L. F. (1981). A psychiatric consultation service for hospitalized children. Psychosomatics 22, 29-33.

Lange, R. J., & Maxwell, E. (1980). Psychiatric consult to children. In J. Neil (Ed.), Practical manual of psychiatric consultation. Baltimore: Williams and Wilkins.

Lewis, M. (1978). Child psychiatric consultation in pediatrics. Pediatrics 62, 359-364.

Pediatric consultation--liaison. Psychiatric Clinics of North America 5, 239-446.

Phillips, S., Sarles, R. M., & Friedman, S. B. (1980). Consultation and referral when, why, and how. Pediatric Annals 9, 269-275.

Ravenscroft, K. (1982). Psychiatric consultation to the child with acute physical trauma. American Journal of Orthopsychiatry 52, 298-307.

Reinhart, J. B. (1979). Direct consultation on a pediatric service. In J. D. Noshpitz (Ed.), Basic handbook of child psychiatry (Vol. 1, pp. 648-654). New York: Basic Books.

Rice, H. W., & Greenberg, L. W. (1982). A pediatric-child psychiatry liaison program on postpartum unit of a community hospital. Journal of Developmental and Behavioral Pediatrics 3, 201-205.

Rothenberg, M. B. (1968). Child psychiatry-pediatrics liaison. Journal of the American Academy of Child Psychiatry 7, 492-509.

Rothenberg, M. B. (1979). Child psychiatry-pediatrics consultation-liaison services in the hospital setting: A review. General Hospital Psychiatry 1, 281-286.

Sack, W., Cohen, S., & Grout, C. (1977). One year's survey of child psychiatry consultations in a pediatric hospital. Journal of the American Academy of Child Psychiatry 16, 716-727.

Schowalter, J. E. (1979). Hospital consultation as therapy. In J. D. Noshpitz (Ed.), Basic handbook of child psychiatry (Vol. 3, pp. 365-375). New York: Basic Books.

Schowalter, J. E., & Solnit, J. (1966). Child psychiatry consultation in a general hospital emergency room. Journal of the American Academy of Child Psychiatry 5, 534-549.

Silber, T. J., & Bagado, P. (1983). Pediatrician and psychiatrist as co-therapists. Adolescence 18, 331-337.

Simonds, J. F. (1977). Psychiatric consultations for 112 pediatric inpatients. Southern Medical Journal 70, 980-984.

Solnit, A. J., & Start, M. H. (1961). Mourning and the birth of a defective child. In R. S. Eissler, et al. (Eds.), Psychoanalytic study of the child (Vol. 16, pp. 523-537). New York: International Universities Press.

Stocking, M., Rothney, W., Grosser, G., & Goodwin, R. (1972). Psychopathology in pediatric hospital--implications for community health. American Jurnal of Pediatrics 36, 551-563.

Work, H. H. (1978). The burned out missionary. Pediatrics 62, 425-427.

Wrate, R. M., & Kolvin, I. (1978). A child psychiatry consultation service to pediatricians. Developmental Medicine and Child Neurology 20, 347-356.

2. Training in Consultation Liaison

Fritz, G. K., & Bergman, A. S. (1984). Consultation-liaison training of child psychiatrists: Results of a survey. General Hospital Psychiatry 6, 25-29.

Hickson, L., & Mann, E. M. (1985-1986). The relationship between attitudinal and behavioral change in pediatric residents in a psychiatric liaison teaching program: A pilot study. International Journal of Psychiatry and Medicine 15, 61-73.

Reinhart, J. B. (1982). Disorders of the gastrointestinal tract in children: Consultation-liaison experience. Psychiatric Clinics of North America 5, 387-397.

Rogers, R. R., & Rasof, B. (1975). A teaching drill in child psychiatry. American Journal of Psychiatry 132, 158-163.

Sadler, J. E. (1982). Childhood asthma from the point of view of the liaison child psychiatrist. Psychiatric Clinics of North America 5, 333-342.

Schowalter, J. (1977). Psychological reactions to physical illness and hospitalization in adolescents. Journal of the American Academy of Child Psychiatry 16, 500-516.

Schowalter, J. E. (1970). Death and the pediatric house officer. Pediatrics 76, 706-710.

Stabler, B., & Whitt, J. K. (1980). Pediatric psychology: Perspectives and training implications. Journal of Pediatric Psychology 5, 245-251.

Strafford, M. A., Griffiths, S. P., & Gersony, W. M. (1982). Coarctation of the aorta: A study of delayed detection. Pediatrics 69, 1-10.

3. Methods of Pediatric Consultation

Anders, T. (1977). Child psychiatry and pediatrics: The state of the relationship. Pediatrics 60(4), 313-321.

Anders, T. F., & Niehans, M. (1982). Promoting the alliance between pediatrics and child psychiatry. Psychiatric Clinics of North America 5, 388-395.

Fritz, G. K., & Bergman, A. S. (1985). Child psychiatrists seen through pediatricians' eyes: Results of a national survey. Journal of the American Academy of Child Psychiatry 24, 81-86.

Froese, A. P. (1976-1977). Pediatric referrals to psychiatry: II. Fears relating to delays in referral. International Journal of Psychiatry and Medicine 7, 249-253.

Goldbloom, R. B. (1975). Editorial: The lost art of consultation--the wish for the return of striped trousers. Pediatrics 56, 347-348.

Graham, P. (1984). Pediatric referral to a child psychiatrist. Diseases of Children 59, 1103-1105.

Greene, C. M. (1984). Mutual collaboration between child psychiatry and pediatrics: Resistances and facilitation. Journal of Developmental and Behavioral Pediatrics 6, 315-318.

Greenspan, S. I., Nover, R. A., & Brunt, C. H. (1976). The child psychiatrist and day care. Theoretical and clinical aspects of consultation. Journal of the American Academy of Child Psychiatry 15, 108-130.

Haggerty, R. J. (1974). II. The pediatrician and the child psychiatrist--a basis for cooperation. Rhode Island Medical Journal 57, 412-415, 442.

Hodas, G. R., & Honig, P. J. (1983). An approach to psychiatric referrals in pediatric patients. Psychosomatic complaints. Pediatrics 22, 167-172.

Kronz, K. K., et al. (1989). Management of diabetes in pediatric resident continuity clinics. Journal of the American Academy of Child and Adolescent Psychiatry 143, 1173-1179.

Kupst, M. J., & Schulomann, J. L. (1988). Long-term coping with pediatric leukemia, a six year follow-up study. Journal of Pediatric Psychology 13, 7-22.

LeBaron, S., & Zeltzer, L. (1985). Pediatrics and psychology: A collaboration that works. Journal of Developmental and Behavioral Pediatrics 6, 157-161.

Lewis, M. (1978). Child psychiatric consultation in pediatrics. Pediatrics 62, 359-364.

Lloyd, G. G. (1980). Whence and whither 'liaison' psychiatry? [Editorial]. Psychological Medicine 10, 11-14.

Minuchin, S. (1975). A conceptual model of psychosomatic illness in children. Archives of General Psychiatry 32, 1031.

Schowalter, J. E. (1979). Hospital consultation as therapy. In J. D. Noshpitz (Ed.), Basic handbook of child psychiatry (Vol. 3, pp. 365-375). New York: Basic Books.

Sherman, M. (1982). Communicating: A practical guide for the liaison psychiatrist. Psychiatric Clinics of North America 5, 271-281.

Stern, R. C. (1989). The primary care physician and the patient with cystic fibrosis. Journal of Pediatrics 114, 31-36.

Taintor, Z., Spikes, J., Gise, L. H., & Strain, J. J. (1979). Recorded psychiatric consultations: A preliminary report. General Hospital Psychiatry 1, 139-149.

Whitt, J. K., Hunter, R. S., Dykstra, W., Lauria, M. M., Stabler, B., & Taylor, W. (1981-1982). Pediatric liaison psychiatry: A forum for understanding separation and loss. International Journal of Psychiatry and Medicine 11, 59-68.

Work, H. (1978). The burned out missionary. Pediatrics 62, 399-427.

4. Treatment of Psychological Aspects of Physical Illness

Burke, S. O., Costello, E. A., & Handley-Derry, M. H. (1989). Maternal stress and repeated hospitalizations of children who are physically disabled. Children's Health Care 18, 82-90.

Cromer, B. A., & Tarnowski, K. J. (1989). Noncompliance in adolescents: A review. Journal of Developmental and Behavioral Pediatrics 10, 207-215.

Fritz, G. K., Steiner, H., Hillyard, J., & Lewiston, N. (1981). Pediatric and psychiatric collaboration in the management of childhood asthma. Clinical Pediatrics 20, 772-776.

Grossman, M. L. (1975). The psychosocial approach to the medical management of patients with cystic fibrosis. Clinical Pediatrics 14, 830-833.

Hollingsworth, C. E., Simons, J. Q., & Crumley, K. F. (1979). Psychiatric aspects of physical illness in children. In D. P. Cantwell (Ed.), Clinical child psychiatry. New York: Spectrum Publications.

Kazak, A., Reber, M., & Carter, A. (1988). Structural and qualitative aspects of social networks in families with young chronically ill children. Journal of Pediatric Psychology 13, 171-182.

Reinhart, J. B. (1982). Disorders of the gastrointestinal tract in children: Consultation-liaison experience. Psychiatric Clinics of North America 5, 387-397.

Rosenbaum, P. L., Armstrong, R. W., & King, S. M. (1989). Determinants of children's attitudes towards disability: A review of evidence. Children's Health Care 17, 32-39.

Sadler, J. E. (1982). Childhood asthma from the point of view of the liaison child psychiatrist. Psychiatric Clinics of North America 5, 333-343.

Sajwaj, T., Libet, J., & Agras, S. (1974). Lemon-juice therapy: The control of life-threatening rumination in a six-month-old infant. Journal of Applied Behavior Analysis 7, 557-563.

Schowalter, J. (1977). Psychological reactions to physical illness and hospitalization in adolescents. Journal of the American Academy of Child Psychiatry 16, 500-516.

Shagena, M., Sandler, H., & Perrin, E. (1988). Concepts of illness and perception of control in healthy children and in children with chronic illnesses. Journal of Developmental and Behavioral Pediatrics 9, 252-256.

Stoddard, F. J., et al. (1989). Psychiatric outcome of burned children and adolescents. Journal of the American Academy of Child and Adolescent Psychiatry 143, 589-595.

Strafford, M. A., Griffiths, S. P., & Gersony, W. M. (1982). Coarctation of the aorta: A study of delayed detection. Pediatrics 69, 159-163.

Wallander, J. L., et al. (1989). Disability parameters, chronic strain and adaptation of physically handicapped children and their mothers. Journal of Pediatric Psychology 14, 23-42.

Werder, D. S., & Sargent, J. D. (1984). A study of childhood headache using biofeedback as a treatment alternative. Headache 24, 122-126.

Wille, S. (1986). Comparison of desmopressin and enuresis alarm for nocturnal enuresis. Archives of Disease in Childhood 61, 30-33.

Williams, J. A., Hurst, M. K., & Stokes, T. F. (1983). Peer observation in decreasing uncooperative behavior in young dental patients. Behavior Modification 7, 225-242.

Winton, A. S., & Singh, N. N. (1983). Suppression of pica using brief-duration physical restraint. Journal of Mental Deficiency Research 27, 93-103.

Yager, J., et al. (1988). Attitudes toward mental illness prevention in routine pediatric practice. Journal of the American Academy of Child and Adolescent Psychiatry 143, 1087-1090.

5. Use of Play and Games--Therapy with Children in a Pediatric Ward

Abramson, R. M., Hoffman, L., & Johns, C. A. (1979). Play group psychotherapy for early latency-age children on an inpatient psychiatric unit. International Journal of Group Psychotherapy 29, 383-392.

Adams, M. A. (1976). A hospital play program: Helping children with serious illness. American Journal of Orthopsychiatry 46, 416-424.

Beiser, H. R. (1979). Formal games in diagnosis and therapy. Journal of the American Academy of Child Psychiatry 18, 480-491.

Harter, S. (1977). A cognitive-developmental approach to children's expression of conflicting feelings and a technique to facilitate such expression in play therapy. Journal of Consulting and Clinical Psychology 45, 417-432.

Irwin, E. C. (1977). Play, fantasy, and symbols: Drama with emotionally disturbed children. American Journal of Psychotherapy 31, 426-436.

Irwin, E. C. (1985). Puppets in therapy: An assessment procedure. American Journal of Psychotherapy 39, 389-400.

Schiffer, M. (1977). Activity-interview group psychotherapy: Theory, principles, and practice. International Journal of Group Psychotherapy 27, 377-388.

6. Behavioral Treatment of Childhood Illness

Alexander, A. B., Cropp, G. J., & Chai, H. (1979). Effects of relaxation training on pulmonary mechanics in children with asthma. Journal of Applied Behavior Analysis 12, 27-35.

Altman, K., Grahs, C., & Friman, P. (1982). Treatment of unobserved trichotillomania by attention-reflection and punishment of an apparent covariant. Journal of Behavior Therapy and Experimental Psychiatry 13, 337-340.

Altman, K., Haavik, S., & Higgins, S. T. (1983). Modifying the self-injurious behavior of an infant with spina bifida and diminished pain sensitivity. Journal of Behavior Therapy and Experimental Psychiatry 14, 165-168.

Anderson, L., Dancis, J., & Alpert, M. (1978). Behavioral contingencies and self-mutilation in Lesch-Nyhan disease. Journal of Consulting and Clinical Psychology 46, 529-536.

Ayllon, T., Garber, S. W., & Allison, M. G. (1977). Behavioral treatment of childhood neurosis. Psychiatry 40, 315-322.

Azrin, N. H., Nunn, R. G., & Frantz-Renshaw, S. E. (1982). Habit reversal vs. negative practice treatment of self-destructive oral habits (biting, chewing or licking of the lips, cheeks, tongue or palate). Journal of Behavior Therapy and Experimental Psychiatry 13, 49-54.

Barmann, B. C., Croyle-Barmann, C., & McLain, B. (1980). The use of contingent-interrupted music in the treatment of disruptive bus-riding behavior. Journal of Applied Behavior Analysis 13, 693-698.

Barrett, T. E. (1985). Clinical application of behavioral social skills training with children. Psychological Reports 57, 1183-1186.

Baumeister, A. A., & Baumeister, A. A. (1978). Suppression of repetitive self-injurious behavior by contingent inhalation of aromatic ammonia. Journal of Autism and Childhood Schizophrenia 8, 71-77.

Bean, A. W., & Roberts, M. W. (1981). The effect of time-out release contingencies on changes in child noncompliance. Journal of Abnormal Child Psychology 9, 95-105.

Belcastro, F. P. (1979). Use of behavior modification with hearing-impaired subjects. American Annals of the Deaf 124, 820-824.

Blagg, N. R., & Yule, W. (1984). The behavioral treatment of school refusal--a comparative study. Behavior Research and Therapy 22, 119-127.

Blanchard, E. B., & Andrasik, F. (1982). Psychological assessment and treatment of headache: Recent developments and emerging issues. Journal of Consulting and Clinical Psychology 50, 859-879.

Blechman, E. A., Taylor, C. J., & Schrader, S. M. (1981). Family problem solving versus home notes as early intervention with high-risk children. Journal of Consulting and Clinical Psychology 49, 919-926.

Bogdanov, O. V., Smetankin, A. A., Inin, Y. S., & Khakhan, Y. V. (1983). Voluntary control of heart rate by external feedback in normal children and children with infantile cerebral palsy. Human Physiology 9, 319-322.

Bollard, J. (1982). A 2-year follow-up of bedwetters treated by dry-bed training and standard condition. Behavior Research and Therapy 20, 571-580.

Bornstein, M. R., Bellack, A. S., & Hersen, M. (1977). Social-skills training for unassertive children: A multiple-baseline analysis. Journal of Applied Behavior Analysis 10, 183-195.

Bornstein, P. H., Balleweg, B. J., McLellarn, R. W., Wilson, G. L., Sturm, C. A., Andre, J. C., & van den Pol, R. A. (1983). The "bathroom game": A systematic program for the elimination of encopretic behavior. Journal of Behavior Therapy and Experimental Psychiatry 14, 67-71.

Bornstein, P. H., Sturm, C. A., Retzlaff, P. D., Kirby, K. L., & Chong, H. (1981). Paradoxical instruction in the treatment of encopresis and chronic constipation: An experimental analysis. Journal of Behavior Therapy and Experimental Psychiatry 12, 167-170.

Brown, R. T., Wynne, M. E., & Medenis, R. (1985). Methylphenidate and cognitive therapy: A comparison of treatment approaches with hyperactive boys. Journal of Abnormal Child Psychology 13, 69-87.

Brownell, K. D., & Stunkard, A. J. (1978). Behavioral treatment of obesity in children. American Journal of Diseases of Children 132, 403-412.

Bryant, L. E., & Budd, K. S. (1984). Teaching behaviorally handicapped preschool children to share. Journal of Applied Behavior Analysis 17, 45-56.

Buell, G., & Snyder, J. (1981). Assertiveness training with children. Psychological Reports 49, 71-80.

Bull, M., & LaVecchio, F. (1978). Behavior therapy for a child with Lesch-Nyhan syndrome. Developmental Medicine and Child Neurology 20, 368-375.

Bull, R. W., Lindquist, B. E., & Schroeder, D. H. (1980). Television puppet skits as a tool for modeling children's behavior. Hospital and Community Psychiatry 31, 706-707.

Camp, B. W., Blom, G. E., Hebert, F., & van Doorninck, W. J. (1977). "Think aloud": A program for developing self-control in young aggressive boys. Journal of Abnormal Child Psychology 5, 157-169.

Carr, E. G., & Newsom, C. (1985). Demand-related tantrums. Conceptualization and treatment. Behavior Modification 9, 403-426.

Carstens, C. (1982). Behavioral treatment of functional dysphagia in a 12-year-old boy. Psychosomatics 23, 195-196.

Christie, D. J., Dewitt, R. A., Kaltenbach, P., & Reed, D. (1984). Using EMg biofeedback to signal hyperactive children when to relax. Exceptional Children 50, 547-548.

Clement, P. W., Anderson, E., Arnold, J., Butman, R., Fantuzzo, J., & Mays, R. (1978). Self-observation and self-reinforcement as sources of self-control in children. Biofeedback and Self Regulation 3, 247-267.

Conners, C. K. (1979). Application of biofeedback to treatment of children. Journal of the American Academy of Child Psychiatry 18, 143-153.

Corral-Romero, M. A., & Bustamante-Balcarcel, A. (1982). Biofeedback rehabilitation in seventh nerve paralysis. Annals of Otology, Rhinology and Laryngology 91, 166-168.

Cracco, A., Belloli, G. P., & Ronconi, G. F. (1984). Sound alarms and conditioning therapy in the treatment of childhood enuresis: A study of 180 cases. Pediatria Medica e Chirurgica 6, 681-689.

Cullinan, D., Epstein, M. H., & Silver, L. (1977). Modification of impulsive tempo in learning disabled pupils. Journal of Abnormal Child Psychology 5, 437-444.

Czyzewski, M. J., Barrera, R. D., & Sulzer-Azaroff, B. (1982). An abbreviated overcorrection program to reduce self-stimulatory behaviors. Journal of Behavior Therapy and Experimental Psychiatry 13, 55-62.

Dahl, J., Melin, L., Brorson, L. O., & Schollin, J. (1985). Effects of a broad-spectrum behavior modification treatment program on children with refractory epileptic seizures. Epilepsia 26, 303-309.

Dahlquist, L. M., Gil, K. M., Armstong, F. D., Ginsberg, A., & Jones, B. (1985). Behavioral management of children's distress during chemotherapy. Journal of Behavior Therapy and Experimental Psychiatry 16, 325-329.

Daniel, W. H. (1982). Management of chronic rumination with a contingent exercise procedure employing topographically dissimilar behavior. Journal of Behavior Therapy and Experimental Psychiatry 13, 149-152.

Dash, J. (1981). Rapid hypno-behavioral treatment of a needle phobia in a five-year-old cardiac patient. Journal of Pediatric Psychology 6, 37-42.

de Vriendt, X., & Ruel, J. M. (1980). Simultaneous use of psychotherapy based on the analytic and behavioral schools Neuropsychiatrie de l'Enfance et de l'Adolescence 28, 243-246.

Delamater, A. M., Rosenbloom, N., Conners, C. K., & Hertweck, L. (1983). The behavioral treatment of hysterical paralysis in a ten-year-old boy. A case study. Journal of the American Academy of Child Psychiatry 22, 73-79.

Diamond, S., & Montrose, D. (1984). The value of biofeedback in the treatment of chronic headache: A four-year retrospective study. Headache 24, 5-18.

Dorsey, M. F., Iwata, B. A., Ong, P., & McSween, T. E. (1980). Treatment of self-injurious behavior using a water mist: Initial response suppression and generalization. Journal of Applied Behavior Analysis 13, 343-353.

Duker, P. C. (1981). Treatment of food refusal by the overcorrective functional movement training method. Journal of Behavior Therapy and Experimental Psychiatry 12, 337-340.

Egel, A. L. (1981). Reinforcer variation: Implications for motivating developmentally disabled children. Journal of Applied Behavior Analysis 14, 345-350.

Epstein, L. H., Wing, R. R., Steranchak, L., Dickson, B., & Michelson, J. (1980). Comparison of family-based behavior modification and nutrition education for childhood obesity. Journal of Pediatric Psychology 5, 25-36.

Fielding, D. (1980). The response of day and night wetting children and children who wet only at night to retention control training and the enuresis alarm. Behavior Research and Therapy 18, 305-317.

Finley, W. W., Rainwater, A. J., & Johnson, G. (1982). Effect of varying alarm schedules on acquisition and relapse parameters in the conditioning treatment of enuresis. Behavior Research and Therapy 20, 69-80.

Finney, J. W., Russo, D. C., & Cataldo, M. F. (1982). Reduction of pica in young children with lead poisoning. Journal of Pediatric Psychology 7, 197-207.

Forehand, R., Rogers, T., McMahon, R. J., Wells, K. C., & Griest, D. L. (1981). Teaching parents to modify child behavior problems: An examination of some follow-up date. Journal of Pediatric Psychology 6, 313-322.

Fox, J. E., & Houston, B. K. (1981). Efficacy of self-instructional training for reducing children's anxiety in an evaluative situation. Behavior Research and Therapy 19, 509-515.

Frankel, F., & Simmons, J. Q. (1985). Behavioral treatment approaches to pathological unsocialized physical aggression in young children. Journal of Child Psychology and Psychiatry and Allied Disciplines 26, 525-551.

Freschi, D. F., & DiLeo, P. D. (1982). Treatment of self-abusive behaviors using positive intervention with an autistic boy. Exceptional Children 49, 77-78.

Friedling, C., & O'Leary, S. G. (1979). Effects of self-instructional training on second- and third-grade hyperactive children: A failure to replicate. Journal of Applied Behavior Analysis 12, 211-219.

Friedman, S. (1980). Self-control in the treatment of Gilles de la Tourette's syndrome: Case study with 18-month follow-up. Journal of Consulting and Clinical Psychology 48, 400-402.

Gittelman-Klein, R., Klein, D. F., Abikoff, H., Katz, S., Gloisten, A. C., & Kates, W. (1976). Relative efficacy of methylphenidate and behavior modification in hyperkinetic children: An interim report. Journal of Abnormal Child Psychology 4, 361-379.

Griffiths, P., Meldrum, C., & McWilliam, R. (1982). Dry-bed training in the treatment of nocturnal enuresis in childhood: A research report. Journal of Child Psychology and Psychiatry and Allied Disciplines 23, 485-495.

Hall, M. D. (1983). Using relaxation imagery with children with malignancies: A developmental perspective. American Journal of Clinical Hypnosis 25, 143-149.

Haynes, S. N., Wilson, C. C., Jaffe, P. G., & Britton, B. T. (1979). Biofeedback treatment of atopic dermatitis: Controlled case studies of eight cases. Biofeedback and Self Regulation 4, 195-209.

Hill, L. D. (1985). Contributions of behavior modification to cerebral palsy habilitation. Physical Therapy 65, 341-345.

Hinshaw, S. P., Henker, B., & Whalen, C. K. (1984). Self-control in hyperactive boys in anger-inducing situations: Effects of cognitive-behavioral training and of methylphenidate. Journal of Abnormal Child Psychology 12, 55-77.

Hock, R. A., Rodgers, C. H., Reddi, C., & Kennard, D. W. (1978). Medico-psychological interventions in male asthmatic children: An evaluation of physiological change. Psychosomatic Medicine 40, 210-215.

Horn, W. F., Chatoor, I., & Conners, C. K. (1983). Additive effects of dexedrine and self-control training. A multiple assessment. Behavior Modification 7, 383-402.

Jackson, H. J., & King, N. J. (1981). The emotive imagery treatment of a child's trauma-induced phobia. Journal of Behavior Therapy and Experimental Psychiatry 12, 325-328.

Jay, S. M., Elliott, C. H., Ozolins, M., Olson, R. A., & Pruitt, S. D. (1985). Behavioral management of children's distress during painful medical procedures. Behavior Research and Therapy 23, 513-520.

Jones, D. P., & Verduyn, C. M. (1983). Behavioral management of sleep problems. Archives of Disease in Childhood 58, 442-444.

Kauffman, J., Hallahan, D. P., & Ianna, S. (1977). Suppression of a retardate's tongue protrusion by contingent imitation: A case study. Behavior Research and Therapy 15, 196-197.

Keating, J. C., Butz, R. A., Burke, E., & Heimberg, R. G. (1983). Dry bed training without a urine alarm: Lack of effect of setting and therapist contact with child. Journal of Behavior Therapy and Experimental Psychiatry 14, 109-115.

Kellerman, J. (1979). Behavioral treatment of night terrors in a child with acute leukemia. Journal of Nervous and Mental Disease 167, 182-185.

Kelley, M. L., Jarvie, G. J., Middlebrook, J. L., McNeer, M. F., & Drabman, R. S. (1984). Decreasing burned children's pain behavior: Impacting the trauma of hydrotherapy. Journal of Applied Behavior Analysis 17, 147-158.

Kelton, A., & Belar, C. D. (1983). The relative efficacy of autogenic phrases and autogenic-feedback training in teaching hand warming to children. Biofeedback and Self Regulation 8, 461-475.

King, N. J. (1980). The behavioral management of asthma and asthma-related problems in children: A critical review of the literature. Journal of Behavioral Medicine 3, 169-189.

Klesges, R. C., Malott, J. M., & Ugland, M. (1984). The effects of graded exposure and parental modeling on the dental phobias of a four-year-old girl and her mother. Journal of Behavior Therapy and Experimental Psychiatry 15, 161-164.

Koepke, J. M., & Thyer, B. A. (1985). Behavioral treatment of failure-to-thrive in a two-year-old. Child Welfare 64, 511-516.

Kohen, D. P., Olness, K. N., Colwell, S. O., & Heimel, A. (1984). The use of relaxation-mental imagery (self-hypnosis) in the management of 505 pediatric behavioral encounters. Journal of Developmental and Behavioral Pediatrics 5, 21-25.

Koles, M. R., & Jenson, W. R. (1985). Comprehensive treatment of chronic fire setting in a severely disordered boy. Journal of Behavior Therapy and Experimental Psychiatry 16, 81-85.

Kotses, H., & Glaus, K. D. (1981). Applications of biofeedback to the treatment of asthma: A critical review. Biofeedback and Self Regulation 6, 573-593.

LaVecchio, F. (1980). Behavioral treatment of Lesch-Nyhan syndrome. Developmental Medicine and Child Neurology 22, 405-407.

Labb:e, E. L., & Williamson, D. A. (1984). Treatment of childhood migraine using autogenic feedback training. Journal of Consulting and Clinical Psychology 52, 968-976.

Ladouceur, R., & Martineau, G. (1982). Evaluation of regulated-breathing method with and without parental assistance in the treatment of child stutterers. Journal of Behavior Therapy and Experimental Psychiatry 13, 301-306.

Masek, B. J., Russo, D. C., & Varni, J. W. (1984). Behavioral approaches to the management of chronic pain in children. Pediatric Clinics of North America 31, 1113-1131.

McAuley,- R. (1982). Training parents to modify conduct problems in their children. Journal of Child Psychology and Psychiatry and Allied Disciplines 23, 335-342.

Minderaa, R. B., & Wit, J. M. (1983). Behavior therapy of obese children. and results 21 months after treatment. International Journal of Obesity 7, 143-152.

Nakanishi, D. A., & Anderson, D. R. (1982). Behavioral treatment of psychogenic vomiting among children--a review and case example. Journal of Psychosocial Nursing and Mental Health Services 20, 17-20.

Olness, K., & MacDonald, J. (1981). Self-hypnosis and biofeedback in the management of juvenile migraine. Journal of Developmental and Behavioral Pediatrics 2, 168-170.

Overholser, J., & Beck, S. (1985). Assessing generalization of treatment effects and self-efficacy in the modification of eating styles in obese children. Addictive Behavior 10, 145-152.

Page, T. J., Finney, J. W., Parrish, J. M., & Iwata, B. A. (1983). Assessment and reduction of food stealing in Prader-Willi children. Applied Research in Mental Retardation 4, 219-228.

Parker, L. H., & Cinciripini, P. M. (1984). Behavioral medicine with children: Applications in chronic disease. Progress in Behavior Modification 17, 135-165.

Peterson, L. (1984). The "safe at home" game. Training comprehensive prevention skills in latchkey children. Behavior Modification 8, 474-494.

Poster, E. C., & Betz, C. L. (1983). Allaying the anxiety of hospitalized children using stress immunization techniques. Issues in Comprehensive Pediatric Nursing 6, 227-233.

Prytula, R. E., Joyner, K. B., & Schnelle, J. F. (1981). Utilizing the school to control head-banging behavior of a child at home. Psychological Reports 48, 887-894.

Rekers, G. A., & Mead, S. (1979). Early intervention for female sexual identity disturbance: Self-monitoring of play behavior. Journal of Abnormal Child Psychology 7, 405-423.

Richman, N., Douglas, J., Hunt, H., Lansdown, R., & Levere, R. (1985). Behavioral methods in the treatment of sleep disorders--a pilot study. Journal of Child Psychology and Psychiatry and Allied Disciplines 26, 581-590.

Rinchuse, D. J., & Rinchuse, A. S. (1986). Overcoming fingersucking habits. Journal of Clinical Orthodontics 20, 46-47.

Rolider, A., & Van Houten, R. (1985). Treatment of constipation-caused encopresis by a negative reinforcement procedure. Journal of Behavior Therapy and Experimental Psychiatry 16, 67-70.

Rubin, R. M. (1983). Behavior modification for orthodontic cooperation. Journal of Clinical Orthodontics 17, 322-325.

Schroeder, S. R., Kanoy, R. C., Mulick, J. A., Rojahn, J., Thios, S. J., Stephens, M., & Hawk, B. (1982). Environmental antecedents which affect management and maintenance of programs for self-injurious behavior. Monographs of the American Association on Mental Deficiency 92, 105-59.

Scott, E. A. (1977). Treatment of encopresis in a classroom setting: A case study. British Journal of Educational Psychology 47, 199-202.

Sellick, K. J., & Peck, C. L. (1981). Behavioral treatment of fear in a child with cerebral palsy using a flooding procedure. Archives of Physical Medicine and Rehabilitation 62, 398-400.

Shapiro, S. R. (1985). Enuresis: Treatment and overtreatment. Pediatric Nursing 11, 203-207, 214.

Slifer, K. J., Iwata, B. A., & Dorsey, M. G. (1984). Reduction of eye gouging using a response interruption procedure. Journal of Behavior Therapy and Experimental Psychiatry 15, 369-375.

Smeets, P. M., Lancioni, G. E., Ball, T. S., & Oliva, D. S. (1985). Shaping self-initiated toileting in infants. Journal of Applied Behavior Analysis 18, 303-308.

Sreenivasan, U., Manocha, S. N., & Jain, V. K. (1979). Treatment of severe dog phobia in childhood by flooding: A case report. Journal of Child Psychology and Psychiatry and Allied Disciplines 2, 255-260.

Suter, S, & Loughry-Machado, G. (1981). Skin temperature biofeedback in children and adults. Journal of Experimental Child Psychology 32, 77-87.

Talbot, M. L., & Junkala, J. (1981). The effects of auditorally augmented feedback on the eye-hand coordination of students with cerebral palsy. American Journal of Occupational Therapy 35, 525-528.

Tansey, M. A. (1985). Brainwave signatures--an index reflective of the brain's functional neuroanatomy: Further findings on the effect of EEG sensorimotor rhythm biofeedback training on the neurologic precursors of learning disabilities. International Journal of Psychophysiology 3, 85-99.

Tharp, R. G., & Gallimore, R. (1985). The logical status of metacognitive training. Journal of Abnormal Child Psychology 13, 455-466.

Thompson, G. A., Iwata, B. A., & Poynter, H. (1979). Operant control of pathological tongue thrust in spastic cerebral palsy. Journal of Applied Behavior Analysis 12, 325-333.

Varni, J. W., & Banis, H. T. (1985). Behavior therapy techniques applied to eating, exercise, and diet modification in childhood obesity. Journal of Developmental and Behavioral Pediatrics 6, 367-372.

Varni, J. W., Bessman, C. A., Russo, D. C., & Cataldo, M. F. (1980). Behavioral medicine of chronic pain in children: Case study. Archives of Physical Medicine and Rehabilitation 61, 375-379.

Varni, J. W., Gilbert, A., & Dietrich, S. L. (1981). Behavioral medicine in pain and analgesia management for the hemophilic child with factor VIII inhibitor. Pain 11, 121-126.

Wakefield, M. A., Woodbridge, C., Steward, J., & Croke, W. M. (1984). A treatment programme for faecal incontinence. Developmental Medicine and Child Neurology 26, 613-616.

Waranch, H. R., & Keenan, D. M. (1985). Behavioral treatment of children with recurrent headaches. Journal of Behavior Therapy and Experimental Psychiatry 16, 31-38.

Weinstein, A. G. (1984). Crying-induced bronchospasm in childhood asthma: Combined pharmacologic and behavioral management. Deleware Medical Journal 56, 473-476.

PART V

COMMUNITY MENTAL HEALTH AND CONSULTATION

A. Community Mental Health

Section Editor:

Irving N. Berlin, M.D.
Professor of Psychiatry and Pediatrics
University of New Mexico School of Medicine
Albuquerque, New Mexico

1. Historical Aspects of Epidemiological Research

Armstrong, H. E., Jr., Ishiki, D., Heiman, J., Mundt, J., & Womack, W. (1984). Service utilization by black and white clientele in an urban community mental health center: Revised assessment of an old problem. Community Mental Health Journal 20, 269-281.

Birch, H. G. (1964). The problem of "brain damage" in children. In H. G. Birch (Ed.), Brain damage in children: The biological and social aspects (pp. 3-12). Baltimore: Williams and Wilkins.

Cantwell, D. P., & Carey, W. B. (1974). Prevalence of psychiatric disorder in a pediatric clinic for military dependent children. Journal of Pediatrics 85, 711-716.

Cassel, J. (1966). Social class and mental disorders: An analysis of the limitations and potentialities of current epidemiological approaches. In K. S. Miller & C. M. Grigg (Eds.), Mental health and the lower classes (pp. 42-53). Tallahassee: Florida State University.

Cravioto, J., deLicardie, E. R., & Birch, H. G. (1966). Nutrition, growth and neurointegrative development: An experimental and ecological study. Pediatrics 38, 319-372.

Goldberg, I. D., Roshmann, K. J., McInerny, T. K., & Burke, J. D., Jr. (1984). Mental health problems among children seen in pediatric practice: Prevalence and management. Pediatrics 73, 278-293.

Gruenberg, E. M., & Leighton, A. H. (1965). Epidemiology and psychiatric training. In S. E. Goldston (Ed.), Concepts of community psychiatry: A framework for training. (pp. 109-115). Bethesda, Md.: National Institute of Mental Health.

Joint Commission on Mental Health of Children. (1970). Crisis in child mental health: Challenge for the 1970's. New York: Harper and Row.

Mirowsky, J., & Ross, C. E. (1983). The multidimensionality of psychopathology in a community sample. American Journal of Community Psychology 11, 573-591.

Noll, G. A., & Dubinsky, M. (1985). Prevalence and predictors of depression in a suburban county. Journal of Community Psychology 13, 13-19.

Pasamanick, B., & Knobloch, H. (1960). Brain behavior: Session II. Symposium, 1959. II. Brain damage and reproductive casualty. American Journal of Orthopsychiatry 30, 298-305.

Thoits, P. (1982). Life stress, social support and psychological vulnerability: Epidemiological considerations. Journal of Community Psychology 10, 341-362.

Waldron, S., Jr. (1976). The significance of childhood neurosis for adult mental health: A follow-up study. American Journal of Psychiatry 133, 532-538.
Werner, E. E., Bierman, J. M., & French, F. E. (1971). The children of Kauai. Honolulu: University of Hawaii Press.

2. Historical Aspects of the Community Mental Health Movement and Community Mental Health Centers

Barrera, M., & Ainlay, S. L. (1983). The structure of social support: A conceptual and empirical analysis. Journal of Community Psychology 11, 133-143.
Bindman, A. J., & Klebanoff, L. B. (1960). Administrative problems in establishing a community mental health program. American Journal of Orthopsychiatry 30, 696-711.
Block, M., & Zautra, A. (1981). Satisfaction and distress in a community: A test of the effects of life events. American Journal of Community Psychology 9, 165-180.
Caplan, G. (1961). An approach to community mental health. New York: Grune & Stratton.
Joint Commission on Mental Illness and Health. (1961). Action for mental health. New York: Basic Books.
Klerman, G. L. (1969). Mental health and the urban crisis. American Journal of Orthopsychiatry 39, 818-826.

3. Principles of Community Mental Health Center Function

Bennett, M. J., & Gavalya, A. S. (1982). Prepaid comprehensive mental health services for children. Journal of the American Academy of Child Psychiatry 21, 486-491.
Berlin, I. N. (1969). Resistance to change in mental health professionals. American Journal of Orthopsychiatry 39, 109-115.
Bertalanffy, L. von (1968). General system theory. New York: G. Braziller.
Black, B. J. (1964). Psychiatric rehabilitation in the community. In L. Bellak (Ed.), Handbook of community psychiatry and community mental health (pp. 248-264). New York: Grune & Stratton.
Caplan, G. (1964). The role of pediatricians in community mental health (with particular reference to the primary prevention of mental disorders in children). In L. Bellak (Ed.), Handbook of community psychiatry and community mental health (pp. 287-299). New York: Grune & Stratton.
Coren, H. Z., & McKale, M. A. (1985). Community mental health unraveling: The folly of cost containment. American Journal of Orthopsychiatry 55, 618-619.
Eisdorfer, C., Altrocchi, J., & Young, R. F. (1968). Principles of community mental health in a rural setting: The Halifax County program. Community Mental Health Journal 4, 211-220.
Fishman, J. R., & McCormack, J. (1970). Mental health without walls: Community mental health in the ghetto. American Journal of Psychiatry 126, 1461-1467.

Freed, H. M., & Miller, L. (1971). Planning a community mental health program: A case history. Community Mental Health Journal 7, 107-117.

Gardner, C. S., Hurt, S. W., Maltman, G., Greenberg, R., & Holtzman, S. R. (1985). Clinic turmoil and staff transitions. American Journal of Orthopsychiatry 55, 439-445.

Hume, P. B. (1966). General principles of community psychiatry. In S. Arieti (Ed.), American handbook of psychiatry (Vol. 3, pp. 515-541). New York: Basic Books.

Lafollette, J., & Pilisuk, M. (1981). Changing models of community mental health services. Journal of Community Psychology 9, 210-223.

Leopold, R. L. (1971). Urban problems and the community mental health center: Multiple mandates, difficult choices. I. Background and current status. American Journal of Orthopsychiatry 41, 144-149.

Mitchell, C. M. (1983). The dissemination of social intervention: Process and effectiveness of two types of paraprofessional change agents. American Journal of Community Psychology 11, 723-739.

Okin, R. L. (1984). How community mental health centers are coping. Hospital and Community Psychiatry 35, 1118-1125.

Raeburn, J. M., & Seymour, F. W. (1979). A simple systems model for community programs. Journal of Community Psychology 7, 290-297.

Rieman, D. W. (1976). Strengthening board-staff collaboration in community mental health programs (Vol. 36). Columbia: Missouri University.

Schwebel, A. I., Kershaw, R., Reeve, S., Hartung, J. G., & Reeve, W. (1973). A community organization approach to implementation of comprehensive health planning. American Journal of Public Health 63, 675-680.

Serrano, A. C., & Gibson, G. (1973). Mental health services to the Mexican-American community in San Antonio, Texas. American Journal of Public Health 63, 1055-1057.

Stretch, J. J. (1967). Community mental health: The evolution of a concept in social policy. Community Mental Health Journal 3, 5-12.

4. Community Mental Health Centers Programs

a. Training

Bumpass, E. R., Brix, R. J., & Preston, D. (1985). A community-based program for juvenile firesetters. Hospital and Community Psychiatry 36, 529-533.

D'Augelli, J. F., & Weener, J. M. (1978). Training parents as mental health agents. Community Mental Health Journal 14, 14-25.

DeShong, B. R. (1979). Training community staff to serve children discharged from a state hospital. Hospital and Community Psychiatry 30, 13, 17-18.

Lefley, H. P. (1984). Cross-cultural training for mental health professionals: Effects on the delivery of services. Hospital and Community Psychiatry 35, 1127-1229.

McLennan, J. P. (1984). Helping beliefs inventory: Brief screening measure for training volunteer applicants in counseling. Psychological Reports 56, 843-846.

Melick, M. E., & Fisher, I. E. (1983). The outcomes of mental health training programs: A review of the literature. Journal of Allied Health 12, 287-302.

Rieger, N. I., & Devries, A. G. (1977). A model training program for child mental health specialists. Hospital and Community Psychiatry 28, 690-693.

b. Treatment

Bird, H. W., & Schuham, A. I. (1978). Meeting families' treatment needs through a family psychotherapy center. Hospital and Community Psychiatry 29, 175-178.

Brierley, E. (1984). A child clinical psychologist in the community. A perceived need effectively met? Practitioner 228, 855-859.

Cutler, D. L., & Madore, E. (1980). Community-family network therapy in a rural setting. Community Mental Health Journal 16, 144-155.

Goeller, D., & Jones, E. (1981). An innovative approach to the delivery of behavioral services in Worcester County. Maryland Nurse April, 4-6.

Jordan, D. D. (1985). Impact of an alternatives program on client utilization of services in a county mental health system. Hospital and Community Psychiatry 36, 1291-1296.

Kellam, S. G., & Schiff, S. K. (1966). The Woodlawn Mental Health Center: A community mental health center model. Social Service Review 40, 255-263.

Kiesler, F. (1969). More than psychiatry: A rural program. In M. F. Shore & F. V. Mannion (Eds.), Mental health and the community: Problems, programs, and strategies (pp. 103-120). New York: Behavioral Publications.

Knesper, D. J., & Carlson, B. W. (1985). Employment of child and adult psychiatrists in community mental health centers. Journal of the American Academy of Child Psychiatry 24, 647-652.

Lamb, H. R. (1980). Structure: The neglected ingredient of community treatment. Archives of General Psychiatry 37, 1224-1228.

Looff, D. H. (1969). Appalachian public health nursing: Mental health component in eastern Kentucky. Community Mental Health Journal 5, 295-303.

Mitchell, J. R., & Smith, M. S. (1981). Adolescents' use of mental health services in a comprehensive treatment facility: Age, sex and mode of entry. American Journal of Public Health 71, 1329-1332.

Stage, T. B., & Keast, T. J. (1966). A psychiatric service for Plains Indians. Hospital and Community Psychiatry 17, 74-76.

Turner, C. (1980). Resources for help in parenting. Child Welfare 59, 179-188.

5. Special Settings for Community Mental Health Centers

a. Treatment

Albin, R. S. (1982). Children of psychotic mothers may benefit from home care. Psychiatric News 17, 11-17.

Berlin, I. N. (1975). Some models for reversing the myth of child treatment in community mental health centers. Journal of the American Academy of Child Psychiatry 14, 76-94.

Blinder, B. J., Young, W. M., Fineman, K. R., & Miller, S. J. (1978). The children's psychiatric hospital unit in the community: I. Concept and development. American Journal of Psychiatry 135, 848-851.

Christ, A. E., Adler, A. G., Merling, B., & Gershansky, I. (1981). Brooklyn Kings County Hospital child psychiatric study, 1957-1977: A longitudinal comparison of court-remanded and psychiatrically admitted children. Journal of the American Academy of Child Psychiatry 20, 777-791.

Corney, R. H. (1984). The mental and physical health of clients referred to social workers in a local authority department and a general practice attachment scheme. Psychological Medicine 14, 137-144.

Davidson, W. S., II, & Wolfred, T. R. (1977). Evaluation of a community-based behavior modification program for prevention of delinquency: The failure of success. Community Mental Health Journal 13, 296-306.

Halpern, W. I., Kissel, S., & Gold, J. (1978). Day treatment as an aid to mainstreaming troubled children. Community Mental Health Journal 14, 319-326.

Jacobson, A. M., Goldberg, I. D., Burns, B. J., Hoeper, E. W., Hankin, J. R., & Hewitt, K. (1980). Diagnosed mental disorder in children and use of health services in four organized health care settings. American Journal of Psychiatry 137, 559-565.

Lamb, H. R. (1980). Structure: The neglected ingredient of community treatment. Archives of General Psychiatry 37, 1224-1228.

Perlmutter, R. A., Schwartz, A. J., & Reifler, C. B. (1985). The college student psychiatric emergency: II. Diagnosis and disposition. Journal of American College Health 33, 152-158.

Prevost, J. A. (1982). Youthful chronicity: Paradox of the 80s. Hospital and Community Psychiatry 33, 173.

Rhodes, W. C., & Gibbins, S. (1972). Community programming for the behaviorally deviant child. In H. C. Quay & J. S. Werry (Eds.), Psychopathological disorders of childhood (pp. 348-387). New York: Wiley.

Rickel, A. U. (1986). Prescriptions for a new generation: Early life interventions. American Journal of Community Psychology 14, 1-15.

Rosen, P. M., Peterson, L., & Walsh, B. W. (1980). A community residence for severely disturbed adolescents: A cognitive-behavioral approach. Child Welfare 59, 15-25.

Schoenfeld, P., Halevy-Martini, J., Hemley-VanderVelden, E., & Ruhf, L. (1985). Network therapy: Outcome study of twelve social networks. Journal of Community Psychology 13, 281-287.

Seltzer, M. M., & Krauss, M. W. (1984). Family, community residence, and institutional placements of a sample of mentally retarded children. American Journal of Mental Deficiency 89, 257-266.

Shore, M. F. (1981). Non-traditional mental health services for youth in six European countries: Some general observations. Adolescence 16, 195-201.

Stephenson, J. N., Moberg, P., Daniels, B. J., & Robertson, J. F. (1984). Treating the intoxicated adolescent. A need for comprehensive services. Journal of the American Medical Association 252, 1884-1888.

Walker, P. W., & Brook, B. D. (1981). Community homes as hospital alternatives for youth in crisis. Journal of Psychiatric Nursing and Mental Health Services 19, 17-19.

Weinstein, A. S., & Cohen, M. (1984). Young chronic patients and changes in the state hospital population. Hospital and Community Psychiatry 35, 595-600.

Winsberg, B. G., Bialer, I., Kupietz, S., Botti, E., & Balka, E. B. (1980). Home versus hospital care of children with behavior disorders. A controlled investigation. Archives of General Psychiatry 37, 413-418.

b. Chronic Patient Care

Davis, E. B., Egri, G., & Caton, C. L. (1984). Outcomes of care systems for chronic patients. Journal of the National Medical Association 76, 67-73.

Intagliata, J., & Baker, F. (1984). A comparative analysis of the young adult chronic patient in New York State's community support system. Hospital and Community Psychiatry 35, 45-50.

Sargent, J., & Liebman, R. (1985). Childhood chronic illness: Issues for psychotherapists. Community Mental Health Journal 21, 294-311.

c. Hard-to-Reach Populations

Sabatino, D. A., Heald, J. E., Rothman, S. G., & Miller, T. L. (1978). Destructive norm-violating school behavior among adolescents: A review of protective and preventive efforts. Adolescence 13, 675-686.

Severy, L. J., & Whitaker, J. M. (1984). Memphis-Metro youth diversion project: Final report. Child Welfare 63, 269-277.

Shanok, S. S., & Lewis, D. O. (1977). Juvenile court versus child guidance referral: Psychosocial and parental factors. American Journal of Psychiatry 134, 1130-1133.

Whitaker, J. M., Severy, L. J., & Morton, D. S. (1984). A comprehensive community-based youth diversion program. Child Welfare 63, 175-181.

d. Dealing with Physical and Sexual Abuse

Anderson, L. M., & Shafer, G. (1979). The character-disordered family: A community treatment model for family sexual abuse. American Journal of Orthopsychiatry 49, 436-445.

Coolsen, P. (1980). Community involvement in the prevention of child abuse and neglect. Children Today 9, 5-8.

Gentry, T., & Brisbane, F. L. (1982). The solution for child abuse rests with the community. Children Today 11, 22-24.

Miller, C. C. (1981). Primary prevention of child mistreatment: Meeting a national need. Child Welfare 60, 11-23.

Sefcik, T. R., & Ormsby, N. J. (1978). Establishing a rural child abuse/neglect treatment program. Child Welfare 57, 187-195.

e. Dealing with Substance Abuse

Galanter, M., Gleaton, T., Marcus, C. E., & McMillen, J. (1984). Self-help groups for parents of young drug and alcohol abusers. American Journal of Psychiatry 141, 889-891.

Masterton, G. (1979). The management of solvent abuse. Journal of Adolescence 2, 65-75.

6. Community Mental Health Centers--Community Involvement

a. Minority Involvement and Programs

Baker, F., & Perkins, D. V. (1984). Program maturity and cost analysis in the evaluation of primary prevention programs. Journal of Community Psychology 12, 31-42.

Beiser, M., & Attneave, C. L. (1982). Mental disorders among native American children: Rates and risk periods for entering treatment. American Journal of Psychiatry 139, 193-198.

Beiser, M., Shore, J. H., Peters, R., & Tatum, E. (1985). Does community care for the mentally ill make a difference? A tale of two cities. American Journal of Psychiatry 142, 1047-1052.

Kellam, S. G., Branch, J. D., Agrawal, K. C., & Grabill, M. E. (1972). Woodlawn Mental Health Center: An evolving strategy for planning in community mental health. In S. E. Golann & C. Eisdorder (Eds.), Handbook of community mental health (pp. 711-727). New York: Appleton-Century-Crofts.

Kellam, S. G., & Schiff, S. K. (1968). An urban community mental health center. In L. F. Duhl & R. L. Leopold (Eds.), Mental health and urban social policy (pp. 112-138). San Francisco: Jossey-Bass.

Kraft, S. P., & DeMaio, T. J. (1982). An ecological intervention with adolescents in low-income families. American Journal of Orthopsychiatry 52, 131-140.

Martinez, C. (1973). Community mental health and the Chicano movement. American Journal of Orthopsychiatry 43, 595-601.

Perlmutter, R. A., & Jones, J. E. (1985). Problem solving with families in psychiatric emergencies. Psychiatric Quarterly 57, 23-32.

Reeves, K. (1986). Hispanic utilization of an ethnic mental health clinic. Journal of Psychosocial Nursing and Mental Health Services 24, 23-26.

Schiff, S. K. (1970). Community accountability and mental health services. Mental Hygiene 54, 205-214.

Schore, J. H., & Nicholls, W. M. (1975). Indian children and tribal group homes: New interpretations of the Whipper Man. American Journal of Psychiatry 132, 454-456.
Spurlock, J. (1986). Development of self-concept in Afro-American children. Hospital and Community Psychiatry 37, 66-70.

b. Rural Programs

Jerrell, J. M., & DiPasquale, S. A. (1984). Staffing patterns in rural health services for children and adolescents. Community Mental Health Journal 20, 212-222.
Thompson, C. M. (1985). Characteristics associated with outcome in a community mental health partial hospitalization program. Community Mental Health Journal 21, 179-188.

c. Evaluation of Community Participation

Adams, P. L. (1976). Local community change for service to children. Child Psychiatry and Human Development 7, 22-30.
Darley, P. J. (1974). Who shall hold the conch? Some thoughts on community control of mental health programs. Community Mental Health Journal 10, 185-191.
D'Augelli, A. R., & Vallance, T. R. (1982). The helping community: Issues in the evaluation of a preventive intervention to promote informal helping. Journal of Community Psychology 10, 199-209.
Ellsworth, R. B. (1978). Community treatment for young psychiatric patients: A case study in program evaluation. Evaluation and the Health Professionals 1, 66-80.
Hester, P. (1977). Evaluation and accountability in a parent-implemented early intervention service. Community Mental Health Journal 13, 261-267.
Holder, H. D. (1969). Mental health and the search for new organizational strategies: A systems proposal. Archives of General Psychiatry 20, 709-717.
Landsberg, G., & Hammer, R. (1978). Involving community representatives in CMHC evaluation and research. Hospital and Community Psychiatry 29, 245-247.
Lorefice, L. S., & Borus, J. F. (1984). Consumer evaluation of a community mental health service, II: Perceptions of clinical care. American Journal of Psychiatry 141, 1449-1452.
Lorefice, L. S., Borus, J. F., & Keefe, C. (1982). Consumer evaluation of a community mental health service, I: Care delivery patterns. American Journal of Psychiatry 139, 1331-1334.
Munk-Jurgensen, P. (1985). Cumulated need for psychiatric service as shown in a community psychiatric project. Psychological Medicine 15, 629-635.
Niebuhr, R. (1971). Without consensus there is no consent. Center Magazine 4, 2-9.
Nolan, W. (1981). Getting a timely evaluation from your local mental health facility. Journal of Learning Disabilities 14, 81-110.

Pratt, M. W., Luszcz, M. A., & Brown, M. E. (1980). Measuring dimensions of the quality of care in small community residences. American Journal of Mental Deficiency 85, 188-194.

Reiff, R., & Riessman, F. (1968). The indigenous nonprofessional: A strategy of change in community action and community mental health programs. Community Mental Health Journal Monograph Series 1, 1-32.

Rotberg, J., Forness, S. R., Lynch, E. W., Gardner, T. P., Urbano, R., & Bender, M. (1982). Status of interagency cooperation between interdisciplinary clinics or hospitals and the public schools. Child Psychiatry and Human Development 12, 153-159.

Sonis, W. A., & Costello, A. J. (1981). Evaluation of differential data sources. Application of the diagnostic process in child psychiatry. Journal of the American Academy of Child Psychiatry 20, 597-610.

Sorensen, J. L., Kantor, L., Margolis, R. B., & Galano, J. (1979). The extent, nature, and utility of evaluating consumer satisfaction in community mental health centers. American Journal of Community Psychology 7, 329-337.

Thorne, M. Q., Jr. (1975). PSRO-future impact on community mental health centers. Community Mental Health Journal 11, 389-393.

Turkat, D., & Buzzell, V. (1982). Psychosocial rehabilitation: A process evaluation. Hospital and Community Psychiatry 33, 848-850.

d. Rights of Children

Kriechman, A. M. (1985). A school-based program of mental health services. Hospital and Community Psychiatry 36, 876-878.

Mearig, J. S. (1982). Ethical implications of the children's rights movement for professionals. American Journal of Orthopsychiatry 52, 518-529.

Miller, C. C. (1981). Primary prevention of child mistreatment: Meeting a national need. Child Welfare 60, 11-23.

Westman, J. C. (1973). The legal rights of adolescents from a developmental perspective. In J. C. Schoolar (Ed.), Current issues in adolescent psychiatry (pp. 252-262). New York: Brunner/Mazel.

Worsfold, V. L. (1974). A philosophical justification of children's rights. Harvard Education Review 44, 142-157.

7. Community Mental Health Centers and Child Mental Health Professional Participation

a. Work with Families and Parents

Beach, W. B. (1975). The child psychiatrist attempts to introduce community psychiatry into a state mental health program. Journal of the American Academy of Child Psychiatry 14, 66-75.

Blinzinsky, M. (1982). Parents anonymous and the private agency: Administrative cooperation. Child Welfare 61, 305-311.

Fine, P. (1973). Family networks and child psychiatry in a community health project. Journal of the American Academy of Child Psychiatry 12, 675-689.

Galanter, M., Gleaton, T., Marcus, C. E., & McMillen, J. (1984). Self-help groups for parents of young drug and alcohol abusers. American Journal of Psychiatry 141, 889-891.

Harrison, S. I., McDermott, J. F., Schrager, J., & Showerman, E. R. (1970). Social status and child psychiatric practice: The influence of the clinician's socioeconomic origin. American Journal of Psychiatry 127, 652-658.

Malone, C. A. (1967). Child psychiatric services for low socioeconomic families. Journal of the American Academy of Child Psychiatry 6, 332-345.

Press-Rigler, M., Kent, J. T., Croot, P., & Finnila, M. (1980). Parent aides: An intervention program in cases of child abuse and neglect. Journal of the Association for the Care of Children in Hospitals 8, 64-68.

Rafferty, F. T. (1967). Child psychiatry service for a total population. Journal of the American Academy of Child Psychiatry 6, 295-308.

Schaughency, E. A., & Lahey, B. B. (1985). Mothers' and fathers' perceptions of child deviance: Roles of child behavior, parental depression, and marital satisfaction. Journal of Consulting and Clinical Psychology 53, 718-723.

Sneddon, J., Kerry, R. J., & Bant, W. P. (1981). The psychiatric mother and baby unit. A three-year study. Practitioner 225, 1295-1300.

Turner, C. (1980). Resources for help in parenting. Child Welfare 59, 179-188.

b. Work with Preschool Children

Anderson, D. R., Long, A., Leathers, E., Denny, B., & Hilliard, D. (1981). Documentation of change in problem behaviors among anxious and hostile-aggressive children enrolled in a therapeutic preschool program. Child Psychiatry and Human Development 11, 232-240.

Baumann, E. H. (1976). A day treatment program for severely disturbed young children. Hospital and Community Psychiatry 27, 174-179.

Rutter, M. (1982). Psychological therapies in child Psychiatry: Issues and prospects. Psychological Medicine 12, 723-740.

c. Work with School Age Children

Klebanoff, L. B., & Bindman, A. J. (1962). The organization and development of a community mental health program for children.: A case study. American Journal of Orthopsychiatry 32, 119-132.

Marcus, S. D., Fox, D., & Brown, D. (1982). Identifying school children with behavior disorders. Community Mental Health Journal 18, 249-256.

Michelson, L. (1981). Psychotherapeutic outcome for children in a community mental health center: Psychological, demographic, and treatment predictors. Psychological Reports 48, 323-326.

Roshmann, K. J., Babisian, H. M., Goldberg, I. D., & Zastowny, T. R. (1982). The increasing number of children using psychiatric services: Analysis of a cumulative psychiatric case register. Pediatrics 70, 790-801.

Warren, M. Q. (1988). The "impossible" child, the difficult child, and other assorted delinquents: Etiology, characteristics and incidence. Canadian Psychiatric Association Journal 23, 41-60.

d. Work with Adolescents

1) In Clinics

Berkman, I. P., & Rosenblum, L. (1982). Serving high school students in need: A look at restrengthening the linkage between the school and community referral sources. Adolescence 17, 465-470.

Reinherz, H., Heywood, M., & Camp, J. (1976). Shared perspectives: A community counseling center for adolescents. Adolescence 11, 167-179.

Shorts, I. D. (1985). The prediction of in-programme failure among delinquent youths in anon-residential community-based programme. British Journal of Clinical Psychology 24, 301-302.

Whitaker, J. M., Severy, L. J., & Morton, D. S. (1984). A comprehensive community-based youth diversion program. Child Welfare 63, 175-181.

2) In Courts

Alessi, N. E., McManus, M., Grapentine, W. L., & Brickman, A. (1984). The characterization of depressive disorders in serious juvenile offenders. Journal of Affective Disorders 6, 9-17.

Halpern, W. I., Arkins, V., Mitchell, N., Freeling, N., & Healy, B. (1981). Continuity of mental health care to youth in the juvenile justice network. Hospital and Community Psychiatry 32, 114-117.

Mearing, J. S. (1982). Ethical implications of the children's rights movement for professionals. American Journal of Orthopsychiatry 52, 518-529.

Modlin, H. C., Porter, L., & Benson, R. E. (1976). Mental health centers and the criminal justice system. Hospital and Community Psychiatry 27, 716-719.

8. Training of Child Mental Health Professionals

Berlin, I. N. (1970). From confrontation to collaboration. American Journal of Orthopsychiatry 40, 473-480.

Malone, C. A. (1975). The impact of community mental health centers on child psychiatry training. Journal of the American Academy of Child Psychiatry 14, 32-48.

Meijer, A. (1977). Child psychiatry in a community health centre. Israel Annals of Psychiatry and Related Disciplines 15, 232-244.

Michelman, J. D. (1983). Child psychiatry in an HMO. A critical review. Minnesota Medicine 66, 52-57.

Rexford, E. N. (1969). Children, child psychiatry, and our brave new world. Archives of General Psychiatry 20, 25-37.
Shapiro, A. H., & Ash, L. C. (1977). Child psychiatry in northwestern Ontario: A community model. Canadian Journal of Public Health 68, 291-295.
Silver, L. B. (1977). Difficulties in integrating child and adolescent training and service in a community mental health center. Hospital and Community Psychiatry 28, 26-30.

9. Community Mental Health Centers and Prevention

a. Primary Prevention

Anthony, E. J. (1962). Primary prevention with school children. In H. H. Barten & L. Bellak (Eds.), Progress in community mental health (Vol. 2, pp. 131-158). New York: Grune & Stratton.
Berlin, I. N. (1967). Preventive aspects of mental health consultation to schools. Mental Hygiene 51, 34-40.
Berlin, I. N. (1972). Prevention of mental and emotional disorders of childhood. In B. B. Wolman (Ed.), Manual of child psychopathology (pp. 1088-1109). New York: McGraw-Hill.
Bloom, B. L. (1979). Prevention of mental disorders: Recent advances in theory and practice. Community Mental Health Journal 15, 179-191.
Bolman, W. M. (1967). An outline of preventive psychiatric programs for children. Archives of General Psychiatry 17, 5-8.
Bolman, W. M., & Westman, J. C. (1967). Prevention of mental disorder: An overview of current programs. American Journal of Psychiatry 123, 1058-1068.
Bowlby, J. (1951). Maternal care and mental health. Geneva: World Health Organization.
Brown, B. S. (1967). Definition of mental health and disease. In A. M. Freedman & H. I. Kaplan (Eds.), Comprehensive textbook of psychiatry (pp. 1516-1520). Baltimore: Williams and Wilkins.
Caplan, G., & Grunebaum, H. (1967). Perspectives on primary prevention: A review. Archives of General Psychiatry 17, 331-346.
Carbonara, N. T. (1961). Techniques for observing normal child behavior. Pittsburgh: University of Pittsburgh Press.
Comer, J. P. (1985). The Yale-New Haven primary prevention project: A follow-up study. Journal of the American Academy of Child Psychiatry 24, 154-160.
Cowen, E. L. (1980). The wooing of primary prevention. American Journal of Community Psychology 8, 258-284.
Felner, R. D., Ginter, M., & Primavera, J. (1982). Primary prevention during school transitions: Social support and environmental structure. American Journal of Community Psychology 10, 277-290.
Gottlieb, B. J. (1975). The contribution of natural support systems to primary prevention among four social subgroups of adolescent males. Adolescence 10, 207-220.

Hess, R., & Hermalin, J. (1983). Innovations in prevention. New York: Haworth Press.

Johnson, D. L., & Brekenridge, J. N. (1982). The Houston parent-child development center and the primary prevention of behavior problems in young children. American Journal of Community Psychology 10, 305-316.

Leon, R. L. (1968). Some implications for a preventive program for American Indians. American Journal of Psychiatry 125, 232-236.

Lindemann, E., & Dawes, L. G. (1952). The use of psychoanalytic constructs in preventive psychiatry. In R. S. Eissler, et al. (Eds.), Psychoanalytic study of the child (Vol. 7, pp. 429-448). New York: International Universities Press.

Offord, D. R. (1982). Primary prevention: Aspects of program design and evaluation. Journal of the American Academy of Child Psychiatry 21, 225-230.

Parrish, V., & Hester, P. (1980). Controlling behavioral techniques in an early intervention program. Community Mental Health Journal 16, 175-269.

Signell, K. A. (1983). Starting prevention work. Community Mental Health Journal 19, 144-163.

Stone, N. W., Pendleton, V. M., Vaill, M. B., Slatin, M., Mitcham, C., & Georgette, F. (1982). Primary prevention in mental health: A Head Start demonstration model. American Journal of Orthopsychiatry 52, 360-363.

Velasquez, J. S., & Lyle, C. G. (1985). Day versus residential treatment for juvenile offenders: The impact of program evaluation. Child Welfare 64, 145-156.

Waldfogel, S., & Gardner, G. E. (1961). Intervention in crises as a method of primary prevention. In G. Caplan (Ed.), Prevention of mental disorders in children (pp. 207-322). New York: Basic Books.

Wyatt, G. E., Bass, B. A., Powell, G. J., & Lim, P. (1983). Parents' and medical student therapists' perceptions of child mental health services. A teaching program in prevention and early intervention. Child Psychiatry and Human Development 13, 139-152.

Yee, T. T., & Lee, R. H. (1977). Based on cultural strengths. A school primary prevention program for Asian-American youth. Community Mental Health Journal 13, 239-248.

b. Secondary Prevention

Balser, B. H., Wacker, E., Gratwick, M., Mumford, R. S., Clinton, W., & Balser, P. (1965). Predicting mental disturbance in early adolescence. American Journal of Psychiatry 121, xi-xix.

Barnes, K. E. (1975). Secondary prevention. The utilization of public health nurses as agents of behavioral change in the community. American Journal of Public Health 65, 1099-1101.

Becker, D., & Margolin, F. (1967). How surviving parents handled their young children's adaptation to the crisis of loss. American Journal of Orthopsychiatry 37, 753-757.

Berlin, I. N. (1967). Secondary prevention. In A. M. Freedman & H. I. Kaplan (Eds.), Comprehensive textbook of psychiatry (pp. 1541-1548). Baltimore: Williams and Wilkins.

Bry, B. H. (1982). Reducing the incidence of adolescent problems through preventive intervention: One- and five-year follow-up. American Journal of Community Psychology 10, 265-276.

Burdsal, C., & Buel, C. L. (1980). A short term community based early stage intervention program for behavior problem youth. Journal of Clinical Psychology 36, 226-241.

Burks, H. L., & Harrison, S. I. (1962). Aggressive behavior as a means of avoiding depression. American Journal of Orthopsychiatry 32, 416-422.

Chess, S., & Thomas, A. (1972). Differences in outcome with early intervention in children with behavior disorders. In M. Roff, L. N. Robins, & M. Pollock (Eds.), Life history research in psychopathology (Vol. 2, pp. 35-46). Minneapolis: University of Minnesota Press.

Coolsen, P. (1980). Community involvement in the prevention of child abuse and neglect. Children Today 9, 5-8.

Eisenberg, L., & Gruenberg, E. M. (1969). The current status of secondary prevention in child psychiatry. In A. J. Bindman & A. D. Spiegel (Eds.), Perspectives in community mental health (pp. 250-262). Chicago: Aldine.

Farie, A. M., Cowen, E. L., & Smith, M. (1986). The development and implementation of a rural consortium program to provide early preventative mental health services. Community Mental Health Journal 22, 94-103.

George, N. M., Braun, B. A., & Walker, J. M. (1982). A prevention and early intervention mental health program for disadvantaged pre-school children. American Journal of Occupational Therapy 36, 99-106.

Guttmacher, A. F. (1967). Unwanted pregnancy: A challenge to mental health. Mental Hygiene 51, 512-516.

Hester, P. (1977). Evaluation and accountability in a parent-implemented early intervention service. Community Mental Health Journal 13, 216-267.

Ilfeld, H. Z., Edwards, D. W., & Yarvis, R. M. (1982). Secondary prevention: Serendipitous therapeutic effects for parents of child patients. Journal of Community Psychology 10, 33-39.

Jason, L. A., DeAmicis, L., & Carter, B. (1978). Preventive intervention programs for disadvantaged children. Community Mental Health Journal 14, 272-278.

John, V. P. (1963). Mental health programs for the socially deprived, urban child--1962 panel. II. The intellectual development of slum children: Some preliminary findings. American Journal of Orthopsychiatry 33, 813-822.

Klein, D. C., & Lindemann, E. (1961). Preventive intervention in individual and fmaily crisis situations. In G. Caplan (Ed.), Prevention of mental disorders in children (pp. 283-306). New York: Basic Books.

Leighton, D. C., Harding, J. S., Macklin, D. B., Macmillan, A. M., & Leighton, A. H. (1963). The character of danger. New York: Basic Books.

Livingood, A. B., Daen, P., & Smith, B. D. (1983). The depressed mother as a cource of stimulation for her infant. Journal of Clinical Psycholgoy 39, 369-375.

McConville, B. J. (1982). Secondary prevention in child psychiatry: An overview with ideas for action. Canada's Mental Health 30, 4-7.

Mechanic, D. (1962). The concept of illness behavior. Journal of Chronic Diseases 15, 189-194.

Minuchin, S. (1982). Reflections on boundaries. American Journal of Orthopsychiatry 52, 655-663.

Parks, C. A. (1982). Combining prevention and remediation services in a church-related agency. Child Welfare 61, 289-296.

Provence, S. (1985). On the efficacy of early intervention programs. Journal of Developmental and Behavioral Pediatrics 6, 363-366.

Rahe, R. H., Meyer, M., Smith, M., Kjaer, G., & Holmes, T. H. (1964). Social stress and illness onset. Journal of Psychosomatic Research 8, 35-44.

Rickel, A. U., & Lampi, L. (1981). A two-year follow-up study of a preventive mental health program for preschoolers. Journal of Abnormal Child Psychology 9, 455-464.

Rickel, A. U., Smith, R. L., & Sharp, K. C. (1979). Description and evaluation of a preventive mental health program for preschoolers. Journal of Abnormal Child Psychology 7, 101-112.

Rutter, M., Birch, H. G., Thomas, A., & Chess, S. (1964). Temperamental characteristics in infancy and the later development of behavioural disorders. British Journal of Psychiatry 110, 651-661.

Schiff, S. K., & Kellam, S. G. (1967). A community-wide mental health program of prevention and early treatment in first grade. Psychiatric Research Reports of the American Psychiatric Association 21, 92-102.

Scott, J. P. (1962). Critical periods in behavioral development. Science 138, 949-958.

Shaw, N. R. (1974). Teaching young mothers their role. Nursing Outlook 22, 695-698.

Signell, K. A. (1983). Starting prevention work. Community Mental Health Journal 19, 144-163.

Skeels, H. M. (1966). Adult status of children with contrasting earlylife experiences: A follow-up study. Monographs of the Society for Research in Child Development (Vol. 31). Chicago: University of Chicago Press.

Srole, L., Langner, T. S., Michael, S. T., Opler, M. K., & Rennie, T. A. C. (1962). The midtown Manhattan study. Vol. 1. Mental health in the metropolis. New York: McGraw-Hill.

Wyatt, G. E., Bass, B. A., Powell, G. E., & Lim, P. (1983). Parents' and medical student therapists' perceptions of child mental health services. A teaching program in prevention and early intervention. Child Psychiatry and Human Development 13, 139-152.

1) Mother-Child Relations

Ainsworth, M. D. (1962). The effects of maternal deprivation: A review of findings and controversy in the context of research strategy. In M.D. Ainsworth, Deprivation of maternal care: A reassessment of its effects (pp. 97-165). Geneva: World Health Organization.

Bibring, G. L., Dwyer, T. F., Huntington, D. S., & Valenstein, A. F. (1961). A study of the psychological process in pregnancy and of the earliest mother-child relationship. I. Some prepositions and comments. In R. S. Eissler, et al. (Eds.), Psychoanalytic study of the child (Vol. 16, pp. 9-24). New York: International Universities Press.

Braun, S. J. (1965). The well baby clinic: Its prospects for building ego strength. American Journal of Public Health 55, 1889-1898.

Bullard, D. M., Glasser, H. H., Heagarty, M. C., & Pivchik, E. (1967). Failure to thrive in the "neglected" child. American Journal of Orthopsychiatry 37, 680-690.

Danieli, Y. (1981). The group project for holocaust survivors and their children. Children Today 10, 11-33.

Heller, M. (1975). Preventive mental health services for families new to the community. Hospital and Community Psychiatry 26, 493-494.

Korner, A. F., & Grobstein, R. (1966). Visual alertness as related to soothing in neonates: Implications for maternal stimulation and early deprivation. Child Development 37, 867-876.

Robertson, J. (1962). Mothering as an influence on early development: A study of well-baby clinic records. In R. S. Eissler, et al. (Eds.), Psychoanalytic study of the child (Vol. 17, pp. 245-264). New York: International Universities Press.

Sayegh, Y., & Dennis, W. (1965). The effect of supplementary experiences upon the behavioral development of infants in institutions. Child Development 36, 81-90.

Schaefer, E. S., & Bayley, N. (1963). Maternal behavior, child behavior, and their intercorrelations from infancy through adolescence. Monographs of the Society for Research in Child Development (Vol. 28). Chicago: University of Chicago Press.

Spurlock, J. (1985). Assessment and therapeutic intervention of black children. Journal of the American Academy of Child Psychiatry 24, 168-174.

2) Nutrition and Organic Disease

Cravioto, J., DeLicardie, E. R., & Birch, H. G. (1966). Nutrition, growth and neurointegrative development: An experimental and ecologic study. Pediatrics 38, 319-372.

Winick, M. (1968). Changes in nucleic acid and protein content of the human brain during growth. Pediatric Research 2, 352-355.

3) Learning and School Experience

Berlin, I. N. (1966). Consultation and special education. In I. Philips (Ed.), Prevention and treatment of mental retardation (pp. 279-293). New York: Basic Books.

Biber, B. (1955). Schooling as an influence in developing healthy personality. In R. Kotinsky & H. L. Witmer (Eds.), Community programs for mental health (pp. 158-221). Cambridge: Harvard University Press.

Bower, E. M. (1961). Primary prevention in a school setting. In G. Caplan (Ed.), Prevention of mental disorders in children (pp. 353-377). New York: Basic Books.

Dhadphale, M., Lukwago, M. G., Gajjar, M., & Mutie, D. M. (1983). The contribution of a psychological assessment clinic to school health service. East African Medical Journal 60, 760-765.

George, N. M., Braun, B. A., & Walker, J. M. (1982). A prevention and early intervention mental health program for disadvantaged pre-school children. American Journal of Occupational Therapy 36, 99-106.

Gualtieri, C. T., Koriath, U., Van Bourgondien, M., & Saleeby, N. (1983). Language disorders in children referred for psychiatric services. Journal of the American Academy of Child Psychiatry 22, 165-171.

Irigon, F. F., Sarno, M., Sera, J., & Westgard, R. (1981). Child development centers program: An effective school-based mental health service. Child Welfare 60, 569-577.

Kellam, S. G., & Schiff, S. K. (1967). Adaptation and mental illness in the first-grade classrooms of an urban community. Psychiatric Research Reports of the American Psychiatric Association 21, 79-91.

Kriechman, A. M. (1985). A school-based program of mental health services. Hospital and Community Psychiatry 36, 876-878.

Lillie, M. D., & Armstrong, H. E., Jr. (1982). Contributions to the development of psychoeducational approaches to mental health service. American Journal of Occupational Therapy 36, 438-443.

Rickel, A. U., & Lampi, L. (1981). A two-year follow-up study of a preventive mental health program for preschoolers. Journal of Abnormal Child Psychology 9, 455-464.

Silver, A. A., & Hagin, R. A. (1972). Profile of a first grade: A basis for preventive psychiatry. Journal of the American Academy of Child Psychiatry 11, 645-674.

Tolan, P. H., & Lounsbury, J. W. (1982). Community mental health ideology presented in high school health textbooks: A content analysis. Community Mental Health Journal 18, 286-296.

White, R. W. (1959). Motivation reconsidered: The concept of competence. Psychological Review 66, 297-333.

Wolkind, S. N., & Everitt, B. (1974). A cluster analysis of the behavioral items in the pre-school child. Psychological Medicine 4, 422-427.

Zax, M, & Cowen, E. L. (1967). Early identification and prevention of emotional disturbance in a public school. In E. L. Cowen, E. A. Gardner, & M. Zax (Eds.), Emergent approaches to mental health problems (pp. 331-351). New York: Appleton-Century-Crofts.

4) Adolescent Issues

Abend, S. M., Kachalsky, H., & Greenberg, H. R. (1968). Reactions of adolescents to short-term hospitalization. American Journal of Psychiatry 124, 949-954.

Aldrich, A. (1984). Community care for late adolescents. Journal of Adolescence 7, 205-215.

Berkman, I. P., & Rosenblum, L. (1982). Serving high school students in need: A look at restrengthening the linkage between the school and community referral sources. Adolescence 17, 465-470.

Bien, N. Z., & Bry, B. H. (1980). An experimentally designed comparison of four intensities of school-based prevention programs for adolescents with adjustment problems. Journal of Community Psychology 8, 110-116.

Bumpass, E. R., Brix, R. J., & Preston, D. (1985). A community-based program for juvenile firesetters. Hospital and Community Psychiatry 36, 529-533.

Gibbs, J. T. (1984). Black adolescents and youth: An endangered species. American Journal of Orthopsychiatry 54, 6-21.

Gurry, S. E. (1985). Severely disturbed adolescents in community care. Adolescence 20, 265-279.

Kraft, S. P., & DeMaio, T. J. (1982). An ecological intervention with adolescents in low-income families. American Journal of Orthopsychiatry 52, 131-140.

Kvaraceus, W. C. (1961). Forecasting delinquency: A three-year experiment. Exceptional Children 27, 429-435.

Lende, E., Gilmore, E., & Cavenaugh, N. (1980). Vivamos! A summer program for teenage parents. Children Today 9, 9-12.

London, K. (1981). Mainstreaming the adolescent mother. Issues in Health Care of Women 3, 7-22.

Machalow, R. (1981). Review of the literature: Follow-up of psychiatrically hospitalized adolescents. Adolescence 17, 789-799.

Silber, E., Hamburg, D. A., Coelho, G. V., Murphey, E. B., Rosenberg, M., & Pearlin, L. I. (1961). Adaptive behavior in competent adolescents: Coping with the anticipation of college. Archives of General Psychiatry 5, 354-365.

Young, S. (1981). Aspects of social support networks among institutionalized adolescents. Adolescence 16, 123-137.

c. Tertiary Prevention

Berlin, I. N., Boatman, M. J., Sheimo, S. L., & Szurek, S. A. (1950). Adolescent alternation of anorexia and obesity. Workshop. American Journal of Orthopsychiatry 21, 387-419.

Caplan, G., Mason, E. A., & Kaplan, D. (1965). Four studies of crisis in parents of prematures. Community Mental Health Journal 1, 149-161.

Green, M., & Solnit, A. J. (1964). Reactions to the threatened loss of a child. A vulnerable child syndrome. Pediatric management of the dying child, Part III. Pediatrics 34, 58-66.

Lindemann, E. (1944). Symptomatology and management of acute grief. American Journal of Psychiatry 101, 141-148.

Schwartz, L. H., Snider, J., & Schwartz, J. E. (1967). Psychiatric case report of nutritional battering with implications for community agencies. Community Mental Health Journal 3, 163-169.

Sperling, M. (1950). Mucous colitis associated with phobias. Psychoanalytic Quarterly 19, 318-326.

Sperling, M. (1951). The neurotic child and his mother: A psychoanalytic study. American Journal of Orthopsychiatry 21, 351-362.

10. Community Mental Health Centers--Evaluation

Angrosino, M. V. (1978). Applied anthropology and the concept of the underdog: Implications for community mental health planning and evaluation. Community Mental Health Journal 14, 291-299.

Bergen, B. J. (1965). Professional communities and the evaluation of demonstration projects in community mental health. American Journal of Public Health 55, 1057-1066.

Dowell, D. A., & Ciarlo, J. A. (1983). Overview of the community mental health centers program from an evaluation perspective. Community Mental Health Journal 21, 52-57.

Dush, D. M. (1985). Standardizing the outcome data in program evaluation. Community Mental Health Journal 19, 95-128.

Fairchild, H. H., & Wright, C. (1984). A social-ecological assessment and feedback-intervention of an adolescent treatment agency. Adolescence 19, 263-275.

Fiester, A. R. (1978). The ACCES system: A procedure for evaluating children's services at community mental health centers. Community Mental Health Journal 14, 224-232.

Flaherty, E. W., & Olsen, K. (1978a). An assessment of the utility of federally required program evaluation in community mental health centers (Vol. I). Philadelphia: Philadelphia Health Management Corporation.

Flaherty, E. W., & Olsen, K. (1978b). An assessment of the utility of federally required program evaluation in community mental health centers (Vol. II). Philadelphia: Philadelphia Health Management Corporation.

Friedman, S., Jeger, A. M., & Slotnick, R. S. (1982). Social ecological assessment of mental health treatment environments: Towards self-evaluation. Psychological Reports 50, 631-638.

Gillespie, D. F., & Seaberg, J. R. (1977). Individual problem rating: A proposed scale. Administration in Mental Health 5, 21-29.

Gruenberg, E. M. (Ed.). (1966). Evaluating the effectiveness of mental health services. New York: Milbank Memorial Fund.

Hargreaves, W. A., Atkison, C., & Orensen, J. E. (1977). Resource materials for community mental health program evaluation (2nd ed.). San Francisco: Langley Porter Institute.

Kaplan, J. M., & Smith, W. G. (1977). The use of attainment scaling in the evaluation of a regional mental health program. Community Mental Health Journal 13, 188-193.

Kuldau, J. M., & Dirks, S. J. (1977). Controlled evaluation of a hospital-originated community transitional system. Archives of General Psychiatry 34, 1331-1340.

Lebow, J. (1982). Models for evaluating services at community mental health centers. Hospital and Community Psychiatry 33, 1010-1014.

Lemoine, R. L., & Carney, A. (1984). The Louisiana mental health client-outcome evaluation project: An initial progress report. Community Mental Health Journal 20, 90-100.

Loeb, M. B. (1968). Evaluation as accountability: A basis for resistance to planning for community mental health services. In L. M. Roberts, N. S. Greenfield, & M. H. Miller (Eds.), Comprehensive mental health: The challenge of evaluation (pp. 249-258). Madison: University of Wisconsin Press.

Lorei, T. W., & Caffey, E. M., Jr. (1978). Goal definition by staff consensus: A contribution to the planning, delivery, and evaluation of mental health services. Journal of Consulting and Clinical Psychology 46, 1284-1290.

Maher, C. A. (1980). Evaluating school-community prevention programs: The program analysis and review system. Journal of Community Psychology 8, 276-283.

Offord, D. R. (1982). Primary prevention: Aspects of program design and evaluation. Journal of the American Academy of Child Psychiatry 21, 225-230.

Palmer, B. B., & Linn, L. (1979). An evaluation of traditional and alternative mental health facilities. Journal of Community Psychology 7, 324-327.

Reardon, D. F. (1977). A model for communicating about program evaluation. Journal of Community Psychology 5, 350-358.

Schain, R. J., Gardella, D., & Pon, J. (1982). Five-year outcome of children admitted to a state mental hospital. Hospital and Community Psychiatry 33, 847-848.

Schuman, L. M. (1968). Research methodology and potential in community health and preventive medicine. Annals of the New York Academy of Sciences 107(2), 471-808.

Skorupka, P. C., & Cooley, S. J. (1983). The development of a partial hospitalization program evaluation tool. International Journal of Partial Hospitalization 2, 57-66.

Suchman, E. A. (1967). Evaluative research: Principles and practice in public service and social action programs. New York: Russell Sage Foundation.

Walsh, J. A. (1984). Evaluative research in community mental health. Journal of Mental Health Administration 11, 13-15.

Weissberg, R. P., Cowen, E. L., Lotyczewski, B. S., & Gesten, E. L. (1983). The primary mental health project: Seven consecutive years of program outcome research. Journal of Consulting and Clinical Psychology 51, 100-107.

Zalkind, D., Zelon, H., Moore, M., & Kaluzny, A. (1977). A practical reporting and evaluation system for intervention programs: Guiding principles and potential uses. American Journal of Public Health 67, 370-373.

Zusman, J. (1976). Can program evaluation be saved from its enthusiasts? American Journal of Psychiatry 133, 1300-1305.

Zusman, J., & Ross, E. R. R. (1969). Evaluation of the quality of mental health services. Archives of General Psychiatry 20, 352-357.

B. Mental Health Consultation

Irving N. Berlin, M.D., Section Editor

1. History

Abramovitz, A. B. (1958). Methods and techniques of consultation. American Journal of Orthopsychiatry 28, 126-133.

Aldrich, C. K. (1968). A specialized training program for residents in psychiatry. In W. M. Mendel & P. Solomon (Eds.), The psychiatric consultation (pp. 26-32). New York: Grune & Stratton.

Berlin, I. N. (1964). Learning mental health consultation: History and problems. Mental Hygiene 48, 257-266.

Blumberg, A. (1956). A nurse consultant's responsibility and problems. American Journal of Nursing 56, 606-608.

Caplan, G. (1956). Mental health consultation in school. In G. Caplan (Ed.), Elements of a community mental health program (pp. 77-85). New York: Milbank Memorial Fund.

Coleman, J. V. (1947). Psychiatric consultation in case work agencies. American Journal of Orthopsychiatry 17, 533-539.

Covner, B. G. (1947). Principles for psychological consulting with client organization. Journal of Consulting Psychology 11, 227-244.

Gibson, R. W. (1954). The psychiatric consultant and the juvenile court. Mental Hygiene 38, 462-467.

Green, R., & Hamovitch, M. B. (1962). Education of social workers for mental health consultation. American Journal of Orthopsychiatry 32(2), 225-226.

Maddux, J. F. (1953). Psychiatric consultation in a rural setting. American Journal of Orthopsychiatry 23, 775-784.

Rosenfeld, J. M., & Caplan, G. (1954). Techniques of staff consultation in an immigrant children's organization in Israel. American Journal of Orthopsychiatry 24, 42-62.

2. Group Consultation

Altrocchi, G., Spielberger, D., & Schafer, E. (1965). Mental health consultation with groups. Community Mental Health Journal 1, 127-134.

Blumberg, A. (1959). A selected annotated bibliography on the consultant relationship in groups. Journal of Social Issues 15, 68-74.

Bradford, L. P. (1947). The use of psychodrama for group consultants. Sociatry 1, 192-197.

Gibb, J. R., & Lippitt, R. (1959). Consulting with groups and organizations. Journal of Social Issues 15, 1-74.

Kevin, D. (1963). Use of the group method in consultation. In L. Rapaport (Ed.), Consultation in social work practice (pp. 69-84). New York: National Association of Social Workers.

Mackey, R. A., & Hassler, F. R. (1966). Group consultation with school personnel. Mental Hygiene 50, 416-420.

Rieman, D. W. (1963). Group mental health consultation with public health nurses. In L. Rapaport (Ed.), Consultation in social work practice (pp. 85-98). New York: National Association of Social Workers.

3. Consultation in the Schools

Adams, R. S., & Weinick, H. M. (1966). Consultation: An inservice training program for the school. Journal of the American Academy of Child Psychiatry 5, 479-489.

Berkowitz, I. H. (1970). Mental health consultation to school personnel: Attitudes of school administrations and consultant priorities. Journal of School Health 40, 348-354.

Berkowitz, I. H., & Seliges, J. S. (1985). Expanding mental health interventions in schools. Dubuque, Iowa: Kendall/Hunt.

Berlin, I. N. (1956). Some learning experiences as psychiatric consultant in the schools. Mental Hygiene 40, 215-236.

Berlin, I. N. (1962). Mental health consultation in school as a means of communicating mental health principles. Journal of the American Academy of Child Psychiatry 1, 671-680.

Berlin, I. N. (1966a). Consultation and special education. In I. Philips (Ed.), Prevention and treatment of mental retardation (pp. 279-293). New York: Basic Books.

Berlin, I. N. (1966b). School child guidance services: Retrospect and prospect. Psychology in the Schools 3, 229-236.

Berlin, I. N. (1967). Preventive aspects of mental health consultation in schools. Mental Hygiene 51, 34-40.

Bronkowski, R. J. (1968). Mental health consultation and operation head start. American Psychologist 23, 769-773.

Caplan, G. (1956). Mental health consultation in schools. In G. Caplan (Ed.), Elements of a community mental health program (pp. 77-85). New York: Milbank Memorial Fund.

Edelsohn, G. A., & Williams, V. C. (1985). Child psychiatry consultation to a public high school: A developmental perspective. Journal of Child and Adolescent Psychotherapy 2(2), 105-109.

Fisher, L. (1973). Training in school consultation. In W. L. Claiborn & R. Cohen (Eds.), School intervention (pp. 76-93). New York: Behavioral Publications.

Hirschowitz, R. G. (1966). Psychiatric consultation in the schools: Socio-cultural perspectives. Mental Hygiene 50, 218-225.

Idol, L. (1988). A rationale and guidelines for established special education programs. Special Issues. Dimensions of School Consultation Practice/Remedial and Special Education 9(6), 48-58.

Marks, F., & Pennycock, W. (1986). The value of psychiatric consultation to a tutorial class teacher. Maladjustment and Therapeutic Education 4(1), 54-59.

Parker, B. (1962). Some observations on psychiatric consultation with nursery school teachers. Mental Hygiene 46, 559-566.

4. Consultation to Courts and Police

Berlin, I. N. (1964). Mental health consultation with a juvenile probations department. Crime and Delinquency 10, 67-73.

Burkhart, B. R., & King, G. D (1981). Blindmen and elephants: A case study of consultation with police. Journal of Community Psychology 9, 133-139.

Chwast, J. (1965). Mental health consultation with street gant workers. In W. E. Reckless & C. L. Newman (Eds.), Interdisciplinary problems in criminology (pp. 13-21). Columbus, Ohio: American Society of Criminology.

Elkins, A. M., & Papanek, G. O. (1966). Consultation with the police: An example of community psychiatry practice. American Journal of Psychiatry 123, 531-535.

Goldin, G. D. (1967). The psychiatrist as a court consultant: A challenge to community psychiatry. Community Mental Health Journal 3, 396-398.

Goy, G. L. (1982). Consultant to the court in infant-toddler custody cases. Infant Mental Health Journal 3(2), 126-134.

Soskis, D. (1983). Behavioral scientists and law enforcement personnel: Working together on the problem of terrorism. Behavioral Sciences and the Law 1(2), 47-58.

Susselman, S. (1969). Interrelationship of the correctional worker, the offender and the legal structure. In S. A. Szurek & I. N. Berlin (Eds.), The antisocial child: His family and his community (pp. 134-148). Palo Alto: Science and Behavior Books.

Tolan, P. H., Perry, M. S., & Jones, T. (1987). Delinquency prevention: An example of consultation in rural community mental health. Journal of Community Psychology 4, 43-50.

5. Consultation to Welfare Agencies

Bernard, R. W. (1954). Psychiatric consultation in the social agency. Child Welfare 33, 3-8.

Caplan, G. (1955). The role of the social worker in preventive psychiatry. Medical Social Work 4, 144-159.

Coleman, J. R. (1953). The contribution of the psychiatrist to the social worker and to the client. Mental Hygiene 37, 249-255.

Davis, W. E. (1957). Psychiatric consultation: The agency viewpoint. Child Welfare 36, 4-9.

Decker, J. H., & Itzin, F. (1956). An experience in consultation with public assistance. Social Case Work 27, 327-334.

6. Rural Consultation

Eisdorfer, C., Altrocchi, J., & Young, R. F. (1968). Principles of community mental health in a rural setting: The Halifax County program. Community Mental Health Journal 4, 211-220.

Marshall, P., Coleman, L., Daedler, R., & LaBaw, W. (1970). Rural community consultation in child psychiatric training. American Journal of Orthopsychiatry 40(2), 294-295.

7. Training in Mental Health Consultation

Altman, M. (1972). A child psychiatrist steps into the classroom: A report of a training experience. Journal of the American Academy of Child Psychiatry 11, 231-242.

Berlin, I. N. (1965). Mental health consultation in schools: Who can do it and why. Community Mental Health Journal 1, 19-22.

Bernard, V. W. (1964). Role and functions of child psychiatrists in social and community psychiatry: Implications for training. Journal of the American Academy of Child Psychiatry 3, 165-176.

Caplan, G. (1965). Problems of training in mental health consultation. In S. E. Galdston (Ed.), Concepts of community psychiatry (No. 131g, pp. 91-108). Bethesda, Md.: Public Health Service Publication.

Curtis, M. J., & Zins, J. E. (1988). Effects of training in consultation and instructor feedback on acquisition of consultation skills. Journal of the School of Psychology 26(2), 185-190.

Eisdorfer, C., & Batton, L. (1972). The mental health consultant as seen by his consultees. Community Mental Health Journal 8, 171-177.

Leon, R. L. (1960). Participant-directed experience as a method of psychiatric teaching and consultation. Mental Hygiene 44, 375-381.

Magee, J. J., & Pierce, D. (1986). When the supervisor serves as participating consultant for both client and social worker. Clinical Supervisor 4(4), 85-89.

Meyers, J. (1984). Training in consultation. American Journal of Community Psychology 12(2), 233-239.

Parker, B. (1961). The value of supervision in training psychiatrists for mental health consultation. Mental Hygiene 45, 94-100.

Polk, W. J., & MacLennan (1975). Experiences in training of mental health consultants. In F. V. Mannino, et al. (Eds.), The practice of mental health consultation (pp. 131-143). Adelphi, Md.: National Institute of Mental Health.

Rogawski, A. S. (1968). Teaching consultation techniques in a community agency. In W. M. Mendel & P. Solomon (Eds.), The psychiatric consultation (pp. 65-85). New York: Grune & Stratton.

Signell, K. A., & Scott, P. A. (1972). Training in consultation: A crisis of role transition. Community Mental Health Journal 8(2), 149-160.

Thigpen, J. S. (1979). Perceptual differences in the supervision of paraprofessional mental health workers. Community Mental Health Journal 15(2), 139-149.

8. Theoretical Aspects of Mental Health Consultation

Baer, D. M. (1970). The consultation process model as an irrational state of affairs. Psychology in the Schools 7(4), 341-344.

Batman, R. H. (1968). consultation as an educational technique in psychiatric nursing. Mental Hygiene 52(4), 617-621.

Berlin, I. N. (1966). Transference and countertransference in community psychiatry. Archives of General Psychiatry 15, 165-172.

Berlin, I. N. (1969). Mental health consultation for school social workers: A conceptual model. Community Mental Health Journal 5, 280-288.

Berlin, I. N. (1979). Resistance to mental health consultation directed at change in public institution. Community Mental Health Journal 15(2), 119-129.

Bindiman, A. G. (1959). Mental health consultation: Therapy and practice. Journal of Consulting Psychology 23, 473-482.

Bowman, P. H. (1959). The role of the consultant as a motivator of action. Mental Hygiene 43, 105-110.

Brown, D., & Schulte, A. C. (1987). A social learning model of consultation. Professional Psychology Research and Practice 18(3), 283-287.

Caplan, A. (1970). The theory and practice of mental health consultation. New York: Basic Books.

Caplan, G. (1963). Type of mental health consultation. American Journal of Orthopsychiatry 33, 470-481.

Deloughoy, G. L., & Gebbie, K. M. (1973). Categories of cases presented to mental health consultants by health agencies. American Journal of Public Health 63, 1048-1054.

Ferguson, C. K. (1968). Concerning the nature of human systems and the consultant's role. Journal of Applied Behavioral Science 4, 179-193.

Gilmore, T. N., & Krantz, J. (1985). Projective identification in the consulting relationship: Exploring the unconscious dimensions of a client system. Human Relations 38(12), 1147-1159.

Gorman, J. F. (1963). Some characteristics of consultation: Theory and practice. In L. Rapaport (Ed.), Consultation in social work practice (pp. 21-31). New York: National Association of Social Workers.

Glidwell, J. C. (1959). The entry problem in consultation. Journal of Social Issues 15, 51-59.

Griffith, C. R., & Libo, L. M. (1968). Mental health consultants: Agents of community change. San Francisco: Jossey-Bass.

Gutkini, T. B. (1986). Consultees' perceptions of variables relating to outcomes of school based consultation interaction. School Psychology Review 15(3), 375-382.

Hollister, W. G. (1962). Some administrative aspects of consultation. American Journal of Orthopsychiatry 32, 224-225.

Jarvis, P. E., & Nelson, S. E. (1967). Familiarization: A vital step in mental health consultation. Community Mental Health Journal 3, 343-348.

Karp, H. N., & Karls, J. M. (1966). Combining crisis therapy and mental health consultation. Archives of General Psychiatry 14, 536-542.

Klein, D. C. (1959). Consultation processes as a method of improving teaching. Boston University: Human relations research and technical notes, No. 69.

Krell, H. L., & Okin, J. C. L. (1984). Countertransference issues in child abuse and neglect. American Journal of Forensic Psychiatry 5(1), 5-16.

Libo, L. M. (1966). Multiple functions for psychologists in community consultation. American Psychologist 21, 530-534.

Lippitt, G. L. (1960). Organization climate and individual growth: The consultative process at work. Personnel Administrator 23, 19-43.

Maitland, R. F., Fine, M. J., & Tracy, D. B. (1985). The effects of an interpersonally based problem-solving process on consultation outcomes. Journal of School Psychology 23(8), 337-345.

Mannino, F. V. (1964). Developing consultation relationships with community agents. Mental Hygiene 48, 356-362.

Mannino, F. V., & Shore, M. F. (1975). Effecting change through consultation. In F. V. Mannino, et al. (Eds.), The practice of mental health consultations (pp. 25-48). Adelphi, Md.: National Institute of Mental Health.

MacLennan, B. W. (1975a). Program development and gaining access in the community: Mental health consultation in the schools. In F. V. Mannino, et al. (Eds.), The practice of mental health consultations (pp. 61-74). Adelphi, Md.: National Institute of Mental Health.

MacLennan, B. W. (1975b). Some problems in consultation. In F. V. Mannino, et al. (Eds.), The practice of mental health consultations (pp. 148-156). Adelphi, Md.: National Institute of Mental Health.

MacLennan, B. W., Quinn, R. D., & Schroeder, D. (1975). The scope of community mental health consultation. In F. V. Mannino, et al. (Eds.), The practice of mental health consultations (pp. 3-24). Adelphi, Md.: National Institute of Mental Health.

Osterweil, Z. O. (1987). A structural process of problem definition in school consultation. School Counselor 34(5), 345-352.

Spencer, E. C., & Croley, N. T. (1963). Administrative consultation. In L. Rapaport (Ed.), Consultation in social work practice (pp. 51-68). New York: National Association of Social Workers.

Streviger, L. A. (1961). Consultation: Some expectations, principles and skills. Social Work 6, 85-90.

Talbott, J. A. (1988). The elements of community consultation. New Directions for Mental Health Services 37, 69-84.

Valenstein, A. F. (1955). Some principles of psychiatric consultation. Social Case Work 36, 253-256.
West, J. F., & Cannon, G. (1988). Essential collaborative consultation competencies for regular and special education. Journal of Learning Disabilities 21(1), 56-63.
Witt, G. C., & Martens, B. K. (1988). Problems with problem solving consultation: An analysis of assumptions, methods and goals. School Psychology Review 17(2), 211-226.

9. Miscellaneous References

Berlin, I. N. (1977). Some lessons learned in 25 years of mental health consultation. In S. C. Plog & P. G. Ahmed (Eds.), Principles and techniques of mental health consultation (pp. 23-48). New York: Plenum Press.
Collins, M., Fleet, L., Pool, J., & Wood, M. (1985). Consultancy in pastoral care. Educational and Child Psychology 2(1), 53-59.
Greenspan, S. I., Nover, R. A., & Brunt, C. H. (1975). Mental health consultation to early child care. In F. V. Mannino, et al. (Eds.), The practice of mental health consultation (pp. 105-130). Adelphi, Md.: National Institute of Mental Health.
Mouw, M. L., & Haylett, C. H. (1967). Mental health consultation in a public health nursing service. American Journal of Nursing 67, 1447-1450.
Perkins, G. L. (1958). Psychiatric consultation in residential treatment: The consultant's view. American Journal of Orthopsychiatry 28, 266-275.
Pergamenter, R. (1982). Crisis intervention with child-care personnel in an Israeli border kibbutz. Clinical and Community Psychology: Stress and Anxiety 8, 355-360.
Small, R. H. (1987). Psychiatric consultation to community based military child protection teams. Military Medicine 152(5), 223-227.
Smith, K. (1984). A heart with skill to listen: Consultation to a child minding project. Journal of Social Work Practice 1(3), 55-68.

PART VI

RESEARCH

Research

Coeditors:

Donald J. Cohen, M.D.
Professor of Psychiatry and Pediatrics
Director, Yale Child Study Center
Yale University School of Medicine
New Haven, Connecticut

James F. Leckman, M.D.
Associate Professor
Yale University School of Medicine
New Haven, Connecticut

Associate Editors:

George Anderson, Ph.D.
Yale University School of Medicine
New Haven, Connecticut

Joel Bregman, M.D.
Yale University School of Medicine
New Haven, Connecticut

David Pauls, Ph.D.
Yale University School of Medicine
New Haven, Connecticut

Mark Riddle, M.D.
Yale University School of Medicine
New Haven, Connecticut

John Stevenson, M.D.
Yale University School of Medicine
New Haven, Connecticut

Kenneth Towbin, M.D.
Yale University School of Medicine
New Haven, Connecticut

Larry Vitulano, Ph.D.
Yale University School of Medicine
New Haven, Connecticut

Fred Volkmar, M.D.
Yale University School of Medicine
New Haven, Connecticut

Gwen Zahnes, Ph.D.
Yale University School of Medicine
New Haven, Connecticut

A. Methodology in Clinical Research

Achenbach, T. M. (1978). Psychopathology of childhood: Research problems and issues. Journal of Consulting and Clinical Psychology 46, 759-776.

Allen, P. A., & Waters, W. E. (1982). Development of an ethical committee and its effects on research design. Lancet 1, 1233-1236.

Altman, D. G. (1980). Statistics and ethics in medical research. VI. Presentation of results. British Medical Journal 281, 1542-1544.

Anderson, D. L., & Tyre, T. E. (1982). Thoughts on the conduct of behavioral research in the medical setting. QRB. Quality Review Bulletin 8, 7-9.

Austin, J. H. (1979). The varieties of chance in scientific research. Medical Hypotheses 5, 737-742.

Austin, M. A., Criqui, M. H., & Barrett-Connor, E. (1981). The effect of response bias on the odds ration. American Journal of Epidemiology 114, 137-143.

Barlow, D. H., & Hayes, S. C. (1979). Alternating treatments of design: One strategy for comparing the effects of two treatments in a single subject. Journal of Applied Behavior Analysis 12, 199-210.

Barnard, K. E. (1985a). Seeking approval of conducting research. MCN; American Journal of Maternal Child Nursing 10, 292.

Barnard, K. E. (1985b). Studying patterns of behavior. MCN; American Journal of Maternal Child Nursing 10, 358.

Barrett, J. (1981). Psychiatric diagnoses (research diagnostic criteria) in symptomatic volunteers. Archives of General Psychiatry 38, 153-157.

Bartko, J. J., & Carpenter, W. T. (1976). On the methods and theory of reliability. Journal of Nervous and Mental Disease 163, 307-317.

Bath, K. (1974). The use of intensive individual designs in community research. Community Mental Health Journal 10, 418-425.

Berkson, G., & Landesman-Dwyer, S. (1977). Behavioral research on severe and profound mental retardation (1955-1974). American Journal of Mental Deficiency 81, 428-454.

Berwin, T. B. (1982). Consent to randomized treatment. Lancet 2, 919-921.

Birnbrauer, J. S. (1974). Design and interpretation of studies of single subjects. American Journal of Mental Deficiency 79, 191-203.

Blaney, P. H. (1975). The use of medical controls in research with psychiatric populations. Comprehensive Psychiatry 16, 375-377.

Blatt, S. J. (1975). The validity of projective techniques and their research and clinical contribution. Journal of Personality Assessment 39, 327-343.

Research

Burch, P. R. (1983). The surgeon general's "epidemiologic criteria for causality." A critique. Journal of Chronic Diseases 36, 821-836.

Burke, J. D., Pincus, H. A., & Pardes, H. (1986). The clinician-researcher in psychiatry. American Journal of Psychiatry 143, 968-975.

Byar, D. P., Simm, R. M., & Friedenwald, W. T. (1976). Randomized clinical trials: Perspectives on some recent ideas. New England Journal of Medicine 295, 74-80.

Chassan, J. B. (1981). Some notes on the foundations and scope of intensive design. Psychiatry 44, 34-38.

Cicchetti, D. V. (1967). Assessing inter-rater reliability for rating scales: Resolving some basic issues. British Journal of Psychiatry 129, 452-456.

Cohen, L. H., & Suchy, K. R. (1979). The bias in psychotherapy research evaluation. Journal of Clinical Psychology 35, 184-187.

Cole, P. (1979). the evolving case control study. Journal of Chronic Diseases 32, 15-27.

Collins, B. E., Henker, B., & Whalen, C. (1979). A mixed crossover and parallel group design in psychopharmacological research--example B. Psychopharmacology Bulletin 15, 40-42.

Davis, C. E. (1976). The effect of regression to the mean in epidemiologic and clinical studies. American Journal of Epidemiology 104, 493-498.

DeMyer, M. K. (1975). Research in infantile autism: A strategy and its results. Biological Psychiatry 10, 433-452.

Diamond, G. A., & Forrester, J. S. (1983). Clinical trials and statistical verdicts: Probable grounds for appeal. Annals of Internal Medicine 98, 358-394.

DeMascio, A., Klerman, G. L., Weissman, M. M., Prusoff, B. A., Neu, C., & Moore, P. (1979). A control group for psychotherapy research in acute depression: One solution to ethical and methodologic issues. Journal of Psychiatric Research 15, 189-197.

Dohrenwend, B. S., & Dohrenwend, B. P. (1978). Some issues in research on stressful life events. Journal of Nervous and Mental Disease 166, 7-15.

Donner, A. (1985). A regression approach to the analysis of data arising from cluster randomization. International Journal of Epidemiology 14, 322-326.

Donovick, P. J., & Horowitz, G. P. (1982). On the choice of subject populations for research in neurobehavioral toxicology. Journal of Toxocology and Environmental Health 10, 1-9.

Eaves, L. J. (1978). Twins as a basis for the causal analysis of human personality. Progress in Clinical and Biological Research 24A, 151-174.

Edelheit, H. (1976). Complementarity as a rule in psychological research. Jackson, Freud and the mind/body problem. International Journal of Psycho-Analysis 57, 23-36.

Edlund, M. J., Craig, T. J., & Richardson, M. A. (1985). Informed consent as a form of volunteer bias. American Journal of Psychiatry 142, 624-627.

Edlund, M. J., Overall, J. E., & Rhoades, H. M. (1985). Beta, or type II error in psychiatric controlled clinical trials. Journal of Psychiatric Research 19, 563-567.

Eisenberg, L., & Kleimann, A. (1980). The relevance of social science for medicine. New York: Reidel.

Elkins, H. B., Pagnotto, L. D., & Brugsch, H. G. (1972). Confusion concerning "normal" values in biologic analysis. New England Journal of Medicine 286, 1268-1269.

Elveback, L. R. (1972). How high is high? A proposed alternative to the normal range. Mayo Clinic Proceedings 47, 93-97.

Endicott, J., & Spitzer, R. L. (1975). Designing mental health studies: The case for experimental design. Hospital and Community Psychiatry 26, 737-739.

Fann, W. E., Stafford, J. R., Malone, R. L., Frost, J. D., & Richman, B. W. (1977). Clinical research techniques in tardive dyskinesia. American Journal of Psychiatry 134, 759-762.

Feinstein, A. R. (1972a). The need for humanised science in evaluating medication. Lancet 2, 421-423.

Feinstein, A. R. (1972b). Why clinical epidemiology? Clinical Research 20, 821-825.

Feinstein, A. R. (1974). Clinical biostatistics. XXVI. Medical ethics and the architecture of clinical research. Clinical Pharmacology and Therapeutics 15, 316-334.

Feinstein, A. R. (1979a). Clinical biostatistics. XLVII. Scientific standards vs. statistical associations and biologic logic in the analysis of causation. Clinical Pharmacology and Therapeutics 25, 481-492.

Feinstein, A. R. (1979b). Clinical biostatistics. XLVIII. Efficacy of different research structures in preventing bias in the analysis of causation. Clinical Pharmacology and Therapeutics 26, 129-141.

Feinstein, A. R. (1981). Clinical biostatistics. LVI. "The t test" and the basic ethos of parametric statistical inference (conclusion). Clinical Pharmacology and Therapeutics 30, 133-146.

Fleiss, J. L. (1975). Measuring agreement between two judges on the presence or absence of a trait. Biometrics 31, 651-659.

Fleiss, J. L. (1986). The design and analysis of clinical experiments. New York: Wiley.

Frank, J. D. (1974). Therapeutic components of psychotherapy. A 25-year progress report of research. Journal of Nervous and Mental Disease 159, 325-342.

Freiman, J. A., Chalmers, T. C., & Smith, H. (1978). The importance of beta, the type II error and sample size in the design and interpretation of the randomized control trial. New England Journal of Medicine 299, 690-694.

Garmezy, N. (1974). Children at risk: The search for the antecedents of schizophrenia. Part II: Ongoing research programs, issues, and intervention. Schizophrenia Bulletin 55, 125.

Giller, E., & Strauss, J. (1984). Clinical research: A key to clinical training. American Journal of Psychiatry 141, 1075-1077.

Glenn, N. D. (1981). Age, birth cohorts, and drinking: An illustration of the hazards of inferring effects from cohort data. Journal of Gerontology 36, 362-369.

Goodwin, D. W. (1977). Genetic and experiential antecedents of alcoholism: A prospective study. Alcoholism 1, 259-265.

Research

Gordis, L. (1979). Assuring the quality of questionnaire data in epidemiologic research. American Journal of Epidemiology 109, 21-24.

Gore, S. M. (1981). Assessing clinical trials--double-blind trials. British Medical Journal 283, 122-124.

Gottschalk, L. A. (1974). The application of a method of content analysis to psychotherapy research. American Journal of Psychotherapy 28, 488-499.

Graham, S. (1974). The sociological approach to epidemiology. American Journal of Public Health 64, 1046-1049.

Grant, I., Sweetwood, H., Gerst, M. S., & Yager, J. (1978). Scaling procedures in life events research. Journal of Psychosomatic Research 22, 225-230.

Gray, G. H., Cooke, R. A., & Tannenbaum, A. S. (1978). Research involving human subjects. Science 201, 1094-1101.

Grinker, R. R. (1981). Planning for a schizophrenia research program: A prototype. Schizophrenia Bulletin 7, 181-195.

Grove, W. M., & Andreasen, N. C. (1982). Simultaneous tests of many hypotheses in exploratory research. Journal of Nervous and Mental Disease 170, 3-8.

Guze, S. B. (1976). Editorial: Research and psychiatric training. Biological Psychiatry 11, 265-266.

Halperin, S., Nehrke, M. F., Hulicka, I. M., & Morganti, J. B. (1976). Partitioning chi-square the analysis of contingency tables with repeated measurements. Experimental Aging Research 2, 105-118.

Hanlon, T. E., Blatchley, R. J., & Kurland, A. A. (1975). Effects of control techniques on therapeutic outcome in a controlled clinical trial. International Pharmacopsychiatry 10, 169-176.

Harris, T., & Brown, G. W. (1985). Interpreting data in aetiological studies of affective disorder: Some pitfalls and ambiguities. British Journal of Psychiatry 147, 5-15.

Heinicke, C. M., & Strassmann, L. H. (1975). Toward more effective research on child psychotherapy. Journal of the American Academy of Child Psychiatry 14, 561-588.

Helmchen, H., & Muller-Oerlinghausen, B. (1975). The inherent paradox of clinical trials in psychiatry. Journal of Medical Ethics 1, 168-173.

Herschberg, R. I., Harper, D., & Leichner, P. (1980). Research in psychiatry: Residents' attitudes and use. Journal of Medical Education 55, 540-541.

Hewett, S. (1976). Research on families with handicapped children--an aid or an impediment to understanding? Birth Defects Original Articles Series 12, 35-46.

Hills, A. B., & Armitage, P. (1979). The two-period cross-over clinical trial. British Journal of Clinical Pharmacology 8, 7-20.

Horn, M. J., Green, M., Carney, R., & Erickson, M. T. (1975). Bias against genetic hypotheses in adoption studies. Archives of General Psychiatry 32, 1365-1367.

Howard, J., & Friedman, L. (1981). Protecting the scientific integrity of a clinical trial: Some ethical dilemmas. Clinical Pharmacology and Therapeutics 29, 561-570.

Howard, K. I., Krause, M. S., & Orlinsky, D. E. (1986). The attrition dilemma: Toward a new strategy for psychotherapy research. Journal of Consulting and Clinical Psychology 54, 106-110.

Hrubec, Z. (1981). Methodologic problems in matched-pair studies using twins. Progress in Clinical and Biological Research 69(C), 1-7.

Hughes, J. R., & Krahn, D. (1985). Blindness and the validity of the double-blind procedure. Journal of Clinical Psychopharmacology 5, 138-142.

Hulley, S. B. (1978). Symposium on CHD prevention trials: Design issues in testing life style intervention. American Journal of Epidemiology 108, 85-86.

Hutchinson, T. A., Boyd, N. F., & Feinstein, A. R. (1979). Scientific problems in clinical scales, as demonstrated in the Karnofsky index of performance status. Journal of Chronic Diseases 32, 661-666.

Imber, S. D., Glanz, L. M., Elkin, I., Sotsky, S. M., Boyer, J. L., & Leber, W. R. (1986). Ethical issues in psychotherapy research. Problems in a collaborative clinical trials study. American Psychologist 41, 137-146.

Innes, J. M. (1979). Attitudes towards randomized control group experimental designs in the field of community welfare. Psychological Reports 44, 1207-1213.

Jason, J., Anderek, N., & Marks, J. (1982). Child abuse in Georgia: A method to evaluate risk factors and reporting bias. American Journal of Public Health 72, 1353-1358.

Jones, E. (1974). Social class and psychotherapy: A critical review of research. Psychiatry 37, 307-320.

Jonsen, A. R., Siegler, M., & Winslade, W. J. (1982). Clinical ethics. New York: Macmillan.

Kappauf, W. E. (1976). Critique of the use of covariance adjustments for CA and MA in comparative studies of retarded and nonretarded persons. American Journal of Mental Deficiency 81, 240-247.

Karch, F. E., & Lasagna, L. (1975). Adverse drug reactions: A clinical review. Journal of the American Medical Association 234, 1236-1241.

Kelly, D. D. (1974). The experimental imperative: Laboratory analyses of aggressive behaviors. Research Publications- Associations for Research in Nervous and Mental Disease 52, 21-41.

Kemp, R. (1977). Controversy in scientific research and tactics of communication. Sociological Review 25, 515-534.

Kernberg, O. F. (1976). Some methodological strategic issues in psychotherapy research: Research implications of the Menninger Foundations's Psychotherapy Research Project. Proceedings of the American Psychopathology Association 64, 23-38.

Kety, S. S. (1976). Studies designed to disentangle genetic and environmental variables in schizophrenia: Some epistemological questions and answers. American Journal of Psychiatry 133, 1134-1137.

Kidd, K. K., & Matthysee, S. (1978). Research designs for the study of gene-environment interactions in psychiatric disorders. Report of a Foundation Fund for Research in Psychiatry panel. Archives of General Psychiatry 35, 925-932.

Kistner, J., & Robbins, F. (1986). Brief report: Characteristics of methods of subject selection and description in research on autism. Journal of Autism and Developmental Disorders 16, 77-82.

Kokes, R. F., Fremouw, W., & Strauss, J. S. (1977). Lost subjects. Source of bias in clinical research. Archives of General Psychiatry 34, 1363-1365.

Kolata, G. B. (1980). Love canal: False alarm caused by botched study. Science 208, 1239-1242.

Koran, L. M. (1975). The reliability of clinical methods, data and judgments. New England Journal of Medicine 293, 642-646.

Kramer, M. (1976). Issues in the development of statistical and epidemiological data for mental health services research. Psychological Medicine 6, 185-215.

Kramer, M. S., & Feinstein, A. R. (1981). Clinical biostatistics: LIV. The biostatistics of concordance. Clinical Pharmacology and Therapeutics 29, 111-123.

Krause, M. S., & Howard, K. I. (1976). Program evaluation in the public interest: A new research methodology. Community Mental Health Journal 12, 291-300.

Lader, M. (1976). Assessment of drugs in schizophrenia. Basic trial design. British Journal of Clinical Pharmacology 3, 375-379.

Lester, D. (1977). Longitudinal studies on alcoholism: Three proposals. Alcoholism 1, 249-250.

Levine, J. (1974). Guidelines for the conduct of clinical trials. FDA guidelines for psychotropic drugs. Psychopharmacology Bulletin 10, 70-91.

Levine, R. J., & Lebacqz, K. (1979). Some ethical considerations in clinical trials. Clinical Pharmacology and Therapeutics 25, 728-741.

Lewine, R. R. (1978). Choosing control groups in the study of schizophrenic subtypes. Schizophrenia Bulletin 4, 244-247.

Lewine, R. R., Watt, N. F., & Grubb, T. W. (1981). High-risk-for-schizophrenia research: Sampling bias and its implications. Schizophrenia Bulletin 7, 273-280.

Lion, J. R., & Monroe, R. R. (1975). Editorial: Clinical research of the violent individual. Journal of Nervous and Mental Disease 160, 75.

Lipton, E. L. (1976). Psychoanalytic child development research and the practice of general psychiatry. International Journal of Psycho-Analysis 57, 113-126.

Little, J. W. (1976). An overview of the legal aspects of human experimentation and research. Journal of Forensic Sciences 21, 427-440.

Lykken, D. T., Tellegen, A., & DeRubeis, R. (1978). Volunteer bias in twin research: The rule of two-thirds. Social Biology 25, 1-9.

Madle, R. A., Neisworth, J. T., & Kurtz, P. D. (1980). Biasing of hyperkinetic behavior ratings by diagnostic reports: Effects of observer training and assessment method. Journal of Learning Disabilities 13, 35-38.

Mahoney, M. J. (1976). Discussion: Behavior therapy. Some critical comments. Proceedings of the American Psychopathology Association 64, 127-131.

Mansell, J. (1985). Time sampling and measurement error: The effect of interval length and sampling pattern. Journal of Behavior Therapy and Experimental Psychiatry 16, 245-251.

Martin, R. L. (1985). Methodological and conceptual problems in the study of mortality in psychiatry. Psychiatric Developments 3, 317-333.

May, P. R., & Van Putten, T. (1974). Treatment of schizophrenia. II. A proposed rating scale of design and outcome for use in literature surveys. Comprehensive Psychiatry 15, 267-275.

Meinert, C. L. (1981). Organization of multicenter clinical trials. Controlled Clinical Trials 1, 305-313.

Michelson, L., Mannarino, A., Marchione, K., Kazdin, A. E., & Costello, A. (1985). Expectancy bias in behavioral observations of therapeutic outcome: An experimental analysis of treatment and halo effects. Behavior Research and Therapy 23, 407-414.

Mills, M. J., Hsu, L. C., & Berger, P. A. (1980). Informed consent: Psychotic patients and research. Bulletin of the American Academy of Psychiatry and the Law 8, 119-132.

Mintz, J. (1983). Integrating research evidence: A commentary on meta-analysis. Journal of Consulting and Clinical Psychology 51, 71-75.

Moser, J. (1977). Community response to alcohol-related problems: A WHO research proposal. Alcoholism 1, 267-270.

Neale, J. M., & Weintraub, S. (1975). Children vulnerable to psychopathology: The Stony Brook high-risk project. Journal of Abnormal Child Psychology 3, 95-113.

Offord, D. R., & Jones, M. B. (1976). The proband-sibling design in psychiatry, with two technical notes. Canadian Psychiatric Association Journal 21, 101-107.

O'Leary, K. D., & Borkovec, T. D. (1978). Conceptual, methodological, and ethical problems of placebo groups in psychotherapy research. American Psychologist 33, 821-830.

O'Leary, K. D., & Turkewitz, H. (1978). Methodological errors in marital and child treatment research. Journal of Consulting and Clinical Psychology 46, 747-758.

Olsen, D. M., Kane, R. L., & Proctor, P. H. (1976). A controlled trial of multiphasic screening. New England Journal of Medicine 294, 925-930.

Patkai, P. (1974). Laboratory studies of psychological stress. International Journal of Psychiatry and Medicine 5, 575-585.

Paykel, E. S. (1983). Methodological aspects of life events research. Journal of Psychosomatic Research 27, 341-352.

Poling, A., Cleary, J., & Monaghan, M. (1980). The use of human observers in psychopharmacological research. Pharmacology, Biochemistry and Behavior 13, 243-246.

Poling, A., Grossett, D., Karas, C. A., & Breuning, S. E. (1985). Medication regimen: A subject characteristic rarely reported in behavior modification studies. Applied Research in Mental Retardation 6, 71-77.

Pryce, I. G. (1978). Clinical research upon mentally ill subjects who cannot give informed consent. British Journal of Psychiatry 133, 366-369.

Rabin, C. (1981). The single-case design in family therapy evaluation research. Family Process 20, 351-366.

Reid, D. D. (1975). International studies in epidemiology. American Journal of Epidemiology 102, 469-476.

Reiss, D., & Wyatt, R. J. (1975). Family and biologic variables in the same etiologic studies of schizophrenia: A proposal. Schizophrenia Bulletin 14, 64-81.

Repp, B. H. (1981). On levels of description in speech research. Journal of the Acoustical Society of America 69, 1462-1464.

Rohsenow, D. J., & Marlatt, G. A. (1981). The balanced placebo design: Methodological considerations. Addictive Behavior 6, 107-122.

Rosner, B. (1979). The analysis of longitudinal data in epidemiologic studies. Journal of Chronic Disease 32, 163-173.

Roth, L. H., & Appelbaum, P. S. (1983). Obtaining informed consent for research with psychiatric patients. The controversy continues. Psychiatric Clinics of North America 6, 551-565.

Sackett, D. L. (1980). Editorial: The competing objectives of randomized trials. New England Journal of Medicine 303, 1059-1060.

Sarason, I. G., Smith, R. E., & Diener, E. (1975). Personality research: Components of variance attributable to the person and the situation. Journal of Personality and Social Psychology 32, 199-204.

Sartorius, N. (1980). The research component of the WHO mental health programme. Psychological Medicine 10, 175-185.

Sells, S. B. (1976). New data source for drug-abuse epidemiology research. Journal of Clinical Psychology 32, 199-200.

Sethi, B. B., & Prakash, R. (1981). Cultural factors in the organization of multicentre trials. Modern Problems of Pharmacopsychiatry 16, 21-36.

Shader, R. I. (1976). Discussion: Sources of variance in studies of drugs and other therapies. Proceedings of the American Psychopathology Association 64, 294-312.

Shaffer, H., & Gambino, B. (1983-1984). Addictions paradigms III. From theory-research to practice and back. Advances in Alcohol and Substance Abuse 3, 135-152.

Shakow, D. (1977). Some thoughts about schizophrenia research in the context of high risk studies. Psychological Issues 10, 316-334.

Shapiro, D. A., & Shapiro, D. (1983). Comparative therapy outcome research: Methodological implications of meta-analysis. Journal of Consulting and Clinical Psychology 51, 42-53.

Shapiro, T. (1978-1979). On the verification of psychoanalytic concepts by extraclinical techniques. International Journal of Psychoanalytic Psychotherapy 7, 586-601.

Shrout, P. E., & Fleiss, J. L. (1979). Intraclass correlations: Uses in assessing rater reliability. Psychological Bulletin 86, 420-428.

Silverman, L. H. (1975). An experimental method for the study of unconscious conflict: A progress report. British Journal of Medical Psychology 48, 291-298.

Siris, S. G., Docherty, J. P., & McGlashan, T. H. (1979). Intrapsychic structural effects of psychiatric research. American Journal of Psychiatry 136, 1561-1571.

Staats, A. W. (1977). Experimental-longitudinal methods in assessment, research, and treatment. Journal of Abnormal Child Psychology 5, 323-333.

Stewart, R. S., Barsky, A. J., & Stewart, R. M. (1978). Dynamic interactions affecting psychiatric research in a comprehensive health clinic. Journal of the American Medical Women's Association 33, 470, 472, 477-478.

Stone, W. N., Green, B. L., Gleser, G. C., Whitman, R. M., & Foster, B. B. (1975). Impact of psychosocial factors on the conduct of combined drug and psychotherapy research. British Journal of Psychiatry 127, 432-439.

Strauss, G. D., Yager, J., & Offer, D. (1980). Research training in psychiatry: A survey of current practices. American Journal of Psychiatry 137, 727-729.

Strauss, M. E. (1978). The differential and experimental paradigms in the study of cognition in schizophrenia. Journal of Psychiatric Research 14, 316-320.

Stricker, G. (1977). Implications of research for psychotherapeutic treatment of women. American Psychologist 32, 14-22.

Syme, S. L. (1974). Behavioral factors associated with the etiology of physical disease. A social epidemiological approach. American Journal of Public Health 64, 1043-1045.

Taves, D. R. (1971). Minimization: A new method of assigning patients to treatment groups. Clinical Pharmacology and Therapeutics 15, 443-453.

Temple, N. J. (1985). Simplicity--the key to fruitful medical research. Medical Hypotheses 17, 139-145.

Thompson, W. D., Kelsey, J. L., & Walter, S. D. (1982). Cost and efficiency in the choice of matched and unmatched case-control study designs. American Journal of Epidemiology 116, 840-851.

Tizard, J. (1978). Research in special education. Special Education: Forward Trends 5, 23-26.

Tsai, L. Y., & Beisler, J. M. (1984). Research in infantile autism: A methodological problem in using language comprehension as the basis for selecting matched controls. Journal of the American Academy of Child Psychiatry 23, 700-703.

Uhlenhuth, E. H., Glass, R. M., & Fischman, M. W. (1979). Multiple crossover designs with an antianxiety agent and an antidepressant. Psychopharmacology Bulletin 15, 37-40.

van Praag, H. M. (1975). Neuroleptics as a guideline to biological research in psychotic disorders. Comprehensive Psychiatry 16, 7-22.

Walsh, R. N. (1980). On the necessity for a shift in emphasis from means-oriented to problem-oriented research in developmental psychobiology. Developmental Psychobiology 13, 231-239.

Watson, J. P. (1975). An experimental method for the study of unconscious conflict. British Journal of Medical Psychology 48, 299-301.

Westheimer, R. (1975). Evaluation criteria and psychotherapy research. Psychotherapy and Psychosomatics 25, 236-238.

Wilson, A. (1976). Multivariate analysis: Data reduction and treatment evaluation. British Journal of Psychiatry 128, 404-407.

Wodarski, J. S., Feldman, R. A., & Pedi, S. J. (1974). Objective measurement of the independent variables: A neglected methodological aspect in community-based behavioral research. Journal of Abnormal Child Psychology 2, 239-244.

Zelen, M. (1979). A new design for randomized clinical trials. New England Journal of Medicine 300, 1242-1245.

Zifferblatt, S. M., & Wilbur, C. S. (1978). A psychological perspective for double-blind trials. Clinical Pharmacology and Therapeutics 23, 1-10.

B. Epidemiology Research

Achenbach, T. M. (1980). DSM III: In light of empirical research on the classification of child psychopathology. Journal of the American Academy of Child Psychiatry 19, 395-412.

Ahlburs, D. A., & Schapiro, M. O. (1984). Socioeconomic ramifications of changing cohort size: An analysis of U. S. postwar suicide rates by age and sex. Demography 21(1), 97-108.

Alexander, G. R., Massey, R. M., Gibbs, T., & Altekruse, J. M. (1985). Firearm-related fatalities: An epidemiologic assessment of violent death. American Journal of Public Health 75(2), 165-168.

Barnes, R. A., Ennis, J., & Schober, R. (1986). Cohort analysis of Ontario suicide rates, 1877-1976. Canadian Journal of Psychiatry 31(3), 208-213.

Boudreault, M., & Thivierge, J. (1986). The impact of temperament in a school setting: An epidemiological study. Canadian Journal of Psychiatry 31(6), 499-504.

Cooper, P. J., & Fairburn, C. G. (1983). Binge-eating and self-induced vomiting in the community: A preliminary study. British Journal of Psychiatry 142, 139-144.

Copelan, A. R. (1985). Teenage suicide--the five-year Metro Dade County experience from 1979 until 1983. Forensic Science International 28(1), 27-33.

Cornely, P., & Bromet, E. (1986). Prevalence of behavior problems in three-year-old children living near Three Mile Island: A comparative analysis. Journal of Child Psychology and Psychiatry and Allied Disciplines 27(4), 486-498.

Cosand, B. J., Bourque, L. B., & Kraus, J. F. (1982). Suicide among adolescents in Sacramento County, California, 1950-1979. Adolescence 17(68), 917-930.

Crowther, J. H., Bond, L. A., & Rolf, J. E. (1981). The incidence, prevalence, and severity of behavior disorders among preschool-aged children in day care. Journal of Abnormal Child Psychology 9(1), 23-42.

Davis, R. (1979). Black suicide in the seventies: Current trends. Suicide and Life-Threatening Behavior 9(3), 131-140.

Earls, F. (1980). The prevalence of behavioral problems in 3-year-old children. Journal of the American Academy of Child Psychiatry 19(3), 439-452.

Earls, F. (1982). Application of DSM-III in an epidemiological study of preschool children. American Journal of Psychiatry 139(2), 242-243.

Eisenberg, L. (1984). The epidemiology of suicide in adolescents. Pediatric Annals 13(1), 47-54.

Eme, R. F. (1979). Sex differences in childhood psychopathology: A review. Psychological Bulletin 86(3), 574-595.

Flaherty, M. G. (1983). The national incidence of juvenile suicide in adult jails and juvenile detention centers. Suicide and Life-Threatening Behavior 13(2), 85-94.

Foutenberry, J. D. (1985). Gasoline sniffing. American Journal of Medicine 79(6), 740-744.

Gould, M. S., Wunsch-Hitzik, R., & Dohrenwend, B. (1981). Estimating the prevalence of childhood psychopathology: A critical review. Journal of the American Academy of Child Psychiatry 20, 462-476.

Graham, P., Monck, E., Dobbs, B., & Richman, N. (1984). Epidemiological study of psychiatric disorder in adolescent girls: Preliminary communication. Journal of the Royal Society of Medicine 77(5), 387-389.

Graham, P. J. (1978). Epidemiologic perspective on maladaptation in children: Neurological, familial, and social factors. Journal of the American Academy of Child Psychiatry 17(2), 197-208.

Hingson, R., Merrigan, D., & Heeren, T. (1985). Effects of Massachusetts raising its legal drinking age from 18 to 20 on deaths from teenage homicide, suicide, and nontraffic accidents. Pediatric Clinics of North America 32(1), 221-232.

Holborow, P. L., Berry, P., & Elkins, J. (1984). Prevalence of hyperkinesis: A comparison of three rating scales. Journal of Learning Disabilities 17(7), 411-417.

Holinger, P. C. (1981). Self-destructiveness among the young: An epidemiological study of violent deaths. International Journal of Social Psychiatry 27(4), 277-282.

Holinger, P. C., & Offer, D. (1982). Prediction of adolescent suicide: A population mode. American Journal of Psychiatry 139(3), 302-307.

Hoppe, S. K., & Martin, H. W. (1986). Patterns of suicide among Mexican American and Anglos, 1960-1980. Social Psychiatry 21(2), 83-88.

Humphrey, J. A., & Kupferer, H. J. (1982). Homicide and suicide among the Cherokee and Lumbee Indians of North Carolina. International Journal of Social Psychiatry 28(2), 121-128.

Kagan, D. M., & Squires, R. L. (1984). Eating disorders among adolescents: Patterns and prevalence. Adolescence 19(73), 15-29.

Kroft, S. B., Ratzlaff, H. C., & Perks, B. A. (1986). Intelligence and early academic underachievement. British Journal of Clinical Psychology Part 2, 147-148.

Ladame, F., & Jeanneret, O. (1982). Suicide in adolescence: Some comments on epidemiology and prevention. Journal of Adolescence 5(4), 355-366.

Lambert, N. M., Sandoval, J. H., & Sassone, D. M. (1978). Prevalence estimates of hyperactivity in school children. Pediatric Annals 7(5), 330-338.

Lester, D. (1982). The distribution of sex and age among completed suicides: A cross-national study. International Journal of Social Psychology 28(4), 256-260.

Links, P. S. (1983). Community surveys of the prevalence of childhood psychotic disorders: A review. Child Development 54, 531-548.

McCarron, M. M., Schulze, B. W., Thompson, G. A., Conder, M. C., & Goetz, W. A. (1981). Acute phencyclidine intoxication: Incidence of clinical findings in 1,000 cases. Annals of Emergency Medicine 10(5), 237-242.

McClure, G. M. (1986). Recent changes in suicide among adolescents in England and Wales. Journal of Adolescence 9(2), 135-143.

McDermott, P. A. (1980). Prevalence and constituency of behavioral disturbance taxonomies in regular school population. Journal of Abnormal Child Psychology 8(4), 523-536.

McGee, R., Silva, P. A., & Williams, S. (1984). Behavior problems in a population of seven-year-old children: Prevalence, stability and types of disorder--a research report. Journal of Child Psychology and Psychiatry and Allied Disciplines 25(2), 251-259.

McGuire, J., & Richman, N. (1986a). The prevalence of behavioral problems in three types of preschool groups. Journal of Child Psychology and Psychiatry and Allied Disciplines 27(4), 455-472.

McGuire, J., & Richman, N. (1986b). Screening for behavior problems in nurseries: The reliability and validity of the preschool behavior checklist. Journal of Child Psychology and Psychiatry and Allied Disciplines 27(1), 7-32.

O'Malley, P. M., Bachman, J. G., & Johnston, L. D. (1984). Period, age, and cohort effects on substance use among American youth. American Journal of Public Health 74(7), 682-688.

Phillips, D. P., & Carstensen, L. L. (1986). Clustering of teenage suicides after television news stories about suicide. New England Journal of Medicine 315(11), 685-689.

Ramsey, R., & Bagley, C. (1985). The prevalence of suicidal behaviors, attitudes and associated social experiences in an urban population. Suicide and Life-Threatening Behavior 15(3), 151-167.

Richman, N., Stevenson, J. E., & Graham, P. J. (1975). Prevalence of behavior problems in 3 year old children: An epidemiological study of a London borough. Journal of Child Psychology and Psychiatry and Allied Disciplines 16, 277-287.

Salk, L., Lipsitt, L. P., Sturner, W. Q., Reilly, B. M., & Levat, R. H. (1985). Relationship of maternal and perinatal conditions to eventual adolescent suicide. Lancet 1(129), 624-627.

Shaffer, D., & Fisher, P. (1981). The epidemiology of suicide in children and young adolescents. Journal of the American Academy of Child Psychiatry 20(3), 545-565.

Sievers, M. L., Cynamon, M. H., & Bittker, T. E. (1975). Intentional isoniazid overdosage among southwestern American Indians. American Journal of Psychiatry 132(6), 662-665.

Solomon, M. I., & Hellon, C. P. (1980). Suicide and age in Alberta, Canada, 1951 to 1977. A cohort analysis. Archives of General Psychiatry 37(5), 511-513.

Stiffman, A. R., Jung, K. G., & Feldman, R. A. (1986). A multivariate risk model for childhood behavior problems. American Journal of Orthopsychiatry 56(2), 204-211.

Stott, D. H. (1978). Epidemiological indicators of the origins of behavior disturbance as measured by the Bristol social adjustment guides. Genetic Psychology Monographs 48, 201-215.

Tizard, B., & Rees, J. (1975). The effect of early institutional rearing on the behavior problems and affectional relationships of four-year-old children. Journal of Child Psychology and Psychiatry and Allied Disciplines 16(1), 61-73.

Werner, E. E., & Smith, R. S. (1979). An epidemiologic perspective in some antecedents and consequences of childhood mental health problems and learning disabilities. A report from the Kauai longitudinal study. Journal of the American Academy of Child Psychiatry 18, 292-306.

Werner, E. E., & Smith, R. S. (1981). Vulnerable, but invincible: A longitudinal study of resilient children and youth. New York: McGraw-Hill.

C. General Overview of Child Psychiatric Research

Anders, T. F. (1982). The child psychiatrist and research. Journal of the American Academy of Child Psychiatry 21, 570-571.

Cohen, D. J., Bruun, R., & Leckman, J. F. (Eds.). (1988). Tourette syndrome and tic disorders: Clinical understanding and treatment. New York: Wiley.

Comings, D. E., & Comings, B. G. (1987). A controlled study of Tourette syndrome: I. Attention-deficit disorder, learning disorders and school problems. American Journal of Human Genetics 41, 701-741.

Edlund, M. J., Overall, J. E., & Rhoades, H. M. (1985). Beta, or type II error in psychiatric controlled clinical trials. Journal of Psychiatric Research 19, 563-567.

Kovacs, M., Feinberg, T. L., Paulauskas, S., Finkelstein, R., Pollock, M., & Crouse-Novak, M. (1985). Initial coping responses and psychosocial characteristics of children with insulin-dependent diabetes mellitus. Journal of Pediatrics 106, 827-834.

Leckman, J. F., Riddle, M. A., Berrettini, W. H., Anderson, G. M., Hardin, M. T., Chappell, P., Bissett, G., Nemeroff, C. B., Goodman, W. K., & Cohen, D. J. (1988). Elevated CSF levels of dynorphin, A [1-8] in Tourette's syndrome. Life Sciences 43, 88-93.

Leckman, J. F., Riddle, M. A., Hardin, M. T., Ort, S. I., Swartz, K. L., Stevenson, J., & Cohen, D. J. (1989). The Yale global tic severity scale: Initial testing of a clinician-rated scale of tic severity. Journal of the American Academy of Child and Adolescent Psychiatry 28, 566-573.

Lewis, D. O. (1983). Neuropsychiatric vulnerabilities and violent juvenile delinquency. Psychiatric Clinics of North America 6, 707-714.

McDermott, J. F., McGuire, C., & Berner, E. S. (1977). A study of board certification in child psychiatry as a valid indicator of clinical competence. Journal of the American Academy of Child Psychiatry 16, 517-528.

Michelson, L., Mannarino, A., Marchione, K., Kazdin, A. E., & Costello, A. (1985). Expectancy bias in behavioral observations of therapeutic outcome: An experimental analysis of treatment and halo effects. Behavior Research and Therapy 23, 407-414.

Rapoport, J. L. (1985). DSM-III-R and pediatric psychopharmacology. Psychopharmacology Bulletin 21, 803-806.

Robertson, M. M. (1989). The Gilles de la Tourette syndrome: The current status. British Journal of Psychiatry 154, 147-169.

Shapiro, A. K., Shapiro, E. S., Young, J. G., & Feinberg, T. E. (Eds.). (1988). Gilles de la Tourette syndrome. New York: Raven Press.

D. Nosologic Issues

Ainsworth, M. D. (1969). Object relations, dependency and attachment: A theoretical review. Child Development 40, 969-1025.

Campbell, M., Anderson, L., & Meier, M. (1978). A comparison of haldiporal and behavior therapy and their interaction in autistic children. Journal of the American Academy of Child Psychiatry 17, 640-655.

Cantor, S., Evans, J., & Pezzot-Pearce, P. (1982). Childhood schizophrenia: Present but not accounted for. American Journal of Psychiatry 139, 758-762.

Cohen, D. J., Volkmar, F. R., & Paul, R. (1986). Issues in the classification of pervasive developmental disorders: History and current status of nosology. Journal of the American Academy of Child Psychiatry 25, 158-161.

Dahl, E. K., Cohen, D. J., & Provence, S. (1986). Clinical and multivariate approaches to the nosology of pervasive developmental disorders. Journal of the American Academy of Child Psychiatry 25, 170-180.

Demyer, M. K., Hingtgen, J. N., & Jackson, R. K. (1981). Infantile autism reviewed: A decade of research. Schizophrenia Bulletin 7, 388-451.

Green, W. H., Campbell, M., Hardesty, A. S., Grega, D. M., Padron-Gayol, M., Shell, J., & Erelenmeyere-Kimling, L. (1984). A comparison of schizophrenic and autistic children. Journal of the American Academy of Child Psychiatry 23, 399-409.

Mahler, M. (1952). On child psychoses and schizophrenia: Autistic and symbiotic infantile psychoses. In R. S. Eissler, et al. (Eds.), Psychoanalytic study of the child (Vol. 7, pp. 286-305). New York: International Universities Press.

Mikkelsen, E. (1982). Efficacy of neuroleptic medication in pervasive developmental disorders of childhood. Schizophrenia Bulletin 8, 320-328.

Rutter, M. (1972). Child schizophrenia reconsidered. Journal of Autism and Childhood Schizophrenia 2, 315-338.

Rutter, M., & Shaffer, D. (1980). DSM-III: A step forward or back in terms of the classification of childhood psychiatric disorder? Journal of the American Academy of Child Psychiatry 19, 371-394.

Wolff, S., & Barlow, A. (1979). Schizoid personality in childhood: A comparative study of schizoid, autistic, and normal children. Journal of Child Psychology and Psychiatry and Allied Disciplines 20, 29-46.

E. Psychotherapy Research

Cicchetti, D. V., & Ryan, E. R. (1976). A reply to Beutler et al.'s study: Some sources of variance in accurate empathy ratings. Journal of Consulting and Clinical Psychology 44, 858-861.

DeWitt, K. N. (1978). The effectiveness of family therapy: A review of outcome research. Archives of General Psychiatry 35, 549-561.

Gill, M. M., & Hoffman, I. Z. (1982). A method for studying the analysis of aspects of the patients's experience of the relationship in psychoanalysis and psychotherapy. Journal of the American Psychoanalytic Association 30, 137-167.
Gunderson, J. G. (1978). Patient-therapist matching: A research evaluation. American Journal of Psychiatry 135, 1193-1197.
Heinicke, C. M., & Strassmann, L. H. (1975). Toward more effective research on child psychotherapy. Journal of the American Academy of Child Psychiatry 14, 561-588.
Koss, M. P., Butcher, J. N., & Strupp, H. H. (1986). Brief psychotherapy methods in clinical research. Journal of Consulting and Clinical Psychology 54, 60-67.
Shaffer, D. (1984). Notes on psychotherapy research among children and adolescents. Journal of the American Academy of Child Psychiatry 23, 552-561.
Strupp, H. H. (1980). Success and failure in time-limited psychotherapy. With special reference to the performance of a lay counselor. Archives of General Psychiatry 37, 831-841.
Strupp, H. H. (1986). Psychotherapy. Research, practice, and public policy (how to avoid dead ends). American Psychologist 41, 120-130.

F. Family Research

Barkley, R. A. (1981). The use of psychopharmacology to study reciprocal influences in parent-child interaction. Journal of Abnormal Child Psychology 9, 303-310.
Barkley, R. A., & Cunningham, C. E. (1979). The effects of methylphenidate on the mother-child interactions of hyperactive children. Archives of General Psychiatry 36, 201-208.
Baron, M., Gruen, R., Asnis, L., & Kane, J. (1983). Familial relatedness of schizophrenia and schizotypal states. American Journal of Psychiatry 140, 1437-1442.
Doane, J. A. (1978). Family interaction and communication deviance in disturbed and normal families. Questions of strategy: Rejoinder to Jacob and Grounds. Family Process 17, 389-394.
Jacobs, J. W. (1982). The effect of divorce on fathers: An overview of the literature. American Journal of Psychiatry 139, 1235-1241.
Vaughn, C. E., Snyder, K. S., Jones, S., Freeman, W. B., & Falloon, I. R. (1984). Family factors in schizophrenic relapse. Replication in California of British research on expressed emotion. Archives of General Psychiatry 41, 1169-1177.
Wolkind, S., & Coleman, E. Z. (1983). Adult psychiatric disorder and childhood experiences. The validity of retrospective data. British Journal of Psychiatry 143, 188-191.

PART VII

Training in Child and Adolescent Mental Health

A. Training in Child and Adolescent Psychiatry

Section Editor:

David B. Pruitt, M.D.
Director, Division of Child and Adolescent Psychiatry
Associate Professor of Psychiatry and Pediatrics
University of Tennessee College of Medicine
Memphis, Tennessee

Associate Editors

Richard Angell, M.D.
Assistant Professor
Director of Child Psychiatry Training
Oregon Health Sciences University
Portland, Oregon

David Inwood, M.D.
Assistant Professor
Director of Training
Child and Adolescent Psychiatry
New York University, SUNY
Downstate Medical Center
Brooklyn, New York

1. General Review of Training Issues

Adams, P. (1975). The ideal training program in child psychiatry. Journal of the American Academy of Child Psychiatry 14(2), 228-243.

Appelbaum, A. S., Stone, W. E., Johnson, J. H., & Heck, D. H. (1978). Research training in psychiatric residency programs: A survey. Texas Reports on Biology and Medicine 36, 17-23.

Barker, P. (1982). Training standards for career child psychiatrists. Canadian Journal of Psychiatry 27, 543-545.

Beresin, E. V., & Borus, J. F. (1989). Child psychiatry fellowship training: A crisis in manpower and recruitment. American Journal of Psychiatry 146, 759-763.

Berlin, I. N. (1967). A history of child psychiatry training. In S. A. Szurek & I. N. Berlin (Eds.), Training in therapeutic work with children. The Langley Porter child psychiatry series (Vol. 2, pp. 285-294). Palo Alto: Science and Behavior Books.

Berlin, I. N. (1976). Bibliography for training in child psychiatry [Official publication of the American Academy of Child Psychiatry]. New York: Human Sciences Press.

Berlin, I. N. (1977). Child psychiatry perspectives: Professional competence, public confidence, and children's rights. Journal of the American Academy of Child Psychiatry 16(4), 748-752.

Binger, C. (1973). Training in child psychiatry for general residents. Journal of the American Academy of Child Psychiatry 12, 425-440.

Bloom, J. D., Kinzie, J. D., & Shore, J. H. (1980). Residency curriculum in forensic psychiatry. American Journal of Psychiatry 137, 730-732.

Blotcky, M. J. (1975). Discounting psychotherapy in training programs: Throwing out the baby. Hospital and Community Psychiatry 26, 760.

Child and adolescent psychiatry recruitment. (1989). [Special Issues]. Academic Psychiatry 13(4).

Cohen, R. L., & Dulcan, M. K. (Eds.). (1987). Basic handbook for training in child and adolescent psychiatry. Springfield, Ill.: Charles C. Thomas.

Havilind, M. G., Dial, T. H., & Pincus, H. A. (1988). Characteristics of senior medical students planning to specialize in child psychiatry. Journal of the American Academy of Child and Adolescent Psychiatry 27(4), 404-407.

Pruitt, D. B. (1985). The interface between academic training and investor owned hospitals. Psychiatric Annals 15(8), 121-129.

Reichsman, F. (1975). Teaching psychosomatic medicine to medical students, residents and postgraduate fellows. International Journal of Psychiatry and Medicine 6, 307-316.

Rutter, M. (1986). Child psychiatry: Looking 30 years ahead. Journal of Child Psychology and Psychiatry and Allied Disciplines 27, 803-840.

Sabin, J. E., & Sharfstein, S. S. (1975). Integrating community psychiatry into residency training. Hospital and Community Psychiatry 26, 289-292.

Schowalter, J. E. (1989). Child psychiatry program directors' rating of residency experiences. Journal of the American Academy of Child and Adolescent Psychiatry 28(1), 124-129.

Shulman, L. (1981). Learning dynamic psychotherapy in psychiatric training. American Journal of Psychiatry 138, 167-171.

Solyom, A. E., & Greenman, G. W. (1980). Training and primary intervention: Clinical experience with infants and their families as an obligatory part of the child psychiatrist's training. Infant Mental Health Journal 1(2), 76-88.

Spiegel, D., & Grunebaum, H. (1977). Training versus treating the psychiatric resident. American Journal of Psychotherapy 31, 618-625.

Strauss, G. D., Yager, J., & Offer, D. (1980). Research training in psychiatry: A survey of current practices. American Journal of Psychiatry 137, 727-729.

Sugarman, S. (1984). Integrating family therapy training into psychiatry residency programs: Policy issues and alternatives. Family Process 23, 23-32.

Szurek, S., & Berlin, I. (1966). The question of therapy for the trainee in the psychiatric training program. Journal of the American Academy of Child Psychiatry 5, 155-165.

Thompson, T. L., & Thomas, M. R. (1985). Teaching psychiatry to primary care internists. General Hospital Psychiatry 7, 210-213.

Wallerstein, R. (1980). Psychoanalysis and academic psychiatry--bridges. In A. Solnit, et al. (Eds.), Psychoanalytic study of the child (Vol. 35, pp. 419-448). New Haven: Yale University Press.

2. Overview of Training Goals

Borus, J. F. (1983). Teaching residents the administrative aspects of psychiatric practice. American Journal of Psychiatry 140, 444-448.

Bowden, C., & Barton, D. (1975). Goals of medical student psychiatric education. Journal of Medical Education 50, 257-263.

Bowden, C. L., Humphrey, F. J., & Thompson, M. G. (1980). Priorities in psychiatric residency training. American Journal of Psychiatry 137, 1243-1246.

Bowden, C. L., Sledge, W. H., Humphrey, F. J., & Kromer, M. (1983). Educational objectives in psychiatric residency training: A survey of training directors and residents. American Journal of Psychiatry 140, 1352-1355.

Brown, H., & Zinberg, N. (1982). Difficulties in the integration of psychological and medical practices. American Journal of Psychiatry 139(12), 1576-1582.

Buckley, P. (1982). Teaching dynamic psychotherapy: A longitudinal study. American Journal of Psychiatry 139(12), 1607-1609.

Campbell, J. (1975). Child psychiatry. Training: View from a fellow. Journal of the American Academy of Child Psychiatry 14, 210-215.

Collins, J. L., Mathura, C. B., & Risher, D. L. (1984). Training psychiatric staff to treat a multicultural patient population. Hospital and Community Psychiatry 35, 372-376.

Ekstein, R., & Wallerstein, R. (1958). The teaching and learning of psychotherapy. New York: Basic Books.

Fauman, B. J. (1983). Psychiatric residency training in the management of emergencies. Psychiatric Clinics of North America 6, 325-334.

Solnit, A. J., & Michels, R. (1988). Resolved: Child and adolescent psychiatry should stand separate from general psychiatry. Journal of the American Academy of Child Psychiatry 27(5), 658-661.

3. Training Curriculae

Fauman, B. J. (1985). Psychiatric residency training in the consideration of alternatives to hospitalization. Psychiatric Clinics of North America 8, 609-615.

Fine, S., Penfold, P. S., & Krell, R. (1982). Biases of teachers and trainees in child psychiatry. Canadian Journal of Psychiatry 27, 553-555.

Foulks, E. F. (1980). The concept of culture in psychiatric residency education. American Journal of Psychiatry 137, 811-816.

Friedman, S. B. (1982). Alternate pathways to training in child psychiatry. Journal of Nervous and Mental Disease 170, 191-192.

Glick, I. D., & Epstein, L. J. (1977). Increasing learning during the psychiatric residency. Comprehensive Psychiatry 18, 545-550.

Granet, R. B., Kalman, T. P., & Sacks, M. H. (1980). From supervisee to supervisor: An unexplored aspect of the psychiatrist's education. American Journal of Psychiatry 137, 1443-1446.

Greden, J. F. (1979). Child psychiatry education for general residents. American Journal of Psychiatry 136, 213-216.

Greenman, G. W., Benson, R., Grapentine, L., Legg, C., & Sherik, I. (1978). The role of infant observation in child psychiatry training. American Journal of Psychiatry 10, 1174-1178.

Harbin, H. T. (1980). Family therapy training for psychiatric residents. American Journal of Psychiatry 137, 1595-1598.

Harrison, S. I., & Delano, G. (1976). The status of prevention in the education of child psychiatrist. Child Psychiatry and Human Development 7(1), 3-21.

Janzen, C. L., Phillips, I., & Malloy, M. (1981). Child psychiatry education in early child development: Description of a training program. Child Psychiatry and Human Development 11(3), 158-166.

Jellinek, M. S. (1982). Sounding board. The present status of child psychiatry in pediatrics. New England Journal of Medicine 306, 1227-1230.

White, H. S., & Bennett, M. B. (1981). Training psychiatric residents in chronic care. Hospital and Community Psychiatry 32, 339-343.

Winokur, G. (1980). What to do? Or what do we owe our residents? Biological Psychiatry 15, 599-611.

Wyatt, D. J. (1979). Training child psychiatrists to teach sex education. Journal of Medical Education 54(6), 505-507.

Yager, J., & Pasnau, R. O. (1976). The educational objectives of a psychiatric residency program. American Journal of Psychiatry 133, 217-220.

4. Options and Requirements in Training

Kates, N. S., & Lesser, A. L. (1985). The resident as a teacher: A neglected role. Canadian Journal of Psychiatry 30, 418-421.

Kernberg, P. F. (1978). Use of latency-age groups in the training of child psychiatrists. International Journal of Group Psychotherapy 28(1), 95-108.

Leblanc, J. (1985). Is it still necessary to teach community psychiatry to the psychiatric resident? Canadian Journal of Psychiatry 30, 107-110.

Lewis, M. (1975). A model for a graduate education program in child psychiatry. Journal of the American Academy of Child Psychiatry 14(2), 216-227.

Lomax, J. W. (1986). The proposed curriculum on suicide care for psychiatry residency. Suicide and Life-Threatening Behavior 16, 56-64.

Looney, J. G., Ellis, W., Benedek, E., & Schowalter, J. (1985). Training in adolescent psychiatry for general psychiatry residents: Elements of a model curriculum. In S. C. Feinstein, et al. (Eds.), Adolescent psychiatry: Developmental and clinical studies (Vol. 12, pp. 94-114). Chicago: University of Chicago Press.

Malone, C. A. (1974). Observations on the role of family therapy in child psychiatry training. Journal of the American Academy of Child Psychiatry 13(3), 437-458.

Mansheim, P. (1981). Advantages of providing mental retardation training to first-year residents. Hospital and Community Psychiatry 32, 347-348.

Meijer, A. (1983). Psychodynamic perspectives of training in child psychiatry. Psychiatric Quarterly 55, 261-267.

Nemiah, J. C. (1981). On learning psychotherapy. American Journal of Psychiatry 138, 216-217.

Pattison, E. M. (1976). Teaching mental health administration to psychiatric residents. Administration in Mental Health 4, 54-59.

5. Methods of Training

Agbayewa, M. O., & Leichner, P. P. (1985). Effects of a psychiatric rotation on psychiatric knowledge and attitudes towards psychiatry in rotating interns. Canadian Journal of Psychiatry 30, 602-604.

Bair, J. P., & Greenspan, B. K. (1986). TEAMS: Teamwork training for interns, residents, and nurses. Hospital and Community Psychiatry 37, 633-635.

Beiser, H. R. (1971). Pre-testing as a teaching tool in a child psychiatry clerkship. Journal of the American Academy of Child Psychiatry 10(3), 444-463.

Bieniek, C., Barton, G., & Benedek, E. (1981). Training female mental health professionals: Sexual countertransference issues. Journal of the American Medical Women's Association 36, 131, 134-136, 138-139.

Borus, J. F. (1983). Teaching residents the administrative aspects of psychiatric practice. American Journal of Psychiatry 140, 444-448.

Borus, J. F., & Groves, J. E. (1982). Training supervision as a separate faculty role. American Journal of Psychiatry 139, 1339-1342.

Brown, J. T., & O'Shanick, G. J. (1981). Psychiatric education of the internist: A teaching conference approach. Psychosomatics 22, 1038-1043.

Buckley, P., Conte, H. R., Plutchik, R., & Karasu, T. B. (1981). Psychotherapy skill profiles of psychiatric residents. Journal of Nervous and Mental Disease 169, 733-737.

Cohen, R. J., & DeBetz, B. (1977). Responsive supervision of the psychiatric resident and clinical psychology intern. American Journal of Psychoanalysis 37, 51-64.

De la Torre, J. (1974). Use and misuse of cliches in clinical supervision. Archives of General Psychiatry 31, 302-306.

Malmquist, C., & Soth, N. (1984). A review of psychiatric literature for residency training programs, 1980s. Bulletin of the Medical Library Association 72, 287-294.

Pinney, E. L., Wells, S. H., & Fisher, B. (1978). Group therapy training in psychiatric residency programs: A national survey. American Journal of Psychiatry 135, 1505-1508.

Pruitt, D. B., McColgan, E. B., Pugh, R. L., & Kiser, L. J. (1981). Approaches to psychotherapy supervision. Journal of Psychiatric Education 22, 179-183.

Roman, M., & Porter, K. (1978). Combining experiential and didactic aspects in a new group therapy training approach. International Journal of Group Psychotherapy 28, 371-387.

Scher, M. (1981). Gender issues in psychiatric supervision. Comprehensive Psychiatry 22, 179-183.

Solomon, S., Saravay, S. M., & Steinberg, H. (1980). Supervision in liaison and consultation psychiatry. General Hospital Psychiatry 2, 294-299.

Taintor, Z., Morphy, M., Seiden, A., & Val, E. (1983). Psychiatric residency training: Relationships and value development. American Journal of Psychiatry 140, 778-780.

6. Training Settings

Brantley, J. T., Wise, T. N., & Ahmed, S. W. (1985). Consultation-liaison fellowships: Effect on internists' attitudes toward psychiatric consultation. Psychosomatics 26, 18-20, 25-27.

Chess, S. (1970). The child psychiatrist's role in mental retardation. Journal of Special Education 4(2), 149-155.

Cohen-Cole, S. A., Haggerty, J., & Raft, D. (1982). Objectives for residents in consultation psychiatry: Recommendations of a task force. Psychosomatics 23, 699-703.

Looney, J. G., Ellis, W., Benedek, E., & Schowalter, J. (1985). Training in adolescent psychiatry for general psychiatry residents: Elements of a model curriculum. In S. C. Feinstein, et al. (Eds.), Adolescent psychiatry: Developmental and clinical studies (Vol. 12, pp. 94-114). Chicago: University of Chicago Press.

Rothenberg, M. (1979). Child psychiatry-pediatrics consultation service in hospital setting. General Hospital Psychiatry 1(4), 281-286.

Shafii, M. (1979). The development of an acute short-term inpatient child psychiatric setting: A pediatric-psychiatric model. American Journal of Psychiatry 136(4), 427-429.

7. Trainees' Views of Training

Berlin, I. N. (1978). Training in child psychiatry. The generation gap--another view. Psychiatric Opinion 15(8), 40-42.

Berlin, I. N., & Christ, A. E. (1969). The unique role of the child psychiatry trainee on an inpatient or day care unit. Journal of the American Academy of Child Psychiatry 8(2), 247-258.

Binger, C. (1974). Training in child psychiatry for general residents. Journal of the American Academy of Child Psychiatry 12, 425-440.

Buckley, P., Karasu, T. B., & Charles, E. (1979). Common mistakes in psychotherapy. American Journal of Psychiatry 136, 1587-1589.

Butts, N. T., & Cavenar, J. O. (1979). Colleagues' responses to the pregnant psychiatric resident. American Journal of Psychiatry 136, 1587-1589.

Campbell, H. D. (1982). The prevalence and ramifications of psychopathology in psychiatric residents: An overview. American Journal of Psychiatry 139, 1405-1411.

Campbell, J. (1975). Child psychiatry. Training: View from a fellow. Journal of the American Academy of Child Psychiatry 14, 210-215.

Cotton, P. G., & Pruett, K. D. (1975). The affective experience of residency training in community psychiatry. American Journal of Psychiatry 132, 267-270.

Fine, S., Penfold, P. S., & Krell, R. (1982). Biases of teachers and trainees in child psychiatry. Canadian Journal of Psychiatry 27, 553-555.

Foulks, E. F. (1980). The concept of culture in psychiatric residency education. American Journal of Psychiatry 137, 811-816.

Garetz, F. K., Raths, O. N., & Morse, R. H. (1976). The disturbed and the disturbing psychiatric resident. Archives of General Psychiatry 33, 446-450.

Garfinkel, B. D., Golombek, H., & Garfinkel, P. E. (1976). Training in child and adolescent psychiatry: Selection, academic performance and outcome. Canadian Psychiatric Association Journal 21, 151-153.

Griffith, E. E., & Delgado, A. (1979). On the professional socialization of black residents in psychiatry. Journal of Medical Education 54, 471-476.

Henn, R. F. (1978). Patient suicide as part of psychiatric residency. American Journal of Psychiatry 135, 745-747.

Hickson, L., & Mann, E. M. (1985-1986). The relationship between attitudinal and behavioral change in pediatric residents in a psychiatric liaison teaching program: A pilot study. International Journal of Psychiatry and Medicine 15, 61-73.

Kass, F., Charles, E., & Buckley, P. (1980). Two-year follow-up of a peer review training program for residents. American Journal of Psychiatry 137, 244-245.

Kay, J. (1981). When psychiatric residents treat medical students: A passage through idealization and overidentification. General Hospital Psychiatry 3, 89-94.

Kessler, M. D., Hellekson-Emery, C., & Wilder, J. F. (1982). The psychiatric chief resident: Does gender make a difference? American Journal of Psychiatry 139, 1610-1613.

Lieberman, C. (1981). Problems of women psychiatric residents. Psychiatric Quarterly 53, 175-177.

Lycaki, H., Josef, N. C., & Chapin, K. (1983). Sex bias in the training of psychiatric residents. Journal of the American Medical Women's Association 38, 105-107.

Margolis, J. A. (1977). The role of the child psychiatrist in peer review. Hospital and Community Psychiatry 28(12), 898-900.

McCready, J. R., & Waring, E. M. (1986). Interviewing skills in relation to psychiatric residency. Canadian Journal of Psychiatry 31, 317-322.

Mrazek, A., & Prugh, D. (1980). Critical incidents in child psychiatry training. Journal of the American Academy of Child Psychiatry 19(2), 311-319.

Neilsen, A. C. (1979). The magnitude of declining psychiatric career choice. Journal of Medical Education 54, 632-637.

Paris, J. (1981). Intellectuality and emotionality in psychiatric residents. Canadian Journal of Psychiatry 26, 159-161.

Pasnau, R. O., & Russell, A. T. (1975). Psychiatric resident suicide: An analysis of five cases. American Journal of Psychiatry 132, 402-406.
Potter, R. L. (1983). Resident, woman, wife, mother: Issues for women in training. Journal of the American Medical Women's Association 38, 98-102.
Schacher, R. J. (1985). Evaluating attitudes of child psychiatry residents to psychotropic medication: Implications for training. Canadian Journal of Psychiatry 30, 348-352.
Scher, M. (1981). Gender issues in psychiatric supervision. Comprehensive Psychiatry 22, 179-183.
Schultz, S. L., & Russell, A. T. (1984). The emotionally disturbed child psychiatry trainee. Journal of the American Academy of Child Psychiatry 23, 226-232.
Sherwood, E., Greenblatt, M., & Pasnau, R. O. (1986). Psychiatric residency, role models, and leadership. American Journal of Psychiatry 143, 764-767.
Silver, L., & Brunstetter, R. (1977). Governmental peer review of training programs in child psychiatry. American Journal of Psychiatry 134, 11-14.
Steinhauer, P. D. (1982). Training in child psychiatry: Some problems, areas of controversy and some attempted solutions. Canadian Journal of Psychiatry 27, 546-548.
Stewart, D. E., & Robinson, G. E. (1985). Combining motherhood with psychiatric training and practice. Canadian Journal of Psychiatry 30, 28-34.
Waring, E. M. (1977). A preventative approach to emotional illness in psychiatric residents. Psychiatric Quarterly 49, 303-315.
Waring, E. M. (1983). Psychopathology in psychiatric residents [Letter]. American Journal of Psychiatry 140, 821-822.
Zimmer, B. (1985). Cultural phenomenology and residency training revisited: A personal account. International Journal of Social Psychiatry 31, 188-193.

8. Supervision of Training

Doyle, B. B., & Balsley, E. (1979). Supervision of the resident as a teacher. Journal of Medical Education 54, 338-339.
Drucker, J. J., Klass, D. B., & Strizich, M. (1978). Supervision and the professional development of the psychiatric resident. American Journal of Psychiatry 135, 1516-1519.
Dunlop, S. R. (1978). Using a moot court experience in the education of psychiatric residents. Bulletin of the American Academy of Psychiatry and the Law 6, 423-432.
Enelow, M. L. (1982). Psychoanalysis and training residents in psychiatry at Tulane medical school. Journal of the American Academy of Psychoanalysis 10, 137-145.
Forgotson, J. H., & Sweeny, T. J. (1977). Use of videotapes to teach child psychiatry to medical students. Journal of Medical Education 52(4), 351-353.
Goodrich, W. (1972). Changes in child psychiatry training required by developmental-adaptive theory. Journal of Nervous and Mental Disease 154(3), 213-220.

Granet, R. B., Kalman, T. P., & Sacks, M. H. (1980). From supervisee to supervisor: An unexplored aspect of the psychiatrist's education. American Journal of Psychiatry 137, 1443-1446.

Greben, S. E. (1985). Dear Brutus: Dealing with unresponsiveness through supervision. Canadian Journal of Psychiatry 30, 48-53.

Harrison, S. I. (1978). Expanding the role of supervision in child psychiatric education. Child Psychiatry and Human Development 9, 40-55.

Kates, N. S., & Lesser, A. L. (1985). The resident as a teacher: A neglected role. Canadian Journal of Psychiatry 30, 418-421.

Kinzie, J. D., & Jurgensen, R. A. (1976). Modes of experience and psychiatric education. American Journal of Psychotherapy 30, 276-288.

9. Evaluation of Training

Barker, P. (1982). Training standards for career child psychiatrists. Canadian Journal of Psychiatry 27, 543-545.

Borus, J., & Yager, J. (1986). Ongoing evaluations in psychiatry: The first step toward quality. American Journal of Psychiatry 143(11), 1415-1419.

Colenda, C. C. (1985). A survey of 10 psychiatry residency training programs on procedures for evaluating residents. Journal of Medical Education 60, 886-888.

Eaton, J. S. (1980). Is there life after evaluation? Journal of Psychiatric Education 4, 79-85.

Jampala, V. C., Sierles, F. S., & Taylor, M. A. (1986). Consumers' views of DSM-III: Attitudes and practices of U.S. psychiatrists and 1984 graduating psychiatric residents. American Journal of Psychiatry 143, 148-153.

Kandler, H., Plutchik, R., Conte, H., & Siegel, B. (1975). Prediction of performance of psychiatric residents: A three-year follow-up study. American Journal of Psychiatry 132, 1286-1290.

Kaplan, S. L., Rosman, B. L., Liebman, R., & Honig, P. (1979). Predicting performance in a child psychiatry program for pediatric residents. Journal of Medical Education 54, 42-50.

Kass, F., Charles, E., & Buckley, P. (1980). Two-year follow-up of a peer review training program for residents. American Journal of Psychiatry 137, 244-245.

Lingas, J., Cohen, S. N., & Angell, R. (1976). Survey of the evaluation methods used in child psychiatry training programs. Canadian Psychiatric Association Journal 21, 157-161.

McDermott, J. F. (1975). Certification of the child psychiatrist: What is special about the specialist. Journal of the American Academy of Child Psychiatry 14(2), 196-203.

McDermott, J. F., McGuire, C., & Berner, E. S. (1977). A study of board certification in child psychiatry as a valid indicator of clinical competence. Journal of the American Academy of Child Psychiatry 16(3), 517-528.

Mrazek, D., & Prugh, D. (1980). Critical incidents in child psychiatric training. Journal of the American Academy of Child Psychiatry 19(2), 311-319.

Pfeifer, C. M., Rogeness, G. A., Rubin, R. L., & Serrano, A. C. (1979). Effects of a program for evaluating child psychiatry fellows. Journal of the American Academy of Child Psychiatry 136(7), 967-969.

Silver, L. B., Brunstetter, R., Renshaw, D., & Comer, J. (1977). Governmental peer review of training programs in child psychiatry. American Journal of Psychiatry 134, 11-14.

Simmons, J. E. (1975). The training of child psychiatrists: Is quantitative and qualitative improvement possible. Journal of the American Academy of Child Psychiatry 14(2), 193-195.

Strauss, G. D., Yager, J., Liston, E. H., & Strauss, G. E. (1981). Testing psychiatric knowledge with in-house examinations. American Journal of Psychiatry 138, 636-641.

Strauss, G. D., Yager, J., & Liston, E. H. (1984). A comparison of national and in-house examinations of psychiatric knowledge. American Journal of Psychiatry 141, 882-884.

Williams, J. B., Spitzer, R. L., & Skodol, A. E. (1985). DSM-III in residency training: Results of a national survey. American Journal of Psychiatry 142, 755-758.

Yager, J. (1975). The clinical experience worksheet. Journal of Medical Education 50, 1061-1062.

10. Training in Administration and Ethics

Barton, W. E., & Barton, G. M. (1983). Mental health administration: Principles and practice. New York: Human Sciences Press.

Bloch, S., & Chodoff, P. (1981). Psychiatric ethics. New York: Oxford University Press.

Gruskey, O., & Miller, G. (1981). The sociology of organizations: Basic studies. New York: The Free Press.

Gutheil, T. G., & Appelbaum, P. S. (1982). Clinical handbook of psychiatry and the law. New York: McGraw-Hill.

The principles of medical ethics, with annotations especially applicable to psychiatry. (1981). Washington, D.C.: American Psychiatric Association.

Talbott, J. A., & Kaplan, S. R. (1982). Psychiatric administration: A comprehensive text for the clinician-executive. New York: Grune & Stratton.

Woy, J. R., Lund, D. A., & Attkisson, C. C. (1978). Quality assurance in human service program evaluation. In C. C. Attkisson, J. R. Woy, & D. A. Lund (Eds.), Evaluation of human service programs. New York: Academic Press.

B. Training and Practice in Child and Adolescent Psychiatric Nursing

Section Editor:

Deane L. Critchley, Ph.D., R.N., C.S., F.A.A.N.
Associate Clinical Professor
Department of Psychiatry
University of New Mexico School of Medicine
Albuquerque, New Mexico

1. Education in Nursing in Child and Adolescent Mental Health

American Nurses Association. (1985). Standards of child and adolescent psychiatric and mental health nursing [Pamphlet]. American Nursing Association Publication Council on Psychiatric Mental Health Nursing PMH-7, 1-27.

Cannon, M. T. (1978). Clinical and administrative issues of a child psychiatric nurse's role in a community hospital. Journal of Psychiatric Nursing and Mental Health Services 16(2), 29-32.

Chamberlain, J. G. (1988). Challenges for child psychiatric mentalhealth nursing. Journal of Child and Adolescent Psychiatric and Mental Health Nursing 1(1), 66-71.

Critchley, D. L. (1987). Clinical supervision as a learning tool for student therapists in milieu settings. Journal of Psychosocial Nursing and Mental Health Services 25(8), 18-22.

Denyes, M. J. (1983). Nursing research related to school age children and adolescents. Annual Review of Nursing Research 1, 27-53.

Dumas, R. G. (1983). Social, economic and political factors and mental illness. Journal of Psychosocial Nursing and Mental Health Services 21(3), 31-35.

Feldstein, M. A. (1984). Supervising graduate students in family therapy. Perspectives in Psychiatric Care 22(3), 93-98.

Frutiger, A. D., & Eakes, G. B. (1985). The developmental evaluation center as a clinical setting for mental health nursing students. Perspectives in Psychiatric Care 23(1), 27-32.

Gilbert, M. T. (1977). Child abuse. Nursing Mirror 144(19), 50-51.

Hamilton, W. (1977). Role of the nurse in child psychiatry. Nursing Mirror 144(21), 29-32.

Harnett, N. E. (1989). Conduct disorder in childhood and adolescence: An update. Journal of Child and Adolescent Psychiatric and Mental Health Nursing 2(2), 74-77.

Heinlein, D. (1980). The nurse's role in helping to assess learning disabilities in the school setting. Journal of School Health 50(1), 15-17.

Holland, C. J., Daly, R. M., & Capanzano, C. T. (1978). The student nurse as therapeutic consultant. International Journal of Nursing Studies 15(3), 153-157.

Koehler, M. F. (1981). Child psychiatric nursing option. Nursing Outlook 29, 174-177.

Krowchuk, H. V. K. (1989). Child abuser stereotypes: Consensus among clinicians. Nursing Research 2(1), 35-39.

Misener, T. R. (1986). Toward a nursing definition of child maltreatment using seriousness vignettes. Advances in Nursing Science 8(4), 1-14.

Pothier, P. C. (1984). Child psychiatric nursing. Journal of Psychosocial Nursing and Mental Health Services 22(3), 10-13, 17-21.

Pothier, P. C. (1988a). Child mental health: Problems and policy. Archives of Psychiatric Nursing 2(3), 165-169.

Pothier, P. C. (1988b). Graduate preparation in child and adolescent psychiatric mental health nursing. Archives of Psychiatric Nursing 2(3), 170-172.

Pothier, P. C. (1989). Impact of privatization of psychiatric care on children and adolescents. Archives of Psychiatric Nursing 3(3), 123-124.

Pothier, P. C., Norbeck, J. S., & Laliberte, M. (1985). Child psychiatric nursing: The gap between need and utilization. Journal of Psychosocial Nursing and Mental Health Services 23(7), 18-23.

Thomas, S. P., & Wilt, D. (1986). Mental health nursing clinical specialization: Extinction or adaptation. Issues in Mental Health Nursing 8(1), 1-13.

2. Nursing Roles in Child and Adolescent Mental Disorders

Burgess, A. W., Hartman, C. R., Wolbert, W. A., & Grant, C. A. (1987). Child molestation: Assessing impact in multiple victims, Part I. Archives of Psychiatric Nursing 1(1), 33-39.

Cooney, K. M. (1978). Nursing care of emotionally abused and deprived children. Issues in Comprehensive Pediatric Nursing 3(3), 54-62.

Deering, C. G. (1987). Developing a therapeutic alliance with the anorexia nervosa client. Journal of Psychosocial Nursing and Mental Health Services 25(3), 11-13, 17.

Elvik, S. L. (1987). From disclosure to court: The facets of sexual abuse. Journal of Pediatric Health Care 1(3), 136-140.

Fleming, J. W., et al. (1988-1989). Color drawings: A means of identifying problems of children. Journal of National Black Nurses Association 3(1), 36-84.

Gilead, M. P., & Mulaik, J. S. (1983). Adolescent suicide: A response to developmental crisis. Perspectives in Psychiatric Care 21(3), 94-101.

Long, K. A. (1985). Are children too young for mental disorders. American Journal of Nursing 85(11), 1254-1257.

Macherski, H. (1978). Nursing care study: A teenage homosexual. I'm Jack, I'm 14, I'm gay. Nursing Mirror 147(14), 29-32.

Moore, D. S., Erickson, P. I., & Wurgel, M. (1984). Adolescent pregnancy and parenting: The role of the nurse. Topics in Clinical Nursing 6(3), 72-82.

Pont, V. E. (1988). The angry adolescent. Journal of Psychosocial Nursing and Mental Health Services 26(12), 15-17.

Quinn, D. (1977). The conduct disordered child--a psychiatric nursing approach. Nursing Times 73(12), 426-427.

Siemon, M. (1978). Mental health in school-aged children. Part II. Maternal-Child Nursing Journal 3(4), 211-217.
Valente, S. M. (1987). Assessing suicide risk in the school-aged child. Journal of Pediatric Health Care 1(1), 14-20.
Walshe-Brennan, K. S. (1976). Teenage violence in psychiatric wards. Nursing Mirror 143(13), 63-64.

3. Multiple Nursing Roles in Child and Adolescent Psychiatric Nursing

Allen, H. (1981). Problem children: The nonconformists--dealing with violent behavior on a children's psychiatric ward. Nursing Mirror 152, 33-35.
Bakke, K. (1981). Ethical dilemmas: Institutionalizing a severely disabled child. Pediatric Nursing 7(6), 27-29.
Barker, P. (1980). Behavior therapy in psychiatric and mental handicap nursing. Journal of Advanced Nursing 5(1), 55-69.
Bessill, E. A. (1978). Diagnostic labels: Do they determine nursing care. Issues in Comprehensive Pediatric Nursing 3(3), 1-10.
Brady, M. (1987). Practice management exchange--children of alcoholics. Journal of Pediatric Health Care 1(1), 45-47.
Brown, E. (1981). Multidisciplinary assessment of learning problems--school nurse's role. Journal of School Health 51(9), 595-596.
Brown, F. E. (1980). Juvenile prostitution: A nursing perspective. Journal of Pyschiatric Nursing and Mental Health Services 18(12), 32-34.
Bumbalo, J. A., & Siemon, M. K. (1983). Nursing assessment and diagnosis: Mental health problems of children. Topics in Clinical Nursing 5(1), 41-54.
Burgess, A. W., & Brinbaum, H. J. (1982). Youth prostitution. American Journal of Nursing 82(5), 832-844.
Clark, C. C. (1977). Psychotherapy with the resistant child. Perspectives in Psychiatric Care 15(3), 122-125.
Clark, D. A., & Long, K. A. (1979). Nurses as health educators with emotionally disturbed children. Perspectives in Psychiatric Care 17(4), 167-173.
Clarke, B. A. (1983). Improving adolescent parenting through participant modeling and self evaluation. Nursing Clinics of North America 18(2), 303-311.
Cooney, K. M. (1978). Nursing care of emotionally abused and deprived children. Comprehensive Pediatric Nursing 3, 54-62.
Cormier, P. P. (1979). Identification of typologies derived from child behaviors in the hospital as predictors of psychological upset. Journal of Pyschiatric Nursing and Mental Health Services 17(6), 28-35.
Cowherd, M. (1977). One child's reaction to acute pain. Nursing intervention. Nursing Clinics of North America 12(4), 639-643.
Critchley, D. L. (1979a). The adverse influence of psychiatric diagnostic labels on the observation of child behavior. American Journal of Orthopsychiatry 49, 157-160.
Critchley, D. L. (1979b). Mental status examinations with children and adolescents: A developmental approach. Nursing Clinics of North America 14(3), 429-441.

Critchley, D. L (1981). The child as patient: Assessing the effects of family stress and disruption on the mental health of the child. Perspectives in Psychiatric Care 19(5-6), 144-155.

Cvejic, H., & Smith, A. (1979). The evolution of a school-based mental health program using a nurse as a mental health consultant. Journal of School Health 49(1), 36-39.

Denny, S. (1982). Therapeutic play--the nurse's role. New Zealand Nursing Journal 75(6), 3-4.

Dudding, G. (1980). Behavioral pediatrics in nursing: A behavior modification approach. Current Practice in Pediatric Nursing 3, 114-135.

Dunn, K. L. (1977). Using reality orientation on behavior problems in an adolescent girl. Journal of Pyschiatric Nursing and Mental Health Services 15(5), 23-25.

Engle, N. S., & Lau, A. D. (1983). Nursing care for the adolescent urban nomad. Maternal-Child Nursing Journal 8(1), 74-77.

Federation, S. (1986). Sexual abuse: Treatment modalities for the younger child. Journal of Psychosocial Nursing and Mental Health Services 24(7), 21-24.

Foster, P. H., Lanier, M. W., & Whitworth, J. M. (1980). The role of nurses in child abuse prevention and treatment. Journal of Pyschiatric Nursing and Mental Health Services 18(2), 24-28.

Garot, P. A. (1986). Therapeutic play: Work of both child and nurse. Journal of Pediatric Nursing 1(2), 111-116.

Harden, A. (1989). Children in crisis: A response to schools. Journal of Child and Adolescent Psychiatric and Mental Health Nursing 2(2), 68-69.

Howard, A. C. (1986). Developmental play ages of physically abused and non-abused children. American Journal of Occupational Therapy 40(10), 691-695.

Kelley, S. J. (1984). The use of art therapy with sexually abused children. Journal of Psychosocial Nursing and Mental Health Services 22(12), 12-18.

Knecht, L. D. (1981). Consent and confidentiality: Legal issues in adolescent health care for the school nurse. Journal of School Health 51(9), 606-609.

Kreitzer, M. (1981). Legal aspects of child abuse: Guidelines for the nurses. Nursing Clinics of North America 16(1), 149-160.

Long, K. A. (1985). Pitfalls to avoid and positive approaches in the nurse-adolescent relationship. Perspectives in Psychiatric Care 23(1), 22-26.

Lynn, M. R. (1987). Projective techniques in research and practice with the pediatric client. Part III. Journal of Pediatric Nursing 2(2), 129-131.

Manov, A., & Lowther, L. (1983). A health care approach for hard-to-reach adolescent runaways. Nursing Clinics of North America 18(2), 333-342.

McElroy, E., Roginis, B., & Shaefer, S. J. (1979). Symposium on child psychiatric nursing: Sudden infant death syndrome: A framework for preventive mental health. Nursing Clinics of North America 14(3), 391-403.

McElroy, E. M. (Ed.). (1979). Symposium on child psychiatric nursing. Nursing Clinics of North America 14(3), 389-482.

Mellencamp, A. (1981). Adolescent depression: A review of the literature with implications for nursing care. Journal of Psychosocial Nursing and Mental Health Services 19(9), 15-20.

Nalepka, C., O'Toole, R., & Turbett, J. P. (1981). Nurses and physicians' recognition and reporting of child abuse. Issues in Comprehensive Pediatric Nursing 5(1), 33-44.

Neaver, B. M., & McCarthy, P. (1981). Sexual misuse of children: An emergency department nursing perspective. Journal of Emergency Nursing 7(2), 59-62.

Opel, N. D., et al. (1988). Mental health needs of children in school. Journal of Child and Adolescent Psychiatric and Mental Health Nursing 1(1), 31-35.

Rodgers, B. M. (1986). Nursing management of a depressed child with a chronic physical illness. Psychiatric Nursing Forum 3(1), 4-8, 10-14.

Ross, D. C., Meinster, M. O., & Gingrich, L. J. (1978). A program for expanding the mental health function of the school nurse. Journal of School Health 48(3), 157-159.

Rubin, R. L. (1986). Assisting adolescents toward mental health. Nursing Clinics of North America 21(3), 439-450.

Sahin, S. T. (1979). the nurse and the early identification of young children at risk. International Journal of Nursing Studies 16(2), 141-149.

Salmonsen, L. E. (1988). Social maladaption to first grade and teen drug abuse. School Nursing 4(4), 8-14.

Scavnicky-Mylant, M. M. (1986). The use of drawings in the assessment and treatment of children of alcoholics. Journal of Pediatric Nursing 1(3), 178-194.

Triplett, J. E., & Arneson, S. W. (1978). Children of alcoholic parents: A neglected issue. Journal of School Health 48(10), 596-599.

Varley, C. K. (1985). A clinical nurse specialist's role in the comprehensive management of attention deficit disorder. Children's Health Care 13(3), 139-142.

Volmut, J. A. (1979). Fantasy in the nursing of children. Perspectives in Psychiatric Care 17(5), 211-217.

Webb, T. E., Adams, M. R., & Vandevere, C. A. (1983). Listening reliably to psychosocial concerns of youth. Journal of Psychosocial Nursing and Mental Health Services 21(6), 25-28.

Webster-Stratton, C. (1983a). Intervention approaches to conduct disorders in young children. Nursing Practice 8(5), 23-24, 29, 33-34.

Webster-Stratton, C. (1983b). Recognizing and assessing conduct disorders in children. Maternal-Child Nursing Journal 8(5), 330-335.

Wilkinson, T. (1979). The problem and the values of objective nursing observation in psychiatric nursing care. Journal of Advanced Nursing 4, 151-159.

Wynne, E. (1987). Storytelling in therapy and counseling. Children Today 16(2), 11-15.

4. Group and Family Therapy

Bappert, K. G. (1989). Intervention strategies with multiproblem families: A psychoanalytical approach--disturbed infant-mother interactions, Part I. Journal of Community Health Nursing 6(1), 15-23.

Bingham, A., & Bargar, J. (1985). Children of alcoholic families: A group treatment approach for latency age children. Journal of Psychosocial Nursing and Mental Health Services 23(12), 13-15.

Bishop, S. M. (1988). The primacy of the family in child and adolescent psychiatric mental health nursing. Journal of Child and Adolescent Psychiatric and Mental Health Nursing 1(2), 45-49.

Cain, A. O. (1986). Family therapy: One role of the clinical specialist in psychiatric nursing. Nursing Clinics of North America 21(3), 483-492.

Cronin-Stubbs, D. (1978). Family crisis intervention: A study. Journal of Psychiatric Nursing and Mental Health Services 16(1), 36-44.

Critchley, D. L. (1982a). Interventions with disorganized parents of disturbed children. Issues in Mental Health Nursing 4(3), 199-215.

Critchley, D. L. (1982b). Therapeutic group work with abused preschool children. Perspectives in Psychiatric Care 20(2), 79-85.

Danziger, S. (1982). Major treatment issues and techniques in family therapy with the borderline adolescent. Journal of Psychosocial Nursing and Mental Health Services 20(1), 27-34.

Davis, K. E. (1988). Interparental violence: The children as victims. Issues in Comprehensive Pediatric Nursing 11(5/6), 291-302.

de Chesnay, M. (1984). Father-daughter incest: Issues in treatment and research. Journal of Psychosocial Nursing and Mental Health Services 22(9), 8-11, 15-16.

Deering, C. G., et al. (1989). Adopted children in psychotherapy. Archives of Psychiatric Nursing 3(2), 79-85.

Duffey, M. (1979). Factors contributing to the development of a cohesive adolescent psychotherapy group. Journal of Psychiatric Nursing and Mental Health Services 17(1), 21-24.

Feetham, S. L. (1984). Family research: Issues and directions for nursing. Annual Review of Nursing Research 2, 3-25.

Gilbert, C. M. (1988). Children in women's shelters: A group intervention using art. Journal of Child and Adolescent Psychiatric and Mental Health Nursing 1(1), 7-13.

Gilbert, C. M. (1989). Sibling incest. Journal of Child and Adolescent Psychiatric and Mental Health Nursing 2(2), 70-73.

Gilliss, C. L. (1983). The family as a unit of analysis: Strategies for the nurse researcher. Advances in Nursing Science 5(3), 50-59.

Goren, S. (1979). A systems approach to emotional disorders of children. Nursing Clinics of North America 14(3), 457-465.

Gross, D. (1989). Children of the mentally ill. Journal of Psychosocial Nursing and Mental Health Services 27(8), 14-19.

Hetherington, S. E. (1988). Children of alcoholics: An emerging mental health issue. Archives of Psychiatric Nursing 2(4), 251-255.

Hubbard, G. B. (1989). Mothers' perceptions of incest: Sustained disruption and turmoil. Archives of Psychiatric Nursing 3(1), 34-40.

Jaffe, P., Wolfe, D., Wilson, S., et al. (1985). Critical issues in the assessment of children's adjustment to witnessing family violence. Canada's Mental Health 33(4), 15-19.

Jerrett, M. D., & Ross, M. M. (1982). Learning to nurse: The family as the unit of care. Journal of Advanced Nursing 7(5), 461-468.

Jones, S. L., & Dimond, M. (1982). Family theory and family therapy models: Comparative review with implications for nursing practice. Journal of Psychosocial Nursing and Mental Health Services 20(10), 12-19.

Killeen, M. R. (1988a). Self-concept of children of alcoholics: Family influences. Part I. Journal of Child and Adolescent Psychiatric and Mental Health Nursing 1(1), 25-30.

Killeen, M. R. (1988b). Self-concept of children of alcoholics: Family influences. Part II. Journal of Child and Adolescent Psychiatric and Mental Health Nursing 1(2), 77-81.

King, J., McSwain, K., & Reid, S. (1986). A nursing family assessment program. Canadian Journal of Psychiatric Nursing 27(3), 12-14.

Lansky, M. R., McVey, G. G., Wendahl, N., et al. (1978). Family treatment training for psychiatric nurses: A report on serial in-service workshops. Journal of Psychiatric Nursing and Mental Health Services 16, 19-22.

Minarik, P. A. (1984). The psychiatric liaison nurse's role with families in acute care. Nursing Clinics of North America 19(1), 161-172.

Moss, N. G. (1984). Child therapy groups in the real world. Journal of Psychosocial Nursing and Mental Health Services 22(3), 43-48.

Rauch, S. P., Brack, C. J., & Orr, D. P. (1987). School-based short-term group treatment for behaviorally disturbed young adolescent males: A pilot intervention. Journal of School Health 57(1), 19-22.

Scharer, K. (1979a). Nursing intervention with abusive and neglectful families within the community. Maternal-Child Nursing Journal 8(2), 85-94.

Scharer, K. (1979b). Nursing therapy with abusive and neglectful families. Journal of Psychiatric Nursing and Mental Health Services 17(9), 12-16.

Shufer, S. (1977). Communicating with young children. Teaching via the play discussion group. American Journal of Nursing 77(12), 1960-1962.

Sideleau, B. F., & Light, N. (1981). Family treatment for the disturbed child? Perspectives in Psychiatric Care 19(2), 78-80.

Smith, J. B. (1984). Care of the hospitalized abused child and family. A framework for nursing intervention. Nursing Clinics of North America 16(1), 127-137.

Whall, A. L. (1981). Nursing theory and the assessment of families. Journal of Psychiatric Nursing and Mental Health Services 19(1), 30-36.

Williams, K., & Baeker, M. (1983). Use of small group with chronically ill children. Journal of School Health 53(3), 205-207.

Williams, P. D., Elder, J. H., & Griggs, C. (1987). The effects of family training and support on child behavior and parent satisfaction. Archives of Psychiatric Nursing 1(2), 89-97.

Zimmerman, M. L., Wolbert, W. A., Burgess, A. W., & Hartman, C. R. (1987). Art and group work: Interventions for multiple victims of child molestation, Part II. Archives of Psychiatric Nursing 1(1), 40-46.

5. Residential and Inpatient Treatment

Barlow, D. J. (1989). Therapeutic holding: Effective intervention with the aggressive child. Journal of Psychosocial Nursing and Mental Health Services 27(1), 10-14.

Beat, P. A., & Barbee, M. A. (1986). Breaking barriers: The pediatric CNS on the child psychiatric inpatient unit. Journal of Psychosocial Nursing and Mental Health Services 24(5), 29-33.

Bonier, R. J. (1982). Staff countertransference in an adolescent milieu treatment setting. In S. C. Feinstein, et al. (Eds.), Adolescent psychiatry: Developmental and clinical studies (Vol. 10, pp. 382-390). Chicago: University of Chicago Press.

Buchanan, D. M., & Rogers, A. S. (1980). A comprehensive adolescent treatment program: An inpatient interdisciplinary approach. Journal of Psychiatric Nursing and Mental Health Services 18(7), 42-45.

Cannon, M. T. (1978). Clinical and administrative issues of a child psychiatric nurse's role in a community hospital. Journal of Psychiatric Nursing and Mental Health Services 16, 29-32.

Critchley, D., & Berlin, I. (1979). Day treatment of young psychotic children and their parents: Interdisciplinary issues and problems. Child Psychiatry and Human Development 9(4), 227-237.

Critchley, D., & Berlin, I. (1981). Parent participation in milieu treatment of young psychotic children. American Journal of Orthopsychiatry 51(1), 149-155.

Erickson, W. D., & Realmuto, G. (1983). Frequency of seclusion in an adolescent psychiatric unit. Journal of Clinical Psychiatry 44(7), 238-241.

Freeberg, S., Kiner, D., & Walker, B. (1976). Nursing care in a combined adolescent medical-psychiatric unit. Journal of Psychiatric Nursing and Mental Health Services 14(11), 13-15.

Galle, M. A. (1979). Point systems vs. level system: Effects on adolescent psychiatric nursing staff. Free Associations 6, 3-4.

Gentilin, J. (1987). Room restriction: A therapeutic prescription. Journal of Psychosocial Nursing and Mental Health Services 25(7), 12-16.

Gross, D. (1979). Helping children deal with loss in a psychiatric setting. Journal of Psychiatric Nursing and Mental Health Services 17(1), 17-20.

Hogarth, T. (1985). Providing a therapeutic milieu on an inpatient adolescent unit. Ohio Nurse's Review 60(4), 7-9.

Johnson, S. (1982). Residential treatment for emotionally disturbed children and adolescents: A review of the literature. Canada's Mental Health 30, 5-8.

Kalogjera, I. J., et al. (1989). Impact of therapeutic management on the use of seclusion and restraint with disruptive adolescent inpatients. Hospital and Community Psychiatry 40(3), 280-285.

Miller, D., et al. (1989). Use of a holding technique to control the violent behavior of seriously disturbed adolescents. Hospital and Community Psychiatry 40(5), 520-524.

Mulvihill, D. L. (1983). Milieu therapy in a children's unit. Canadian Journal of Psychiatric Nursing 24(4), 17-18.

Pearson, G. S. (1988). The latency age child in out-of-home placement: Treatment considerations. Journal of Child and Adolescent Psychiatric and Mental Health Nursing 1(2), 82-88.

Rowe, J. (1988). Attachment theory and the milieu treatment of children. Journal of Child and Adolescent Psychiatric and Mental Health Nursing 1(2), 66-71.

Scharer, K. M. (1979). Helping disturbed children change there passive-aggressive behavior through milieu therapy. American Nursing Association Publication NP-59, 275-292.

Scharer, K. M. (1982). Developing an outcome audit for a child psychiatric inpatient unit. Journal of Psychosocial Nursing and Mental Health Services 20(11), 27-34.

Smith, C., & Murphy, K. E. (1984). Developing a children's inpatient psychiatric unit. Journal of Psychosocial Nursing and Mental Health Services 22(3), 31-36.

6. Depression

Koversky, R. S. (1989). Loneliness and distrubed grief: A comparison of parents who lost a child to suicide or accidental death. Archives of Psychiatric Nursing 3(2), 86-96.

Mellencamp, A. (1981). Adolescent depression: A review of the literature, with implications for nursing care. Journal of Psychosocial Nursing and Mental Health Services 19, 15-20.

Nelms, B. C., & Brody, M. A. (1980). Assessment and intervention: The depressed school-age child. Pediatric Nursing 6(4), 15-19, 47.

Newbern, V. B. (1989). Sexual victimization of child and adolescent patients. Image-The Journal of Nursing Scholarship 21(1), 10-13.

Valente, S. M. (1988). Children, adolescents and nuclear war anxiety. Journal of Child and Adolescent Psychiatric and Mental Health Nursing 1(1), 36-41.

Wiley, L. (1980). Nursing care of a suicidal adolescents. Nursing 80(10), 56-59.

7. Cultural Aspects

Beard, M. T. (1980). Interpersonal trust, life events and coping in an ethnic adolescent population. Journal of Psychiatric Nursing and Mental Health Services 18(11), 12-20.

Levinson, R. M., Graves, W. L., & Holcombe, J. (1984). Cross-cultural vairations in the definition of child Absue: Nurses in the United States and the United Kingdom. International Journal of Nursing Studies 21(1), 35-44.

Santora, D., & Starkey, P. (1982). Research studies in American Indian suicides. Journal of Psychosocial Nursing and Mental Health Services 20(8), 25-29.

Tamez, E. G. (1981). Familisim, Machismo and child rearting practices mong Mexican Americans. Journal of Psychosocial Nursing and Mental Health Services 19(9), 21-25.

C. Training in Social Work--Mental Health--Treatment of Children, Adolescents, and Families

Section Editor:

Henry C. Maier, Ph.D.
Emeritus Professor of Social Work
University of Washington School of Social Work
Seattle, Washington

1. Social Work Training

Aldgate, J., Maluccio, A., & Reeves, C. (Eds.). (1989). Adolescents in foster families. Chicago: Lyseum.

Anthony, E. J.,& Cohler, B. J. (1987). The invulnerable child. New York: Guilford Press.

Ashway, J. A. (1984). A therapist's pregnancy: An opportunity for conflict resolution and growth in the treatment of children. Clinical Social Work Journal 12(1), 3-17.

Bergoff, J. (1989). The role of attachment in female adolescent development. Child and Adolescent Social Work Journal 6(2), 115-125.

Bizynaki, M. N. (1985). The effects of maternal depression on children. Clinical Social Work Journal 13(2), 103-116.

Bloom, M. (1979). Life-span development. New York: Macmillan.

Boyer, P. A. (1986a). The role of the family therapist in supporting services to families with handicapped children. I. Clinical Social Work Journal 14(3), 150-161.

Boyer, P. A. (1986b). The role of the family therapist in supporting services to families with handicapped children. II. Clinical Social Work Journal 14(3), 250-261.

Brandell, J. (1985). Using children's anlogenic stories in dynamic clinical assessment. Child and Adolescent 2(3), 181-190.

Carter, E., & McGoldrick, M. (1980). The family life cycle: A framework for family therapy. New York: Gardner Press.

Cooper, S., & Wasserman, L. (1977). Children in treatment. New York: Brunner/Mazel.

Cozzarelli, L. A., & Silin, M. W. (1984). Therapeutic intervention with families with psychotic young children. Clinical Social Work Journal 12(2), 140-151.

Daro, D. (1988). Confronting child abuse: Research for effective program design. New York: The Free Press.

Dodds, J. (1985). A child psychotherapy primer. New York: Human Sciences Press.

Feiring, C., & Lewis, M. (1989). The social networks of girls and boys from early through middle childhood. In D. Belle (Ed.), Children's social networks and social supports (pp. 115-125). New York: Wiley.

Frank, M. (1984). A child's brain. New York: Haworth Press.

Freeman, D. S. (1981). Techniques of family therapy. New York: Jason Aronson.

Freeman, E. M. (1987). Interaction of pregnancy, loss and developmental issues in adolescents. Social Casework 68(1), 39-46.

Garbarino, J., & Stott, F. M. (Eds.). (1989). What children can tell us. San Francisco: Jossey-Bass.

Gilligan, C. (1987). Adolescent development reconsidered [The Tenth Annual Gisela Konopka Lecture Monograph]. St. Paul, Minn.: Center for Youth Development and Research, University of Minnesota.

Gizynaki, M. N. (1985). The effects of maternal depression on children. Clinical Social Work Journal 13(2), 103-116.

Holman, A. (1983). Family assessment: Tools for understanding and intervention. Beverly Hills: Sage Publications.

Houter, D. K. (1981). To silence one's self: A brief analysis of the literature on adolescent suicide. Child Welfare 60(1), 2-10.

Jenson, J. M., & Whittaker, J. K. (1987). Parental involvement in children's residential treatment. Children and Youth Services Review 9, 81-100.

Jewett, C. (1982). Helping children cope with separation and loss. Cambridge: Harvard Common Press.

Kubler-Ross, E. (1985). Death and dying. New York: Collier.

Laird, J., & Hartman, A. (1985). A handbook of child welfare. New York: The Free Press.

Lieberman, F. (1984). Children, adolescent, and social work. Child and Adolescent Social Work Journal 1(1), 3-17.

Lockland, L. L. (1989). Facing the unknown: Children and adolescents with AIDS. Social Work 34(3), 215-221.

Maas, H. S. (1980). The child's responsibility to society. Vancouver, B.C.: Butterworth.

Maas, H. S. (1984). People in context: Social development from birth to old age. Englewood Cliffs, N.J.: Prentice Hall.

Maier, H. W. (1965). Adolescenthood. Social Casework 46(1), 3-9.

Maier, H. W. (1976). Teaching for competence in the delivery of direct services. New York: Council on Social Work Education.

Maier, H. W. (1987). Developmental group care of children and youth. New York: Haworth Press.

Norman, J. S. (1980). Short term treatment with the adolescent client. Social Casework 61(2), 74-82.

Palmbo, J. (1982). Critical review of the concept of the borderline child. Clinical Social Work Journal 10(4), 246-264.

Robinson, J. (1988). Clinical treatment of black families: Issues and strategies. Social Work 34(4), 313-329.

Sandler, I. N., Miller, P., Short, J., & Wolshik, S. A. (1989). Social support as a protective factor for children in stress. In D. Belle (Ed.), Children's social networks and social supports (pp. 207-307). New York: Wiley.

Seligman, E. (1983). The family with a handicapped child: Understanding and treatment. New York: Grune & Stratton.

Sherradon, M., & Adamek, M. (1985). Treating unemployed adolescents. Social Casework 66(5), 467-474.

Sullivan, T. (1983). Native children in treatment: Clinical, social, and cultural issues. Journal of Child Care 1(5), 75-94.

Turner, F. J. (1989). Child psychopathology: A social work perspective. New York: The Free Press.

Warmtrod, M. T. (1986). Counseling bereaved children: Stages with the process. Social Casework 67(6), 351-358.

Watson, H., & Levine, M. (1989). Psychotherapy and mandated reporting o child abuse. American Journal of Orthopsychiatry 59(2), 246-256.

Werner, E. E. (1989). High-risk children in young adulthood: A longitudinal study from birth to 32 years. American Journal of Orthopsychiatry 59(1), 72-81.

2. Social Support in Mental Health

Cansler, D. (1986). Review of the Millon adolescent personality inventory. Journal of Counseling and Development 64, 469-471.

Cohen, S., & Wills, T. A. (1985). Stress, social support, and the buffering hypothesis. Psychological Bulletin 98, 310-357.

Dean, A., Lin, N., & Ensel, W. M. (1981). The epidemiological significance of social support systems in depression. In R. G. Simmons (Ed.), Research in community and mental health (pp. 77-109). Greenwich, Conn.: JAI Press.

DeAraujo, G., Van Arsde, P. P., Holmes, T. H., & Dudley, D. L. (1973). Life change, coping ability and chronic intrinsic asthma. Journal of Psychosomatic Research 17, 359-363.

Federal Bureau of Investigation. (1986). Uniformed crime reports of the United States. Washington, D.C.: Government Printing Office.

Haynes, A., Feinleib, M., & Kannel, W. (1980). The relationship of psychosocial factors to coronary heart disease in the Framingham study. III. Eight year incidence of coronary heart disease. American Journal of Epidemiology 111, 37-58.

Hollingshead, A. B., & Redlich, R. C. (1958). Social class and mental illness. New York: Wiley.

Israel, B. A. (1982). Social networks and health status: Linking theory, research and practice. Patient Counselling and Health Education 4, 65-79.

Johnson, J. H., & Sarason, I. G. (1979). Moderator variables in stress research. In I. G. Sarason & C. D. Spielberger (Eds.), Stress and anxiety (Vol. 6, pp. 151-167). Washington, D.C.: Hemisphere.

Justice, B., & Swenson, K. (1980). Social assets and personal and social functioning. Journal of Personality 106, 277-286.

Kessler, R. C., & McLeod, J. D. (1985). Social support and mental health in community samples. In S. Cohen & S. L. Syme (Eds.), Social support and health (pp. 219-240). New York: Academic Press.

Lewis, D. O., Shanok, S. S., Grant, M., & Ritvo, E. (1983). Homicidally aggressive young children: Neuropsychiatric and experiential correlates. American Journal of Psychiatry 140, 148-153.

Millon, T., Green, C. J., & Meagher, R. B. (1984). Millon adolescent personality inventory manual. Minneapolis, Minn.: Interpretative Scoring Systems.

Mulligan, M. A. (1977). An investigation of factors associated with violent modes of conflict resolution in the family. Unpublished master's thesis. University of Rhode Island, Providence, Rhode Island.

Pedhazur, E. J. (1982). Multiple regression in behavioral research (2nd ed.). New York: Holt, Rinehart, & Winston.

Romig, D. A. (1978). Justice for our children. Lexington, Mass.: Heath.

Rutter, M., & Giller, H. (1984). Juvenile delinquency: Trends and perspective. New York: Guilford Press.

Sarason, B. R., Sarason, I. G., Hacker, T. A., & Basham, R. B. (1985). Concomitants of social support: Social skills, physical attractiveness, and gender. Journal of Personality and Social Psychology 49, 469-480.

Sarason, I. G., Levine, H. M., Basham, R. B., & Sarason, B. R. (1983). Assessing social support: The social support questionnaire. Journal of Personality and Social Psychology 44, 127-139.

Sarason, I. G., & Sarason, B. R. (1982). Concomitants of social support: Attitudes, personality characteristics, and life experiences. Journal of Personality 50, 331-344.

Sarason, I. G., & Sarason, B. R. (1984). Social support as a stable personal characteristic. Unpublished manuscript, University of Washington, Seattle.

Shamsie, S. J. (1982). Antisocial adolescents: Our treatments do not work--where do we go from here? In S. Chess & A. Thomas (Eds.), Annual progress in child psychiatry and child development (pp. 631-347). New York: Brunner/Mazel.

Steinmetz, S. K. (1971). Occupation and physical punishment: A response to Straus. Journal of Marriage and the Family 33, 664-666.

Steinmetz, S. K. (1974). Occupation environment in relation to physical punishment and dogmatism. In S. Steinmetz & M. Straus (Eds.), Violence in the family (pp. 167-172). New York: Harper and Row.

Steinmetz, S. K. (1977). The cycle of violence: Assertive, aggressive and abusive family interaction. New York: Praeger.

Straus, M. A. (1971). Some social antecedents of physical punishment: A linkage theory interpretation. Journal of Marriage and the Family 33, 658-663.

Straus, M. A. (1979). Measuring intrafamily conflict and violence: The conflict tactics (CT) scales. Journal of Marriage and the Family 41, 75-88.

Straus, M. A., Gelles, R. J., & Steinmetz, S. K. (1980). Behind closed doors: Violence in the American family. New York: Anchor Press.

Turner, R. J. (1983). Direct, indirect, and moderating effects of social support on psychological distress and associated conditions. In H. B. Kaplan (Ed.),

Psychosocial stress: Trends in theory and research (pp. 105-115). New York: Academic Press.

Vega, S. (1987). Suka: In solitude standing (Recording). New York: A & M Records,Social Work and Humanities Division.

Wan, T. T. H., & Weissert, W. G. (1981). Social support networks, patient status and institutionalization. Research on Aging 3, 240-256.

PART VIII

FORENSIC CHILD PSYCHIATRY

Forensic Child Psychiatry

Editor:

Elissa P. Benedek, M.D.
Director of Training and Research
Center for Forensic Psychiatry
Ann Arbor, Michigan

Associate Editor:

Diane Schetky, M.D.
Center for Forensic Psychiatry
Ann Arbor, Michigan

A. General References

Benedek, E. (1983). Psychiatry and juvenile law. Psychiatric Clinics of North America 6, 695-705.

Diamond, B. L. (1983). The psychiatrist as expert witness. Psychiatric Clinics of North America 6, 597-609.

Lewis, D. O. (1983). Neuropsychiatric vulnerabilities and violent juvenile delinquency. Psychiatric Clinics of North America 6, 707-714.

Schetky, D., & Benedek, E. P. (1980). Child psychiatry and the law (Vol. 1). New York: Brunner/Mazel.

B. History of Forensic Psychiatry

Bazelon, D. (1974). Psychiatrists and the adversary process. Scientific American 230, 18-25.

Benedek, E., & Selzer, M. (1977). Lawyer's use of psychiatry. American Journal of Psychiatry 134(4), 435-436.

Freud, A. (1958). Child observation and prediction of development. In R. S. Eissler, et al. (Eds.), Psychoanalytic study of the child (Vol. 13, pp. 92-124). New York: International Universities Press.

Perr, I. (1977). Cross examination of the psychiatrist, using publications. Bulletin of the American Academy of Psychiatry and the Law 5, 327-331.

Pollock, S. (1974). The role of psychiatry in the rule of la. Psychiatric Annals 4, 8-15.

Poythress, N. (1977). Mental health expert testimony: Current problems. Journal of Psychiatry and Law 5, 201-227.

C. Ethics and Forensic Child Psychiatry

Appelbaum, P. S. (1984). Psychiatric ethics in the courtroom. Bulletin of the American Academy of Psychiatry and the Law 12, 225-231.

Ciccone, J. R., & Clements, C. D. (1984). The ethical practice of forensic psychiatry: A view from the trenches. Bulletin of the American Academy of Psychiatry and the Law 12, 263-277.

Perlin, M. L (1983). Recent developments in mental health law. Psychiatric Clinics of North America 6, 539-549.

Stone, A. A. (1984). The ethical boundaries of forensic psychiatry: A view from the ivory tower. Bulletin of the American Academy of Psychiatry and the Law 12, 209-219.

D. Physical and Sexual Child-Adolescent Abuse and the Courts

De Francis, V. (1963). The battered child--a role for the juvenile court, the legislature and the child welfare agency. Juvenile Court Judges Journal 14, 27-29, 33.

Kempe, C. H. (1968). Some problems encountered by welfare departments in the management of the battered child syndrome. In R. E. Helfer & C. H. Kempe (Eds.), The battered child (pp. 169-171). Chicago: University of Chicago Press.

Pollock, C., & Steele, B. (1972). A therapeutic approach to the parents. In C. H. Kempe & R. E. Helfer (Eds.), In helping the battered child and his family (pp. 3-21). Philadelphia: Lippincott.

Steele, B. F., & Pollock, C. B. (1968). A psychiatric study of parents who abuse infants and small children. In R. E. Helfer & C. H. Kempe (Eds.), The battered child (pp. 103-147). Chicago: University of Chicago Press.

E. Child Sexual Abuse--Forensic Issues

Benedek, E. P. (1982). The role of the child psychiatrist in court cases involving child victims of sexual assault [Editorial]. Journal of the American Academy of Child Psychiatry 21, 519-520.

Benedek, E. P., & Schetky, D. H. (1985). Allegations of child sexual abuse in child custody and visitation disputes. In D. H. Schetky & E. P. Benedek (Eds.), Emerging issues in child psychiatry and the law (pp. 145-156). New York: Brunner/Mazel.

Claman, L., Harris, J. C., Bernstein, B. E., & Lovitt, R. (1986). The adolescent as a witness in a case of incest. Assessment and outcome. Journal of the American Academy of Child Psychiatry 25, 457-461.

Densen-Gerber, J., & Lothian, J. (1985). Emerging issues at the interface of law and medicine concerning children of the 1980's. In D. H. Schetky & E. P. Benedek (Eds.), Emerging issues in child psychiatry and the law (pp. 323-346). New York: Brunner/Mazel.

Eth, S., & Pynoos, R. (Eds.) (1985). Post-traumatic stress disorder in children. Washington, D.C.: American Psychiatric Association Press.

Faller, C. K. (1984). Is the child victim of sexual abuse telling the truth? Child Abuse and Neglect 8, 473-481.

Finkelhor, D., & Hotaling, G. T. (1984). Sexual abuse in the National Incidence study of child abuse and neglect: And appraisals. Child Abuse and Neglect 8, 23-33.

Goodman, G. S. (Ed.). (1984). The child as a witness [Special issue]. Journal of Social Issues 40(2), 1-7.

Goodwin, J., Sahd, D., & Rada, R. (1978). Incest hoax: False accusations, false denials. Bulletin of the American Academy of Psychiatry and the Law 6(3), 269-276.

Kaplan, S., & Kaplan, S. (1981). The child's accusation of sexual abuse during a divorce and custody struggle. Hillside Journal of Clinical Psychiatry 3(1), 81-95.

Marin, B. V., Holmes, D. L., Guth, M., & Kovac, P. (1979). The potential of children as eyewitnesses. A comparison of children and adults on eyewitness tasks. Law and Human Behavior 3(4), 295-305.

Nurcombe, B. (1986). The child as witness: Competency and credibility. Journal of the American Academy of Child Psychiatry 25, 473-480.

Yates, A., Beutler, L. S., & Crago, M. (1985). Drawings by child victims of incest. Child Abuse and Neglect 9, 183-189.

F. Termination of Parental Rights

Golstein, J., Freud, A., & Solnit, A. (1973). Beyond the best interests of the child. New York: The Free Press.

Levine, R. (1975). Foundations for drafting a model statute to terminate parental rights: A select bibliography. Juvenile Justice August, 42-56.

Schetky, D., Angell, R., Morrison, C. V., & Sack, W. H. (1979). Parents who fail: A study of 51 cases of termination of parental rights. Journal of the American Academy of Child Psychiatry 18, 366-383.

Wald, M. (1976). State intervention on behalf of neglected children: Standards for removal of children from their homes, monitoring the children in foster care and termination of parental rights. Stanford Law Review 28(4), 523-705.

G. Adoption

Baran, A., Pannor, R., & Sorosky, A. D. (1976). Open adoption. Social Work 21, 97-100.

Bernard, V. W. (1974). Adoption. In S. Arieti (Ed.), American handbook of psychiatry (2nd ed.). (Vol. 1, pp. 514-534). New York: Basic Books.

Cantwell, D. P. (1976). Genetic factors in the hyperkinetic syndrome. Journal of the American Academy of Child Psychiatry 15, 214-223.

Cantwell, D. P. (1978). Hyperactivity and antisocial behavior. Journal of the American Academy of Child Psychiatry 17, 252-262.

Derdeyn, A. P. (1977). A case for permanent foster placement of dependent, neglected, and abused children. American Journal of Orthopsychiatry 47, 604-614.

Derdeyn, A. P., & Wadlington, W. J. (1977). Adoption: The rights of parents versus the beat interests of their children. Journal of the American Academy of Child Psychiatry 16, 238-255.

Gill, M. M. (1978). Adoption of older children: The problems faced. Social Casework 59, 272-278.

Goldstein, J. (1975). Why foster care--for whom for how long? In R. S. Eissler, et al. (Eds.), Psychoanalytic study of the child (Vol. 30, pp. 647-662). New York: International Universities Press.

Johnson, A. M., & Szurek, S. A. (1952). The genesis of antisocial acting out in children and adults. Psychoanalytic Quarterly 21, 323-343.

Kent, K. G., & Ritchie, J. L. (1976). Adoption as an issue in casework with adoptive parents. Journal of the American Academy of Child Psychiatry 15, 510-522.

Lewis, D. O. (1976). Delinquency, psychomotor epileptic symptoms, and paranoid ideation: A triad. American Journal of Psychiatry 133, 1395-1398.

Lewis, D. O., Balla, D., Lewis, M., & Gore, R. (1975). The treatment of adopted versus neglected delinquent children in the court: A problem of reciprocal attachment. American Journal of Psychiatry 132, 142-145.

Lewis, D. O., Pincus, J. H., Shanok, S. S., & Glaser, G. H. (1982). Psychomotor epilepsy and violence in an incarcerated adolescent population. American Journal of Psychiatry 139, 882-887.

Lewis, D. O., & Shanok, S. S. (1977). Medical histories of delinquents and nondelinquents: An epidemiological study. American Journal of Psychiatry 134, 1020-1025.

Lewis, D. O., Shanok, S. S., & Balla, D. A. (1979). Perinatal difficulties, head and face trauma, and child abuse in the medical histories of seriously disturbed children. American Journal of Psychiatry 136, 419-423.

Robins, L. N., West, P. A., & Herjanic, B. L. (1975). Arrests and delinquency in two generations: A study of black urban families and their children. Journal of Child Pyschology and Psychaitry and Allied Disciplines 16, 125-140.

Silver, L. B. (1970). Frequency of adoption in children with the neurological learning disability syndrome. Journal of Learning Disabilities 3, 11-14.

Walsh, E. D., & Lewis, F. S. (1969). A study of adoptive mothers in a child guidance clinic. Social Casework 50, 587-594.

H. Evaluation of Juvenile Offenders

Rutter, M., & Giller, H. (1983). Juvenile delinquency: Trends and perspectives. London: Penguin Books.

I. Child Murderers

Adams, K. A. (1974). The child who murders. Criminal Justice and Behavior 1, 51-61.

Bender, L. (1959). Children and adolescents who have killed. American Journal of Psychiatry 116, 510-513.

Carek, D. J., & Watson, A. S. (1964). Treatment of a family involved in fratricide. Archives of General Psychiatry 11, 533-542.

Duncan, J. W., & Duncan, G. M. (1971). Murder in the family. American Journal of Psychiatry 127, 1498-1502.

Easson, W. M., & Steinhilber, R. M. (1961). Murderous aggression by children and adolescents. Archives of General Psychiatry 4, 1-9.

Malmquist, C. P. (1971). Premonitory signs of homicidal aggression in juveniles. American Journal of Psychiatry 128, 461-465.

Sendi, I. B., & Blomgren, P. G. (1975). A comparative study of predictive criteria in the predisposition of homicidal adolescents. American Journal of Psychiatry 132, 423-427.

Tooley, K. (1975). The small assassins. Journal of the American Academy of Child Psychiatry 14, 306-318.

J. The Child as Witness

Panneton, C. D. (1977). Children, commitment and consent: A constitutional crisis. Family Law Quarterly 10, 295-334.

Pynoos, R., & Eth, S. (1984). The child as criminal witness to homicide. Journal of Social Issues 40, 87-108.

Pynoos, R., & Eth, S. (1986). Witness to violence: The child interview. Journal of the American Academy of Child Psychiatry 25, 306-319.

Terr, L. (1983a). Chowchilla revisited: The effects of psychic trauma four years after a schoolbus kidnapping. Journal of the American Academy of Child Psychiatry 40, 1543-1550.

Terr, L. (1983b). Time sense following psychic trauma: A clinical study of ten adults and twenty children. American Journal of Orthopsychiatry 53, 244-261.

K. Competency to Consent

Gaylin, W. (1979). Who speaks for the helpless--the question of proxy consent. Journal of the American Academy of Child Psychiatry 18, 419-436.

Grisso, J. T., & Vierling, L. (1978). Minors' consent to treatment: A developmental perspective. Professional Psychology 9, 412-427.

Holmes, D. S., & Uric, R. G. (1975). Effects of preparing children for psychotherapy. Journal of Consulting and Clinical Psychology 43, 311-318.

Keith-Spiegel, P. (1976). Children's rights as participants in research. In G. P. Koocher (Ed.), Children's rights and the mental health professions (pp. 53-81). New York: Wiley.

Lewis, C. (1981). How adolescents approach decisions: Changes over grades seven to twelve and policy implications. Child Development 52, 538-544.

Lewis, C. E., Lewis, M. A., Lorimer, A., & Palmer, B. B. (1977). Child-initiated care: The sue of school nursing services by children in an "adult-free" system. Pediatrics 60, 499-507.

Meisel, A., Roth, L. H., & Lidz, C. W. (1977). Toward a model of legal doctrine of informed consent. American Journal of Psychiatry 134, 284-289.
Melton, G. B. (1983a). Decision making by children: Psychological risks and benefits. In G. B. Melton, G. P. Koocher, & M. J. Saks (Eds.), Children's competence to consent. New York: Plenum Press.
Melton, G. B. (1983b). Toward "personhood" for adolescents: Autonomy and privacy as values in public policy. American Psychologist 38, 99-103.
Melton, G. B. (1984). Developmental psychology and the law: The state of the art. Journal of Family Law 22, 445-482.
Roth, L. H., Meisel, A., & Lidz, S. W. (1977). Tests of competency to consent to treatment. American Journal of Psychiatry 134, 279-284.
Tapp, J. L., & Kohlberg, L. (1971). Developing senses of law and legal justice. Journal of Social Issues 27, 65-91.
Weithorn, L. A. (1983). Developmental factors and competence to make informed treatment decisions. In G. B. Melton (Ed.), Legal reforms affecting child and youth services (pp. 85-100). New York: Haworth Press.
Weithorn, L. A., & Campbell, S. B. (1982). The competency of children and adolescents to make informed treatment decisions. Child Development 53, 1589-1598.

L. Commitment

Amaya, M., & Burlingame, W. V. (1981). Judicial review of psychiatric admissions: The clinical impact on child and adolescent inpatients. Journal of the American Academy of Child Psychiatry 20, 761-776.
Appelbaum, P. S., & Gutheil, T. G. (1979). Rotting with their rights on: Constitutional theory and clinical reality in drug refusal by psychiatric patients. Bulletin of the American Academy of Psychiatry and the Law 7, 306-315.
Roth, L. G. (1980). Mental health commitment: The state of the debate, 1980. Hospital and Community Psychiatry 31, 385-396.

M. General Literature in Forensic Child Psychiatry

Appelbaum, P. S. (1985a). The role of the mental health professional in court. Hospital and Community Psychiatry 36, 1043-1044, 1046.
Appelbaum, P. S. (1985b). Tarasoff and the clinician: Problems in fulfilling the duty to protect. American Journal of Psychiatry 142, 425-429.
Ash, P., & Guyer, M. (1984). court implementation of mental health professionals' recommendations in contested child custody and visitation cases. Bulletin of the American Academy of Psychiatry and the Law 12, 137-147.
Atwell, A. E., Moore, U. S., Nielsen, E., & Levite, Z. (1984). Effects of joint custody on children. Bulletin of the American Academy of Psychiatry and the Law 12, 149-157.
Bazelon, D. L. (1978). The role of the psychiatrist in the criminal justice system. Bulletin of the American Academy of Psychiatry and the Law 6, 139-146.

Benedek, E. P. (1974). Forensic psychiatry training for child psychiatrists. Bulletin of the American Academy of Psychiatry and the Law 2, 262-265.

Bernet, W. (1983). The therapists's role in child custody disputes. Journal of the American Academy of Child Psychiatry 22, 180-183.

Ciccone, J. R., & Barry, D. J. (1978). The experience of using DSM-III in a court clinic setting: I. Basic changes in the methodology of psychiatric diagnosis. Bulletin of the American Academy of Psychiatry and the Law 6, 23-25.

Derdeyn, A. P. (1976). A consideration of legal issues in child custody contests: Implications for change. Archives of General Psychiatry 33, 165-171.

Dix, G. E. (1978). Participation by mental health professionals in capital murder sentencing. International Journal of Law and Psychiatry 1, 283-308.

Ennis, B. J. (1974). Emerging legal rights for the mentally handicapped. Bulletin of the American Academy of Psychiatry and the Law 2, 185-193.

Eth, S. (1983). Adolescent separation-individuation and the court. Bulletin of the American Academy of Psychiatry and the Law 11, 231-238.

Eth, S., Levine, M. L., & Lyon-Levine, M. (1984). Ethical conflicts at the interface of advocacy and psychiatry. Hospital and Community Psychiatry 35, 665-666.

Garmise, R., Guggenheim, P. D., & Schuster, R. (1984). Diagnostic and statistical manual-III: A perspective from family court. Journal of Forensic Sciences 29, 1127-1139.

Goodwin, J., Sahd, D., & Rada, R. T. (1978). Incest hoax: False accusations, false denials. Bulletin of the American Academy of Psychiatry and the Law 6, 269-276.

Halleck, S. L. (1984). The ethical dilemmas of forensic psychiatry: A utilitarian approach. Bulletin of the American Academy of Psychiatry and the Law 12, 279-288.

Lewis, M. (1974). The latency child in a custody conflict. Journal of the American Academy of Child Psychiatry 13, 635-647.

McGrath, J. J. (1985). Toward unity: The joint statement of the American Medical Association and the American Psychiatric Association regarding the insanity defense [Editorial]. American Journal of Psychiatry 142, 1058-1059.

Monahan, J. (1984). The prediction of violent behavior: Toward a second generation of theory and policy. American Journal of Psychiatry 141, 10-15.

Monahan, J., & Ruggiero, M. (1980). Psychological and psychiatric aspect of determinate criminal sentencing. International Journal of Law and Psychiatry 3, 143-154.

Moore, M. (1983). The relevance of philosophy to law and psychiatry. International Journal of Law and Psychiatry 6, 177-192.

Perlin, M. L. (1976). Rights of the mentally handicapped. Bulletin of the American Academy of Psychiatry and the Law 4, 77-86.

Roth, L. H., & Meisel, A. (1977). Dangerousness, confidentiality, and the duty to warn. American Journal of Psychiatry 134, 508-511.

Schetky, D. H., & Colbach, E. M. (1982). Countertransference on the witness stand: A flight from self? Bulletin of the American Academy of Psychiatry and the Law 10, 115-121.

Shah, S. A. (1975). Dangerousness and civil commitment of the mentally ill: Some public policy considerations. American Journal of Psychiatry 132, 501-505.

Shah, S. A. (1978). Dangerousness: A paradigm for exploring some issues in law and psychology. American Psychologist 33, 224-238.

Shanok, S. S., & Lewis, D. O. (1977). Juvenile court versus child guidance referral: Psychosocial and parental factors. American Journal of Psychiatry 134, 1130-1133.

Weiner, B. A. (1984). Ethical issues in forensic psychiatry: From an attorney's perspective. Bulletin of the American Academy of Psychiatry and the Law 12, 253-261.

PART IX

Ethics in Child and Adolescent Psychiatry

Ethics in Child and Adolescent Psychiatry

Editor:

Norbert Enzer, M.D.
Professor of Psychiatry and Pediatrics
Division of Child Psychiatry
Michigan State University School of Medicine
East Lansing, Michigan

EDITOR'S NOTE: This section on Ethics is new to the bibliography with this edition. It should be explicitly understood that, with the exception of the Code of Ethics of the American Academy of Child and Adolescent Psychiatry, the inclusion of material in this listing does not imply an endorsement of the views expressed by the authors.

Some of these references address ethical and moral issues in medicine in general, pediatrics, or adult psychiatry but, nevertheless, may prove valuable in the consideration of ethics in child mental health. Many topics are addressed but no claims can be made for comprehensiveness. Rather, the list is intended to provide some historical perspective and examples of more current thinking. It is hoped that these references may stimulate discussion and provide examples of the definition of moral issues and ethical problem solving.

A. An Overview of Ethics in Child Psychiatry and Psychiatry

Applebaum, P. S. (1982). Confidentiality in psychiatric treatment. In L. Grinspoon (Ed.), Psychiatry 1982: The American Psychiatric Association's annual review of psychiatry (pp. 327-350). Washington, D.C.: American Psychiatric Association.

Bartholome, W. E. (1980). The child patient: Do parents have the right to decide? In W. E. Bartholome (Ed.), The law-medicine relation: A philosophical exploration (pp. 271-277). Boston: Reidel.

Bazelon, D. L (1974). "The problem child"--whose problem? Journal of the American Academy of Child Psychiatry 13, 193-201.

Beauchamp, T. L., & Childress, J. F. (1983). Principles of biomedical ethics. Oxford: Oxford University Press.

Busse, E. W. (1984). Ethics and psychiatry--old and new issues. American Journal of Psychiatry 141, 410-411.

Chodoff, P. (1984). Involuntary hospitalization of the mentally ill as a moral issue. American Journal of Psychiatry 141, 384-389.

Ciccone, J. R., & Clements, C. (1984). Forensic psychiatry and applied clinical ethics: Theory and practice. American Journal of Psychiatry 141, 395-399.

Code of ethics. (1980). Washington, D.C.: American Academy of Child and Adolescent Psychiatry.

Committee on Child Psychiatry, Group for the Advancement of Psychiatry. (1989). How old is old enough? The ages of rights and responsibilities. New York: Brunner/Mazel.

Eichelman, B., Wikler, D., & Hartwig, A. (1984). Ethics and psychiatric research: Problems and justification. American Journal of Psychiatry 141, 400-405.

Eisenberg, L (1966). Discussion of Dr. Solnit's paper, "Who deserves child psychiatry? A study in priorities." Journal of the American Academy of Child Psychiatry 5, 17-25.

Englehardt, H. T., Jr., & Rie, M. A. (1988a). Morality for the medical-industrial complex: A code of ethics for the medical-industrial complex. New England Journal of Medicine 319, 1088-1089.

Englehardt, H. T., Jr., & Rie, M. A. (1988b). Morality for the medical-industrial complex: Practicing medicine within a hierarchy: Whose agent is the physician, after all? New England Journal of Medicine 319, 1086-1087.

Enzer, N. B. (1985). Ethics in child psychiatry--an overview. In D. H. Schetky & E. P. Benedek (Eds.), Emerging issues in child psychiatry and the law (pp. 3-21). New York: Brunner/Mazel.

Eth, S., & Schowalter, J. E. (1989). Debate forum resolved: There is no special developmental consideration in adolescence mitigating against capital punishment for those who committed murder under eighteen years of age. Journal of the American Academy of Child and Adolescent Psychiatry 28(5), 450-454.

Fink, P. J. (1989). Presidential address: On being ethical in an unethical world. American Journal of Psychiatry 146(9), 1097-1104.

Gaylin, W. (1979). Who speaks for the helpless? Journal of the American Academy of Child Psychiatry 18, 419-436.

Gaylin, W. (1982). The "competence" of children: No longer all or none. Journal of the American Academy of Child Psychiatry 21, 153-162.

Ginsberg, L. H. (1973). An examination of the civil rights of mentally ill children. Child Welfare 52, 14-25.

Kett, J. F. (1984). The search for a science of infancy. Hastings Center Report 4, 34-39.

Lakin, M. (1988). Ethical issues in the psychotherapies. New York: Oxford University Press.

Lewis, M. (1985). Organ transplants, research and children. In D. H. Schetky & E. P. Benedek (Eds.), Emerging issues in child psychiatry and the law (pp. 44-56). New York: Brunner/Mazel.

Macklin, R. (1977). Consent, coercion and conflict. Perspectives in Biology and Medicine 20, 360.

Melton, G. B. (Ed.). (1989). Reforming the law: Impact of child development research. New York: Guilford Press.

Melton, G. B., Koocher, G. P., & Saks, J. J. (Eds.). (1983). Children's competence to consent. New York: Plenum Press.

Mercer, J. R. (1974). A policy statement on assessment procedures and the rights of children. Harvard Educational Review 44, 121-133.

Miller, C. A. (1984). The health of children, a crisis of ethics. Pediatrics 73, 550-558.

Miller, D., & Burt, R. A. (1977). Children's rights on entering therapeutic institutions. American Journal of Psychiatry 134, 153-156.

Moore, R. S., & Hofmann, A. D. (1982). American Academy of Pediatrics conference on consent and confidentiality. In R. S. Moore & A. D. Hofman (Eds.), Adolescent health care [Monograph]. Philadelphia: American Academy of Pediatrics.

Morison, R. S. (1984). The biological limits on autonomy. Hastings Center Report 4, 43-49.

Pardes, H., Kaufman, C. A., Pincus, H. A., & West, A. (1989). Genetics and psychiatry: Past discoveries, current dilemmas, and future directions. American Journal of Psychiatry 146(4), 435-443.

Polier, W. (1975). Professional abuse of children: Responsibility for the delivery of services. American Journal of Orthopsychiatry 45, 357-364.

Racusin, R. J., & Relsman, J. K. (1986). Reporting child abuse: The ethical obligations to inform parents. Journal of the American Academy of Child Psychiatry 25, 485-489.

Rexford, E. N. (1966). Discussion of Dr. Solnit's paper, "Who deserves child psychiatry? A study in priorities." Journal of the American Academy of Child Psychiatry 5, 24-34.

Roth, L. H. (1982). Competency to consent to or refuse treatment. In L. Grinspoon (Ed.), Psychiatry 1982: The American Psychiatric Association's annual review of psychiatry (pp. 350-360). Washington, D.C.: American Psychiatric Association.

Schetky, D. H., & Benedek, E. P. (Eds.). (1985). Emerging issues in child psychiatry and the law. New York: Brunner/Mazel.

Schowalter, J. E. (1978). The minor's role in consent for mental health treatment. Journal of the American Academy of Child Psychiatry 17, 505-515.

Sider, R. C. (1984). The ethics of therapeutic modality choice. American Journal of Psychiatry 141, 390-394.

Solnit, A. J. (1966). Who deserves child psychiatry? A study in priorities. Journal of the American Academy of Child Psychiatry 5, 1-16.

Weithorn, L. A. (1985). Children's capacities for participation in treatment decision-making. In D. H. Schetky & E. P. Benedek (Eds.), Emerging issues in child psychiatry and the law (pp. 22-36). New York: Brunner/Mazel.

B. Ethics and the Treatment of Children

Eisenberg, L. (1975). The ethics of intervention: Acting amidst ambiguity. Journal of Child Psychology 16, 93-104.

Panneton, J. P. (1977). Children, commitment and consent: A constitutional crisis. Family Law Quarterly 10, 295-334.

Perr, I. N. (1976). Confidentiality and consent in psychiatric treatment of minors. Journal of Legal Medicine 4, 9-13.

C. Ethics in Child Psychiatric Practice

American Psychiatric Association. (1975). Task force on confidentiality as it relates to third parties: Position statement on the role of confidentiality in volunteer military drug abuse programs. American Journal of Psychiatry 132, 362.

Annas, G. J. (1976). Confidentiality and the duty to warn. Hastings Center Report 6, 6-8.

Appelbaum, P. S. (1985). Tarasoff and the clinician: Problems in fulfilling the duty to protect. American Journal of Psychiatry 142(4), 425-429.

Appelbaum, P. S., Kapen, G., Lidz, C., & Roth, L. H. (1984). Confidentiality: An empirical test of the utilitarian perspective. Bulletin of the American Academy of Psychiatry and the law 12(2), 109-116.

Beck, J. C. (1982). When the patient threatens violence: An empirical study of clinical practice after Tarasoff. Bulletin of the American Academy of Psychiatry and the Law 10(3), 189-201.

Cavenar, J. O., Rhoads, E. J., & Sullivan, J. L. (1980). Ethical and legal aspects of supervision. Bulletin of the Menninger Clinic 44(1), 15-22.

Coyne, J. C. (1976). The place of informed consent in ethical dilemmas. Journal of Consulting and Clinical Psychology 44(6), 1015-1016.

Dalton, E., & Hopper, K. (1976). Ethical issues in behavior control: Preliminary examination. Man and medicine. Journal of Values and Ethics in Health Care 2, 1-40.

DiMascio, A. (1979). A control group for psychotherapy research in acute depression: One solution to ethical and methodologic issues. Journal of Psychiatric Research 15(3), 189-197.

Dulchin, J., & Segal, A. J. (1982a). The ambiguity of confidentiality in a psychoanalytic institute. Psychiatry 45(1), 13-25.

Dulchin, J., & Segal, A. J. (1982b). Third-party confidences: The uses of information in a psychoanalytic institute. Psychiatry 45(1), 27-37.

Everstine, L. (1980). Privacy and confidentiality in psychotherapy. American Psychologist 35(9), 828-840.

Fieldsteel, N. D. (1982). Ethical issues in family therapy. In M. Rosenbaum (Ed.), Ethics and values in psychotherapy: A guidebook (pp. 258-268). New York: The Free Press.

Gansheroff, N., Boszormenyi-Nagy, I., & Matrullo, J. (1977). Clinical and legal issues in the family therapy record. Hospital and Community Psychiatry 28(12), 911-913.

Glenn, C. M. (1980). Ethical issues in the practice of child psychotherapy. Professional Psychology 11(4), 613-619.

Gumper, L. L., & Sprenkle, D. H. (1981). Privileged communication in therapy: Special problems for the family couples therapist. Family Process 20(1), 11-23.

Hale, W. D. (1976). Responsibility and psychotherapy. Psychotherapy: Theory, Research and Practice 13, 298-302.

Hines, P. M., & Hare-Mustin, R. T. (1978). Ethical concerns in family therapy. Professional Psychology 9(1), 165-171.

Karasu, T. B. (1980). The ethics of psychotherapy. American Journal of Psychiatry 137(12), 1502-1512.

Karoly, P. (1975). Ethical considerations in the application of self-control techniques. Journal of Abnormal Psychology 84, 175-177.

Ledermann, E. K. (1982). Ethics in psychiatry--the patient's freedom and bondage. Journal of Medical Ethics 8(4), 191-194.

Lief, H. I. (1982). Ethical problems in sex therapy. In M. Rosenbaum (Ed.), Ethics and values in psychotherapy: A guidebook (pp. 269-296). New York: The Free Press.

Margolin, G. (1982). Ethical and legal considerations in marital and family therapy. American Psychologist 37(7), 788-801.

Mclemore, C. W., & Court, J. H. (1977). Religion and psychotherapy--ethics, civil liberties, and clinical savvy: A critique. Journal of Consulting and Clinical Psychology 45, 1172-1175.

Melton, G. B. (1981). Effects of a state law permitting minors to consent to psychotherapy. Professional Psychology 12(5), 647-654.

Messenger, C. B., & McGuire, J. M. (1981). The child's conception of confidentiality in the therapeutic relationship. Psychotherapy: Theory, Research and Practice 18(1), 123-130.

Michels, R. (1976). Professional ethics and social values. International Review of Psychoanalysis 3(4), 377-384.

O'Leary, K. D., & Borkovec, T. D. (1978). Conceptual, methodological, and ethical problems of placebo groups in psychotherapy research. American Psychologist 33(9), 821-830.

Pleune, F. G. (1979). On confidentiality: Whose right to decide? Journal of the American College Health Association 26(4), 195-199.

Popiel, D. J. (1980). Confidentiality in the context of court referrals to mental health professionals. American Journal of Orthopsychiatry 50(4), 678-685.

Re, P. (1979). Confidentiality and patient's records: Balancing the interests of society and the individual. Journal of Psychiatry and Law 7(1), 49-70.

Redlich, F., & Pope, K. S. (1980). Ethics of mental health training [Editorial]. Journal of Nervous and Mental Disease 168(12), 709-714.

Rosner, B. L. (1980). Psychiatrists, confidentiality and insurance claims. Hastings Center Report 10(6), 5-7.

Schopp, R. F., & Quattrocchi, M. R. (1984). Tarasoff, the doctrine of special relationships, and the psychotherapist's duty to warn. Journal of Psychiatry and Law 12(1), 13-37.

Schowalter, J. E. (1978). The minor's role in consent for mental health treatment. Journal of the American Academy of Child Psychiatry 17(3), 505-513.

Serban, G. (1981). Sexual activity in therapy: Legal and ethical issues. American Journal of Psychotherapy 35(1), 76-85.

Sider, R. C., & Clements, C. D. (1982). Family or individual therapy: The ethics of modality choice. American Journal of Psychiatry 139(11), 1455-1459.

Slovenko, R. (1977). Group psychotherapy: Privileged communication and confidentiality. Journal of Psychiatry and Law 5(3), 405-466.

Smith, W. H. (1978). Ethical, social, and professional issues in patient's access to psychological test reports. Bulletin of the Menninger Clinic 42(2), 150-155.

Stone, A. A. (1983). Sexual misconduct by psychiatrists: The ethical and clinical dilemma of confidentiality. American Journal of Psychiatry 140(2), 195-197.

Visotsky, H. (1978). Recommendations for protecting patient's records. American Journal of Forensic Psychiatry 1(1), 21-27.

D. Treatment of the Hyperactive Child

MBD, drug research and the schools: A conference on medical responsibility and community control. (1976). Hastings Center Report 6, 1-23.

Miller, L. G. (1977). Genetic disease and social pathology. Ethics in Science and Medicine 4, 29-50.

Padway, L. (1978). Federal regulation of Ritalin in the treatment of hyperactive children. Ecology Law Quarterly 7, 457-495.

Springmeyer, D. W. (1979). Hyperactive children and the use of psychoactive drugs: Treatment or coercive behavior management? Journal of Contemporary Law 5, 215-231.

E. Ethics in Working with Retarded Children

Annas, G. J. (1982). Mandatory PKU screening: The other side of the looking glass. American Journal of Public Health 72(12), 1401-1403.

Faden, R. R., Chwalow, A. J., Holtzman, N. A., & Horn, S. D. (1982). A survey to evaluate parental consent as public policy for neonatal screening. American Journal of Public Health 72(12), 1347-1352.

Fost, N. (1982). Passive euthanasia of patients with Down's syndrome. Archives of Internal Medicine 142, 2295.

Gunn, M. J., & Smith, J. C. (1985). Case and the right to life of Down's syndrome child. Criminal Law Review 1985, 705-715.

Lister, J. (1975). Private rights and the public good--sterilization of minors--comment or report? New England Journal of Medicine 293(22), 1135-1137.

Shepperdson, B. (1983). Abortion and euthanasia of Down's syndrome children --the parents' view. Journal of Medical Ethics 9(3), 152-157.

Smith, G. F. (1984). The rights of infants with Down's syndrome. Journal of the American Medical Association 251, 229.

Walters, L., & Gaylin, W. (1976). Sterilizing the retarded child. Hastings Center Report 6(2), 13-15.

F. Use of Aversive Conditioning--Ethical Issues

Goldiamond, I. (1974). Toward a constructional approach to social problems: Ethical and constitutional issues raised by applied behavior analysis. Behaviorism 2, 1-84.

Koocher, G. P. (1976). Civil liberties and aversive conditioning for children. American Psychologist 31, 94-95.

Logan, D. L., & Turnage, J. R. (1975). Ethical considerations in the use of faradic aversion therapy. Behavioral Engineering 3, 29-34.

Noll, R. B., & Seagull, A. A. (1982). Beyond informed consent: Ethical and philosophical considerations in using behavior modification or play therapy in the treatment of enuresis. Journal of Clinical Child Psychology 11, 44-49.

G. Ethical Issues in Various Medical-Psychological Situations

Binger, C. M. (1973). Jimmy--a clinical case presentation of a child with a fatal disease. In E. J. Anthony & C. J. Koupernik (Eds.), The child in his family: The impact of disease and death (pp. 171-188). New York: Wiley.

Denkowski, K. M., & Denkowski, G. C. (1982). Client-counselor confidentiality: An update of rationale, legal status, and implications. Personnel and Guidance Journal 60, 371-375.

Duncan, S. L. (1979). Ethical problems in advising contraception and sterilization. Practitioner 233, 237-242.

Fost, N. (1981). Counseling families who have a child with a severe congenital anomaly. Pediatrics 67, 321-324.

Grunebaum, H., & Abernathy, V. (1975). Ethical issues in family planning for hospitalized psychiatric patients. American Journal of Psychiatry 132, 236-240.

Messenger, C. B., & McGuire, J. M. (1981). The child's conception of confidentiality in the therapeutic relationship. Psychotherapy: Theory, Research and Practice 18, 123-130.

Trachtman, G. M. (1974). Ethical issues in school psychology. School Psychology Digest 3, 4-15.

Wilson, J. M. (1978). Should the patient be told the truth? Patient Counselling and Health Education 1, 70-74.

H. The Determination of Individual Rights

Bartholome, W. G., & Arras, J. (1985). Imperiled newborns raise moral doubts. Hastings Center Report 15, 46-47.

Bernstein, D. M., & Simons, R. G. (1974). The adolescent kidney donor: The right to give. American Journal of Psychiatry 131, 1338-1343.

Berwick, D. M., & Komaroff, A. L. (1982). Cost effectiveness of lead screening. New England Journal of Medicine 306, 1392-1398.

Gillon, R. (1985). To what do we have moral obligation and why? II. British Medical Journal 290, 1734-1736.

Glantz, L. H. (1983). The role of personhood in treatment decision made by courts. Milbank Memorial Fund Quarterly. Health and Society 61, 76-100.

Stevens, J. C. (1984). Must the bearer of a right have the concept of that to which he has a right? Ethics 95, 68-74.

PART X

Creativity in Children and Adolescents

Creativity in Children and Adolescents

Editor:

E. J. Anthony, M.D.
Clinical Professor of Psychiatry
George Washington School of Medicine
and
Director of Psychotherapy
Chestnut Lodge
Rockville, Maryland

Associate Editor:

Irving N. Berlin, M.D.
Professor of Psychiatry and Pediatrics
Senior Consultant in Child Psychiatry
University of New Mexico School of Medicine
Albuquerque, New Mexico

A. Historical Aspects of Creativity in Children

Barron, F. (1955). The disposition toward originality. Journal of Abnormal and Social Psychology 51, 478-485.

Berlin, I. N. (1960). Aspects of creativity and the learning process. American Imago 17, 83-99.

Getzels, J. W., & Jackson, P. W. (1962). Creativity and intelligence: Explorations with gifted students. New York: Wiley.

Ghiselin, B. (Ed.). (1955). The creative process. New York: Mentor.

Guilford, J. P. (1967). Creativity: Yesterday, today, and tomorrow. Journal of Creative Behavior 1, 3-14.

Hamilton, J. W. (1969). Object loss, dreaming, and creativity: The poetry of John Keats. In R. S. Eissler, et al. (Eds.), Psychoanalytic study of the child (Vol. 24, pp. 488-531). New York: International Universities Press.

Maddi, S. R. (1965). Motivational aspects of creativity. Journal of Personality 33, 330-347.

Nagera, H. (1967). The concepts of structure and structuralization: Psychoanalytic usage and implications for a theory of learning and creativity. In R. S. Eissler, et al. (Eds.), Psychoanalytic study of the child (Vol. 22, pp. 77-86). New York: International Universities Press.

Robbins, M. D. (1969a). On the psychology of artistic creativity. In R. S. Eissler, et al. (Eds.), Psychoanalytic study of the child (Vol. 24, pp. 227-232). New York: International Universities Press.

Robbins, M. D. (1969b). On the psychology of artistic creativity. In R. S. Eissler, et al. (Eds.), Psychoanalytic study of the child (Vol. 24, pp. 233-241). New York: International Universities Press.

Robbins, M. D. (1969c). On the psychology of artistic creativity. In R. S. Eissler, et al. (Eds.), Psychoanalytic study of the child (Vol. 24, pp. 241-251). New York: International Universities Press.

Stein, M. K., & Heinze, S. J. (1960). Creativity and the individual: Summaries of selected literature in psychology and psychiatry. Glencoe, Ill.: The Free Press.

Ward, W. C. (1968). Creativity in young children. Child Development 39, 737-754.

B. General References on Creativity

Albaum, G. (1977). Birth order and creativity: Some further evidence. Psychological Reports 40, 792-794.

Brenman-Gibson, M. (1976). Notes on the study of the creative process. Psychological Issues 9, 326-357.

Corbin, E. I. (1974). The autonomous ego functions in creativity. Journal of the American Psychoanalytic Association 22, 568-587.

Flach, F. F. (1980). Psychobiologic resilience, psychotherapy, and the creative process. Comprehensive Psychiatry 21, 510-518.

Martindale, C., & Hasenfus, N. (1978). EEG differences as a function of creativity, stage of the creative process, and effort to be original. Biological Psychology 6, 157-167.

Martindale, C., & Hines, D. (1975). Creativity and cortical activation during creative, intellectual and EEG feedback tasks. Biological Psychology 3, 91-100.

Modlin, H. C. (1979a). Creativity. A conference sponsored by the Spencer Foundation of Chicago: Introduction. Bulletin of the Menninger Clinic 43, 291-293.

Modlin, H. C. (1979b). Creativity in clinical practice. Bulletin of the Menninger Clinic 43, 379-388.

Pruyser, P. W. (1979). An essay on creativity. Bulletin of the Menninger Clinic 43, 294-353.

Richards, R. L. (1981). Relationships between creativity and psychopathology: An evaluation and interpretation of the evidence. Genetic Psychology Monographs 103, 261-324.

Rotenberg, V. S. (1985). Sleep dreams, cerebral dominance and creation. A new approach to the problem. Pavlovian Journal of Biological Science 20, 53-58.

Simon, H. A. (1983). Discovery, invention, and development: Human creative thinking. Proceedings of the National Academy of Sciences of the United States of America 80, 4569-4571.

C. Views of the Creative Process in Children and Adolescents

Argulewicz, E. N., Mealor, D. J., & Richmond, B. O. (1979). Creative abilities of learning disabled children. Journal of Learning Disabilities 12, 21-24.

Bender, L. (1976). Comprehensive view of the creative process in psychopathological art. The process of creativity. Conferences in Psychiatry 19, 177-181.

Creativity in Children and Adolescents

Eisenstadt, J. M. (1978). Parental loss and genius. American Psychologist 33, 211-223.

Ford, B. G., & Ford, R. D. (1981). Identifying creative potential in handicapped children. Exceptional Children 48, 115-122.

Gottschalk, L. A. (1981). Psychoanalytic contributions to the generation of creativity in children. Psychiatry 44, 210-229.

Jakab, I. (1979). Creativity and mental illness. Bulletin of the Menninger Clinic 43, 365-378.

Kestenbaum, C. J. (1985). The creative process in child psychotherapy. American Journal of Psychotherapy 39, 479-489.

Kolb, L. C. (1982). Assertive traits fostering social adaptation and creativity. Psychiatric Journal of the University of Ottawa 7, 217-225.

Manosevitz, M., Fling, S., & Prentice, N. M. (1977). Imaginary companions in young children: Relationships with intelligence, creativity and waiting ability. Journal of Child Psychology and Psychiatry and Allied Disciplines 18, 73-78.

McDonagh, M. J. (1976). Creative process and its relation to sense of self, separateness, and reality. Perspectives in Psychiatric Care 14, 68-74.

Paget, K. D. (1982). The creative abilities of children with social and emotional problems. Journal of Abnormal Child Psychology 10, 107-112.

Silver, R. A. (1977). The question of imagination, originality, and abstract thinking by deaf children. American Annals of the Deaf 122, 349-354.

Uno, T., Gargiulo, R. M., Sears, J. D., Mauter, M., & Rowe, J. (1977). Creativity in developmentally disabled adolescents. Psychological Reports 40, 1207-1212.

D. Creativity in Adolescents

Anderson, C. M., & Stoffer, G. R. (1979). Creative thinking and juvenile delinquency: A study of delinquent and nondelinquent youth on the Torrance tests of creative thinking. Adolescence 14, 221-231.

Gottschalk, L. A. (1981). Psychoanalytic contributions to the generation of creativity in children. Psychiatry 44, 210-229.

Rabinowitz, A., & Engelberg, D. (1984). Parental influence on adolescents' imagination. Journal of Adolescence 7, 277-284.

Rosenthal, D. A., & Conway, M. (1980). Adolescents' creativity and non-conformity in school. Psychological Reports 47, 668.

Schwartzman, J. (1982). Creativity, pathology, and family structure: A cybernetic metaphor. Family Process 21, 113-127.

Shaw, J. A. (1981). Adolescence, mourning, and creativity. Adolescent Psychology 9, 60-77.

Workman, E. A., & Stillion, J. M. (1974). The relationship between creativity and ego development. Journal of Psychology 88, 191-195.

PART XI

Films and Videos with Commentary

Films and Videos with Commentary

Editors:

Paul N. Graffagnino, M.D.
Clinical Professor of Psychiatry
Associate Clinical Professor of Pediatrics
University of Connecticut School of Medicine
Farmington, Connecticut

David Scott May, M.D.
Assistant Clinical Professor of Psychiatry
University of California School of Medicine
Los Angeles, California

Consultant to the Editors:

Edward A. Mason, M.D.
Associate Clinical Professor of Psychiatry
Harvard Medical School
Director, Documentaries for Learning
Boston, Massachusetts

A. Sources of Films and Videos

EDITOR'S NOTE: Many sources are transferring older films to video tapes. The reader is advised to contact these sources directly for updated information and for complete catalogs. (Throughout this section, the letter "V" indicates video, and the letter "F" indicates film.)

AACAP	American Academy of Child and Adolescent Psychiatry Central Office Library 3615 Wisconsin Avenue Washington, D.C. 20016 (202) 966-7300
ABCN	ABC News 7 W. 66th Street New York, New York 10023 (212) 887-7777
AMA	American Medical Association Video Clinic Library Division of Marketing 535 North Dearborn Street Chicago, Illinois 60610

AMC	Albany Medical College Department of Pediatrics Albany, New York 12208
B	Bellefaire 22001 Fairmont Boulevard Cleveland, Ohio 44118
BBCTV	British Broadcasting Company - T.V. 630 5th Avenue New York, New York 10020 (212) 581-7100
BF	Britannica Films/Video Encyclopedia Britannica Educational Corp. 524 North Michigan Avenue Chicago, Illinois 60611
BFI	Boston Family Institute 315 Dartmouth Street Boston, Massachusetts 02116 (617) 262-8561
BH	Benhaven 9 St. Ronan Terrace New Haven, Connecticut (203) 624-9819
BM	Brunner/Mazel Pubs. 19 Union Square, West New York, New York 10003 (212) 924-3344
BSML	Behavioral Science Media Laboratory Neuropsychiatric Institute 760 Westwood Plaza Los Angeles, California 90024 (213) 825-0448
BU	Brown University Post Office Box R Providence, Rhode Island 02912

Films and Videos with Commentary

CCDE	Cincinnati Center for Developmental Disorders Children's Hospital Medical Center Corryville, Ohio 45200 (513) 559-4688
CEC	Council for Exceptional Children 1920 Association Drive Reston, Virginia 22091
CES	Continuing Education Seminars Marion Solomon, Ph.D. 1023 Westholme Avenue Los Angeles, California 90024 (800) 621-2131
CF	Coronet Films 108 Wilmont Road Deerfield, Illinois 60015 (800) 621-2131
CFC	Concord Film Council 201 Felixstone Road, Ipswich Suffolk, England IP3 9BJ
CFS	Creative Film Society 14558 Valerio Street Van Nuys, California 91405
CG	Cinema Guild 1697 Broadway New York, New York 10019
CGC	Child Guidance Center c/o Care Video Productions Post Office Box 45132 Cleveland, Ohio 44145 (216) 835-5872
CHD	College of Human Development Department of Family Services Pennsylvania State University University Park, Pennsylvania 16812

CHNMC	Children's Hospital National Medical Center Media Center 111 Michigan Avenue, N.W. Washington, D.C. 20010
CLP	Carole Langer Productions 28 Greene Street New York, New York 10013
CMC	Carle Medical Communications 510 West Main Street Urbana, Illinois 61801 (217) 384-4838
CMH	Children's Memorial Hospital Department of Child Psychiatry 2300 Children's Plaza Chicago, Illinois 60614
CP	Consolidated Productions 9000 Sunset Boulevard, #1020 Los Angeles, California 90069 (213) 275-5719
CTW	Children's Television Workshop One Lincoln Plaza New York, New York 10023
CU	Cornell University Educational Television Center MVR Hall Ithaca, New York 14835
CWR	Case Western Reserve University Health Sciences Communication Center 2119 Abington Road Cleveland, Ohio 44106 (216) 368-3776
DF	Davidson Film, Inc. 231 East Street Davis, California 95616

DL	Documentaries for Learning 74 Fenwood Road Boston, Massachusetts 02115 (617) 566-6793
ECU	Audiovisual Services Center East Carolina University Greenville, North Carolina 27858-4352 (919) 757-6131
EDC	Educational Development Center, Inc. 55 Chapel Street, Suite 309 Newton, Massachusetts 02160
EFVA	Education Foundation for Visual Aids 33 Queen Anne Street London W 1, England
EMTN	Emory Medical Television Network Emory University Atlanta, Georgia 30322 (404) 727-2545
FF	Franciscan Films Post Office Box 6116 San Francisco, California 94101
FL	Filmmakers Library 290 West End Avenue New York, New York 10023
FLRC	Fleischmann Learning Resource Center Stanford University School of Medicine Stanford, California 94305
FLWF	Flower Films and Video 10341 San Pablo Avenue El Cerrito, California 94530 (415) 525-0942
GP	Golden Productions 9022 Leatrice Drive Little Rock, Arkansas 72207

GSA — U.S. Government General Services Administration
National Audiovisual Center
National Archives and Records Service
Washington, D.C. 20409

HCF — Hawthorn Center Films in Child Psychiatry
Hawthorn Center
Northville, Michigan 48167
(313) 349-3000

HCI — Health Communications, Inc.
2119-A Hollywood Boulevard
Hollywood, Florida 33020
(305) 920-9435

HMS — Harvard Medical School
Office of Dean for Administration
Building A, Room 109
25 Shattuck Street
Boston, Massachusetts 06115
(617) 432-1633

HR — Harper and Row Publishers, Inc.
10 East 53rd Street
New York, New York 10022
(212) 207-7000

HSC — Health Sciences Consortium
103 Laurel Avenue
Garrboro, North Carolina 27510
(919) 942-8731

HSV — Health Sciences Videolog
Ohio State University
Columbus, Ohio 43212
(614) 422-3323

IEA — IEA Productions, Inc.
520 East 77th Street
New York, New York 10021
(212) 988-9244

Films and Videos with Commentary

IFB	International Film Bureau, Inc. 332 South Michigan Avenue Chicago, Illinois 60604 (312) 427-4545
IFEX	IFEX Films 201 West 52nd Street New York, New York 10019
IMC	Instructional Media Center Kane Hall DF10 University of Washington Seattle, Washington 98195 (206) 543-9909
IMS,UW	Instructional Media Services University of Washington Seattle, Washington 98195
IU	Medical Television Facility Indiana University School of Medicine Bloomington, Indiana 47405 (812) 855-9343
JBL	J.B. Lippincott Company East Washington Square Philadelphia, Pennsylvania 19105
LP	Lawren Productions, Inc. Post Office Box 666 Mendocino, California 95460 (707) 937-0536
MAC	MAC 1850 High Street Denver, Colorado 80218 (303) 321-2651
MAM	Marquis Academic Media (Mental Health Materials Center) Marquis Who's Who, Inc. 200 East Ohio Street Chicago, Illinois 60611

McH	McGraw-Hill Post Office Box 641 Del Mar, California 92014
McMU	McMaster University 1280 Main Street, West Hamilton, Ontario, Canada L8S4L8 (416) 525-9140
MG	Media Guild Box 881 Solana Beach, California 92075 (714) 755-9191
MRF	Mahler Research Foundation Film Library Box 315 Franklin Lakes, New Jersey 07417
MTI	MTI Films and Video 108 Wilmot Road Deerfield, Illinois 60015 (312) 940-1260
MTPS	Modern Talking Picture Service 2323 New Hyde Park Road New Hyde Park, New York 10040 (516) 437-6300
NAV	National Audiovisual Center National Archives & Records Administration Customer Services Sc. PY 8700 Edgeworth Drive Capital Heights, Maryland 20743-3701 (301) 763-1896
NFBC	National Film Board of Canada 1251 Avenue of the Americas New York, New York 10020
NIMH	National Institute of Mental Health 5600 Fishers Lane Rockville, Maryland 20857 (301) 443-3673

NIU	Northern Illinois University Media Department DeKalb, Illinois 60115
NYSPI	New York State Psychiatric Institute Electronic Textbooks of Psychiatry & Neurology 722 West 168th Street New York, New York 10032
NYU	New York University, Film Library 26 Washington Place New York, New York 10003 (212) 598-2251
OSU	Ohio State University Department of Photography and Cinema Film Distribution Supervisor 156 West 19th Avenue Columbus, Ohio 43210
PBS	PBS Video 475 L'Enfant Plaza, S.W. Washington, D.C. 20024
PCGC	Philadelphia Child Guidance Clinic Attn: Videotape Rentals Two Children's Center 34th Street & Civic Center Boulevard Philadelphia, Pennsylvania 19104
PCR	Psychological Cinema Register Audio-Visual Services/Special Services Building Pennsylvania State University University Park, Pennsylvania 16802
PE	Peach Enterprises, Inc. 4649 Gerald Warren, Michigan 48092 (313) 751-7730
PF	Phoenix Films, Inc. 470 Park Avenue South, #802 New York, New York 10028

PIMC	Psychiatric Institute of Montgomery County Public Information Office 14901 Broschart Road Rockville, Maryland 20850
PMF	Polymorph Films 118 South Street Boston, Massachusetts 02111 (617) 542-2004
PT	Prime Time School Television 40 East Huron Chicago, Illinois 60611 (312) 787-7600
PYF	Pyramid Film & Video Box 1048 Santa Monica, California 90406 (213) 828-7577
SC	Sunburst Communications Room 30, 39 Washington Avenue Pleasantville, New York 10570
SCIS	Science Curriculum Improvement Study University of California Lawrence Hall of Science Berkeley, California 94720
SIU	Medical T.V. Southern Illinois University School of Medicine Post Office Box 3926 Springfield, Illinois 62708
SKF	Smith Kline and French Laboratories Medical Film Center 1500 Spring Garden Street Philadelphia, Pennsylvania 19130
SP	Sandoz Pharmaceuticals Route 10 East Hanover, New Jersey 07936

SUNY	Research Foundation of SUNY SUNY Health Science Center 450 Clarkson Avenue Brooklyn, New York 11203 (718) 270-1155
TCP	Technology for Children Project Department of Education Division of Vocational Education 225 West State Street Trenton, New Jersey 08625
TLV	Time Life Video Distribution Center Post Office Box 644 Paramus, New Jersey 07652 (201) 843-4545
UA	Biomedical Communications University of Arizona Health Services Center Tucson, Arizona 85721 (602) 621-3471
UC	University of Connecticut Health Center Audiovisuals, Stowe Library Farmington, Connecticut 06032 (203) 674-3272
UCEMC	University of California, Extension Media Center 2176 Shattuck Avenue Berkeley, California 94704
UCLA	University of California, Los Angeles Instructional Media Library 46 Powell Street Los Angeles, California 90024 (213) 825-0755
UCOL	Biomedical Communications - Medical Cinematography University of Colorado Denver, Colorado 80202 (303) 556-2875

UEC	University of East Carolina Greenville, North Carolina 27858-4352 (919) 757-6131
UI	University of Illinois Film Center 1325 South Oak Street Champaign, Illinois 61820
UK	University of Kansas Medical Center National Medical Audiovisual Center 39th and Rainbow Boulevard Kansas City, Kansas 66103 (913) 588-1258
UMG	University of Michigan Media Library R 4440 Kresge I, Box 56 Ann Arbor, Michigan 48104-0010 (313) 763-2074
UMN	University of Minnesota Institute of Child Development 51 East River Road Minneapolis, Minnesota 55455
UNC	Medical Television Center Medical Sciences Teaching Labs University of North Carolina School of Medicine Chapel Hill, North Carolina 27599 (919) 966-2611
UND	Child Evaluation & Treatment Program University of North Dakota Medical Center Rehabilitation Hospital 1300 Colombia Road, South Grand Forks, North Dakota 58201 (701) 780-2311
USC	Medical University of South Carolina 171 Ashley Avenue Charleston, South Carolina 29425 (803) 792-3391

UTEX	University of Texas Health Science Center Post Office Box 20036 Houston, Texas 77225 (713) 792-7444
UTOR	University of Toronto Media Centre 121 St. George St. Ontario, Canada M5S1A1
UUMC	Parent to Parent Room 2C 57E University of Utah Medical Center 50 North Medical Drive Salt Lake City, Utah 84132
UWF	Human Resource Video Library Department of Social Work The University of West Florida 11000 University Parkway Pensacola, Florida 32515-5751
UWMRC	University of Wisconsin Mental Retardation Center Madison, Wisconsin 53792
VCU	Virginia Commonwealth University Box 568 Richmond, Virginia 23298 (804) 786-0347
VN	Video Nursing, Inc. 2645 Girard Avenue Evanston, Illinois 60201
WD	Walt Disney Educational Media Company 500 South Buena Vista Street Burbank, California 91521 (800) 423-2555
WGBH	PBS Boston 125 Western Avenue Alston, Massachusetts 02134

WP Wombat Productions
Little Lake, Glendale Road
Post Office Box 70
Ossining, New York 10562
(914) 762-0011

WPIC Western Psychiatric Institute and Clinic
3811 O'Hara Street
Pittsburgh, Pennsylvania 15213

WRMC Walter Reed Medical Center
6900 Georgia Avenue, N.W.
Washington, D.C. 20307-5001
(202) 576-3501

WSU Wayne State University
Center for Instructional Technology
77 West Caulfield Avenue
Detroit, Michigan 48202

B. History of Child and Adolescent Mental Health

<u>The American workplace</u> F
(1980) Source: UCLA

History, social. This film examines work and working conditions in the early days of U.S. history; the changes due to mechanization; beginnings, growth and accomplishments of unions; the changes in status, education, and attitudes of American workers; and what these changes will mean to the nation now and in the future. Associated Press; Prentice Hall Media. (25 mins.)

<u>An Edwardian childhood</u> F
(1968) Source: PYF

History, social. Noted art historian Kenneth Clark gives a humorous, affectionate, and objective account of what life was like for the British upper classes in the decade before the First World War. Family photographs and scenes of the English countryside evoke impressions of an era of wealth and luxury, not irrevocably past. Clark's witty and articulate recollections of a privileged childhood provide insight into the social attitudes and activities of Edwardian England. C. Clark, Director. (27 mins.)

Films and Videos with Commentary

George L. Engel, M.D. — V
(1974) — Source: NAV

History, Engel. Sanford Meyerowitz and George Libman Engel, Directors. (61 mins.)

Face to face: Professor Jung — F
(1972) — Source: UI

History, Jung. This film is a personal interview with Carl Gustav Jung at age eighty-four in his home on Lake Zurich, Switzerland. Jung discusses his childhood, his relationship with his father and mother, his years as a student, and how he decided to specialize in psychiatry. Comments on his personal friendship with Freud, the effect of their temperamental differences on their approach to psychology, his study of dreams, and his view on death. John Freeman, Director. (40 mins.)

Freud: The hidden nature of man — F
(1970) — Source: IU

History, Freud. An analysis of Freud's theories of the power of the unconscious; the Oedipus complex; dream analysis; and the ego, superego, and id of the human personality, bringing out Freud's background and personal struggles. Points out the impact his ideas had on man's attitude toward himself, particularly Victorian man's approach to sexuality. Western Civilization: Majesty and Madness Series. (29 mins.)

Grasping/Mother love/Smile of the baby/Anxiety — F
(1940) — Source: BU

History, Gesell. Historically, this is an important film. Dr. Arnold Gesell explains his own work, which has had an enormous influence in the last thirty or thirty-five years. We believe that this film is not quite as it could have been with respect to the commentary, but it is still quite good. (Four films, 16 mins.)

Infantile autism: The invisible wall — V
(1967) — Source: FLRC

History, autism. Dr. Bernard Rimland outlines the symptomatology and presents his theory of infantile autism. Interviews with four mothers of autistic children describe the nature of the disorder on a personal level. Scenes of autistic children in a wide variety of situations at home are included. (27 mins.)

<u>Jean Piaget: Memory and intelligence</u> F
(1971) Source: UI

History, Piaget. This is a documentary of Jean Piaget's lecture-presentation of his work on memory and intelligence, given at the International Congress of Preschool Educational Specialists in Kyoto, Japan, in 1971. In French, with carefully translated English subtitles. (45 mins.)

<u>Life with baby</u> F
(1945) Source: NYU

History, Gesell. In this film, Dr. Arnold Gesell describes his own work, and Dr. Gesell's comments about the Gesell schedules are worth something in the background of a professional. Though it is clearly an "antique" film, it is easy to understand, pleasant to view, and has a good deal of charm to it. It would be of interest primarily to professionals in the field as a historical piece. (18 mins.)

<u>Mother love</u> F
(1960) Source: IU

History, Harlow. Here are recorded the experiments of Dr. Harry Harlow in which he used two newborn rhesus monkeys to study the infant-mother relationship. He created two substitute mothers, one of wire and one of cloth, and tested the monkeys' reactions to them in different situations. He demonstrated through these experiments that the single most important factor in an infant's love for its mother is that of body contact--holding and nestling--and that deprivation of this can cause deep emotional disturbances, even death. Conquest Series, CBS. (26 mins.)

<u>Professor Erik Erikson, Part 1</u> F
(1964) Source: UCEMC

History, Erik Erikson. In this informal session, Professor Erikson discusses his work in depth and talks about various approaches to the background and involvement with psychoanalysis. He explores his theory of the eight stages of psychosocial development. (40 mins.)

<u>Professor Erik Erikson, Part 2</u> F
(1964) Source: UCEMC

History, Erik Erikson. Professor Erikson talks spontaneously about some of his ideas that have helped shape modern psychology. He discusses the libido theory, ego identity, and positive and negative identity. He delves into the concept of existentialism and his fascination with cross-cultural research. (50 mins.)

Sigmund Freud: His office and home, Vienna F
(1938) Source: FL

History, Freud. This film is composed of more than one hundred still photographs taken by Edmund Engelman in 1938, just prior to Freud's leaving 19 Berggasse Strasse in Vienna for London, England. The format of the film is like a travelogue as one pursues each corner of Freud's famous consulting room as well as his living quarters. There is a conscious effort made to emphasize the parallels between Freud's collection and interest in antiquities and the hidden material of the human unconscious. There is also some examination of Freud's library and sculpture that is likely to have influenced his ideas. G. Friedman, Director. (17 mins.)

Step by step F
(1979) Source: PYF

Development, history of childhood. Childhood's past, present, and future come to life imaginatively and symbolically in this visual tone poem. Evocative vignettes focus on childhood's harsh historical realities, today's child at work and play, and tomorrow's hope for all children everywhere. In the universal language of music, rhythm, and art, Step by step asks us all to take the first step toward insuring a positive future for all the children of the world. An award-winning animated film. Faith Hubley, Director. (11 mins.)

The story of Anna O V
(1979) Source: FLWF

History, early psychoanalysis. Terrel Seltzer, Jósef Breuer, and Bertha Pappenheim, Director. (18 mins.)

C. Animal Studies Relevant to Development, Pathology, and Disorder

Aggression--or love? F
(1968) Source: UI

Research, basic. Current animal research into aggression is presented in this film. The role of aggression in the preservation of the species is considered, along with ritual as a substitute for aggression, aggressive behavior as instinctual or learned, and environmental factors which encourage aggression. Animal Secrets Series. (23 mins.)

Animal parents V,F
(1972) Source: PCR

Research, basic. This film looks at patterns of behavior that determine parent-infant relationships and explains the ways in which relationships take on added complexity along the evolutionary scale, from insect to monkey. N. Tinbergen, Director. Behavior and Survival Series. (25 mins.)

Care of the infant: Animal and human F
(1961) Source: UI

Research, basic. This film compares birth, care, and early development of human and animal babies. It draws parallels in the establishment of individual, parental, and group relationships. Besides a human family, the film uses footage of the following African animals: elephant, giraffe, baboon, and wildebeest. (22 mins.)

Childhood of the chimpanzee V,F
(1966) Source: IU

Research, basic. Documents experiments in isolating some of the significant patterns in the young chimpanzee's social behavior. Compares the chimpanzee with man physically and mentally--particularly in early social behavior. Experimental Series. (30 mins.)

Ethology: From newts to newborn F
(1980) Source: PCR

Research, basic. This film illustrates the methods of investigation used to observe and describe the behavior of newts, birds, and human infants. From the Biology, Brain, and Behavior Series. (24 mins.)

The first signs of Washoe V,F
(1984) Source: TLV

Research, basic. A psychologist couple took a baby chimpanzee home and began to teach her American sign language. By the time she was five, the chimpanzee had a vocabulary of 130 words. Another chimp was taught to communicate with a computer. (59 mins.)

Infant development F
(1982) Source: IU

Research, basic. This film examines the behavioral and developmental characteristics of the infant chimpanzee and the effect that the presence of new life has on the rest of the community. It focuses on Flo, a chimpanzee, to emphasize such key points as sucking, protection, and grooming. The film points out the similarities of child rearing habits between the chimpanzee and man. Jane Goodall: Studies of the Chimpanzee Series. (25 mins.)

<u>Primate growth and development: A gorilla's first year</u> F
(1968) Source: IU

Research, basic. In this film, the first year in the life of a lowland gorilla is documented, with particular aspects of physical and behavioral development pointed out as the gorilla passes through the various stages of maturation. The film utilizes screened charts to contrast capabilities and development at a given stage with those of an infant and a chimpanzee. The importance of studying the gorilla is emphasized, since this leads to a greater scientific knowledge of all primates. (22 mins.)

<u>Talk to the animals</u> F
(1978) Source: UCLA

Research, basic. This film looks into research about communication with animals. Sign language is taught to chimpanzees at the Institute for Primate Studies. Lana, a chimpanzee at the Yerkes Primate Center in Atlanta, Georgia, uses a computer to communicate. The same conversation board developed for the Lana project helps a brain-damaged girl at the Georgia Retardation Center to talk. Koko, a gorilla at Stanford University, communicates with people through a typewriter that translates the keys hit by Koko into a voice language. CBS; CRM/McGraw-Hill. (14 mins.)

<u>A touch of sensitivity</u> F
(1979) Source: UI

Research, basic. In this film, studies on touch deprivation in animals and humans are covered. The effects of short- and long-term deprivation on monkeys are shown: body functions are all measurably disturbed, including the immune system. Physical dysfunctions persist, even in reversal of deprivation, and brain damage was evident in the sparsity of dendrites and neurons on tissue examination. Also shown are visits to a psychiatric unit for disturbed adolescents in Britain, where touch therapy has proven the first really effective approach in reducing property damage and violent encounters. The film also considers the role of pets in the recovery of heart attach patients. (50 mins.)

What time is your body? F
(1973) Source: UI

Research, basic. This film presents a summary of research on circadian rhythm of animals and man. Animals, including man, when cut off from any indication of time or when light and dark cycles are extended indefinitely, run to a slightly longer or shorter period than a day--the average being twenty-five hours. How the experiments are planned and controlled, and what has been learned, are explained. (22 mins.)

D. Development, Diagnosis, and Treatment in Maldevelopment

1. Development and Growth

Abby's first two years: A backward look F
(1960) Source: NYU

Development, infant. This film is organized in reverse sequence, i.e., Abby gets younger rather than older as the film progresses. She is shown in routine situations such as feeding, bathing, and play. The dropping away rather than accretion of new skills in locomotion, posture, manipulation, and social relationships has more impact than the usual forward sequence. Vassar College Department of Child Study. Joseph Stone, Dirctor. (30 mins.)

The amazing newborn F
(1945) Source: CWR

Development, growth. This film both demonstrates and describes the highly responsive and adaptive behavior of the newborn. It shows how the newborn is more than a series of reflex arcs. It begins by explaining the six states of arousal put forward by Dr. Peter Wolf. In particular, it examines the capacity of the newborn when it is in the quiet alert state as opposed to the active alert, crying, or sleeping states. The film also shows how the newborn has preferences for high contrast visual patterns, organized human faces, and curved lines. There is a suggestion of imitation and synchrony of movements with the human voice. The adaptive nature of these early responses, the differences depending on the state of the newborn, the length of gestation, and sedating drugs given during delivery are discussed. American Academy of Pediatrics/Ross Laboratories. (25 mins.)

The beginning of life F
(1976) Source: UCLA

Development, growth. This film captures the development of a human embryo from fertilized ovum to birth. With remarkable artistry and innovative camera techniques, acclaimed photographer L. Nilsson catches the ever-growing, self-transforming evolution of a single-cell into a human baby--the story of life repeating itself without end. Benchmark Films. (30 mins.)

Birth of a brain (Naissance du cerveau) F
(1983) Source: UI

Development, growth. In this film, we learn about the types of developmental changes in the brain and their timing from conception through the first two years after birth, using computer graphics, sonograph, and films of living nerve cells to show processes. The emphasis is on their interactive nature, asserting that the brain is actually built through the child's interactions with the surrounding world. Note: includes a live birth sequence. (35 mins.)

The brain and behavior F
(1970) Source: PCR

Development, growth. (22 mins.)

Brazelton neonatal behavioral assessment scale F
(1978) Source: UCLA

Development, growth. This neonatal assessment scale is a forty-item test that attempts to establish the "nature" rather than the "nurture" aspect of the neonate before the environment has come into play, except as far as the intrauterine environment is concerned. It takes into account the neonate's "state" rather than ignoring it, and thus has more appeal as a research tool as well as a clinical assessment scale. The forty items are a mix of neurological reflexes, "social" responses, sensory stimulation, changes in state measures, and measures of self-quieting ability on the part of the neonate. In the first film, a two-day-old neonate is shown going thought the entire battery of tests. In the second film, the examiner demonstrates the differences between three distinct neonates when presented with the same stimuli. In the third film, one is silently taken through all forty items of the test with a scoring booklet as a means to acquire proficiency with this scale. National Spastic Foundation. (Three films: #1, 20 mins.; #2, 20 mins.; #3, 23 mins.)

Child development: the early years V
(1984) Source: NYSPI

Development, infant. In this film, we see the day old's responses and his/her developing sense that what he does can change his environment. There is also the beginning of basic trust, and the demonstration of the three- to four-month old infant preferring the human face and that the mother's face is special. By seven months, the smile can elicit good nurturing maternal response, and there is progress in cognitive as well as object relations development. The fleeting image of mother's face, appearing and reappearing, can lead to object permanence--mother reappears. At seven months, the infant shows stranger anxiety; at thirteen months, object permanence (baby rattle); at twenty-two months, other adults can understand the child's expressive language. The film has an excellent segment explaining the three-year-old's status on object constancy; the child's readiness for nursery school is contingent on having an inner representation of the mother when she is not in sight. The last three segments show the child's phase specific development through verbalization, symbolic play, and fantasy material. An excellent dynamic review, birth to five years. Also available in the same series are a videotape on the school years and one on the adolescent years. C. Kestenberg, Director. (30 mins.)

<u>Eight infants: Tension manifestations in response to perceptual stimulation</u> F
(1968) Source: NYU

Development, growth. The behavior of eight infants, eighteen to twenty-five weeks of age, was systematically examined before and after prolonged perceptual stimulation of the kind to which they are frequently exposed when shown toys, played with vigorously by siblings and visiting relatives, included in family events, etc. The film shows the infants' behavior before, during, and after such stimulation. S. Escalona, Director. (42 mins.)

<u>Expressive movements (affectomotor patterns) in infancy</u> F
(1955) Source: NYU

Development, growth. Bela Mittelman, et al., Directors. (42 mins.)

<u>Fantasies in children</u> F
(1966) Source: WPIC

Development, fantasy. Originally shown on closed-circuit TV as part of the post-graduate education in the University of Pittsburgh School of Medicine, the film features Miss Helen Ross, educator, psychoanalyst, and expert on children. On the panel with her are Marita Kenna, M.D., child psychiatrist, and Ray Greco, M.D., general practitioner. The discussion is on the fantasy world of small children, mostly of pre-school age, concerning their own body image, the meaning of illness, what going to the hospital or the doctor's office means, etc. Emphasis is placed on the need for the adults (parents, physicians, nurses, etc.) to realize the existence of the fantasy world and the need to understand it. University of Pittsburgh School of Medicine. (58 mins.)

Grasping (1969) F Source: NYU

Development, growth. This is an experimental study in motion pictures of the development of the grasping pattern. Grasping develops as a sequence in which motor skills interact progressively with the ever-widening radius of the unfolding of the psyche. Grasping proper is an intentional act. Its earliest predecessor in the development is the clutching reflex, a purely motor pattern present at birth and shown in the first pictures. A learning process adapts this motor pattern to purposeful use. Between grasping proper and clutching reflex, there is also a motor difference shown in the film: the clutching reflex takes place with unopposed thumb, grasping with opposed thumb. Mastery of grasping is achieved when the infant uses the neuromuscular pattern adequately to exploit environmental facilities to gratify its needs. The development takes all of the first year. Film Studies of the Psychoanalytic Research Project on Problems in Infancy Series. R. Spitz, Director. (20 mins.)

Maternal deprivation in young children (1968) F Source: WPIC

Development, check of maternal deprivation on infants. This film is part of the record collected by a French research unit studying the effect of maternal deprivation in young children between one- to two-and-a-half years old. All have been reared in institutions without opportunity for a stable and intimate relationship to one person. All have been displaced several times from institution to institution. For most of these children, capacity for human relationship was seriously impaired. The first part of the film shows some of the disorders that appear in these children; the second shows progress of the children under psychotherapy. (30 mins.)

Motility in parent-child relationships (1956) F Source: NYU

Development, growth. The second film in Dr. Mittelman's series on motility is focused on its important role in the development of interpersonal relationships in the first year and a half of life. Reciprocity between parent and child, involving modes of motility, is the main theme of this film. Maturational aspects are considered under three headings: (1) the pre-personal phase--up to about three months, when humans are important only because they supply flexibly the basic wants of the infant; (2) the general personal phase--roughly three to eight months when people as such are important to the baby; and (3) the specific personal phase--when the child recognizes familiar people, notably the mother, and is shy or anxious with strangers. The newborn infant's motility, at first random activity or reactions to distress, soon includes vigorous manifestations of pleasure. These merge into aggressive behavior and are related to the developments of adaptive patterns of locomotion and manipulation. The film shows how the parents' active response to the baby's motor behavior results in social interchange. (40 mins.)

Newborn F
(1978) Source: FL

Development, infant. Opening with a natural childbirth sequence, this absorbing film tells us that the newborn infant is far from helpless. A number of pediatricians and researchers in neonatal biology report on their findings. Among those heard from are Dr. T. Berry Brazelton, Harvard Medical School; Dr. Lewis Lipsitt, Brown University; Dr. Louis Sanders, Boston University; and Dr. Klaus Minde, Hospital for Sick Children, Toronto. The film's primary emphasis, however, is on the importance of close maternal contact during the first hours after birth, to start the "bonding" process, which is the basis of all subsequent emotional development. Premature babies, too, can benefit from this kind of contact, and the film demonstrates how even incubator babies can receive some forms of maternal nurturing. (28 mins.)

Newly fathers V
(1980) Source: UI

Development, family relations--father's role in child's development. This film features a specialist in early childhood education discussing the key role fathers play in child development. It emmphasizes the dramatic effect of fathers on their children's educational motivation and achievement. Focus on Children Series. (29 mins.)

The psychological birth of the human infant V,F
(1984) Source: MRF

Development. This production, designed strictly for professional audiences, is culled from thousands of hours of taping mothers and their young children in Mahler's eleven-year research study of the separation/individuation process. It explains and depicts each step of the process, from the first stage of differentiation through the fourth stage of "On the way to object and self constancy." John McDevitt, Anni Bergman, and Margaret Mahler narrate. Mahler Research Foundation. (50 mins.)

Psychological hazards of infancy F
(1965) Source: NYU

Developmental, infant. Technically, this is an absolutely first-rate product. This film focuses on the possibilities of emotional injury to humans in the fist years of life. It borrows a great deal of footage from Dr. Rene Spitz's original work on the effects of institutionalization or prolonged separation from mother on young infants. It is clearly possible to devastate a child's future in the first years of his life. J. Stone, Director. (20 mins.)

Right from the start V
(1973) Source: PT

Development, infant. A presentation about parent-infant attachment produced with the consultation of thirteen leaders in the field of infant development, this videotape contains footage of T. Berry Brazelton, John Kennel, and Marshall Klaus, Bernice Weissbourd and Selma Frailberg and her colleagues at the San Francisco Infant-Parent Program, as well as clips from Rene Spitz's films of institutionalized infants and Harlow's studies of maternally deprived monkey. PBS. (60 mins.)

Shaping the personality: The role of mother-child relations in infancy F
(1956) Source: NYU

Development. This films illustrates forms of mother-child relations and their influence on the child. A brief anamnesis of the mother's pregnancy is compared with her behavior during breast feeding in an attempt to present the biological and psychological factors which will decide the future attitude of the mother to her child. Five mothers, breast feeding their children, are successively shown. The first mother, patient, loving, secure; the second, outgoing with mild anxiety; the third, concerned but without hostility; the fourth, rejecting and hostile toward the child; and the fifth, hostile toward an unwanted child. The behavior of the mothers in feeding and play situations is shown to be an expression of their conscious or unconscious wishes of what their children should be like. Five children are shown, illustrating how much the child's personality is a product of the mother's wishes and how much it molds itself to the picture she has of him. Distribution is limited to professional groups. Silent film of historic interest. (20 mins.)

The sleep of babies:
Spontaneous cyclical phenomena during neonate sleep F
(1970) Source: PCR

Sleep. This film records observable behavior of three- to five-day-old infants during sleep by means of normal speed, slowed motion, and stop motion cinephotography. It illustrates methods of classifying and recording various types of behavior during sleep, including body movements, rapid eye movements, respiration, and brain activity, as well as rhythmic patterns of activity which are possible indicators of maturational changes. D. Coleman and J. G. Minard, Directors. (30 mins.)

Study in human development: Part II
Forty two weeks to fifteen months F
(1946) Source: PCR

Development. In this film, we see development at forty-two weeks, twelve months, and fifteen months of age. Emphasis is given to gross motor development and to perceptual-manipulatory reactions to objects including a cup, a spoon, a bell, a hoop, a ball, and a mirror. A child pulls himself up, stands, crawls, mounts stairs, and exhibits walking readiness. At one year of age he is given simple tests for fine manipulation, imitation, and stair climbing. Development of motor skills is further demonstrated for the fifteen-month stage, and early interactions with another child are described photographically. H. D. Behrens, Director. (17 mins.)

Study in human development: Part III
Nineteen months to two years and eight months F
(1946) Source: PCR

Development. In this film, emphasis is on continued gross and fine motor development and the beginnings of cooperative play. The stages shown are nineteen, twenty-four, and thirty-two months. At nineteen months a boy imitates building a block tower, drinks by holding a glass with both hands, and throws a ball; he exhibits handedness, but play is non-cooperative. At two years, a boy walks up stairs but shows hesitation and caution about descents. He marks on paper, but no patterns are made; great increment in motor development is exhibited, but play is still essentially individualistic. The child draws patterns and crude "man" at thirty-two months; he plays more cooperatively with other children and uses a wide variety of toys and play equipment. H. D. Behrens, Director. (19 mins.)

Study in human development: Part IV
Three years to five years F
(1948) Source: PCR

Development. At the third year, we see socially interdependent play, the development of skill in drawing, and typical motor coordination. The fourth year brings finer coordination, greater ability in drawing, and rudimentary musical skills; the application of performance tests for intelligence is shown at this level. During the fifth year, a boy enrolls in kindergarten and begins characteristic social play activities. H. D. Behrens, Director. (18 mins.)

Study of twins: Part I F
(1947) Source: PCR

Development. This series presents the growth and development of identical twin boys, and deals primarily with responses to everyday informal situations; it stresses the differences between developing twins. Illustrated here are motor growth in infancy, especially differences in the rate of development among various parts of the body. Cephalocaudal pattern is emphasized. Sequences are provided at fourteen, twenty-two, twenty-eight, and forty weeks. H. D. Behrens, Director. (17 mins.)

Study of twins: Part II F
(1947) Source: PCR

Development. Here we see twins at twelve, fifteen, eighteen, and twenty-one months of age. They are shown in the getting up, standing, and walking stages, and they also demonstrate certain amounts of independent play and cooperative play. H. D. Behrens, Director. (17 mins.)

Study of twins: Part III F
(1949) Source: PCR

Development. In this film, behavior is recorded at twenty-four, twenty-eight, and thirty-two months. It shows amicable but independent play and the rapidity of the development of motor skills and of the larger muscles. H. D. Behrens, Director. (18 mins.)

Where did I come from? V
(1982) Source: CP

Development. This videotape is an adaptation of the successful book of the same name by Peter Mayle. The videotape starts playfully with more of a cartoon effect of children of different cultures playing, all done as animation. The next section of the videotape illustrates a series of myths and folkstories about where babies supposedly come from, all the way from the stork to a hamburger at a restaurant. About ten minutes into the tape, it begins the section on reproduction by explaining the differences between men and women. This leads to a real but understandable explanation of the functional aspects of these anatomical differences. It leads then into affection between adults, and without actually showing intercourse, to an appropriate and believable discussion (all still in animation) of orgasm, sperm, and fertilization. It moves on to the developing fetus, discussing what has formed by various months of gestation and what can be seen from the outside. It then proceeds to labor and delivery, concluding with why one needs to have, and then sever, the umbilical cord. For children aged five to thirteen. Consolidated Productions. (30 mins.)

The world of three — F
(1965) — Source: NYU

Development, sibling identity. This is a very sensitive and authentic presentation of the sibling rivalry issues. The camera acts as a third-person observer in the home of a three-year-old boy with his parents and new sibling. The perspective of the three-year-old is assumed in several sequences, heightening the viewer's empathy. The boy is followed through his day at home, largely restricted to his bedroom; at the park; in his father's office; and at the dinner table. His behaviors range from curiosity about the baby to a variety of attention-getting tactics and a tantrum. The viewer is particularly struck by the parents' often insensitive responses to the child's behavior. National Film Board of Canada. (28 mins.)

2. Psychiatry--Individuals

Anatomy of youth, with Dr. Margaret Mead — F
(1970) — Source: UI

Psychiatry, individuals. Dr. Margaret Mead is interviewed in an informal setting. Stating that post-Wold War II babies are pioneers in a new world, she comments on their reaction to war, violence, the establishment, authority, dropouts, fashions, and especially the generation gap. Dr. Mead recommends that parents listen to what the youngsters have to say and try to understand what they are all about. (22 mins.)

Dr. Spock: An American institution — F
(1978) — Source: UI

Psychiatry, individuals. A biography of Dr. Spock, whose book, Baby and child care, is second only to the Bible and the works of Shakespeare as the world's all-time best seller. His own children feel that they did not know him very well, as he was too busy when they were small. Now, in his later years, he is renewing family ties. (25 mins.)

3. Development, Cognition, and Play

Aspects of ego development, six weeks to six years;
Individual differences in the growth of competence — F,V
(1984) — Source: NYU

Development, cognition, and play. A by-product of a longitudinal study, this presentation shows a variety of feeding patterns and later handling of construction materials by children, demonstrating dramatic differences in the development of competencies. Sylvia Brody, Director. (40 mins.)

Films and Videos with Commentary

Child's play and the real world F
(1981) Source: DF

Development, cognition, and play. This film takes the viewer into the child's world and shows how play is essential to his development. (20 mins.)

Cognition F
(1972) Source: HR

Development, cognition, and play. Howard Gardner and Jerome Kagan, Directors. (21 mins.)

Cognitive development F
(1973) Source: UI

Development, cognition, and play. Using animation and imaginative special effects, the film presents an overview of Piaget's proposed cognitive stages: sensori-motor, pre-operational, concrete operation, and formal operations. Each stage is discussed in terms of some of the intellectual competencies that human beings are considered to develop from birth through adulthood. A visit to a school where Piagetian theory predominates reveals a free-wheeling "creative" atmosphere with work and play hardly distinguishable. In sharp contract, a visit to another school where behaviorist learning prevails finds psychologists drilling children with specific programmed data. (18 mins.)

Developing social skills through play V
(1980) Source: UCLA

Development, social interaction. This video attempts to recreate an experiment by Dr. Furman demonstrating the difference in social interaction between children of the same age and children of different ages. The influence of younger children on more timid, older playmates is emphasized. Video of children's play (edited) does not include commentary. Supplemented by Furman's article and experimenter's commentary. P. Greenfield, Director. (5 mins.)

Development of the child: A cross-cultural approach to cognition F
(1975) Source: UI

Development, cognition, and play. There is beautiful camera work and a clear sound track in this film directed by Jerome Kagan. It shows children in three settings which differ in their economic status, access to education, and degree of isolation and modernization. These settings are communities in Japan (modern, industrial), Kenya (rural), and Guatemala (isolated, rural). The film tries to make the point of the similarity of the children's cognitive development, despite their widely varying backgrounds. Jerome Kagan, Director. (20 mins.)

Ego development V
(1983) Source: WPIC

Development, play. This is a series of three videotapes that presents close observations of two infant girls during their first year of life. In this study, the concept of ego follows the principles of psychoanalytic psychology and an epigenetic view of development. Part I presents observations of the infants from one to three months of age. Part II presents observations of the infants from four to eight months of age. Part III presents observations of the infants from nine to twelve months of age. Family Communications. (Three tapes: #1, 29 mins; #2, 35 mins.; #3, 54 mins.)

Ego development: The core of a healthy personality F
(1974) Source: UI

Development, play. Bettye Caldwell traces the development of personality using the theories of Erikson. The approach is didactic, but lightened by scenes of babies in a center and through the use of some high quality animation. Caldwell's commentary is careful and thoughtful, given the limited empirical research available in this subject area. Although the narrative extends beyond the birth to the three-year age range, we think this film would be useful for most parent education programs. (19 mins.)

Infancy F
(1970) Source: NYU

Development, cognition, and play. This film focuses on cognitive development in the birth to eighteen-month range. There is a sound introduction to neonatal abilities. The narrative then moves to Kagan's theories of cognitive development. Viewers should be aware that the discussions of Kagan's speculation of cognitive development, which are not necessarily accepted by other researchers, are treated in the same manner as well-established information. (20 mins.)

Learning in infancy F
(1979) Source: BU

Development, cognition, and play. A highly technical presentation of research on infant learning from a specific theoretical approach. (28 mins.)

Object permanence F
(1971) Source: NYU, UCEMC

Development, cognition, and play. This film depicts stages in cognitive development in accordance with Piaget's definitions. It shows the developmental sequence, beginning when infants behave as if an object has ceased to exist when it disappears from view, and continues to the point at which behavior indicates the presence of an internalized mental representation. (23 mins.)

Piaget's developmental theory, classification — V
(1968) — Source: DF

Development, cognition, and play. Robert Karplus and Celia Stendler Lavatelli, Directors. (16 mins.)

Piaget's developmental theory, conservation — V
(1968) — Source: DF

Development, cognition, and play. Celia Stendler Lavatelli and Robert Karplus, Directors. (16 mins.)

Piaget's developmental theory, formal thought — V
(1971) — Source: DF

Development, cognition, and play. Robert Karplus and Rita Peterson, Directors. (30 mins.)

Piaget's developmental theory, the growth of intelligence in the preschool years — V
(1972) — Source: DF

Development, cognition, and play. Celis Stendler Lavatelli and Queenie B. Milles, Directors. (31 mins.)

4. Development--Parent-Child Relations

Attachment behavior — V
(1984) — Source: UMN

Development, parent-child relations. This most effective film demonstrates, by means of the Ainsworth test of attachment behavior, the striking effects of brief, three-minute separations of one-year-olds from their mothers. The procedure is clearly demonstrated in two one-year-old girls. Later, the first girl is shown at age two solving a laboratory problem with the assistance of her mother. D. Sroufe, Director. (30 mins.)

Call me Mama
(1977)

F
Source: PMF

Development, parent-child relations. Miriam Weinstein, a thirty-year-old cinematologist, talks about her responsibilities, feelings, and perceptions of herself as a mother. We see her in various settings with Eli, her eighteen-month-old son. Although background noise from the child's play often drowns out the dialogue, this film should be useful for stimulating discussion in most parent education groups about the demands of motherhood. (14 mins.)

Careers and babies
(1978)

F
Source: PMF

Development, parent-child relations. This film explores the lives, thoughts, and opinions of four women who have made different decisions about the title topic. The four women represent very different lifestyles and points of view, and their comments are interesting. Our only reservation about this film is that the four "types" presented are rather extreme (e.g., one is a "classic" family woman totally devoted to home and motherhood, and another is a politician who has absolutely no time for or interest in having children). The typical parent-to-be or new parent is likely to have more mixed feelings and may have difficulty relating to the principals. (20 mins.)

Feeding and function pleasure in the first year of life
(1968)

F
Source: NYU

Development, parent-child relations. In this film, relationships between types of maternal behavior and maturity of function pleasure of infants is presented. One mother and infant pair from each of seven maternal types is shown. Selections from the feeding scenes of each pair at six weeks, six months, and one year are followed by part of the infant's psychological test performance at age one. Sylvia Brody, Director. Mother-Infant Interaction Series. (42 mins.)

Fetal alcohol education program: Taking a history
Counselling and referral
(1987)

V,F
Source: DL

Development, family relations--maldevelopment and alcohol. These films are designed to train health professionals in educating parents and prospective parents about alcohol and the fetus. E. A. Mason, M.D., Director. (A teaching package of slides and a manual are available from the producers.) (Two films: #1, 9 mins.; #2, 8 mins.)

Grief F
(1953) Source: NYU

Development, parent-child relations. This is an old film, and generally very well done, especially for a silent film. It is a classical work wherein Spitz describes for all to see the devastating consequences of rupturing, or a failure to develop a strong maternal bond in the first three years of live. This film has had a profound impact on many people, both lay and professional, and it resulted in a huge amount of work on maternal deprivation and the mother-child relationship. R. Spitz, Director. (12 mins.)

How babies learn F
(1955) Source: NYU

Development, parent-child relations. This film describes some of the important developmental advances made by babies during the first year of life. All types of infant learning are subject to the influence of the kind of interpersonal and physical environment in which the baby lives. Special attention is given to the importance of the mother-child relationship in enabling children to profit from their learning encounters with infant learning and patterns of family care. Bettye M. Caldwell and Julius B. Richmond, Directors. (35 mins.)

Mother-infant interaction: Forms of feeding at six months F
(1954) Source: NYU

Development, parent-child relations. In this film, we see eight types of interaction, with special attention to relationships between infantile experience at feeding and tension tolerance. Sylvia Brody, Director. Mother-Infant Interaction Series. (42 mins.)

Mother-infant interaction: Forms of feeding at one year F
(1955) Source: NYU

Development, parent-child relations. This film is a study of mother-infant relationships during feeding at the age of one year. Sylvia Brody, Director. Mother-Infant Interaction Series. (39 mins.)

Mother love F
(1957) Source: NYU

Development, parent-child relations. The first part of this film shows the social relations of Johnny to his mother, beginning with the first day of life in the feeding situation. The first feeding is shown, and the mother's attitude toward Johnny is illustrated. Later stages of the development of a close relationship between Johnny and his mother are presented during the nursing situation. The continuation of these relations after weaning and their shifting pattern is shown again in the feeding situation. The influence of the birth of a sibling three years later and the mother's way of dealing with the new situation are presented. In the second part of the film, the loss of mother love is shown in another child. The child's happy behavior so long as she is enjoying her mother's care is described, followed by unhappiness after separation from her mother. Similar stages are shown in three other children. The behavior at the approach of a stranger is presented. The film ends by showing Johnny, the first child shown, whose relations with his mother have been constantly happy ones, in free and boisterous interchanges with a complete stranger. Distribution limited to professional groups. Early silent film of historic interest. Film Studies of the Psychoanalytic Research Project on Problems in Infancy Series. (20 mins.)

<u>Parent child interaction, child's game</u> V
(1981) Source: Medical University, SC

Development, parent-child relations. Arthur W. Ross, Director. (25 mins.)

<u>Resemblances in expressive behavior</u> F
(1955) Source: NYU

Development, parent-child relations. This film shows a variety of examples of mother-infant interaction in which particular modes of maternal behavior have been repeatedly available to the infant's experience during feeding. The typical interaction of each pair suggests that the expressive behavior of the infant is derived, to an important extent, from the maternal behavior. Sylvia Brody, Director. Mother-Infant Interaction Series.

<u>Rock-a-bye baby</u> V,F
(1958) Source: TLV

Development, parent-child relations. In a highly academic fashion, this excellent film examines the phenomenon of maternal deprivation. The work of Rene Spitz and the work of Harry Harlow are highlighted and are accurately portrayed. Time-Life. (30 mins.)

<u>Your baby's first days</u> F
(1980) Source: PMF

Development, parent-child relations. This film shows a class for new mothers at a Seattle hospital. The woman conducting the classes presents information and demonstrates practices related primarily to the physical care of the child in a straightforward and apparently competent manner. Polymorph Films. (21 mins.)

5. Development--Affect

Benjamin V
(1975) Source: UC

Development, affect. This video shows fascinating behavior that has led scientists to claim an astonishing range of abilities for even the very youngest babies. It also demonstrates that children govern a great deal of their parents' behavior towards them. Time-Life. (42 mins.)

Children's aggression: Its origin and control F
(1981) Source: DF

Development, affect. In this film, the basis for normal aggression in young children is examined, along with methods for effectively managing such behavior. (20 mins.)

Emotional ties in infancy F
(1965) Source: NYU

Development, affect. The attachment behaviors and distrust of strangers of nine- to twelve-month-old infants are illustrated. Home-reared and institutionally-reared children are shown. The latter are contrasted in three experimental situations to illustrate degrees of attachment and reactions to strangers. This film is very powerful. J. Stone, Director. (12 mins.)

Jane F
(1975) Source: NYU, WPIC

Development, affect. Jane, aged seventeen months, is placed in temporary foster care after considerable preparation, with many trips to the foster home to ease the transition. The film traces Jane's growing affective concern over the separation, her confusion on being returned to her mother, and the need of the foster mother to make repeated visits to Jane after her return to her mother to avoid Jane having yet another loss reaction. J. Robertson, Director. Young Children in Brief Separation Series. Tavistock Child Development Research Unit. (37 mins.)

John: 17 months--nine days in a residential nursery F
(1967, 1968) Source: NYU, WPIC

Development, affect. This film may be shown separately from Kate (following reference), but the two function well as a pair, since John, a seventeen-month old child, undergoes a major regression when separated from his mother and placed in group care; Kate, on the other hand, though separated twenty-seven days in a comparable circumstance, does well with a familiar but substituted one-to-one foster home relationship. J. Robertson, Director. Young Children in Brief Separation Series. Tavistock Child Development Research Unit. (33 mins.)

Kate: Two year old in foster care F
(1967, 1968) Source: NYU, WPIC

Development, affect. This film may be shown separately from John (preceding reference), but the two function well as a pair, since John, a seventeen-month old child, undergoes a major regression when separated from his mother and placed in group care; Kate, on the other hand, though separated twenty-seven days in a comparable circumstance, does well with a familiar but substituted one-to-one foster home relationship. J. Robertson, Director. Young Children in Brief Separation Series. Tavistock Child Development Research Unit. (45 mins.)

Lucy F
(1975) Source: NYU, WPIC

Development, affect. Lucy is twenty-one months old and is separated from her mother in foster care for nineteen days. Lucy becomes so attached to her foster mother that she needs to be weaned away gradually by the efforts of mother and foster mother. J. Robertson, Director. Young Children in Brief Separation Series. Tavistock Child Development Research Unit. (31 mins.)

A scrapbook experience--building a child's identity F
(1971) Source: UCLA

Development, affect. A social worker helps Gilbert, a latency-aged foster child, develop a sense of identity as he works on his autobiographical scrapbook. In constructing the book, Gilbert has the opportunity to clarify misconception, express his feelings about the past, and explore his fear about the future. He also reveals how he feels about himself and the significant people in his life. County of Los Angeles Department of Adoptions. Image Associates. (16 mins.)

Thomas F
(1975) Source: NYU, WPIC

Development, affect. At two years and four months, Thomas is able to keep his mother in mind during the separation and to talk about her. Daily visits from his father add to his security as his father explains in a way that cannot be done with younger children in this series. The use of doll play by the foster mother is especially interesting as is Thomas' relationship to his foster mother. J. Robertson, Director. Young Children in Brief Separation Series. Tavistock Child Development Research Unit. (38 mins.)

The ties that bind F
(1980) Source: PE

Development, affect. This film addresses itself to the subject of attachment, but more from the perspective of the "bonding" proponents than from long-standing established research. As a result, there are many claims made which are not fully substantiated. Case Western Reserve. (27 mins.)

6. Education--Readiness

From cradle to classroom F
(1976) Source: BU

Education, readiness. These two films were produced for airing on prime time television to examine the growing field of early childhood education. Walter Cronkite provides the narration. Part I provides an overview of several programs and research projects, including those of Merle Karnes, Ira Gordon, Earladeen Badger, O. K. Moore, the Pediatric Institute in Moscow, and Brown University. Part II examines these subjects further. (Two films, 50 mins. each)

It's a whole new world F
(1974) Source: MTPS

Education, readiness. We follow four three-year-olds as they enter nursery school for the first time, and we observe their reactions to socializing in their new world. All are normal children although they display a fascinating variety of individual differences as we get to know them. Adreinne, a delicate but deliberate little blonde, doesn't like to be rushed and is slow to speak up for her rights and needs. Austin is almost completely non-verbal, yet he uses his entire body to express himself. Sarah, a large, slow-moving child, is also lacking in verbal skills, although "no" seems to be her favorite word. Timmy, of Oriental origin, has highly developed social needs but low verbal ability to satisfy them. As these children interact with each other and the rest of the group, we see them beginning to learn limits and to learn to share. The film ends with the narrator's question, "What would you do to help them grow?" (28 mins.)

Jean Piaget V
(1971) Source: DF

Education, readiness. Davidson Films and Jean Piaget, Directors. (45 mins.)

Learning to learn in infancy
(1964)

F
Source: NYU

Education, readiness. Technically, this is an extremely well done (although now somewhat dated) production, originally created to train Head Start staff. The prime focus is on children in centers, demonstrating the intrinsic interest in learning that is shown by all healthy young babies. There is a description of the particular types of learning to be expected, and there are pointers given as to how learning can be encouraged as the child and a staff member go through their ordinary daily experience. (22 mins.)

7. Development--Language and Social Behavior

Child language: Learning without teaching
(1981)

F
Source: DF

Development, language, social behavior. This film introduces the viewer to one of the most involved learning processes a child encounters: mastering the complex system of meanings, grammatical rules, and sounds called language. It shows many of the problems children face while learning to communicate, and reminds adults that a child's language may not necessarily mean what the adult thinks it means. The film shows extensive sequences of actual children talking. Realistic with clear commentary. (20 mins.)

Early words
(1972)

F
Source: UCEMC

Development, language, social behavior. The film consists of a close examination of language development in a single twenty-two-month-old child, using samples of the child's language (mostly one-word utterances) and gestures, along with Jerome Bruner's analyses on the voice over. Production quality is poor in spots. Harvard Center for Cognitive Studies. (22 mins.)

Everybody rides the carousel
(1978)

V,F
Source: IU, PGR

Development, language, social behavior. In this film, the eight stages of life in the phases of personality development as described by psychologist Erik H. Erikson are portrayed. Included are the following stages: newborn, toddler, childhood, school, adolescence, young adulthood, grown-up, and old age. Throughout, the film depicts the ups and downs, positives and negatives, anxieties and stimulations of each stage of life. Pyramid Films. (73 mins.)

Growth and development: Four children--a chronicle of development V
(1976) Source: SUNY

Development, language, social behavior. (Ten video cassettes: 272 mins. total)

How babies learn F
(1954) Source: NYU

Development, language, social behavior. Bettye Caldwell narrates this film, which describes general development during the first years of life. The film stresses the infants's need for attachment to a "special person," using a ten-month-old to illustrate the process. (35 mins.)

Language development F
(1978) Source: McH

Development, language, social behavior. This film outlines the process of expressive language acquisition. Dr. Menlee Oakes narrates the film, citing the work of Dr. Roger Brown on the orderly and predictable sequence of language development; Dr. Ursala Bellugi-Klima on how deaf children learn American sign language; and Dr. David Premack on teaching chimps non-verbal language. The film provides a balanced view of the theoretical field, suggesting the likelihood that both biological and learning-oriented viewpoints are correct in some respects. It also provides an excellent overview of the academic field of expressive language development. (20 mins.)

Social development F
(1960) Source: NYU

Development, language, social behavior. This film provides a reasonable introduction to social development. There are discussions about negativism, parallel play, and cooperative play. However, not enough detail is given, and the narrative moves quickly out of the birth to three-year age range. The film was designed for parents and has many good scenes of children playing. A somewhat faulty soundtrack. Elizabeth Hurlock, Director. (16 mins.)

8. Diagnosis--Psychological Tests

Children's drawing V
(1983) Source: HSC

Diagnosis, psychological tests. This video proposes that having the child patient do figure drawing (or the older child do kinesthetic family drawing) is an economic way to assess ego development, cognitive development, self-image, and personal/social skills and feelings about gender and sexuality. Ample illustrations of the author's points about interpretation are provided. For advanced level professionals. (19 mins.)

Constructing the multi-generational family genogram — V
(1983) — Source: BM

Diagnosis, psychological tests. Stephen Lerner, Director. (30 mins.)

Denver developmental screening test — V
(1975) — Source: UCOL

Diagnosis, psychological tests. William K. Frankenburg, Director. (30 mins.)

The interview for infant development evaluation — V
(1982) — Source: AMC

Diagnosis, psychological tests. Hilda Knobloch, Henry Skoburn, and Bobbi Kamil, Directors. (29 mins.)

Pediatric examination videotapes: Examination of the infant — V
(1978) — Source: JBL

Diagnosis, psychological tests. This tape is of outstanding quality, with a very clear sound track and magnificent close-ups. It consists of three pediatric examinations: a five-month-old, a two-and-a-half-month old, and an eight-month-old. The examinations deal almost exclusively with the physical health aspects of the children and do not cover educational topics to any noticeable degree. (50 mins.)

The psychoeducational profile — V
(1984) — Source: UNC

Diagnosis, psychological tests. Eric Schopler and Robert Jay Reichler, Directors. (22 mins.)

The revised Gesell developmental
and neurological examination in infancy — V
(1982) — Source: AMC

Diagnosis, psychological tests. Hilda Knobloch, Henry Skoburn, and Bobbi Kamil, Directors. (39 mins.)

Films and Videos with Commentary

The revised Gesell developmental and
neurological examination at 18, 24, and 36 months — V
(1982) — Source: AMC

Diagnosis, psychological tests. Hilda Knobloch, Henry Skoburn, and Bobbi Kamil, Directors. (74 mins.)

Some psychiatric aspects of infancy and toddlerhood — V
(1987) — Source: AACAP

Diagnosis, psychological tests. The tape begins with excerpts from Spitz's film Grief and goes on to a review of the present body of knowledge, including what the infant brings to the dyadic experience. Wolff, Brazelton, Sandler, Chess, and Thomas are cited. An excerpt from The amazing newborn is well chosen. Dr. Joseph Marcus makes a number of excellent points, such as the risk of over and under diagnosis. The psychopathology of infancy and early childhood is clearly presented and includes a segment on intervention. The tape concludes with photographs of the chief pioneers. A good overview of the beginnings of infant psychiatry, with a variety of approaches: live families, film clips, and graphics. J. Marcus, Director. University of Chicago. (50 mins.)

Techniques of developmental assessment II — V
(1981) — Source: UNC

Diagnosis, psychological tests. Brian Stabler, Director. (19 mins.)

Within normal limits — V
(1982) — Source: MTI

Diagnosis, psychological tests. This video deals with developmental delays and disabilities. Stressing the need for very early identification and intervention, the question is raised, "by whom?". Neurological assessment is treated accurately and realistically as to its usefulness and its limitations. The plight of the parents is noted, who have discerned many little things about their children, but who are assured by the primary care physicians' reassurance that "it's within normal limits." There are cogent examples of a child's brightness but inability to perform simple visual-motor tasks. A teacher's uncertainty about initiating a referral is demonstrated. This video is important for educating primary pediatric health care staff regarding early detection and intervention. R. Abramovitz and M. Sottnick, Directors. (23 mins.)

9. Diagnosis--Hearing and Visual

Testing hearing in preschool child six months to six years — F
(1973) — Source: NAV

Diagnosis, hearing tests. This movie shows and describes relatively simple hearing testing in younger infants using sounds, such as bells, with localization by the infant as a test of hearing. In the later ages, there is some description of more sophisticated tests using localization. Since there is no other good "quick and easy" screening test for hearing at this age, this approach is acceptable. (20 mins.)

Testing vision in preschool child six months to six years F
(1975) Source: NAV

Diagnosis, visual tests. This movie shows the testing of vision of young infants using graded sizes of balls, toys, etc. at specified distances in an attempt tomeasure the child's visual acuity. It also shows the testing of the subjects and their responses--following, cooing, etc. Other tests for older children are demonstrated as well. Testing for visual acuity in the young child is difficult. The approach is reasonable, although somewhat crude. The movie does not deal well with the problems inherent in testing children at this age (i.e., lack of attention and cooperation). Information about false negativity and positivity is not given. As a crude screening approach, particularly for younger children, this is as good an approach as any. There will be some over-referral, but as long as cooperation and attention are dealt with, it is unlikely that children with significant problems in visual acuity will be missed. (15 mins.)

10. Development--Morals

Introduction to moral development F
(1970) Source: UI

Development, morality. Lawrence Kohlberg and others discuss the origin of moral development theories as well as the six stages of moral development. Theory applications are detailed through visits to both elementary and secondary classrooms. Values and Morality in School Series. (29 mins.)

Moral development F
(1973) Source: UI

Development, morality. This film describes Milgram's experiment. Two persons have volunteered to participate in a learning experiment, one to be the teacher, the other the learner. When the learner answers incorrectly, the teacher is to give him increasingly painful shocks. It turns out that the experiment is actually an investigation of moral development. Harvard psychologist Lawrence Kohlberg believes that there are stages of moral development tied to cognitive development. Learning theorists contend that moral behavior is learned and that reasons for action are irrelevant. The film explores these two viewpoints. (28 mins.)

Moral judgment and reasoning F
(1978) Source: UI

Development, morality. Examines concepts of moral development from three perspectives: psychoanalytical theory, social learning theory, and cognitive developmental theory. A variety of vignettes illustrates the stages of moral development and moral reasoning. (18 mins.)

11. Development and Education

Greensquares to kindergarten F
(1976) Source: PE

Education, readiness. A unique program for educationally "vulnerable" children is thoroughly documented in this charming film. Children with developmental weaknesses who might get into serious trouble when they go to school are helped to acquire some basic skills in pre-primary classes. We observe ten four-year-olds as they receive assistance with motor integration and physical development, tactile awareness, visual-motor integration, visual discrimination, auditory discrimination, conceptual (number) development, language development, and verbal expression. The special education teachers use a variety of materials and illustrate a number of teaching methods, many of which would be equally applicable to teaching normal kindergarten children. (36 mins.)

Peers in middle childhood F
(1975) Source: IFB

Development, school age. Virtually all of this film takes place in a fourth-grade classroom--and for a very good reason. The tenth year is an important time for academic learning and social awareness. Not only are nine-year-olds on the brink of a world of abstract ideas, but they are also mastering learning and social skills that will develop into lifelong patterns. At this age, however, the peer group is the most important thing in their lives. Being different can be frightening. Yet each child is building his own identity with the group. At nine, every victory feeds self-esteem--and every failure is magnified out of proportion. The film also makes clear that children at this age are often good teachers; we watch them sharing information and offering help in solving problems. Mental Health Film Board. (23.5 mins)

Six, seven, and eight-year-olds--society of children F
(1967) Source: NYU

Development, school age. This film depicts the middle years of childhood, with strong allegiance to the group, declaration of independence from adults, and the cleavage of the sexes. It illustrates how children acquire formal and informal skills and knowledge applicable to later stages of development. Part III of A Long Time to Grow Series. (30 mins.)

12. Development--Adolescents

<u>Adolescence: A case study</u> F
(1978) Source: PCR

Development, adolescents. This film is a cognitive developmental focus on a seventeen-year-old girl. (20 mins.)

<u>Adolescence: The winds of change</u> F
(1975) Source: PCR

Development, adolescents. This film presents physical, sexual, and cognitive changes through interviews and didactic techniques. (30 mins.)

<u>Adventures of teenage scientists</u> V,F
(1985) Source: TLV

Development, adolescents. This film probes what it takes to develop the intellectually gifted. NOVA, WGBH. (57 mins.)

<u>Being young</u> F
(1985) Source: UCEMC

Development, adolescents. Produced in honor of International Youth Year (1985), this film is a tribute to the spirit, enthusiasm, and commitment of the world's youth. It focuses on a number of inspiring young people in Peru, Northern Ireland, Japan, Pwanda, the Soviet Union, and the United States. (27 mins.)

<u>The body human. The facts for boys</u> V,F
(1982) Source: TLV

Development, adolescents. Three boys, ages ten to fourteen, talk about male biological functions, burgeoning emotions, and changes in terms of love, family, and responsibilities. Tomorrow Entertainment. (30 mins.)

<u>The body human. The facts for girls</u> V,F
(1982) Source: TLV

Marlo Thomas leads pre-adolescent and adolescent girls in informal discussions about their changing bodies and emotions, their hopes and their fears. Tomorrow Entertainment. (30 mins.)

David
(1980)

F
Source: FL

Development, adolescents. A documentary film about David McFarland, an articulate, personable seventeen-year-old with Down's syndrome. His rich and varied life in his community, including a leading role in a TV drama, is shown. (28 mins.)

Targets
(1987)

V,F
Source: MTI

Development, adolescents. This videotape opens with a teenage boy being hassled by his friends and worried about getting home in time. He ends up speeding because of this rush and his friends' encouragement, and ends up in an apparently fatal accident. The six teenagers with different problems are in a suspended state and are met by a teacher/angel who begins a process of looking at what led to their becoming victims or targets. The issues are (1) dealing with peer pressure, (2) running away, (3) coping with bullying and violence, (4) being beaten up by a boyfriend, (5) having alcoholic parents, and (6) being sexually abused. The second half of the videotape reviews ways that each of these six problems can be handled without becoming a victim. Following this, they return to life and are not killed by the near fatal car accident. (20 mins.)

What guys want
(1985)

F
Source: PMF

Development, adolescents. This is a film in which teenagers of diverse ethnic, racial, and economic backgrounds express their attitudes and feelings about maleness and their male sexual behavior in a remarkably candid and compelling manner. It examines values and helps teens of both sexes understand the consequences of sexual behavior. The teens in the film also talk of "one night stands," commitment and marriage, virginity and peer pressure, their first sexual experience, contraception, and fear of rejection and fatherhood. A. Fiering, Director. (16 mins.)

Whatever happened to Lori Jean Lloyd
(1980)

F
Source: PCR

Development, adolescents. A crisis center and a runaway girl are presented in this film. (27 mins.)

E. Cultural Issues in Child Mental Health

The American Indian speaks F
(1982) Source: BF

Culture. This powerful documentary lets the Indian speak about his people and heritage, about the white man and the future. Visits with the Muskogee Creek, the Sioux, and the Nisqually yield eloquent portraits about life in today's reservations. Highlighting the action are poetic Indian speeches by Academy Award Nominee Chief Dan George. (23 mins.)

Breaking the silence:
The generation after the Holocaust V,F
(1981) Source: CG

Culture. This film is appropriate for survivors and the children of survivors from any major catastrophe, for students of the Holocaust, and for mental health professionals dealing with survivors of major traumas and those interested in intergenerational communication. This film not only admirably explores the impact of the Holocaust one generation later, but it elucidates the forces of guilt, collusion, denial, suppressed anger, and depression that accompany any major trauma and how this is transmitted and handled by the offspring of those suffering the trauma. E. Mason, E. Fogelman, and H. Grunebaum, Directors. (58 mins.)

Cree hunters of Mistassini F
(1974) Source: PCR

Culture. This film documents the hunting culture of the Cree Indians in James Bay, Quebec. Their lifestyle reflects religious beliefs and ecological principles. It follows three families on a hunting trip and illustrates some conflicts between traditional Cree culture and technological development. National Film Board of Canada. (58 mins.)

Dadi's family V
(1978) Source: PBS

Culture. In this video, the viewer looks at the traditionally intricate relationships of a large family in northern India and how it adapts to change. Newly married at the age of sixteen, Dadi went to live in the household of her husband's mother. Now, decades later, she finds herself in charge of the large household and troubled not by social or economic changes, but by internal pressure. This documentary examines a family unit in India and the intricate relationships in an extended family of grandchildren such as Dadi's. (58 mins.)

Four families
(1959)
F
Source: UI

Culture. In a comparison of family life in India, France, Japan, and Canada, Margaret Mead, author-anthropologist, discusses how the upbringing of a child contributes to a distinctive national character. In each case, the film focuses on a one-year-old baby in the family of a farmer of average means. It summarizes the typical national characteristics of the four countries. (60 mins.)

Four families: Parts I and II
(1958)
F
Source: CBC

Culture. This production features four comparable (approximately) rural families. Part I shows an Indian and French family, while Part II shows a Japanese and Canadian family. Each family consists of a baby approximately ten months old, two older siblings, and two parents (the Japanese family also includes the child's paternal grandparents). Each family is filmed in similar settings depicting preparation of food, eating, bathing, division of labor, and layout of the home. Attitudes toward child rearing, including punishment, roles of older children, and toys, are shows. (Two films: 30 mins. each)

Gaucho
(1983)
V,F
Source: TLV

Culture. A fatherless pre-adolescent Puerto Rican boy who lives in New York City's "El Barrio" feels betrayed when his older brother marries and scuttles long-awaited plans to return to Puerto Rico. How the troubled boy, Gaucho, copes with the difficulties in being honest in communication and openness with those who love him is shown. M. Tahse, Director. (47 mins.)

Gift of the black folk
(1978)
F
Source: PYF

Culture. In a striking combination of graphics and historical photographs, this film surveys the lives and accomplishments of three Americans in the struggle for freedom: Denmark Vesey, Harriet Tubman, and Frederick Douglass. Robert Holmes' contemporary symphonic music underscores the film's powerful message. C. Moss, Director. (16 mins.)

The heart of the dragon: Caring V,F
(1984) Source: TLV

Culture. In this film, which focuses on the family of a northern China railway policeman, we see how the family and the neighborhood network look after the young and the old. It shows how ancient tradition and values still function in Chinese society. A.S.H. Films. (57 mins.)

Heritage in black F
(1979) Source: BF

Culture. This film focuses on the black people's 200-year-old struggle to be free. The film also reveals the black man's intense participation in present-day American life--fighting for other people's freedom and making important contributions to science, industry, education, music, labor, and sports. (27 mins.)

Hunters of the seal V,F
(1972) Source: WGBH

Culture. Studies of the nomadic Netsilik Eskimos of Pelly Bay, Canada, explore the impact of modern values on the young Eskimos who are losing the values of their ancestors. (30 mins.)

Living below the line V
(1982) Source: PBS

Culture. Follow "Frontline" through this in-depth study of the United States welfare state. In America, 15.2 percent of the population is trying to survive with some form of government assistance. Almost twenty-five million people are trying to use various agencies and services while trying to subsist during economic hard times. (60 mins.)

The Mexican-American speaks heritage in bronze F
(1986) Source: BF

Culture. Focusing upon Mexican-Americans, this film traces the conquest of the Indians by Spanish conquistadors and the spread of Spanish dominion in the New World. The rule of Spain disappeared, but the heritage of language and of mixed blood and culture remained. Present-day "Latinos"--represented in this film by a cross-section of Spanish-speaking citizens--are now demanding a greater voice in government, education, and the economic life of the nation. (20 mins.)

New options for learning F
(1970) Source: UCLA

Culture. This film portrays novel approaches to urban education. Programs that utilize the enormous facilities of large urban areas are examined, as well as programs aimed at ghetto children, the unmotivated, and the drop-outs. Actual schools and programs are shown which have worked and are working. Institute for the Development of Educational Activities, Inc. (20 mins.)

Rearing kibbutz babies F
(1965) Source: NYU

In this production are extraordinary examples of babies being photographed in their natural environment. The film describes how the children are reared with great professional skill and warmth in one of Israel's outstanding kibbutzim. It is clear that the subject is very carefully dealt with and what we are seeing actually exists. J. Stone, Director. (27 mins.)

Zerda's children F
(1978) Source: UCLA

Culture. Shows Sixto Ramon Zerda's struggle to live and raise his ten children in the Pampas of Argentina. An illiterate isolated serf, Zerda understands his situation with great clarity and never hesitates to speak his mind. He hopes that his children will attain a better life through their education at the public school. Introduced by Henry Fonda. Spanish with English voice over and subtitles. Phoenix Films. Jorge Preloran, Director. (50 mins.)

F. Psychopathology in Childhood and Adolescence

1. Psychopathology--Anxiety Disorders

Afraid of school F
(1965) Source: UI

Psychopathology, anxiety disorders. This film presents a case study of a six-year-old who refuses to attend school. Through discussions with Tommy and his parents, Dr. Taylor Statten learns that Tommy is obsessed with thoughts of dying. This illustrates that school phobia is generally caused by problems in the child and not the school, and the importance of experiences in infancy to a child's emotional development. (18 mins.)

Aggressive child F
(1965) Source: PCR

Psychopathology, anxiety disorders. Through the use of hand puppets in play therapy, a psychiatrist discovers why six-year-old Philip is always in trouble at home and at school because of his fighting. Fighting is actually a mask for deep-seated fears caused by conflict with his parents. After seven months of treatment, Philip learns to express his fears in more direct ways, and his parents become more skilled in handling him. The Disordered Mind Series. (28 mins.)

Dreamspeaker F
(1976) Source: PCR

Psychopathology, anxiety disorders. An emotionally disturbed boy flees an institution and is "adopted" by a gentle old Indian shaman, played by a Nootka Indian dreamspeaker. The Indian's hut becomes a temporary sanctuary for the youth, who responds to his guardian's loving care by expressing real feelings for the first time and by beginning to understand himself in terms of ancient Indian wisdom. Canadian Broadcasting Corporation. (75 mins.)

2. Psychopathology--Psychotic Disorders

Quiet one F
(1948) Source: PCR

Psychopathology, psychotic disorders. This is a classical fictional film that was so convincing that many have called it a documentary. In the streets of Harlem in the late 1940's, Donald, a ten-year-old black child, shows the ghetto's devastating psychological effects. Mentally disturbed, he is sent to Wiltwyck School at Esopus, New York, where counselors and psychiatrists try to help him. Written by James Agee. Sidney Meyers, Director. (66 mins.)

3. Psychopathology--Conduct Disorders

Johnny F
(1983) Source: DL

Psychopathology, conduct disorders in patient management. A nine-year-old boy with a history of aggressive behavior attempts to gain more control of his feelings and find better ways to communicate. He tests the staff with hyperactive and erratic behavior. Several of his frequent tantrums are faithfully reported on film and illustrate problems in the management of this type of disturbance. E. Mason, Director. (32 mins.)

Juvenile law and you V,F
(1986) Source: WD

Psychopathology, conduct disorders. This film follows three separate children from the beginning of their contact with the juvenile authorities to its final disposition. The first case is a sixteen-year-old boy, a repeat juvenile offender who is arrested for purse snatching. His arraignment, contact with his defense attorney and trial are chronicled. The second case is a twelve-year-old boy who is a first-time shoplifting offender. His family situation and court options are documented. The third case is a thirteen-year-old girl who is beaten by her mother's boyfriend. The investigation and judicial handling of this situation is reviewed. All the juvenile authorities and judges are played by actual people who function in these roles. The film presents basic situations realistically. Walt Disney Productions. (28 mins.)

Running to what F
(1979) Source: IU

Psychopathology, conduct disorders. This film looks at the predicament of the teenagers who run away to Fort Lauderdale, Florida. Focusing on the hustling and prostitution that these young people usually turn to as a means of self-support, it shows how many adolescents spend time in prisons or juvenile detention centers. It points out that although the original home conditions may have been rough, the street can be rougher. Interviews with teenagers who have run afoul of the law make the message clear: there are a lot of surprises out in the street, the chances of "making it" are better at home. One of the runaways, it turns out, is serving a life sentence for killing a man who picked him up. NBC. (17 mins.)

What are we doing to our children? Part I--Locked up; locked out F
(1973) Source: PCR

Psychopathology, conduct disorders, antisocial behavior. This is a case study of a ten-year-old from a low-income family in Atlanta, Georgia, whose destructive and antisocial behavior toward neighbors results in his incarceration in a children's treatment center. The legal and emotional struggle among the family is portrayed: the lawyer who wants the boy to go to a country rehabilitation farm, the child's mother who wants to keep him at home, and the judge who is troubled by the lack of constructive alternatives. Comments by child psychiatrist, Dr. Robert Coles. CBS. (30 mins.)

4. Psychopathology--Eating Disorders

Between you and me V
(1984) Source: PCGC

Psychopathology, eating disorders. In this video, we see aspects of the treatment of an anorectic adolescent and her parents. The tape highlights how the enmeshed family system is changed to permit the girl to function as a normal adolescent in the family and with her peers. S. Minuchin, B. Montalvo, and F. Lincoln, Directors. (47 mins.)

Bulimia F
(1987) Source: PCR

Psychopathology, eating disorders. This film examines the effects and dangers of bulimia, an eating disorder in which victims, 95 percent of whom are women, are caught in a cycle of binge-eating, followed by purging themselves through induced vomiting, intense fasting, or abuse of laxatives or diuretics. It interviews psychologists, the parents of bulimics, and recovered bulimics, and includes scenes of group therapy for eating problems. Narrated by Hugh Downs. Produced by ABC. (14 mins.)

Diet unto death: Anorexia nervosa F
(1980) Source: UCEMC

Psychopathology, eating disorders. The underlying causes and possible means of treatment for this widespread emotional disorder, which kills some fifteen thousand adolescent girls in the U.S. each year, is studied. (13 mins.)

The enigma of anorexia nervosa V
(1987) Source: CMC

Psychopathology, eating disorders. This tape was created by a nurse's researcher for nursing education. It deals with the disorder in a hospital setting. Part I: Delusion and discord--overview. Part II: Clinical intervention and rehabilitation. Part III: The battle of wills--typical problems which can arise in nurse/unit. (Three tapes: #1, 18 mins.; #2, 16 mins.; #3, 26 mins.)

The enigma of anorexia nervosa Part I: Delusion and discord V
(1987) Source: CMC

This relatively short videotape reviews the various potential etiological explanations for anorexia nervosa. It goes over the various rationale for biological, psychological, social, and cultural forces that independently and as part of a matrix may lead to anorexia nervosa. It also discusses briefly the basis, both historically and conceptually, for different therapeutic approaches and endocrinological and behavioral therapy. (18 mins.)

Films and Videos with Commentary

Interview with a teenage anorectic patient and her family — V
(1979) — Source: WPIC

Psychopathology, eating disorders. In this video, we see a family case history and an interview by S. Minuchin with the family revealing anorexia as a symptom of the family power struggle. It focuses on the parental difficulty in allowing the patient to mature as a sexual person, to individuate, and to separate. South Beach Psychiatric Center. (120 mins.)

Psychosomatic conditions--obesity — F
(1976) — Source: NYU

Psychopathology, eating disorders. This thirteen-year-old girl is unhappy because she is fat. She is fat because eating helps to relieve her feelings of frustration over a lack of communication between herself and her mother. The girl's parents also receive treatment, and after several months, the family is made aware of the relationship between the girl's unmet emotional needs and her overeating. They learn to communicate more effectively with one another. Dr. V. Rakoff is the psychiatrist who treats the girl and her family. The discussant is Dr. Henry Kravitz. Contemporary Films. The Disordered Mind Series. (28 mins.)

5. Psychopathology--Family Relations

A better beginning — V
(1978) — Source: WPIC

Psychopathology, family relations. The social and emotional components of failure to thrive are identified in this video. Two babies, their parents, and the parent-child interactions are examined. University of Michigan. (37 mins.)

Adapting to parenthood — F
(1975) — Source: PMF

Psychopathology, family relations--post-partum depression. This film follows a young couple through the post-partum period. Feelings are openly expressed by the mother in the hospital and by both parents in the early days at home. Other young parents discuss their initial problems as well. This film is a very realistic presentation of the post-partum period of a very depressed young woman. (20 mins.)

Adapting to parenthood — F
(1976) — Source: PMF

Psychopathology, family relations--stress in families with a newborn infant. A number of new parents speak of their initial problems--sleeplessness and crying babies, interfering grandparents, and frustration and guilt at not feeling the serenity they had anticipated. The film follows a young couple as they adjust to the arrival of their first baby. Family life becomes stressful, and efforts are made to find new ways of communicating feelings. A. Fiering, Director. (20 mins.)

Counselling with parents: Interview III — F
(1967) — Source: PCR

Psychopathology, family relations--children's sensitivities. Parents and teacher discuss the question of sensitivity in children and their reaction to criticism and discipline. James Benjamin, Director. Chico State College: Western Regional Center. Interprofessional Research Commission on Pupil Personnel Services. (35 mins.)

Divorce, for better or for worse — V
(1976) — Source: ABCN

Psychopathology, family relations. James Benjamin, Director. (50 mins.)

Fathers — F
(1980) — Source: UI

Psychopathology, family relations. This films examines, through case histories, three style of fathering. It shows how one father changes his career to overcome his "absentee" style, which he felt cheated himself and his family. Another struggles with a belated sense of responsibility and with his military/authoritarian tendencies. A third takes the prime share of responsibility for care of the baby and seems to enjoy it greatly. (23 mins.)

Growing up together — F
(1975) — Source: NYU

Psychopathology, family relations--unwed teen mothers. This film focuses on the problems of unwed teenage mothers, exploring their feelings as adolescents and their relationships with family and friends. The camera angles are often awkward, and the dialogue is difficult to understand at times. As to the care of the baby, we feel that this film would be useful to train professionals. Children's Home Society. (60 mins.)

New relations — V
(1980) — Source: UI

Psychopathology, family relations--stepparents. In this video, suggestions are made for involving all members of a new family that includes stepchildren in an open communication of feelings: excitement, anxiety, doubt, pain--all of which will serve to diminish tensions and help build the new sets of relationships. Ben Achtenberg, Director. (34 mins.)

Parents of disturbed children V,F
(1974) Source: PCR

Psychopathology, family relations. Parents of emotionally disturbed children participate in a group discussion about their problems. Personal and shared problems in the home are intensified, and the parents tell about being put to the test. The difference in approach between men and women is described; especially notable is one male's difficulty with his son. Martha Stuart, Director. (29 mins.)

The single parent family V
(1981) Source: UI

Psychopathology, family relations in a single parent family. This video dramatizes a readjustment situation in a family with three children whose parents have been divorced just long enough to begin dating someone new. It uses a single day in these lives, including discussion at a single parent meeting, to list and analyze typical problems. (14 mins.)

Stepparenting F
(1980) Source: PMF

Psychopathology, family relations--who is in charge. Stepparents in this film discuss feeling insecure, conflicts over child rearing practices, and confusion as to who has authority over the child. Members of a stepparent support group talk of specific situations they encountered and how they set about overcoming obstacles. Documentary scenes of stepfamily life show weekend visitation and what happens when a reconstituted family may combine "his" children, "her" children, and "their" children for different parts of the week. H. M. Felt, Director. (25 mins.)

A young child is . . . V,F
(1981) Source: LP

Psychopathology, family relations--permission to grow. This film presents children from the age of two months to four-and-one-half years in various forms of their natural activity. It clearly demonstrates play, exploration, learning, and engagement in the environment. Educational Information and Resource Center. (27 mins.)

6. Psychopathology--Miscellaneous

The application of attachment theory to psychopathology V
(1984) Source: CES

Development, parent-child relations. Dr. John Bowlby utilizes his vast research and clinical experiences as he discusses issues of adult psychopathology from the perspective of attachment theory. Dr. Bowlby describes examples from his fifty years of clinical practice as well as discussing cases that are presented to him. There is equal emphasis on both practical treatment implications as well as theoretical issues that are relevant to the practice of psychotherapy. John Bowlby, M.D., Director. (45 mins.)

The hyperactive child — F
(1969) — Source: PCR

Psychopathology, attention disorders. This films shows the hyperactive child in home and school environments. It explains the causes of hyperactivity and discusses professional management by medical and scholastic communities. Ciba Pharmaceutical Company. (34 mins.)

Hyperactivity in children — F
(1973) — Source: HSV

Psychopathology, attention disorders. (18 mins.)

Tourette syndrome: The sudden intruder — V
(1987) — Source: BSML

Psychopathology, tics. The film explores several dimensions of Tourette syndrome. It examines six different individuals with six distinct manifestations of the syndrome. It briefly reviews the historical refinement of the diagnoses. It looks at the confusion in diagnosis and the interplay of psychological and biological forces. It reviews the cardinal features of the syndrome, interviews several prominent researchers in the field, and discusses the "failure to inhibit" theory in some depth. The film goes into some detail about the subjective experience of a child and an adult with this syndrome. It concludes with interviews of two adults with Tourette syndrome who have also achieved success in their chosen careers. B. Addis, Director. (45 mins.)

7. Family Relations

Consultation with a three generation family — V
(1980) — Source: IEA

Family relations--three generations. Carl Alanson Whitaker, Ian Alger, and Hugh James Lurie, Directors. (95 mins.)

Foster parenting F
(1984) Source: UWF

Family relations--foster families. A film useful for the education and screening of foster parents and for training professionals in working with foster parents. (30 mins.)

Having twins F
(1979) Source: PMF

Family relations--problems of parenting twins. This film covers basic information on caring for newborn twins. It shows the delivery of fraternal twins with the attending obstetrician explaining what is going on during labor and delivery. In a filmed discussion group, a number of parents of young twins share their personal experiences and offer helpful suggestions. (22 mins.)

Is my baby okay? V
(1987) Source: IU

Family relations--when faced with a vulnerable infant and toddler. The concept of "the vulnerable child syndrome" elucidated some twenty years ago by Green and Solnit, plus the potential for intervention, are clearly seen in this sensitive presentation through interviews with parents and child over a period of three years. These parents, professionals themselves, talk of their doubts and apprehensions concerning their child's development following cardiac arrest in the early newborn period. The role of the physicians in helping parents through a time of uncertainty, neither being too optimistic nor too pessimistic, carefully watching the child's development in all parameters, physically, cognitively, socially, and psychologically, and continually being sensitive to parents' reaction to the child is demonstrated. A second pregnancy is also discussed and the reaction to it reflects the previous difficult perinatal stress. O. Roeske, Director. (37 mins.)

Parent-to-parent V
(1981) Source: UUMC

Family relations and premature birth. In addition to describing the care of critically ill newborns, this video focuses on parental responses to such a crisis and on the Parent-to-Parent program, which uses "graduate parents" matched for diagnosis, type of delivery, and mother's OB-GYN history and family background, to offer one-to-one support to parents of critically ill infants. The video follows two families as they experience the shock of premature childbirth, the uncertainties of their infant's medical status, and the relief afforded by the opportunity to express their feelings to parents who have been through a similar ordeal. (30 mins.)

Passages in fathering: Sharing my work and myself F
(1984) Source: UWF

Family relations. This film focuses on the identity and role of a father. (28 mins.)

Stepping out: Debolts grow up F
(1980) Source: UI, PYF

Family relations--adopted special children. This film is a celebration and recording of the progress made by the twenty special children, adopted and otherwise, of the famous Debolts. Since the first adoption twenty years ago, eleven of the older children have established their independence. The film shows the daily routine of those still at home, featuring the latest adoptive child, blind and crippled, and his preparation for "mainstreaming." Introduces the first grandchild. (52 mins.)

Team family consultation V
(1976) Source: BFI

Family relations--family consultation. Mary MacGregor and Robert MacGregor, Directors. (60 mins.)

To have and not to hold: Helping the parents of premies cope V
(1978) Source: PMF

Family relations in premature birth. Parents speak candidly about the events surrounding their baby's early birth. They discuss feelings of guilt, apprehension about visiting the Intensive Care Unit, medical setbacks, the problems of single parenting, and fears of their baby's possible death or disability. In addition, the strains on a couple's relationship in these special circumstances are explained, and suggestions given for strengthening communication. By listening to others who have gone through the same experience, parents gain a great deal of valuable information to help them face their problems and cope with the NICU experience. (20 mins.)

Who are the Debolts? F
(1978) Source: PYF

Family relations--adoption and foster care. A portrait of the Debolt family, nineteen special children in foster or adoptive care with one couple. Of different racial backgrounds and with several different types of handicapping conditions, the children's issues are love, courage, finding identity, and becoming a whole person. (72 mins.)

G. Physical and Sexual Abuse Effects on Child and Adolescent Development and Forensic Psychiatry

1. Child Abuse

Child abuse F
(1973) Source: AMA

Child abuse. This film examines the etiologic factors and manifestations of physical and psychological abuse of children; presents to the physician those incongruities and inconsistencies which should arouse suspicion of abuse; discusses elements of an appropriate differential diagnosis; reviews methods of clinical approach to both abused and abuser; highlights legal, social, and psychological aspect of child abuse; and emphasizes establishment of physicians's leadership role as well as an effective liaison with community and social agencies in the management of child abuse. E. Newberger, Director.

Child abuse V
(1977) Source: PCR

Child abuse. This video discusses how physicians and health care professionals can recognize key factors in the identification of child abuse. It emphasizes the importance of early and prompt treatment. C. M. Berlin, Director. (25 mins.)

Child abuse: An overview V
(1976) Source: HSC

Child abuse. In this video, the subjects of physical and sexual abuse and non-organic failure to thrive are covered. It is a concise and direct presentation of the problem, and includes an introduction to three other tapes. Health Sciences Consortium. (24 mins.)

Child abuse: Cradle of violence F
(1976) Source: PCR

Child abuse. Intimate interviews with abusive parents in the areas of child behavior and discipline create an understanding of child abuse and the need to break the cycle. Alternatives to corporal punishment and potential stress situations are presented. (20 mins.)

Physical abuse V
(1981) Source: HSC

Child abuse. This videocassette program with its study guide provides in-depth information on physical abuse of children: its incidence, identification, and treatment. It teaches identification of physical abuse by both physical examination of the victim and interviewing to determine parental characteristics and precipitating events within the family. (14 mins.)

Child abuse: A study in fragmentation — V
(1978) — Source: WPIC

Child abuse. Paulina G. McCullough and Ruth Drescher, Directors. (55 mins.)

Child savers — V
(1985) — Source: CLP

Child abuse. The tape deals with child abuse in a documentary style. We follow along as New York City, borough of Manhattan, child protection workers go out on routine complaints that children are being physically or sexually abused. Some of these are veterans of many years in the work and are articulate about their tasks. Fast paced, highly dramatic, and at times lurid. Public Television. C. Langer, Director. (53 mins.)

If I tell you a secret — V,F
(1984) — Source: LP

Child abuse. This film begins with an introduction by Sandra Baker, the Director of the Sacramento Child Sexual Abuse Center. Following an overview on what to expect and how to establish one's goals in interviewing a child who has been sexually abused, the film has four distinct parts. The first is what information and approach a member of a child protective services department would utilize in doing an interview. The second section is a discussion by a police sergeant who has done fifteen years of interviews of children who have been sexually abused. The third section is a discussion by a pediatrician who outlines both her physical exam and psychological exam, particularly with an eye towards later court appearance. The final section is a discussion by a district attorney and how she conducts her interview and what she anticipates both from the child and from the legal system. S. Baker, Director. (34 mins.)

Incest: The victim nobody believes — V
(1979) — MTI, FLRC

Child abuse. Three young adult women recall their childhood experiences--each a victim of incest from father or stepfather. One was sworn to silence to protect her younger sister only later to find father had relations with her, too. Guilt and love for father delay exposure. They would have welcomed the Hot Line "Does your father bother you, call this number. . ." Supplemental teaching guide offers important advice to the presenter to refrain from asking members of the audience to share personal experiences. Well-edited production. J. G. Mitchell, Director. (23 mins.)

Ordinary people: A film on child abuse — V,F
(1977) — Source: WPIC

Child abuse. This presentation demonstrates that child abusers often seem to be "ordinary people." It shows that there are frequently a multitude of distress signals which health care workers should recognize and heed. (25 mins.)

Prisoners of incest — V
(1984) — BBCTV

Child abuse. This docudrama examines the effects of incest on a family--the secrecy, guilt, fear, and lack of communication that distort the structure of a family's relationships and make the family Prisoners of incest. A family created from the experiences at London's Hospital for Sick Children participate in a typical therapy session. Family members are led through an examination of the problems that exited in the family prior to the incidents of incest. They discuss the stimulus for the father's actions and what effects the situation has had on each member. As the session develops, the revelations of each individual help alleviate the guilt and banish ignorance and fear-induced hatred. Tilman Furniss, Director. BBC, Horizon Series. (50 mins.)

Psychological maltreatment of children — V
(1985) — Source: CHD

Child abuse. James Barbarino and John Merrow, Directors. (19 mins.)

Psychological maltreatment of children: Assault on the psyche — V
(1986) — Source: PCR

Child abuse. Words can hurt, and they can leave psychological scars on an individual just as much as physical abuse. Psychological treatment of children is a dramatized portrayal of the harmful effects parental verbal abuse can have on children. The psychological maltreatment of two children is shown in a living-room vignette, revealing the inner struggle of the parents that gives rise to the abuse, and its disturbing consequences. The program includes interviews with both children and parents that further elucidate the problems of a troubled family. Dr. James Garbarino provides on-camera analysis of the situation and makes recommendations for intervention to help such families. J. Gardino and J. Merrow, Directors. (19 mins.)

Raised in anger: A special program on child abuse V
(1979) Source: IU

Child abuse. Physical, verbal, and emotional abuse of children is a tragic problem of national proportion. Some one million children each year suffer damage at the hands of their parents, people from every sector of society. Edward Asner, host and commentator, introduces several men and women who have been through the experience of abusing their own children. These parents explain how the increasing frustration, isolation, and general stresses of modern living became so unbearable that they found themselves losing control and taking out their guilt and anger on their children. (59 mins.)

The secret burden: How adults face a history of sexual child abuse V
(1984) Source: PIMC

Child abuse. This tape is designed to educate lay and professional audiences about the long-term effects of childhood sexual abuse. It features the real life stories of three women whose "secret burden" led to a host of additional problems in their adult lives, ranging from alcoholism to depression to marital discord. L. L. Kopolow, D. Stern, and I. Olson, Directors. (20 mins.)

Sexual abuse V
(1983) Source: HSC

Child abuse. This videocassette program recognizes the difficulties in diagnosing sexual abuse in children because of the stigma attached to it, which often disrupts usual examining skills. It emphasizes the very complete physical examination that is required, as well as the particular interviewing skill that must be used with both the parents and children of different ages. Treatment information covers steps both to assure a safe home environment and to rehabilitate the parents, but it also recognizes the relapse rate. Reporting responsibilities are also examined. Includes study guide. Health Sciences Consortium. J. R. Hebeler, Director. (18 mins.)

Sound of silence V,F
(1979) Source: MAC

Child abuse. The material in this tape covers the experience of children, adolescents, and adults who grew up in homes with alcoholic adults. Through a combination of brief responses from these children, and adolescents' and adults' didactic presentations, the issues and feelings of being injured by adult alcoholics is illustrated. The main emphasis covers physical and sexual abuse as well as verbal abuse. There is a discussion of the "don't talk rule" whereby the injured person, out of shame, fear, doubts, etc., cannot break the cycle of abuse through bringing it out in the open. Various aspects of sexual abuse that are more specific to homes with alcoholics are explained. The resulting loss of trust and damage from verbal abuse in later years is also explored. C. Black, Director. (26 mins.)

<u>The young victims of sexual abuse: An interview protocol</u> V
(1983) Source: CGC

Child abuse. This videotape shows the viewer how to interview preschool age children using anatomical dolls and an interview protocol to evaluate child sexual abuse. The tape gives professionals a framework in which to work with this age group. Through actual filmed interviews, the tape demonstrates practical tips on how to engage the child's interest, how to handle an uncooperative child, and how to keep control of the interview. The tape stresses the importance of objectivity and non-leading questioning. A study guide will accompany the tape. Cleveland Metropolitan General Hospital. S. White, G. Strom, and G. Santilli, Directors. (38 mins.)

2. Forensic Psychiatry

<u>Child abuse and the law, serious problems and real possibilities</u> V
(1980) Source: UCLA

Forensic psychiatry. Mary J. Spencer and Paul Boland, Directors. (60 mins.)

<u>Child abuse: Nonorganic failure to thrive</u> V
(1977) Source: HSC

Forensic psychiatry. Gerald F. Powell, Director. (21 mins.)

<u>Children of divorce</u> F
(1976) Source: GP

Forensic psychiatry. This film presents a clinical interview, for mental health professionals only, concerning the issues of the effect of divorce on children. (26 mins.)

<u>The effective witness in protective services</u> F
(1982) Source: UWF

Forensic psychiatry. A training film. (25 mins.)

Interviews with a divorced mother, her son, age one and daughter, age 7 — F
(1986) — Source: HSV

Forensic psychiatry. (30 mins.)

Just another missing kid — F
(1984) — Source: UCEMC

Forensic psychiatry. This film is a feature-length investigation of the case of a missing nineteen-year-old who was later found dead. A powerful and sobering documentary with all the suspense of fiction, this is the story of a determined family, frustrated police, unresponsive authorities, hardened criminals, and an old-school private eye. Probing the tragic weaknesses in our judicial system, the film brings the growing problem of missing children into gripping focus. Academy Award winner. Pyramid. (90 mins.)

Juvenile crime: No minor problem
(Parts I and II) — F
(1976) — Source: UWF

Forensic psychiatry. An overview. (40 mins.)

The medical witness and juvenile court — V
(1981) — Source: UA

Forensic psychiatry. Alex Duncan, Director. (36 mins.)

Question of custody — F
(1983) — Source: UWF

Forensic psychiatry. A training film in the Child Welfare Training Series. (42 mins.)

Which mother is mine? — V,F
(1985) — Source: TLV

Forensic psychiatry. A fifteen-year-old was abandoned by her mother when she was very young. She was raised by loving foster parents who are about to adopt her when her natural mother reappears to try to regain custody. Whatever the judge's decision, someone will be hurt. M. Tahse, Director. (47 mins.)

3. Miscellaneous

The battered child: Recognition and management — V
(1975) — Source: FLRC

Psychiatry, individual. Dr. C. Henry Kempe discusses the incidence, recognition, and management of the battered child syndrome. P. F. Wehrle, Director. (30 mins.)

Grief: A peril in infancy — F
(1954) — Source: NYU

Infant neglect. This film shows the effect upon infants of prolonged absence of the mother. A number of babies in a foundling home are shown. It is indicated among infants of less than a year that, if the mother returns after an interval of less than three months, the recovery is rapid. If the absence is prolonged beyond this period, it becomes impossible to achieve contact with the infants, and they become passive. R. Spitz, Director. (25 mins.)

Parents look at genetic counseling — V
(1981) — Source: UMG

Genetics. This video presents comments from parents of handicapped or impaired children who are involved in genetic counseling at the University of Michigan Medical Center. Topics discussed include: how the parents were informed of the condition; their reactions to genetic counseling, both positive and negative, and their plans for future children. D. Baker, Director. (27 mins.)

H. Children in the Hospital--Chronic Illness, Death, and Dying

1. Psychiatry--Training

One day a week — F
(1969) — Source: CMC, NYU

Psychiatry, training. This film illustrates the work of a community psychiatrist and his techniques of community health consultation to a Job Corps Agency in New Bedford, Massachusetts. It portrays one style of consultation to an agency staff. (33 mins.)

Understanding organizational and individual needs — V
(1980) — Source: USC

Psychiatry, training. (22 mins.)

2. Liaison--Various

Dystonia V,F
(1986) Source: BSML

Liaison, neurological disorder. Dystonia musculorum deformans, or dystonia, is a rare neurological disorder that causes the muscles of the body to contract into painfully distorted positions. If often restricts mobility and impairs speech, contributing to serious disability and social isolation. This film documents the experiences of six individuals whose afflictions encompass varying degrees of severity. Included in the documentary are a young man who, despite almost total loss of speech and severely diminished functioning of his limbs, has managed to create an independent and productive lifestyle. Additionally included is a college-bound girl whose severe speech impairment causes tremendous feelings of alienation; a ten-year-old boy whose symptoms have been partially arrested through the use of a spinal cord stimulator device; and an articulate mother and her young daughter, both of whom suffer from dystonia. The film emphasizes the profound adjustments the patients and families need to make to a major physical handicap. C. D. Marsden and J. Waltz, Directors. (29 mins.)

Parents' responses to their children's illnesses V
(1977) Source: UMG

Liaison, chronic illnesses. This video presents a discussion between a University of Michigan Hospital social worker and four parents of chronically ill children. It illustrates parents' responses to their children's illnesses that parallel those of dying patients outlined by Elizabeth Kubler-Ross: denial, anger, bargaining, depression, and acceptance. (27 mins.)

Winning battles, a film about children with cancer V
(1979) Source: FL

Liaison, chronic illnesses. Filmmakers Library, Inc., Director. (8 mins.)

3. Liaison--Hospitalization

The anesthetist/patient interview can make a difference for patients ages 3 to 12 years V
(1979) Source: VCU

Liaison, hospitalization. John T. Beeston, Lawrence D. Egbert, and Raymond Bruce Laravuso, Directors. (38 mins.)

Films and Videos with Commentary

Bone marrows and spinal taps V
(1983) Source: CMC

Liaison, hospitalization. This videotape demonstrates the approach used for cognitive and behavioral control of pain for school age children undergoing a bone marrow aspiration and a spinal tap. It begins with a brief description by the girl, Daniell, who stars through the tape, of her feelings about having leukemia and what it means to undergo painful procedures. Next is the interview and rehearsing of techniques as taught by a clinical psychologist at the clinic. This is followed by practice of these techniques on a doll and finally a mock procedure done on Daniell by the psychologist. The final sequence shows Daniell actually getting the procedures done, including injection of local anesthetic agents and draping the area of the body to be probed. Interspersed is Daniell's frank expressions of her fears. (25 mins.)

The death of a newborn V
(1976) Source: CWR

Liaison, hospitalization. Marshall H. Klaus and Nancy Irvin, Directors. (32 mins.)

Forming an alliance V
(1985) Source: DL

Liaison, hospitalization. Dr. Norman Sherry demonstrates establishing and fostering the important reliance between pediatrician and parent during examinations of three two-year-olds. These are "well-child" visits and are models for family-oriented child care. E. Mason, Director. (25 mins.)

First do no harm: Hospitalization and the developing child F,V
(1981) Source: CHNMC

Liaison, hospitalization. This film includes how hospitals can adapt to meet the psychosocial needs of children and their families. It shows the first moments of a mother with her newborn son, who has a major birth defect; an adolescent "rap" group discussing the death of a patient; a school-age child's frustration with curiosity about chronic illness; fantasy play of pre-schoolers, etc. Treating the mind and body together is stressed. (35 mins.)

Hospitalization in the first decade of life Slides
(1977) Source: McMU

Liaison, hospitalization. Kenneth C. Finkel, Ruth Snider, and C. Vair, Directors. (140 slides)

Parents and staff in a children's ward F
(1971) Source: PCR

Liaison, hospitalization. This film examines a sick child's need for emotional support when in the hospital and the participation of the parents in caring for the child. Included are parents' and staff members' views of their roles, focusing on ways to improve mutual relations. Reenactments of four different situations where parents and nurses come into conflict are presented. H. Lowenstein, Director. (45 mins.)

Pre-op! F
(1980) Source: UI

Liaison, hospitalization. Designed to help prepare a child mentally for surgery, this film dramatizes the story of an over-anxious mother who learns that she is increasing her son's fears with her own. It suggests methods by which parents can diminish their own anxiety and that of the child with openness and facts, and a calm, accepting manner. Footsteps Series. (23 mins.)

Preparation of children for surgery and treatment through planned play V
(1971) Source: USC

Liaison, hospitalization. Barbara Hicks, Director. (30 mins.)

Separations and reunions F
(1968) Source: PCR

Liaison, hospitalization. H. Lowenstein and D. MacCarthy, Directors. (36 mins.)

To prepare a child V,F
(1983) Source: CHNMC

Liaison, hospitalization. A medical center's well-defined preparation program for young children and their families, this film demonstrates preparation for cardiac surgery, a brief hospitalization for ear surgery, and an emergency room visit. (32 mins.)

We won't leave you V
(1975) Source: HMS

Liaison, hospitalization. Edward A. Mason, Director. (17 mins.)

When a child enters the hospital — V
(1980) — Source: PMF

Liaison, hospitalization. Many hospitals are allowing and encouraging parents to remain with their children during a hospital stay. They believe children feel more secure if they are in familiar hands and that nurses benefit from the care and attention parents give. This film chronicles the hospitalization of a young girl undergoing minor surgery and shows how her mother helps. A. Fiering, Director. (16 mins.)

4. Diagnosis

Assessing a young child — F
(1974) — Source: UI

Diagnosis. A physician, teachers, the staff of a special school, and parents measure the strengths and weaknesses of their children. Their goal is to determine the nature of the future schooling each handicapped child requires, by comparing similar data on normal children. All aspects are analyzed: motor skills, development of speech and language, hearing, self-help. BBC. (24 mins.)

Child developmental diagnosis: Part I — V
(1977) — Source: WPIC

Diagnosis. This videotape demonstrates developmental differences in three children with developmental problems. Produced by Western Psychiatric Institute and Clinic for restricted audiences. (60 mins.)

Child developmental diagnosis: Part II — V
(1977) — Source: WPIC

Diagnosis. This videotape demonstrates two adolescent cases: a fifteen-year-old with affective disorder, suicidal behavior, and temporal lobe epilepsy; and an eighteen-year-old with seizure disorder and aggression. Produced by Western Psychiatric Institute and Clinic for restricted audiences. (60 mins.)

5. Death

Death of a sibling: Children describe cancer's impact on the family — V
(1981) — Source: UA

Death. (32 mins.)

I'm still the same person: Teenagers with cancer — V
(1980) — Source: UMG

Death. This video presents interviews with two adolescents--Jenny, who was diagnosed with osteogenic sarcoma resulting in a leg amputation, and Bob, who was diagnosed with Hodgkin's disease. It covers their views of family and friends' responses to their illnesses, hospitalization experiences, effects of chemotherapy, adjustments to the diagnosis and treatment of cancer, and their plans for the future. S. Foley, Director. (29 mins.)

Only one road: Three families coping with childhood cancer — V
(1983) — Source: UMG

Death. Interviews of three children and their families who are past the initial stages of diagnosis and treatment of cancer are presented. The children, Kristie, Faisha, and Jonathan, range in age from five through nine. A special focus of the program is the discussion of the kinds of problems that occur outside the hospital/treatment setting, some of which may be less familiar to health care professionals. Through interviews and actual footage of these families interacting in the home, public school, and hospital settings, their concerns regarding remission of cancer, school problems, long-term effects, survival of the marriage, and handling "left-out" siblings are revealed. The ways of coping with the difficulties are included in the presentation. (53 mins.)

To live until you die — V,F
(1976) — Source: TLV

Death. An intimate portrait of the Swiss-born psychiatrist, Elizabeth Kubler-Ross and her contributions. WGBH/NOVA. (57 mins.)

Where is dead? — F
(1981) — Source: BF

Death. This low-keyed drama deals compassionately, yet realistically, with a subject that young children may be forced to face: the death of a loved one. Six-year-old Sarah plays and fights with her nine-year-old brother, David, in a series of recognizable childhood vignettes. David's sudden death rends the family fabric. Sarah's parents attempt to explain what has happened--with tenderness but without sentimentality. Gradually, the little girl is able to cope with her feelings of sadness, confusion, and fear . . . and life regains most of its earlier joys. John Joseph Hutter, Katherine Burlington, and Franz Farrell, Directors. (19 mins.)

6. Perception--Deafness and Blindness

Blind Sunday — V,F
(1983) — Source: TLV

Perception, deafness, blindness. This video tells the story of a self-reliant high school girl who develops a friendship with a sighted boy. He in turn tries to understand her world. D. Wilson, Director. (31 mins.)

Blindness: Five points of view V,F
(1987) Source: TLV

Perception, deafness, blindness. How five patients who are going blind cope with the condition is explored in this film. WGBH/NOVA. (59 mins.)

Co-twin study: A day in the life of a blind child and her sighted twin sister F
(1965) Source: NIMH

Perception, deafness, blindness. D. A. Pennebaker and Arthur E. Gillman, Directors. (60 mins.)

Deaf like me F
(1980) Source: UI

Perception, deafness, blindness. A deaf girl feels isolated from her peers by her deafness. A young mime performs at her school. He helps her discover a whole new world by teaching her some of his routines. She performs with him and is drawn out of herself. (23 mins.)

Listen (captioned version) F
(1973) Source: GSA

Perception, deafness, blindness. This film documents hearing loss--its psychological meaning, and what can be done to cope with it. Sounds are filtered to approximate how they are heard by persons with different kinds of hearing losses. The film provides an orientation to the problem of hearing loss in today's society. Western Maryland College. (30 mins.)

7. Miscellaneous

Donnie F
(1979) Source: CMH

Prolonged hospitalization. The story of a two-and-one-half year old child who spent two years in an Intensive Care Unit. The film considers the personality development of the child, the impact on the family, and the social issues raised by the hospitalization. J. L. Shulman, Director. (25 mins.)

Mostly I can do more things than I can't F
(1984) Source: CMH

Ethics. A follow-up to the film Donnie, showing him as an eight and one half year old. He is connected by a tube to a respiratory apparatus. He spent the first three-and-one-half years of his life in the hospital in an Intensive Care Unit. This film explores his adjustment to home, as well as funding problems. The child has accomplished remarkable gains in speech and in emotional and personality development. Issues of ethics, values, and the cost of medical care are focused on. J. L. Shulman, Director. (23 mins.)

I. Learning and Learning Disorders

1. Development, Cognition, and Play

Six films on Piaget's development theories of child development — F
(1978) — Source: DF

Development, cognition, play. (1) The growth of intelligence in the preschool years according to Jean Piaget. (2) Conservation--children between the ages of five and twelve are presented in individual interviews with tasks using the standard procedures developed by Piaget. (3) Classification--children are shown at several developmental stages responding to tasks which highlight different mental operations essential to classification such as multiple classification and hierarchical classification. (4) Formal thought--this film illustrates tasks that challenge the thinking of secondary school students. (5) Jean Piaget memory and intelligence--this is a filmed documentary of Jean Piaget presenting his new work on memory and intelligence at the International Congress of Preschool Educational Specialists in Kyoto, Japan. (6) Morality: The process of moral development--this film identifies the process of moral development starting with children age four and continuing to its most complete unfolding in young adults. (68 mins.)

Three cognitive skills: Middle childhood — F
(1978) — Source: IU

Development, cognition, play. This film presents vignettes illustrating the development of three cognitive areas--readiness, memory, and creativity--during ages six through twelve. It shows a variety of factors such as individual intelligence and home environment that affect development of these skills. (21 mins.)

Toying with reality — V
(1980) — Source: IU

Development, cognition, play. This video examines children's playthings. In a child's world, everything he or she comes into contact with is a plaything--toys, people, animals, and events. It observes scenes of spontaneous undirected children's play, including kindergartners building individual structures from a simple set of blocks and ten-year-olds building a fort from a glob of clay. Commentary by the late Dr. Sara Rabinovitch, Dorothy Medhurst, Dr. James Fair, and Patricia MacKay. Learning through Play Series. (30 mins.)

2. Education--Techniques

Combat in the classroom F
(1980) Source: UCLA

Education, techniques. Ed Asner narrates this examination of one of the crucial problems in American public schools: violence. After examining the size and the source of the problem, suggestions and a demonstration on reducing the incidence of violence are given. Dave Bell Associates; MTI Teleprograms. (27 mins.)

Confident teaching F
(1977) Source: LP

Education, techniques. This film demonstrates how the process of self-esteem enhancement can be carried over into the curriculum, with special emphasis on how the teacher can make it work. "The process begins with respect for the child," says one teacher, whose large open classroom is a fine illustration of a functioning democracy. We see children teaching each other, parent volunteers working as aides, and a wide variety of special activities and teaching techniques. All of this material is presented as visual reinforcement for the film's didactic message, which is that four conditions are necessary for the development of a child's self-concept: (1) acceptance, (2) clear structure, (3) clear standards, and (4) integration of experience. A discussion guide is provided with this film. (19 mins.)

Continuous progress learning F
(1971) Source: UCLA

Education, techniques. This film examines a system of education in which children are not grouped by age, but by mental ability. The students learn a system of concepts and skills at their own pace. A concept is unfolded, reinforced, reviewed, rephrased, fortified, revisited, and reconstituted. It requires a careful inventory of students' abilities, adaptation of the physical plant, and having an adaptable faculty and a new approach to learning on the part of administrators. (14 mins.)

David's case: An example F
(1980) Source: IU

Education, techniques. This film demonstrates the procedural steps in reviewing problems between school officials and parents with regard to students: appointing the case conference committee, sharing information, initiation of individual educational plan, placement review, and revised program. It indicates that the appointment of the case conference committee is determined by the child's problems. It discusses a program that will remedy David's academic and social problems. (33 mins.)

Do's and don'ts of tutoring F
(1979) Source: UCLA

Education, techniques. The correct and incorrect approaches and methods in peer tutoring are demonstrated. The film emphasizes that the goal of the student tutor is to help the student develop understanding of the subject. It is useful for student tutors or anyone involved in one-to-one or small group education. Blue Ridge Technical Institute. (30 mins.)

Exceptional times: An historical perspective of special education F
(1979) Source: CEC

Education, techniques. This film is intended to develop an awareness of the struggle for equal humanity that exceptional people have been engaged in for the past century and a half. (25 mins.)

Impact of classroom environment on child development F
(1974) Source: DF

Education, techniques. In this film, three styles of teacher interaction as determinant of children's behavior are demonstrated. It shows ways to handle or avoid problems, encourage social interaction, and stimulate learning among pre-schoolers. (17 mins.)

Learning centers F
(1979) Source: UI

Education, techniques. This film describes learning centers and describes four principle varieties: resource-centered, interest-centered, self-instruction, and activity-centered. It analyzes the use and function of the four types and lists the advantages: greater involvement of the students in the process and of the leader with the student; the presentation of learning as a pleasant experience; the awakening of curiosity and thinking; and the building of self-confidence and of student responsibility, each for his own learning. The Other School System Series. (29 mins.)

Films and Videos with Commentary

Let's look at aggression (1974) — F — Source: MTPS

Education, techniques. At the very beginning of this documentary film, the filmmakers warn us not to expect a picture of a normal nursery school. Instead, they have selected sequences revealing a variety of aggressive and pseudo-aggressive behavior in four-year-olds. The intent is to help teachers and parents learn to observe and understand self-assertive behavior at an objective remove. (In other words, when they're not in the thick of it!) We are also shown some methods that parents and teachers may use to cope with aggression: puppets, for example, allow children to be aggressive in a socially-acceptable and creative way. The vignettes illustrating subtle (and not so subtle) pushy behavior are presented in a fair amount of depth; we can almost read the child's mind before the outburst, and each incident is followed through to show its effect on the other children. (22 mins.)

One at a time--together (1971) — F — Source: UCLA

Education, techniques. This film looks at individually guided education in the elementary school. By examining the school, we see how the system of team teaching, small groups, progressive learning, and non-graded, open classroom approach can function without any additional staff or funds. (19 mins.)

Selecting appropriate leadership styles for instructional improvement (1979) — V — Source: UCLA

Education, techniques. Various types of leadership in the school setting are demonstrated. The film stresses developing leadership style appropriate to the group. ASCD. (33 mins.)

Teachers, parents, children (1973) — F — Source: DF

Education, techniques. This film explains how to construct alliances between families and teachers to ease a child's entrance into school and to support and encourage his or her subsequent growth. (22 mins.)

What a teacher expects: The self-fulfilling prophecy (1971) — F — Source: UCEMC

Education, techniques. How a child's performance in school is affected by the expectations of the teacher is illustrated and discussed by two researchers. NFBC. (26 mins.)

3. Education--Learning Disorders

Adolescence and learning disabilities V
(1974) Source: LP

Education, learning disorders. Carolyn F. Piel, Director. (30 mins.)

Adolescence and learning disabilities F
(1977) Source: LP

Education, learning disorders in adolescence. One of the knottiest problems confronting educators today is the adolescent whose severe learning difficulty interferes with his or her psychological development. What does it do to a boy's self-image to be tagged "disabled" because he can't read? When youngsters pour all their energies into coping with learning problems, how can they be helped to come to grips with their sexuality? How can they become the kind of people who will be able to meet society's demands? In far too many schools, the policy seems to be: "get rid of trouble-makers." However, in a number of places, innovators are developing special programs to help such children. Most of this film consists of demonstrations of these programs by special educators and mental health specialists. We also hear from various students who tell us in their own words how isolated they felt because of their learning disabilities. (25 mins.)

He comes from another room F
(1974) Source: DL

Education, learning disorders, emotional problems. For more than four years, a public school in Needham, Massachusetts, has had a special program for emotionally disturbed children, including a procedure for integrating such children into a regular classroom. In this documentary film, we follow the steps by which Chris and David, two eight-year-old boys, move from their special education classroom into a regular third grade classroom. Much of the success of such a program depends upon the teamwork between the special education teacher, the regular classroom teacher, and the consulting psychiatrist. We are shown several example of the classroom teachers's resourcefulness in using games to encourage rapport and interaction between Chris and David and the rest of the children. Although shy and reluctant to participate at first, they gradually overcome their fears and, at the film's end, seem more secure and socially involved. E. Mason, Director. (28 mins.)

The invisible handicap F
(1976) Source: UI

Education, learning disorders. This film examines dyslexia, which is a disorder which makes reading difficult because visual perception in transmitted to the brain in a jumbled or reversed sequence. This problem is often not recognized for what it is, and children are then misunderstood as slow, clumsy, or retarded. Intelligence is not impaired by this disorder: when special education and an atmosphere of confidence are provided, this disability can be overcome. From "60 Minutes" with Morly Safer. (16 mins.)

Reading disability--dyssymbolia F
(1978) Source: HCF

Education, learning disorders. The film begins by making a distinction between various causes of learning disorders, including dyssymbolia or dyslexia, as well as mental retardation, emotional impairment, limited motivation, and encephalopathies. It further breaks down dyssymbolia into difficulties with acquisition of skill (sensory, specific reading skills, symbolization skills, and general factors), and the application of skill (impulse control, motivation, emotional restraint, and limited opportunity). These distinctions are important as the film goes on to portray the reading difficulties of five very different boys all with I.Q.'s of at least ninety and in most cases over one hundred. Through having the boys read paragraphs, spell, and demonstrate phonic skills, these distinct problems are demonstrated. The film illustrates techniques that can be used to unmask these difficulties. The end of the film covers topics regarding treatment, prognosis, and etiology. R. D. Rabinovitch and F. C. Pasley, Directors. (45 mins.)

Specific learning disabilities: Evaluation V,F
(1984) Source: DF

Education, learning disorders. This film follows two learning disabled children through a series of evaluative tasks to determine their learning strengths and weaknesses. The results are interpreted and optimal patterns of learning are suggested. (28 mins.)

4. Education--Miscellaneous

Footsteps (a series of 20 films) V,F
(1978) Source: NAV

Educational development, public information. In response to the growing public interest in the educational development of very young children, the United States Office of Education has provided funds for the production of a television series on parenting. The initial twenty programs of the series, called Footsteps, are now available for rental or purchase. Detailed discussion guides are also available for purchase. (Twenty films, 30 mins. each)

Max made mischief F
(1985) Source: DL

Development, school age. Max made mischief illustrates a curriculum for teaching literature to young children, which is being developed by Ms. Sonia Landes. In this case, she is using Maurice Sendak's classic children's book, Where the wild things are, in a pilot effort with Emily Graham and her third grade class. The film illustrates the enjoyment of discovery the children find through intensive study, and some of the techniques which can be used as they explore plot structure, the nature of poetry, and the use of illustrations. The children identify with Max's mischievousness and come to understand something about the ways this character uses his mischief and fantasy to deal with his negative feelings and need to be loved by his mother. The teachers discuss their progress between classes and, at the end of the film, are seen meeting with author Maurice Sendak to learn about his intentions in writing the book and his statement that "fantasy only makes sense when rooted ten feet in reality."

J. Autism and Mental Retardation

1. Psychopathology--Developmental Disorders

A boy named Terry Egan F
(1973) Source: UI

Psychopathology, developmental disorders. Eight-year-old Terry Egan is autistic. Autistic children exhibit behavioral patterns such as rocking, language dysfunction, and temper tantrums, and are fascinated with spinning objects. CBS news correspondent Daniel Schorr spent almost a year with the Egan family, observing Terry at home and at school for autistic or emotionally disturbed children. This film is their documentation of a baffling childhood pathology. (52 mins.)

Childhood schizophrenia F
(1972) Source: SP

Psychopathology, developmental disorders. This film begins by discussing some of the problems associated with childhood schizophrenia: undetermined etiology and the need for more effective therapeutic techniques. The film goes on to describe three subtypes of this disorder, as observed by Dr. Finch and his colleagues: early infantile autism, symbiotic psychosis, and borderline psychosis. Three phases of therapy for children with these disorders are also described: (1) breaking through the autistic barrier, (2) developing new ego skills, and (3) working through intra- and inter-psychic conflicts. To illustrate both the clinical picture of these three subtypes of childhood schizophrenia and the techniques employed in their treatment, the film shows several children in various therapeutic situations, e.g., recreational therapy and psychotherapy. S. M. Finch, Director. (44 mins.)

Early infantile autism, the clinical picture through adulthood F
(1968) Source: HCF

Psychopathology, developmental disorders. In the first part of this film, Dr. Pasley discusses the cardinal findings in early infantile autism. Particular reference is make to the Kanner criteria and studies done by Lauretta Bender. Areas of intactness, as well as abnormalities of language, social relationships, and behavior, are both discussed as well as demonstrated through the behavior of three children on film. The children, ages five, eight, and thirteen, exhibit the range of findings in autism. The second part of the film emphasizes the critical differencesbetween adolescent onset psychosis and early childhood psychosis. The film examines the core problems of each, as well as reactive symptoms, restitutive symptoms, and compensatory symptoms. It utilizes five- to ten-minute interviews with three older or grown up autistic individuals, ages sixteen, twenty-one, and forty. The film concludes with a discussion of the life history of those with early childhood autism, with possible etiologies and with exiting treatment. An exceptionally clear film on this subject. R. D. Rabinovitch and F. C. Pasley, Directors. (110 mins.)

Nine diagnostic criteria of psychosis in children V
(1972) Source: FLRC

Psychopathology, developmental disorders. An illustration and description of a widely used set of criteria for diagnosing psychosis in children is shown in this video. It draws on material from the activities of a local treatment center for disturbed children. S. H. Marks, Director. (45 mins.)

Time for Georgia F
(1972) Source: UCEMC

Psychopathology, developmental disorders. This film shows the Pre-schoolers' Workshop, a special nursery-kindergarten school for very young children with learning impairments. It focuses on a four-year-old autistic girl's struggles and triumphs in the class and shows her progress over a six-month period. (14 mins.)

Time's lost children F
(1973) Source: UI

Psychopathology, developmental disorders. An intensive language and behavior modification program for young autistic children is depicted. (30 mins.)

Working with autistic states in children and adults — V
(1986) — Source: CEC

Psychopathology, developmental disorders. Frances Tustin, a highly regarded therapist with more than forty years of experience working with autistic children, discusses in lucid and careful detail her understanding of the use of autistic states as a defense mechanism. In particular, Frances Tustin is able to convey the original and unique blend of psychoanalytic thought as well as intuitive understanding of profoundly defended clients in her work. An advanced level of presentation. D. S. May, Director. (2 tapes, 50 mins. each)

2. Mental Retardation

1972 Special Olympics: "We've Only Just Begun" — F
(1976) — Source: UI

Mental retardation. The courage, determination, and enthusiasm through athletic competition is captured by this film which covers the National Summer Olympics for the mentally retarded. It depicts the grace, agility, skill, and confidence of the contestants. Each event produces victories and defeats, but the end result is victorious because the Special Olympics have opened the door for thousands of mentally retarded young people to take their place in society, with dignity and pride. Pat Lawford, Eunice Shriver, Ethel Kennedy, and Rosey Greer are on hand to present the awards. Without narration, the film is augmented by a popular musical theme, "We've Only Just Begun," sung by the Carpenters. (16 mins.)

Best boy — F
(1979) — Source: IFEX

Mental retardation. The uplifting story of Philly, a fifth-three-year-old retarded man, and his quest for independence under the guidance of his concerned filmmaker/cousin, Ira Wohl, who has recognized that Philly must separate from his elderly parents. Philly's first days in school, his visit to the zoo and to the theater, and his move into a community residence are gently depicted with an emotional spirit. This film won the Academy Award for Best Documentary Feature of 1979. (104 mins.)

Better off dead? — V
(1984) — Source: PBS

Mental retardation. This video investigates the subject of "Baby Doe" that has initiated court fights, legislation, and considerable debate in medical and legal circles over the last few years. As medical technology has advanced to a point where even the most severely damaged infants can be kept alive for even longer periods of time, doctors, lawyers, judges, and especially parents have had to grapple with complex ethical choices about how far to go with medical care for these newborns. PBS. (60 mins.)

Board and care F
(1979) Source: PYF

Mental retardation. This is an Academy Award film and best of the AAMD Region II/USC Film Festival 1980. It focuses on the brief effort to break through to a meaningful relationship on the part of two teenagers with Down's syndrome. (27 mins.)

Children of hope F
(1977) Source: PCR

Mental retardation. A positive look at the future of those born with "Down's syndrome"--a contrast to the unsympathetic label "Mongolian idiot." (15 mins.)

David F
(1980) Source: FL

Psychopathology, mental retardation. A documentary film about David McFarland, an articulate, personable seventeen-year-old with Down's syndrome. His rich and varied life in his community, including a leading role in a TV drama, is shown. (28 mins.)

Down's syndrome V
(1980) Source: UTEX

Mental retardation. Mary Jo Harrod and Jan Marshall Friedman, Directors. (25 mins.)

Hewitt's just different V,F
(1981) Source: TLV

Mental retardation. A normal pre-adolescent boy befriends a sixteen-year-old mentally retarded neighbor boy, Hewitt. The normal boy is forced to take a stand with his baseball team peers who jibe at Hewitt. D. Wilson, Director. (47 mins.)

Mild mental retardation V
(1975) Source: UCLA

Mental retardation. Bernard Towers, Director. (60 mins.)

Mild retardation: A family profile — F
(1982) — Source: PMF

Mental retardation. This film is a developmental study of a young man--now twenty-one years old--who has been followed and filmed for the last eighteen years. The film focuses on family interactions and the young man developing a self-concept of his disability. (15 mins.)

Nesika — V
(1981) — Source: TLV

Mental retardation. A young woman and man, both residents in a hostel for educable retarded young adults, meet and fall in love. They try to announce to the girl's anxious overprotective parents that they should be married. Tisch/Aunet. (15 mins.)

Another love — V,F
(1983) — Source: TLV

Development, adolescents. A young woman and man, both residents in a hostel for educable retarded young adults, meet and fall in love. They try to announce to the girl's anxious overprotective parents that they should be married. Tisch/Aunet. (57 mins.)

One step at a time — V
(1982) — Source: UWMRC

Mental retardation. Jules M. Rosenthal, Director. (27 mins.)

Play therapy with mentally handicapped children — F
(1984) — Source: UWF

Therapeutics, psychotherapy with retarded children. (26 mins.)

Sara has Down's syndrome — F
(1979) — Source: EDC

Development, adolescents. Six-year-old Sara has learned to do many things, thanks to the perseverance of her family. Parents and teenage siblings discuss their feelings. Educational Development Center, Inc. (16 mins.)

Somewhere to go — V,F
(1982) — Source: WPIC

Mental retardation. A film about a "mutual support group" for parents of children with Down's syndrome. Produced at Children's Hospital Medical Center, Boston, it is recommended for professionals and parent and community groups. (25 mins.)

K. Suicide

Preventing teen suicide F
(1985) Source: SC

Suicide. A case study. (30 mins.)

Ronnie's tune F
(1978) Source: WP

Suicide. Through the eyes of an eleven-year-old girl, Julie, we see the effects of a teenager's suicide upon his family. Not merely a bystander, the little girl becomes the catalyst in helping the suicide's mother come to terms with her grief. From Lisa, Julie's summer friend, Julie learns the truth: Ronnie killed himself. Aunt Beth blames herself and Uncle Hal, and the father has left her because of this. Julie runs out into the woods at this news. When Aunt Beth learns that Lisa has informed Julie about all this, she is furious and goes out to look for Julie. When she finds her sitting under a tree, playing Ronnie's tune on his banjo, she is even more upset. But Julie's persistence in preserving her happy memories of Ronnie seem to touch and soften Beth's anger and make her grief less bitter. A charming and poignant story. Thoughtful and thought-provoking for parent groups and lay audiences. G. Feldman, Director. (18 mins.)

Suicide: It doesn't have to happen F
(1976) Source: IU

Suicide. This film presents a teenage girl who has attempted suicide being directed to group therapy by a high school teacher. It shows the girl's parents dealing with the situation and observes group sessions where members discuss problem-solving techniques and symptoms of suicide. A final addition is the perspective of time as the high school teacher comments on his own teenage suicide attempt and his healing process. (24 mins.)

Suicide: The warning signs V,F
(1980) Source: CF

Suicide. The subject of this videotape is teenage suicide. It covers three possible scenarios as it looks at the various warning signs and possible causes of suicide attempts in people fourteen to twenty years of age. Through the use of Gregg, a fifteen-year-old excessive risk taker, through Carol, a sixteen-year-old overachiever, and through Curtis, a black college student who has lost his girlfriend, the common themes and manifestations of suicidal behavior are explored. A clear list of common warning signs, such as statements, changes in sleeping and eating, making final arrangements, accident proneness, and other signs especially relevant to teenagers, are brought out. Suggestions on responses to the potentially suicidal teenager are also discussed. Dr. Jo Ann Myers, a child psychiatrist, discusses the issues in an organized fashion. Discussion guide provided. (24 mins.)

L. Substance Abuse

Alcoholism: Life under the influence — V,F
(1985) — Source: TLV

Psychopathology, substance abuse. This is an interdisciplinary report on the search for scientific understanding of the disease. NOVA, WGBH. (57 mins.)

Angel death — F
(1979) — Source: UCLA

Psychopathology, substance abuse. This is a documentary on PCP, commonly known as "angel dust," and its widespread abuse by young people. It shows the effect of this animal tranquilizer on a jaguar in the zoo, and points out that it has become one of the most dangerous street drugs. The film shows young addicts while high, during a counseling session, in the street, and in hospital emergency rooms, recording both stupor and violence. Narrated by Joanne Woodward and Paul Newman. Begleman/Fields Co. (48 mins.)

Children of denial — V
(1982) — Source: MAC, HCI

Psychopathology, substance abuse. This videotape by the well-known author and therapist, Claudia Black, is a quick but complete look at the issues for adult children of alcoholic parents. There are more than twelve million such children living in homes, and another fifteen million such people who have left home. She identifies the feelings of powerlessness, mistrust, isolation, and difficulty identifying and expressing feelings that are common to such children or grown-up children from alcoholic families. In particular, she addresses the forces on these children and adult children not to remember, not to speak up, and not to take action about their feelings that come from experiences in alcoholic families. At the conclusion of her presentation, she discusses some of the ways to treat this situation. C. Black, Director. (28 mins.)

Cocaine F
(1979) Source: UWF

Psychopathology, substance abuse. This film offers specific treatment modalities for cocaine addiction. Cocaine Symposium Series. (42 mins.)

Cocaine F
(1979) Source: UWF

Psychopathology, substance abuse. Counseling techniques for cocaine addition are presented. Drug Counseling Series. (40 mins.)

Cocaine blues: The myth and reality of cocaine F
(1980) Source: PCR

Psychopathology, substance abuse. More than one-half of the babies born to alcoholic mothers are retarded, victims of permanent fetal damage. This film show symptoms of this form of retardation at birth and development of the children. NBC.

Cocaine diary V,F
(1978) Source: MTI

Psychopathology, substance abuse. This videotape portrays a sixteen-year-old boy with normal relationships and desires who slowly gets drawn into a serious cocaine habit. He is slightly at risk because of mild alienation from his parents and not being a high academic performer. His brother-in-law introduces him to cocaine, an "up" drug, and the false sense of well-being. Over a period of weeks, he alienates his friends, almost gets arrested, wastes his money, has rapid mood shifts, and eventually drives his girlfriend away. It is only when his brother-in-law is revealed as a fraud does he recognize the seriousness of his problems. Accompanied by a useful discussion guide. (24 mins.)

Hope for the children V
(1985) Source: HCI

Psychopathology, substance abuse by parents--effects on children. This videotape is focused on the needs of children ages six to twelve whose parent or parents are chemically dependent and particularly if it involves alcohol. It uses three case example to delineate particular psychological problems and how they manifest themselves in children of this age. It goes through the process of recognizing and diagnosing such problems, ways to enhance children's understanding of this problem, and concrete strategies for mental health professionals for these children. It briefly explains parentification and role reversal, mistrust, social isolation, and loss of self-esteem that often are part of growing up in alcoholic families. It goes into the particular ways these issues will affect children of this age (six to twelve years) and how to work with them since their cognitive abilities and defense mechanisms are distinct from that of teenagers and adults. (28 mins.)

Scag (heroin) F
(1981) Source: BFI

Psychopathology, substance abuse. What it's like to be hooked on heroin comes through clearly and forcefully in the accounts of two young people who have been there and are trying to come back. A black girl from the ghetto and a white boy from suburbia had different reasons for turning to scag and experienced similar sufferings when it wouldn't let them turn away. The girl is off drugs now and struggling to straighten out her life. The boy is still hung up and looking for help. These stories allow viewers to examine the physical, emotional, and social consequences of shooting heroin. (21 mins.)

The summer we moved to Elm Street F
(1968) Source: PCR, McH

Psychopathology, substance abuse. This film describes a ten-year-old girl's reaction to family stress with an alcoholic father, a depressed mother, frequent moves--and her own depression. There are no didactic explanations, but the film can be used to sensitize a group to the child's emotional reactions and perceptions of a difficult situation. National Film Board of Canada. (28 mins.)

Ups/downs (amphetamines and barbiturates) F
(1975) Source: BFV

Psychopathology, substance abuse. This film examines the pep-you-up amphetamines and the slow-you-down barbiturates. Much of the evidence is given by young people. They tell of being trapped on diet pills, pep pills, and speed barbs. How our pill-popping society fosters abuse of these sometimes useful drugs, how severe a user's dependence on them can be, and what's involved in getting free are among the topics explored. (24 mins.)

M. Various Therapies and Diagnostic Processes

1. Diagnosis

Assessment and diagnosis of child psychopathology V
(1976) Source: PCR

Diagnosis. This video presents an overview of a standardized outline of child psychiatric assessment and diagnosis using the Diagnostic and Statistical Manual II/III categories and the classification system recommended by the committee on

Child Psychiatry. Procedures are demonstrated during an evaluation session with a Down's syndrome child and her mother. P. B. Henerson, Director. (26 mins.)

Brief service evaluation model — V
(1983) — Source: SIU

Diagnosis. In this video we are shown a diagnostic evaluation of a four-year-old boy with slow speech development, encopresis, and hyperactivity, together with assessment of his family (parents and older sister). The diagnosis and treatment plan are presented. A group discussion of the evaluation process by a group of medical students on rotation is facilitated by the child psychiatrist who is the diagnostician on the case. A good case is presented for differential diagnosis of emotional conflicts vs. organic developmental deficits. The diagnostic interviews prove to be a beginning of therapy. A well-edited and produced tape. For professional audiences. R. Herrick, Director. (51 mins.)

Family assessment and family treatment — V
(1981) — Source: BFI

Diagnosis, interview. W. Robert Beavers, Director. (45 mins.)

Interviewing children: Assessing mental status — V
(1978) — Source: WPIC

Diagnosis, interview. An integrated approach for developing the interview skills required of health professionals in all disciplines involving the care of children is presented, with emphasis on the clinical dynamics of the interview process. Foundation for Clinical Research in Psychiatry, University of Maryland School of Medicine. (30 mins.)

Interviewing children sounds easy, but . . . — V,F
(1984) — Source: IMS, UW

Diagnosis, interview. A supervising child psychiatrist and medical student talk together about the latter's concern about how to interview a child. The tape employs varied clinical illustrations with "voice over" to convey the rudiments of interviewing young children, particularly during the diagnostic phase. Basic principles, "do's and don'ts," and a humanistic approach are offered to the novice interviewer. Projective techniques are demonstrated, such as Gardner's "Mutual Story Telling" and "Three Wishes," as well as techniques to elicit fantasy. The use of actors detracts somewhat from the authenticity, but the principles presented are sound. H. J. Lurie, Director. (25 mins.)

<u>Interview with a maternally deprived paranoid twelve year old boy</u> V
(1980) Source: HSU

Diagnosis, interview. This video shows a clinical interview with a twelve-year-old boy who reportedly comes from a maternally deprived background. It is reported by the patient that the parents are divorced and that he has not lived with either parent for two years. Though allegedly paranoid, the mental status reveals a schizoid, depressed child with possible developmental delay and a thought disorder. It raises nature vs. nurture issues. (30 mins.)

<u>Referred for underachievement</u> F
(1983) Source: DL

Diagnosis, interview. The intention of this film is to suggest the possibilities of the family session as an intake technique. Afforded a view of the identified patient's total situation, the psychiatrist may be able more readily to observe family processes, to formulate some preliminary hypotheses as to the source of the difficulties, to locate problems as they exist in individual members or groupings within the family, and to learn the ways in which the family members perceive themselves and others. The film offers an interesting and completely spontaneous record that can serve various educational purposes ranging from conveying the atmosphere of one kind of family interview to providing clinical material for practice in understanding family dynamics. E. Mason, Director. (28 mins.)

<u>Structured interview with young children</u> F
(1975) Source: UWF

Diagnosis, interview. (49 mins.)

<u>Structured interview with young children</u> V
(1975) Source: WRMC

Diagnosis, interview. Donald R. Bardill and James A. Granger, Directors. (49 mins.)

2. Therapeutics--Psychotherapy

<u>Aggressive child: A pre-school behavior problem</u> F
(1965) Source: UI

Therapeutics, psychotherapy. This film presents a case study of a six-year-old boy who is in a special school because of fighting. Statements from Philip's mother, the nursery school director and teacher, and the psychiatrists on the case reveal that Philip has become the family dictator by playing a demanding mother and an indulgent father against one another. His aggressive behavior expresses his fear of so much power and his need for unified parental love and disciplines. The film shows play therapy sessions with Philip and counseling sessions with his mother. An evaluation of Philip's progress after seven months of treatment is shown. The Disordered Mind Series. (28 mins.)

Cry help! F
(1983) Source: PCR

Therapeutics, psychotherapy. This film focuses on three mentally disturbed teenagers and their participation in a program which utilizes videotape, self-analysis, psychodrama, and body awareness to help them regain emotional stability and function once again in society. (83 mins.)

Individual treatment with a mentally handicapped child F
(1982) Source: VWF

Therapeutics, psychotherapy. (24 mins.)

3. Therapeutics--Behavior Therapy

The autistic child, a behavioral approach V
(1982) Source: McH

Therapeutics, behavior therapy. William Rose and Paul E. Touchette, Directors. (27 mins.)

Behavior therapy with an autistic child F
(1965) Source: NAV

Therapeutics, behavior therapy. Gerald C. Davison and Leonard Krasner, Directors. (42 mins.)

Changing inappropriate behavior
in psychotic and brain damaged children V
(1972) Source: FLRC

Therapeutics, behavior therapy. Seven children, all with behavioral problems, are shown manifesting inappropriate behaviors. Various treatment methods (primarily modification, but some psychotherapy) are illustrated. S. H. Marks, Director. (25 mins.)

Childhood aggression V
(1977) Source: MG

Therapeutics, behavior therapy. This documentary presents the story of Tim, whose aggressive behavior upset his family and caused problems at school. A shoplifting incident led Tim's parents to seek help. Referred to an experimental child psychotherapy research project, the family was carefully screened to determine whether or not they could manage the behavior modification approach of the project. As it turned out, this highly motivated family quickly acquired the necessary techniques and applied them to one specific behavior pattern that was particularly troublesome. Tim, too, was given an active role in the program, for he was asked what he would like to see changed in his life. One of the most effective devices of this program was "time out"--simply a cessation of arguments and a cooling-off period for everybody. In addition, Tim's cooperative behavior was reinforced by a positive point system. P. Blake, Director. (31 mins.)

Jamie: A behavioral approach to family intervention F
(1976) Source: UI

Therapeutics, behavior therapy. This film outlines the dramatic process as behavior modification is implemented with a five-year-old child. (16 mins.)

Peer-conducted behavior modification F
(1976) Source: MG

Therapeutics, behavior therapy. Phillip R. Black and Paul W. Clement, Directors. (24 mins.)

A primer of pediatric behavior modification V
(1983) Source: CGC

Therapeutics, behavior therapy. Richard F. Rakos, Riley Lipman, and Barbara Hill, Directors. (58 mins.)

Structuring the environment and managing
the behavior of the physically handicapped child V
(1980) Source: UND

Therapeutics, behavior therapy. Doug Knowlton, Director. (14 mins.)

That's what it's all about F
(1973) Source: GSA

Therapeutics, behavior therapy. This film depicts all aspects of the regional intervention program for unmanageable children from initial intake through the various behavior modification modules to the child's return to a normal public school within the community. (29 mins.)

Token economy: Behaviorism applied F
(1972) Source: UI

Therapeutics, behavior therapy. Dr. B. F. Skinner discussed five groups of people within our society who have been classically mistreated: prisoners, psychotics, retardates, old people, and orphans. Dr. Skinner comments on the application of his theories in the education and treatment of these groups, and explains the use of tokens in a program of reinforcement therapy. The film progresses with an interview with Dr. Bernard R. Wagner, head of PACE in Decatur, Illinois, where a token economy is being practiced. Students earn tokens by behaving appropriately. These tokens can be exchanged for desirable material goods or privileges. (21 mins.)

4. Therapeutics--Family Therapy

Affinity V
(1976) Source: PCGC

Therapeutics, family therapy. In this video we see a consultation with the family of an encopretic child. Whitaker joins the family's verbal and nonverbal patterns, enhancing the possible steps out of these patterns the family will move with him. C. Whitaker, Director. (57 mins.)

Anorexia is a Greek word V
(1979) Source: BFI

Therapeutics, family therapy. Salvador Minuchin, Director. (146 mins.)

The case of the dumb delinquent V
(1976) Source: PCGC

Therapeutics, family therapy. Minuchin interviews a thirteen-year-old predelinquent boy and his single mother. Through skillful use of relabeling and reframing, the consultant highlights the complementary pattern that links mother to son and challenges plans for institutional placement. S. Minuchin, Director. (50 mins.)

Families: Alike and different F
(1970) Source: UI

Therapeutics, family therapy. This film illustrates the everyday lives of three six-year-olds living in Japan, America, and Mexico. The photography is beautiful, and the content is appropriate for parents at the high school level on up. (16 mins.)

Family circle V
(1978) Source: IEA

Therapeutics, family therapy. This is a teaching tape that focuses on the use of live videotaping and playback in family therapy sessions. The various possibilities for the use of this tool are explored through active demonstration by Dr. Ian Alger. Through the use of actors and a simulated clinical situation, Dr. Alger plays back sections of the family therapy sessions to the family, demonstrating its ability to capture small gestures, facial expression, and positioning in the room that is often missed both by therapist and family members. Through careful use of this tool, which allows a therapist to emphasize and replay crucial affective and physical communications, he can focus in on patterns of communication, closeness and distance, and defenses and modeling. Dr. Alger demonstrates how with one camera and a playback monitor he shifts the session's focus from the identified problem of a daughter departing for college to relationships of the marital couple and one set of grandparents. J. Lurie and I. Alger, Directors. (27 mins.)

Family therapy consultation V
(1979) Source: IEA

Therapeutics, family therapy. This videotape demonstrates much of the working style of Carl Whitaker, M.D. Dr. Whitaker is engaging a family of three teenage boys and a mother and a father where there is a persistent history of physical abuse directed against the mother by various family members. One can experience first hand Dr. Whitaker's intuitive, rapid-fire interventions as he attempts to engage this family and examine long standing patterns of family interaction. Themes such as the father's lack of discipline as expressed in his poor health from smoking, the mother being willing to be a maid, the role reversals with the parents, and the craziness in this family coming to be "normal" is shown. I. Alger, Director. (30 mins.)

A family with a little fire V
(1981) Source: PCGC

Therapeutics, family therapy. This video depicts therapy with a one-parent family in which the elder daughter sets fires. The son's intervention as a parental child prevents interactions between mother and daughter. Montalvo joins the flow of family patterns in a way that encourages new problem-solving sequences. B. Montalvo, Director. (43 mins.)

Films and Videos with Commentary

A family with Whitaker and Minuchin — V
(1983) — Source: PCGC

Therapeutics, family therapy. Included here are the proceedings from the Whitaker-Minuchin Dialogue in February, 1981, including their interviews with the family of a suicidal preadolescent and excerpts from their ensuing discussion. (Four tapes: 210 mins.)

I'd rather forget it — V
(1985) — Source: PCGC

Therapeutics, family therapy. In this video, we see the use of cotherapy and the combination of pediatrics and psychotherapy in the treatment of a family with an asthmatic child. The video demonstrates the development of a treatment plan to control the child's spiraling illness through hospitalization of the entire family. G. Hodas and N. Betof, Directors. (45 mins.)

Initial family interviews — V
(1982) — Source: IEA

Therapeutics, family therapy. Dr. Ian Alger demonstrates his approach to doing an initial family interview. He explains the three phases of engaging the family, identifying the patterns, and making interventions and establishing goals. He begins by eliciting from family members what it feels like to be in the family as a means of making contact, including the use of humor. He proceeds to identifying patterns, even explicating them out loud to get family reactions to his perceptions. Dr. Alger emphasizes the distinction between family patterns and the family "problem" that may disguise the underlying pattern. He then attempts to draw out of the family member goals that they have in terms of improving the family system. This videotape is technically of a high quality, easy to follow, and demonstrates both abstractly and concretely the approach that Dr. Alger is advocating. I. Alger, Director. (45 mins.)

Just a house, not a home — V
(1977) — Source: PCGC

Therapeutics, family therapy. The video shows excerpts from the treatment of a remarried couple and their adolescent sons from previous marriages. Minuchin explores the complex reaccomodation of coalitions and loyalties that transpires as the original units blend into a new orientation. S. Minuchin and V. Goldner, Directors. (50 mins.)

A modern little Hans — V
(1974) — Source: PCGC

Therapeutics, family therapy. This video shows excerpts and analysis of the treatment of a dog phobia. The tape demonstrates the engagement of the parents in treating their son's problem, the therapist's work with the couple, and his disengagement changed family. M. Barragan and J. Haley, Directors. (60 mins.)

Minuchin interview — V
(1979) — Source: BFI

Therapeutics, family therapy. Frederick J. Duch, Director. (60 mins.)

Pulling together — V
(1981) — Source: PCGC

Therapeutics, family therapy. This video depicts the treatment of an intact family with four children, where the teenage son is threatening violence toward the father. Excellent examples are given of structural treatment with issues of transition. The children are becoming adolescents as the parents are emerging into their own mid-life adolescence. The therapist demonstrates the use of self as an agent for change. C. Hercovici, Director. (48 mins.)

Taming monsters — V
(1975) — Source: PCGC

Therapeutics, family therapy. In this classic consultation, Minuchin joins the family of an "uncontrollable" five-year-old girl, reframes the problem, stages enactments, uses play, and challenges the family's rules for interaction and perception of reality. S. Minuchin, Director. (60 mins.)

5. Therapeutics--Group Therapy

Activity group therapy — F
(1950) — Source: UI

Therapeutics, group therapy. In this film we see the development of a group of emotionally disturbed children in a social club setting with a neutral therapist. It shows gradual improvement in their social adjustment. Filmed with concealed cameras and microphones, the technical deficiencies make this of historical interest only. S. R. Slavson. (54 mins.)

An adolescent group: Social springboard for personal growth — V
(1983) — Source: DL

Therapeutics, group therapy. Camp Wediko, a "summer place for disturbed children," is the setting. The tape shows excerpts from daily group meetings, edited to allow the viewer a sense of the process over time. Additionally, there are a few excerpts from the supervisor's meetings where objectives and appropriate technical interventions are formulated for each child. The tape focuses on two boys, ages thirteen and sixteen. The three-fold purposes of the daily "cabin meetings" are to learn new modes of social skills, self-knowledge, and conflict resolution. The tape demonstrates the usefulness of group process for youngsters who were seriously deficient in social skills, and the use the boys made of feedback from their peers. The tape demonstrates how "contacts" regarding behavioral change are employed. E. Mason, Director. (35 mins.)

Adolescent group therapy: An introduction for parents — V
(1981) — Source: CGC

Therapeutics, group therapy. This is a video for parents with adolescents in a therapy group. (12 mins.)

Broad spectrum behavior therapy in a group — F
(1969) — Source: PCR

Therapeutics, group therapy. Dr. Lazurus demonstrates his active behavioral methods dealing with hostility in the group and using assertive training to replace aggressive behavior. A. A. Lazurus, Director. (29 mins.)

The management of children in groups — V
(1953) — Source: WSU

Therapeutics, group therapy. Fritz Redl, Director. Restricted distribution. (70 mins.)

Management of crisis in adolescent group therapy — V
(1983) — Source: CGC

Therapeutics, group therapy. Riley Lipman, Bette Sherriff, and Edward Carter, Directors. (40 mins.)

Prevention--early intervention — V
(1977) — Source: PCR

Therapeutics, group therapy. This video documents a program in which mother-child groups regularly meet with trained psychoanalytical staff members to learn about childhood behavior patterns. The weekly sessions, where mothers interact with and observe their children, are presented as a method for early diagnosis and prevention of emotional disorders in children. (18 mins.)

6. Therapeutics--Adjunctive Therapies

Functional language structuring. Language training for the autistic through school and work related activities in a residential treatment setting V
(1978) Source: DL

Therapeutics, adjunctive therapies. (28 mins.)

Looking for me F
(1970) Source: UCEMC

Therapeutics, adjunctive therapies. Dance therapist Janet Adler narrates this report of a research project in which she investigated the effects of patterned movement with normal four- and five-year-olds, two autistic children aged two and five, emotionally disturbed children, and adult teachers. The adults are involved in order to enhance their own comfort with themselves. Similarly, the proposition that movement therapy enhances integration of self for disturbed population leads to her effort to awaken or enhance these elements: physical freedom, spontaneity, kinesthetic control and discipline, and, through paired exercises, trust in one's partner through non-verbal communication. Expert technical and aesthetic qualities. (29 mins.)

Stevie's light bulb: Graphic art in child psychiatry F
(1977) Source: HCF

Therapeutics, adjunctive therapies. This film illustrates the potential for art therapy in the diagnosis and treatment of children. It approaches this therapeutic modality both through tracing the drawings of eight children with different diagnoses and ages, as well as through a more systematic analysis of the components of art in a psychiatric setting. Thus, there are sections on: (1) form, (2) affect, (3) themes, (4) defenses, and (5) symbols, with a number of illustrations to develop these areas. Additionally, Stevie and his various artistic productions are examined in the context of his otherwise limited verbal productions and his psychological conflicts. R. B. Rabinovitch and F. B. Pasley, Directors. (76 mins.)

A tape for Sam V
(1984) Source: DL

Therapeutics, adjunctive therapies. This video illustrates the use of an individual videotape prepared for a child, "Sam," by his therapist to review during the long winter months; the videotape is to take the place of the supportive adult therapist and the growth experiencing community that had led to gains for the emotionally disturbed boy in a summer treatment program at Camp Wediko. (15 mins.)

7. Therapeutics--Hospitalization, Residential Treatment

Benhaven's approach to problems in behavior V
(1978) Source: BH

Therapeutics, hospitalization, residential treatment. This video provides an overview of a residential treatment center's program for autistic and multiply handicapped children and adolescents. (20 mins.)

Benhaven's approach to problems in behavior V
(1979) Source: BH

Therapeutics, hospitalization, residential treatment. In this video, we are shown techniques for modifying autistic behavior in home, school, and work environments in a residential home for autistic and neurologically impaired individuals. (20 mins.)

Bruce F
(1983) Source: DL

Therapeutics, hospitalization, residential treatment. The lonely struggle of a suspicious, frightened, and angry thirteen-year-old who is unable to control his impulses is the topic of this film. He fights with everyone, threatens to run away, and explodes in a dramatic cabin group meeting. E. Mason, Director. (26 mins.)

Inpatient adolescents discuss their family life F
(1982) Source: HSV

Therapeutics, hospitalization, residential treatment. (32 mins.)

Randy F
(1983) Source: DL

Therapeutics, hospitalization, residential treatment. Randy is an eleven-year-old, more seriously disturbed than most at Camp Wediko; his beguiling but inconsistent behavior makes care difficult. Four different staff people are seen attempting to help him in various situations and with varying degrees of success. E. Mason, Director. (27 mins.)

Teaching autistic children to play V
(1978) Source: BH

Therapeutics, hospitalization, residential treatment. A structured approach to increasing interaction between autistic children and adults is presented in this video. (20 mins.)

8. Miscellaneous

Beach interview F
(1982) Source: DL

Development, adolescents. Two boys become increasingly upset and demand to leave camp. In the course of a "life space interview," the boys, who normally are able to express their emotions only through action, succeed in verbalizing their resentment and discussing alternative ways of dealing with it. E. Mason, Director. (27 mins.)

Genetic screening: The ultimate preventive medicine? V
(1987) Source: PBS

Genetics and intrauterine diagnosis. What should a woman do if she is told the child she carries is noticeably handicapped: should she abort the fetus or knowingly have the baby? Genetic screening examines this question, the options parents have for prenatal testing of their children, and how genetic counseling has affected some parents. (58 mins.)

Human aggression F
(1976) Source: NIU

Development, adolescent pathology and diagnosis. This film illustrates the expression of aggression in youth gangs, experiments with Bobo the Clown, and discusses the obedience studies of Milgram and the legitimization of aggression in delinquent groups. Harper & Row, Milgram. (24 mins.)

Learning though play: Play space F
(1974) Source: UTOR

Psychiatry, public information. This is a film for parents as audience about the play settings for children. (28 mins.)

Sociobiology: The human animal V
(1984) Source: TLV

Genetics. Are morality and justice embedded in the genetic code? Sociobiology, a new and controversial science, holds that behavior is biologically determined. WGBH/BBC. (57 mins.)

Through the genetic maze V
(1982) Source: PCR

Genetics as a diagnostic tool. (58 mins.)

When teens get pregnant F
(1978) Source: PMF

Development, diagnostic issues in pregnant adolescents. The young girls in When teens get pregnant are real, not actors. The poignant stories they tell are representative of all teens who become pregnant. They speak very openly about their lives before pregnancy, about their families, school, peer pressure to have sex, of the reality of sex as opposed to the fantasy, the differences between their own and their partner's needs and expectation, and the fears and responsibilities introduced into their young lives by a pregnancy. A. Fievius, Director. (18 mins.)

N. Training in Child Mental Health

Consultative medicine V
(1983) Source: EMTN

Psychiatry, training. Michael F. Lubin, Director. (60 mins.)

The day Grandpa died F
(1970) Source: UCEMC

Death. This film is a sensitive dramatized portrayal of a nine-year-old boy's response to the death and funeral of his beloved grandfather, from his initial refusal to accept the fact to his gradual recognition of death as a part of life. Good acting and directing; not mawkish or trite. (11 mins.)

G. Patton, M.D. V
(1984) Source: HSC

Psychiatry, training. This videotape is a take-off on the famous movie, Patton, where General Patton is delivering his famous speech about loyalty and patriotism in front of a huge American flag. What is different is the substitution of medicine and surgery for the instruments of war and disease for the enemy. Thus, in this speech, G. Patton takes to the extreme the idea that medicine, including psychiatry, must be aggressive, invasive, and always involve a direct intervention. G. Patton states that "I never heard of anyone who cured disease by talking to it." Thus, this tape raises many questions about the approach and merits of psychiatry within medicine as viewed from a very action-oriented perspective. An entertaining and challenging film. D. Fidler, Director. (7 mins.)

Management development: Conflict vignettes V
(1978) Source: UEC

Psychiatry, training. Therese Lawler, Director. (23 mins.)

The newborn, parents and you V
(1978) Source:IU

Diagnosis. Richard L. Schreiner, Director. (47 mins.)

Teaching child psychiatrists interventions with children of adult psychiatric patients V
(1978) Source: WPIC

Diagnosis. Dr. Henderson and four chief residents view a tape of Dr. Kupfer interviewing a mother who is diagnosed schizo-affective disorder and discuss the effects of the illness on her nine-year-old son. Produced by Western Psychiatric Institute. For restricted audiences. (25 mins.)

O. Research in Infancy and Childhood

1. Development

Infant reflexes in human motor development V
(1972) Source: LP

Development, growth. This video tape is a systematic review with visual demonstrations of sixteen distinct and infant motor reflexes, of which nine are primitive and seven are postural reflexes. With each reflex the usual time of onset and disappearance is discussed, as well as possible functional aspects to the reflexes, as each reflex is visually presented several times, including during a summary section. Accompanied by study guide and bibliography. Gregory Payne, Director. (23 mins.)

Newborn: Ready for life F
(1979) Source: UCLA, FL

Development, growth. This film, which begins with a natural childbirth sequence, shows how highly developed the newborn responses are to light, sound, and taste, and how he can protect himself against smothering. It demonstrates that various reflexes used later for crawling, walking, and exploring his environment are already present at birth. It emphasizes the bonding process, and features neonatal research of Dr. T. Berry Brazelton, Harvard Medical School; Dr. Lewis Lipsitt, Brown University; Dr. Louis Sanders, Boston University; and Dr. Klaus Minde, Hospital for Sick Children, Toronto. CBC: Filmakers Library. (28 mins.)

Pretending F
(1980) Source: PCR

Development, cognition, play. Children at a day care are presented in this film.

It includes individual and group make-believe, the use of toy props, the role of teacher intervention, and ways that pretending encourages cognitive and linguistic development. Robert Abramovitz and Arthur Greenwald, Directors. (16 mins.)

Right from the start F,V
(1981) Source: PBS

Development, growth. Technically speaking, this is a superb production. Substantial funding was provided by the Harris Foundation, the MacArthur Foundation, and the National Science Foundation, and the quality of sound, camera work, etc. reflects every penny. This film has been shown by the Public Broadcasting System, and it apparently has been designed for commercial television broadcasting as well. (55 mins.)

2. Research--Clinical

Babies respond to a "visual cliff" F
(1980) Source: UCLA

Research, clinical. This film is a re-creation of Rader's experiment "On the nature of the visual-cliff-avoidance response in human infants." Two infants go over the edge when in walkers. The film is to be used in conjunction with the original article and the researcher's comments. P. Greenfield, Director. (10 mins.)

Bayley scales of infant development F
(1968) Source: NYU

Research, clinical. Although this film is worn in parts, the camera work and the sound track are good. The film shows how the Bayley mental scale is administered to children between three and twenty-seven months. It demonstrates sample test items, explaining the purpose for most of them. The film illustrates the difficulties in testing infants and toddlers, especially between the ages of fifteen to twenty-one months, and gives suggestions for engaging and holding a subject's attention. It is not a step-by-step guide, but rather a general education product. Psychological Corp. of NY. (105 mins.)

The brain: The enlightening machine (1) F
(1984) Source: UI

Research, clinical. This film reviews historical descriptions of the brain, pointing out how the vocabulary has often involved an analogy with man's latest invention: pump, switchboard, computer. Animation footage colors a model, showing established loci in the brain having to do with control of touch, sight, movement, and planning. It explains something of how these facts have been determined, introduces an epileptic child and the concept of epilepsy as an "electrical storm" in the brain. The film also examines the effects of Parkinson's, a stroke, and MS. It shows dancer Agnes de Mille's struggle to come back after a stroke. (60 mins.)

The brain: Vision and movement (2) F
(1984) Source: UI

Research, clinical. In this film, we learn about the area in the back of the head that is devoted to the phenomenon of sight. It describes research whose intent is to establish what information the visual cortex actually receives, and how nerve cells decode. It also shows an experiment in which a British art student agrees to wear inversion glasses for a week, trading her adaptation. The interaction between movement and vision are examined, explaining something of how the coordination takes place in the cerebellum. (60 mins.)

The brain: Rhythm and drives (3) F
(1984) Source: UI

Research, clinical. This film examines some of the significances of circadian rhythms: depression, jet lag, and increased accident-proneness on the night shift, for example. It follows a case in which severe winter depression is successfully relieved by light treatment, which seems to have the effect of putting the hypothalamus on a summer schedule. Shown are the internal rhythms evident in sleep patterns using a computerized brain scan whose image on the screen resembles waves on a beach. The film reviews what was learned from a long experiment of living underground, from the removal of a brain tumor in a violent patient, and from an injury caused by an auto accident resulting in hormonal imbalance and impotence. (60 mins.)

The brain: Stress and emotions (4) F
(1984) Source: UI

Research, clinical. This film redramatizes an accident from 1848 in which the foreman of a railroad crew survived an explosion which drove a tamping iron through his brain, severing the cortex from the limbic system and totalling altering his chemistry and behavior. It studies the stress effects on workers in the air traffic control center in Montreal, and shows experiments which compare animals allowed control of stressors to animals without control. How uncontrollable stressful events produce behavioral depression by the depletion of norepinephrine are explained. The film examines panic attacks, and lists several healthful ways to generate endorphins for a feeling of well-being. (60 mins.)

Films and Videos with Commentary

The brain: Learning and memory (5) F
(1984) Source: UI

Research, clinical. In this film, whether the learning/memory process is localized and whether it changes brain structure is investigated. The film reviews evidence and controversy surrounding these questions, and examines amnesia as a phenomenon. It discusses types of change in neuronal connections, and introduces a man who was left, after encephalitis, with global amnesia. (60 mins.)

The brain: The two brains (6) F
(1984) Source: UI

Research, clinical. This film discusses what is known of the specialized functions of the right and left halves of the brain, and of the corpus callosum which connects them. We see a review of how Paul Broca first surmised the left hemisphere's role in language, and the effect of a stroke on the linguistic capability of a forty-five-year-old lawyer. The film examines the biological effect of culture on the organization of language and spatial skills, and the effect of sex differences. (60 mins.)

The brain: Madness (7) F
(1984) Source: UI

Research, clinical. In this film we are introduced to the nature of mental problems in that portion of the population which does not respond to treatment. The film shows interviews with psychiatric patients and their families, and examines evidence of genetic predisposition. The film compares photos of normal brain cells with those of a schizophrenic, and shows how drugs can control, but not cure, some symptoms. (60 mins.)

The brain: States of mind (8) F
(1984) Source: UI

Research, clinical. This film attempts to formulate some ideas of the roles played by the brain's anatomy and chemistry in awareness. It incorporates information derived from sleep research, and shows how PCP destroys the capability of the cortex and hippocampus to govern the limbic system. (60 mins.)

Experimental studies in social climates of groups F
(1953) Source: PCR

Research, clinical. Using a hidden camera, this study illustrates the effects of three types of social organization on attitude and learning of junior high school students: democratic, laissez-faire, and autocratic. K. Lewin, R. Lipp, II, and R. White, Directors. (30 mins.)

Fetal alcoholic syndrome F
(1975) Source: UI

Research, clinical. In this film, we see a discussion of the symptoms and studies of case histories of fetal alcoholic syndrome, a severe form of retardation directly attributed to chronic alcoholism in the mother. Characteristic physical traits are often recognizable at birth--babies are undersized and have narrow slit-like eyes with drooping lids. Development is slow, the amount of brain damage varies, but many of these babies grow up unable to care for themselves. Dr. David Smith of the University of Washington has conducted research into the causes and symptoms of fetal alcohol syndrome, and the film shows experiments relating to Dr. Smith's work being carried out on pregnant mice. (14 mins.)

Finding a place: 3 months-6 months V
(1976) Source: SUNY

Research, clinical. Donna M. Juenker and Jacqueline K. Thompson, Directors. (30 mins.)

The gene engineers V,F
(1988) Source: TLV

Research, clinical. Scientific advances in gene transfer from one animal or plant to another create mutant forms of life with far-reaching consequences--including the possible control of human development. Scientific, moral, and legal questions are explored. NOVA. (57 mins.)

Human experiments: The price of knowledge? V
(1985) Source: PBS

Research, clinical. Since the time of Hippocrates, doctors have sworn an oath that forbids experimentation solely for medical knowledge. However, modern researchers argue that experimentation in pursuit of knowledge can offer benefits to many. Human experiments looks at this sensitive question and dilemmas both doctors and patients face. (58 mins.)

Infancy research methods V,F
(1983) Source: TU, IU

Research, clinical. Four basic methods that have been developed to study the visual and auditory perceptual capabilities of human infants ranging in age from one month to one year are presented. The methods focus upon a variety of overt responses that can be elicited from a subject who cannot be instructed to perform specific tasks. The four methods covered--preference, habituation, eye movements, and conditioning--allow the experimenter certain glimpses at an infant's capabilities. The film explains that each method has certain interpretive limitations and that a combination of methods is the most useful strategy. (18 mins.)

The keys of paradise V,F
(1988) Source: WGBH, TLV

Research, clinical. Endorphins and eukephalins are studied. There are wide-range effects on mood, memory, consciousness, and behavior with implications for treatment of psychiatric patients. NOVA. (57 mins.)

Miracle of life F
(1980) Source: PYF

Research, clinical. The wonder of new life is photographed microscopically in this fascinating study of the reproductive process. With the endoscope lens inserted at the site where life begins, we can witness the living processes of fertilization, cell division, and the growth and development of the fetus to the first heart beat. A stunningly beautiful, unforgettable experience. A technological breakthrough allowing us to see the actual sequence of the formation of new life, this film shows both animal and human fetus development. From the point at which human development is different, the living human fetus is filmed. CineScience. (15 mins.)

Rock-a-bye baby V,F
(1971) Source: TLV

Research, clinical. This film shows the effect of severe maternal deprivation on human and primate development from birth to three years. The psychopathology is clearly presented graphically and through narration. The tape includes material from Harlow's "monkey studies." Research on the premature infant's development need for motion in order to replace the curtailed experience of being carried about in the mother's body is presented, together with a treatment of technique. The infant's need to be touched, handled and cuddled, and moved about is covered as well. Several research projects are shown. (30 mins.)

The secrets of sleep V,F
(1986) Source: WGBH, TLV

Research, clinical. Among the topics covered are sleep states, sleep induced by hypnotics, the jet lag phenomenon, and the importance of dreams and interpreting dreams. (52 mins.)

PART XII

Suggested Reading for Children, Adolescents, and Parents

Suggested Reading

Editor:

Irving N. Berlin, M.D.
Professor of Psychiatry and Pediatrics
University of New Mexico School of Medicine
Albuquerque, New Mexico

A. Children's Books

EDITOR'S NOTE: This book list for children--including many fairy tales--was collected by the staff of the Children's Ward, McAuley Neuropsychiatric Institute, Saint Mary's Hospital, San Francisco, California. It is divided into sections that deal with unconscious elements of aggression, abuse, sibling rivalry, fears and self esteem, night fears and bedtime stories, aloneness, separation, and Oedipal issues.

1. Aggression

Byars, B. (1972). The house of wings. New York: Viking Press. (For grades 4-5).

Gantos, J. (1976). Rotten Ralph. Boston: Houghton Mifflin.

Jack and the Beanstalk (fairy tale).

Lindgren, A. (1979). Emil in the soup tureen. London: Hymlyn Publication Group, Ltd. (For grades 1-3, story of a five-year-old).

Preston, E. M. (1981). The temper tantrum book. Cedar Grove, N.J.: Puffin Books.

Sendak, M. (1963). Where the wild things are. New York: Harper and Row.

Simon, N. (1979). I was so mad. Chicago: Albert Whitman. (For grades K-2).

Udry, J. (1969). Let's be enemies. New York: Harper and Row.

Viorst, J. (1972). Alexander and the terrible, horrible, no good, very bad day. New York: Viking Press. (For grades K-5).

Wells, R. (1973). Noisy Nora. New York: Dial Press, Scholastic Book Services.

Zolotow, C. (1963). The quarreling book. New York: Harper and Row. (For grades 1-3).

Zolotow, C. (1967). The hating book. New York: Harper and Row. (For grades K-2).

2. Abuse

Cinderella (fairy tale).

Daugherty, L. B. (1984). Why me? Help for victims of child sexual abuse. Racine, Wis.: Mother Courage Press.

Dayee, F. S. (1982). Private zone: A book teaching children sexual assault prevention tools. Edmonds, Wash.: Charles Franklin.

Fleishman, P. (1980). Half a moon inn. New York: Harper and Row. (For grades 4-6).

Fontana, V. (1973). Somewhere a child is crying. New York: Macmillan.
Freeman, T. (1982). It's my body. A book to teach young children how to resist uncomfortable touch. Seattle: Parenting Press.
Gordon, S., & Gordon, J. (1984). A better safe than sorry book: A family guide for sexual assault prevention. New York: Fayetteville.
Haddad, J., & Martin, L. H. (1981). What if . . . I say no! Bakersfield, Calif.: M. H. Cap.
Hansel and Gretel (fairy tale).
Hawkins, P. (1986). Children at risk. Bethesda, Md.: Adler and Adler.
Hickman, J. (1983). A very touching book . . . for little people and big people. Durkee, Ore.: McClure-Hindman.
Kraizer, S. K. (1985). The safe child book. New York: Dell Publishing.
Morgan, M. K. (1984). A little bird told me about . . . my feelings. Eugene, Ore.: Equal Justice, Consultants and Educational Products.
Sacks, M. (1976). The December tale. New York: Doubleday.
Schonfield, M. (1983). Talking about touching with preschoolers. Seattle: Seattle Institute for Child Advocacy.
Snow White (fairy tale).
Stowell, J., & Dietzel, M. (1982). My very own book about me. Spokane: Lutheran Social Services of Washington.
Sweet, P. E. (1981). Something happened to me. Racine, Wis.: Mother Courage Press.
Trust your feelings. (1984). Blaine, Wash.: Child Abuse Research and Education Association of B.C.
Wachter, O. (1983). No more secrets for me. Boston: Little, Brown.
Williams, J. (1980). Red flag, green flag people. Fargo, N.D.: Rape and Abuse Crisis Center.

3. Sibling Rivalry/Competition

Amoss, B. (1968). Tom in the middle. New York: Harper and Row. (On being a middle child).
Byars, B. (1971). Go and hush the baby. New York: Viking Press.
Cinderella (fairy tale).
Coleman, H. Diary of a frantic kid sister. New York: Human Sciences Press. (For grades 5-9).
Hoban, R. (1964). A baby sister for Frances. New York: Harper and Row. (For grades K-3).
Keats, E. J. (1967). Peter chair. New York: Harper and Row. (Story of a black family and a new baby).
Mallett, A. (1971). Here comes tag along. New York: Parent's Magazine Press.
Payson, D. (1974). Almost twins. Englewood Cliffs, N.J.: Prentice-Hall.
Scott, A. (1972). On mother's lap. New York: McGraw-Hill. (For grades K-3).
Segal, L. (1970). Tell me a Mitzi. New York: Scholastic Book and Record Companion Series. (Story of a little girl with a brother).

Suggested Reading

Steptoe, J. (1969). Stevie. New York: Harper and Row.
The three feathers (fairy tale)

4. On Being Afraid/Low Self-Esteem

Heide, F. (1970). Giants are very brave people. New York: Parent's Magazine Press. (For grades K-1).
Kraus, R. (1980). Leo the late bloomer. New York: Windmill Books.
Stephenson, D. (1977). How to scare a lion. New York: Windmill Books. (For grades K-3).
The three feathers (fairy tale)
The three languages (fairy tale)

5. Night Fears

Bodecker, A. M., & Kraus, R. (1972). Good night Richard Rabbit. New York: Springfellow Books, Dalton & Co.
Fenner, C. (1979). Tigers in the cellar. New York: Human Sciences Press. (For grades 1-4).
Hoban, R. (1974). Bedtime for Frances. New York: Harper and Row.
Kent, J. (1975). There is no such thing as a dragon. New York: Golden Press.
Mayer, M. (1968). There's a nightmare in my closet. New York: Dial Press.
Waber, B. (1972). Ira sleeps over. Boston: Houghton Mifflin. (For grades K-2).

6. Aloneness/The Feeling of Not Being Seen/Making Friends

Burnett, F. (1981). The secret garden. New York: Dell Publishing, Yearling Books. (For grades 3-5).
Burningham, J. (1978a). Come away from the water, Shirley. New York: Harper and Row.
Burningham, J. (1978b). Time to come out of the bath, Shirley. New York: Harper and Row.
Cecil, E. (1975). Malachi Mudge. New York: Macmillan. (For grades 2-3).
Cohen, M. (1967). Will I have a friend?. New York: Macmillan.
Garrigue, S. (1978). Between friends. New York: Bradberry (Distributed by Elsevier-Dutton).
Heide, F. (1979). The shrinking of treehorn. New York: Dell Publishing.
Hoff, S. (1960). Who will be my friend?. New York: Harper and Row.
Konigsburg, E. L. (1967). Jennifer, Hecate, MacBeth, William McKinley and me, Elizabeth. New York: Atheneum (Aladdin Books). (For grades 4-6).
Steig, W. (1969). Silvester and the magic pebble. New York: Windmill Books. (For grades K-3).
Williams, M. (1975). The velveteen rabbit. New York: Doubleday. (For grades 1-4).

7. Separation

Briengburg, P. (1973). Shawn goes to school. New York: Thomas Y. Crowell.
Hansel and Gretel (fairy tale).
Harner, C. (1978). The single-parent family in children's books. San Francisco: Scarecrow Press.
Newfield, M. (1973). Book for Jodan. New York: Atheneum. (For grades 2-5; subject, divorce).

8. Oedipal Issues

Beauty and the beast (fairy tale, Oedipal-related).
Cinderella (fairy tale, early Oedipal).
The good girl (fairy tale, early Oedipal).
Manheim, R. (Trans.). (1977). Grimms' tales for young and old. New York: Doubleday. (Excellent resources for Oedipal issues).
Rapunzel (fairy tale, early Oedipal).
Snow White (fairy tale, early Oedipal).
The three feathers (fairy tale, Oedipal-related).

9. On Being Different or Unique

de Regniers, B. S. (1974). A little house of your own. New York: Harcourt, Brace and Ward. (On needing your own space and to be alone).
Hazen, B. S. (1974). The gorilla did it. New York: Atheneum.
Jarell, R. (1964). The bat-poet. New York: Macmillan. (Story of a bat who sees things differently from other bats; illustrated by M. Sendak).
Leichman, S. (1973). The boy who could sing pictures. New York: Holt, Rinehart and Winston.
Lionni, Leo. (1973). Frederick. New York: Pinwheel Books (originally published by Pantheon, 1967). (For kindergarten through adults).

10. Developing Moral Judgment and Responsibility

Seuss, Dr. (1975). I had trouble getting to Solla Sollew. New York: Random House. (For grades 1-2).
Stephenson, D. (1971). How to scare a lion. New York: Pinwheel Books.
White, E. B. (1970). The trumpet of the swan. New York: Harper and Row. (For all ages).

11. Affirmation of the Inner World/On Valuing Fantasy as Real

Brock, B. (1970). No flying in the house. New York: Harper and Row. (For grades 2-4).
Kent, J. (1975). There is no such thing as a dragon. New York: Golden Press.

12. On the Need to Distinguish Fantasy from Reality

Ness, E. (1966). Sam, bangs and moonshine. New York: Holt, Rinehart and Winston. (For grades 2-4).
Ness, E. (1970). Exactly alike. New York: Random House. (For grades 1-3).

13. Adoption

Krementz, J. (1982). How it feels to be adopted. New York: Knopf.
Lifton, B. J. (1981). I'm still me. New York: Knopf.
Livingstone, C. (1978). Why was I adopted? Secaucus, N.J.: Lyle Stuart.

14. Death

Buscaglia, L. (1982). The fall of Freddie the leaf. Thorofare, N.J.: SLACK.

15. Development

Long, L., & Linf, T. (1983). The handbook for latchkey children and their parents. New York: Arbor House.
Parkinson, R. W. (1985). Growing up on purpose. Champaign, Ill.: Research Press.

16. Divorce

Boegehold, B. (1985). Daddy doesn't live here anymore. Racine, Wis.: Western Publishing.
Gardner, R. (1977). Boys and girls book about divorce. New York: Bantam Books.
Hazen, B. S. (1983). Two homes to live in: A child's eye view of divorce. New York: Human Sciences Press.
Krasney Brown, L. (1986). Dinosaurs divorce: A guide for changing families. New York: Atlantic Monthly Press.
LeShan, E. (1986). What's going to happen to me? New York: Macmillan.
Lewis, H. C. (1980). All about families the second time around, for boys and girls, their parents and step parents. Atlanta, Ga.: Peachtree Publishers.
Rofes, E. D. (1982). The kids book about divorce. New York: Random House.
Skynner, R., & Cleese, J. (1984). Families and how to survive them. London: Oxford University Press.
Stanek, M., & Mill, E. (1981). I won't go without a father. Chicago: Albert Whitman.
Stenson, J. S. (1979). Now I have a stepparent and it's kind of confusing: A book that explains remarriage to young children. New York: Avon Books.
Vigna, J. (1980). She's not my real mother. Chicago: Albert Whitman.

17. Mental Retardation

Glifton, G. S. (1980). My friend Jacob. New York: E. P. Darfton.
Sobel, H. L. (1977). My brother Steven is retarded. New York: Macmillan.

18. Sexuality

Mayle, P. (1973). Where did I come from? Secaucus, N.J.: Lyle Stuart.

19. Abduction

Meyer, L. D. (1984). Safety zone: A book teaching child abduction prevention rules. Edmonds, Wash.: Charles Franklin.

20. Childhood Disturbance

Elkind, D. (1981). The hurried child. Reading, Mass.: Addison-Wesley.
Minden, H. A. (1982). Two hugs for survival. Toronto: McClelland and Stewart.

B. Books for Adolescents

1. Novels Dealing with the Adolescent Years

Frank, A. (1932). The diary of a young girl. New York: Doubleday.
Green, H. (1964). I never promised you a rose garden. New York: Signet Books.
Mason, B. A. (1985). In country. New York: Harper and Row.
McCorkle, J. (1984). The cheerleader. New York: Penguin Books.
Minot, S. (1986). Monkeys. New York: Pocket Books.
Salinger, J. D. (1977). Catcher in the rye. New York: Bantam Books.

2. Chronic Disease

Ardell, M. (1985). Portrait of an anorexic: A mother and daughter's story. Vancouver, B.C.: Flight Press.
Seligman, A. (1982). Living with Tourette syndrome: A teenager's point of view. New York: Macmillan. (A teenager writes about the experiences of Tourette syndrome and coping with it).

3. Sexual Abuse

Daugherty, L. B. (1984). Why me? Help for the victims of child sexual abuse. Racine, Wis.: Mother Courage Press. (A comprehensive self-help guide for victims of sexual abuse who are now teenagers or adults).

Fay, J. J., & Flerchinger, B. J. (1982). Top secret. Sexual assault information for teenagers only. Renton, Wash.: King County Rape Relief. (An excellent resource for teenagers about sexual assault).

Fortune, M. M. (1984). Sexual abuse prevention: A study for teenagers. New York: United Church.

Mackey, G., & Swan, H. (1983). Dear Elizabeth: The diary of a survivor of sexual abuse. Leawood, Kans.: Children's Institute of Kansas City. (A moving fictional account of a young woman's struggle to cope with her father's sexual abuse).

Terkel, S. N., & Rench, J. E. (1984). Feeling safe, feeling strong: How to avoid sexual abuse and what to do if it happens to you. Minneapolis, Minn.: Lerner.

4. Normal Adolescence

Elkind, D. (1984). All grown up and no place to go. Reading, Mass.: Addison-Wesley.

Turkle, S. (1984). The second self--computers and the human spirit. New York: Simon & Schuster.

5. Stress

Kushner, H. S. (1981). When bad things happen to good people. New York: Schocken Books.

6. Divorce

Richards, A., & Willis, I. (1976). How to get it together when your parents are coming apart. New York: David McKay Co.

C. Books for Parents

1. Autism

Grandin, T., & Scariano, M. M. (1986). Emergence: Labeled autistic. Novato, Calif.: Arena Press.

Park, C. C. (1982). The siege: The first eight years of an autistic child. Boston: Little, Brown.

Schopler, E., & Mesibov, G. B. (1984). The effects of autism on the family. New York: Plenum Press.

Wing, L. (1972). Autism: A guide for parents and professionals. New York: Brunner/Mazel.

Wing, L. (1985). Autistic children. Champaign, Ill.: Research Press.

2. Substance Abuse

Polson, R., & Newton, M. (1984). Not my kid: A parent's guide to kids and drugs. New York: Arbor House.

Seixas, J. S. (1979). Living with a parent who drinks too much. New York: Greenwillow Books.

Woodward, N. H. (1981). Is your child drinking? New York: Putnam.

3. Attention Deficit Disorders and Learning Disabilities

Brutten, M., Richerson, S. O., & Mangel, C. (1973). Something is wrong with my child: A parent's book about children with learning disabilities. New York: Harcourt, Brace Jovanovich.

Cruickshank, W. M., Morse, W. C., & Johns, J. S. (1980). Learning disabilities: The struggle from adolescence toward adulthood. Syracuse, N.Y.: Syracuse University Press.

Gardner, R. (1987). The family book about minimal brain dysfunction. New York: Jason Aronson.

Levick, M. F. (1983). They could not talk so they drew: Children's styles of coping and thinking. Springfield, Ill.: Charles C. Thomas.

Lyons, T. W. (1983). The pelican and after: A novel about emotional disturbance. Richmond, Va.: Prescott, Durrell.

4. Adoption

Gilman, L. (1984). The adoption resource book. New York: Harper and Row.

McNamara, J. (1982). Adopting the child with special needs. Washington, D.C.: North American Council on Adoptable Children.

5. Anorexia Nervosa

Bruch, H. (1979). The golden cage. New York: Vintage Books.

Ardell, M. (1985). Portrait of an anorexic: A mother and daughter's story. Vancouver, B.C.: Flight Press.

6. Chronic Illness/Disabilities

Barach, C. (1983). Help me say it: A parent's guide to speech problems. New York: New American Library.

Featherstone, H. (1980). A difference in the family: Life with a disabled child. New York: Basic Books.

Giddan, J. J., & Giddan, N. S. (1984). Teaching language with pictures. Springfield, Ill.: Charles C. Thomas.

Lagos, J. C. (1974). Seizures, epilepsy and your child. New York: Harper and Row.

Suggested Reading

McCollum, A. T. (1981). The chronically ill child. New Haven, Conn.: Yale University Press.
Ogden, P. W., & Lipsett, S. (1982). The silent garden: Understanding the hearing impaired. New York: St. Martin's Press.

7. Death

Fischoff, J., & Brohl, N. O. (1981). Before and after my child died. Detroit: Emmons-Fairfield.
Grollman, E. A. (1967). Explaining death to children. Boston: Beacon Press.
Stein, S. B. (1974). About dying, an open family book for parents and children together. New York: Walker.

8. Depression and Suicide

Giffin, M., & Felsanthal, C. (1983). A cry for help: Exploring and exploding myths about suicide. New York: Doubleday.
McKnew, D. H., Cytran, L., & Yohaaes, H. (1983). Why isn't Johnny crying: Coping with depression in children. New York: Norton.

9. Child Development

Allen, J. V. (1983). What do I do when . . . ? A handbook for parents and other beleaguered adults. San Ramon, Calif.: Impact Publishers.
Arnold, L. E. (1983). Parents' survival handbook. Sunbury, Ohio: LAMMP Publishing.
Bettelheim, B., & Zelan, K. (1982). On learning to read. New York: Knopf.
Bramnick, L., & Simon, A. (1983). The parents' solution book: Your child from five to twelve. New York: Franklin Watts. (Applying educational principles to building good parent-child relationships during the elementary school years).
Brazelton, T. B. (1969). Infants and mothers. New York: Dell Publishing.
Brooks, J. B. (1981). The process of parenting. Palo Alto, Calif.: Mayfield. (Describes how several major sources have approached many common child-rearing problems and integrates this discussion).
Chess, S., & Thomas, A. (1987). Know your child: An authoritative guide for today's parents. New York: Basic Books.
Coles, R. (1987). The moral life of children. Boston: Houghton Mifflin.
Eden, A. N. (1980). Positive parenting: How to raise a healthier and happier child (from birth to three years). New York: New American Library.
Fassler, J. (1978a). Helping children cope. New York: Macmillan.
Fassler, J. (1978b). Helping children cope: Mastering stress through books and stories. New York: The Free Press.
Fraiberg, S. (1959). The magic years. New York: Scribner's.
Gersh, M. J. (1983). How to raise children at home in your spare time. New York: Briarcliff Manor, Stein and Day. (Gersh, a pediatrician, has written this book for

parents in an attempt to reassure them that raising children is really not all that difficult.).

Gollesmen, D. M. (1982). The powerful parent: A child advocacy handbook. Norwalk, Conn.: Appleton-Century-Crofts.

Hardyman, C. (1983). Dream babies--three centuries of good advice on child care. New York: Harper and Row.

Ilg, F. L., & Ames, L. B. (1981). Child behavior from birth to ten. New York: Harper and Row.

Johnson, D. M. (1983). Children's toys and books. New York: Scribner's.

Kelly, M., & Parsons, E. (1975). The mother's almanac. New York: Doubleday. (This book is unique in the wealth of creative ideas and activities presented for parents of children under six year of age.).

Knippers, O. J. (1984). Kids and common sense. Saratoga, Calif.: R and E.

LeFebre, B. (1983). Raising children for fun and profit. Irvine, Calif.: Rampart. (The focus of the book is on teaching attitudes and values. Topics covered include the nature of freedom, character development, reason instead of violence, and the moral concept.).

Long, L., & Linf, T. (1983). The handbook for latchkey children and their parents. New York: Arbor House.

McDermott, J. F. (1980). Raising Cain (and Abel too). New York: Wyden Books.

Neville, H., & Halaby, M. (1984). No fault parenting. New York: Facts on File.

Powell, D. H. (1986). Teenagers: When to worry and what to do. New York: Doubleday.

Rosner, J. (1983). Myths of child-rearing. New York: Dembner. (Defining and debunking common and destructive myths about raising children).

Salk, L. (1984). What every child would like his parent to know. New York: Simon & Schuster.

Sears, W. (1983). Creative parenting. New York: Dodd, Mead.

Schowalter, J. E., & Anjan, W. R. (1979). The family handbook of adolescence. New York: Knopf.

Siegel-Gorleck, B. (1983). The working parents' guide to child care. Boston: Little, Brown

Stanek, M. (1985). All alive after school. Chicago: Albert Whitman.

Woodbury, M. (1985). Childhood information resources. Arlington, Va.: Information Resources Press.

10. Divorce

Gardner, R. (1977). The parents book about divorce. New York: Doubleday.

Goldstein, S., & Solnit, A. (1984). Divorce and your child: Practical suggestions for parents. New Haven: Yale University Press.

Grollman, E. (Ed.). (1969). Explaining divorce to children. Boston: Beacon Press.

Lewis, H. C. (1980). All about families the second time around, for boys and girls, their parents and step parents. Atlanta, Ga.: Peachtree Publishers.

Sinberg, J. (1978). Divorce is a grown up problem: A book about divorce for young children and their parents. New York: Avon Books.

11. Mental Retardation

Glifton, G. S. (1980). My friend Jacob. New York: E. P. Darfton.
Koch, R., & Koch, K. J. (1974). Understanding the mentally retarded child. New York: Random House.
Menolascino, F. J., & Stark, J. A. (1984). Handbook of mental illness in the mentally retarded. New York: Plenum Press.
Vitello, S. J., & Soskin, R. M. (1984). Mental retardation: Its social and legal context. Englewood Cliffs, N.J.: Prentice-Hall.

12. Sexuality

Calderone, M., & Ramey, J. W. (1982). Talking with your child about sex. New York: Random House.
Girard, L. W. (1983). You were born on your very first birthday. Chicago: Albert Whitman.
Mayle, P. (1973). Where did I come from?. Secaucus, N.J.: Lyle Stuart.

13. Arson

Wooden, W. S., & Berkey, M. L. (1984). Children and arson: America's middle class nightmare. New York: Plenum Press.

14. Sexual Abuse

Adams, C., & Fay, J. (1981). No more secrets: Protecting your child from sexual assault. San Luis Obispo, Calif.: Impact Publishers.
Basset, K. (1980). My very own special body book. Redding, Calif.: Hawthorne.
Krause, E. (1983a). For Pete's sake, tell! Second in a series of books for parents to help children avoid sexual abuse. Oregon City, Oreg.: Krause House.
Krause, E. (1983b). Speak up, say no. A book for adults to help children avoid sexual abuse. Oregon City, Oreg.: Krause House.
Loontjens, L. (1984). Talking to children/talking to parents about sexual assault. Santa Cruz, Calif.: Network.

15. Child Management

Durrell, D. E. (1984). The critical years: A guide for dedicated parents. Oakland, Calif.: New Harbinger.
Fraiberg, S. H. (1984). The magic years: Understanding and handling the problems of early childhood. New York: Scribner's. (This classic book on child-rearing

was originally written almost thirty years ago, yet it is still in print and remains a valuable resource for parents.).
Ginott, H. G. (1959). Between parent and child. New York: Avon.
Ginott, H. G. (1971). Between parent and teenager. New York: Avon.
Patterson, G. R. (1976). Living with children. Champaign, Ill.: Research Press.

16. Childhood Disturbances

Azrin, N. H., & Besalel, V. A. (1979). A parent's guide to bedwetting control. New York: Pocket Books.
Gardner, R. A. (1973). The family book about minimal brain dysfunction. New York: Jason Aronson.
Rutter, M. (1975). Helping troubled children. New York: Plenum Press.
Wolman, B. B. (1978). Children's fears. New York: Grosset & Dunlap.

17. Behavior Therapy in Normal Families

Petterson, G. (1975). Families. Champaign, Ill.: Research Press.